Lecture Notes in Computer Science　　9004

Commenced Publication in 1973
Founding and Former Series Editors:
Gerhard Goos, Juris Hartmanis, and Jan van Leeuwen

More information about this series at http://www.springer.com/series/7412

Daniel Cremers · Ian Reid
Hideo Saito · Ming-Hsuan Yang (Eds.)

Computer Vision – ACCV 2014

12th Asian Conference on Computer Vision
Singapore, Singapore, November 1–5, 2014
Revised Selected Papers, Part II

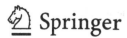 Springer

Editors
Daniel Cremers
Technische Universität München
Garching
Germany

Hideo Saito
Keio University
Yokohama, Kanagawa
Japan

Ian Reid
University of Adelaide
Adelaide, SA
Australia

Ming-Hsuan Yang
University of California at Merced
Merced, CA
USA

Videos to this book can be accessed at
http://www.springerimages.com/videos/978-3-319-16807-4

ISSN 0302-9743   ISSN 1611-3349 (electronic)
Lecture Notes in Computer Science
ISBN 978-3-319-16807-4   ISBN 978-3-319-16808-1   (eBook)
DOI 10.1007/978-3-319-16808-1

Library of Congress Control Number: 2015934895

LNCS Sublibrary: SL6   Image Processing, Computer Vision, Pattern Recognition, and Graphics

Springer Cham Heidelberg New York Dordrecht London

Printed on acid-free paper

Springer International Publishing AG Switzerland is part of Springer Science+Business Media
(www.springer.com)

Preface

ACCV 2014 received a total of 814 submissions, a reflection of the growing strength of Computer Vision in Asia. We note, particularly, that a number of Area Chairs commented very positively on the overall quality of the submissions. The conference had submissions from all continents (except Antarctica, a challenge for the 2016 organizers perhaps) with 64 % from Asia, 20 % from Europe, and 10 % from North America.

The Program Chairs assembled a geographically diverse team of 36 Area Chairs who handled between 20 and 30 papers each. Area Chairs recommended reviewers for papers, and each paper received at least three reviews from the 638 reviewers who participated in the process. Paper decisions were finalized at an Area Chair meeting held in Singapore in September 2014. At this meeting, Area Chairs worked in triples to reach collective decisions about acceptance, and in panels of 12 to decide on the oral/poster distinction. The total number of papers accepted was 227, an overall acceptance rate of 28 %. Of these, 32 were selected for oral presentation.

We extend our immense gratitude to the Area Chairs and Reviewers for their generous participation in the process – the conference would not be possible if it were not for this huge voluntary investment of time and effort. We acknowledge particularly the contribution of 35 reviewers designated as "Outstanding Reviewers" (see page 14 in this booklet for a full list) who were nominated by Area Chairs and Program Chairs for having provided a large number of helpful, high-quality reviews.

The Program Chairs are also extremely grateful for the support, sage advice, and occasional good-natured prompting provided by the General Chairs. Each of them helped with matters that in other circumstances might have been left to the Program Chairs, so that it regularly felt as if we had a team of seven, not four Program Chairs. The PCs are very grateful for this.

Finally, we wish to thank the authors and delegates. Without their participation there would be no conference. The conference was graced with a uniformly high quality of presentations and posters, and we offer particular thanks to the three eminent keynote speakers, Stephane Mallat, Minoru Etoh, and Dieter Fox, who delivered outstanding talks.

Computer Vision in Asia is growing, and the quality of ACCV steadily climbing so that it is now, rightly, considered as one of the top conferences in the field. We look forward to future editions.

November 2014

Daniel Cremers
Ian Reid
Hideo Saito
Ming-Hsuan Yang

Organization

Organizing Committee

General Chairs

Michael S. Brown	National University of Singapore, Singapore
Tat-Jen Cham	Nanyang Technological University, Singapore
Yasuyuki Matsushita	Microsoft Research Asia, China

Program Chairs

Daniel Cremers	Technische Universität München, Germany
Ian Reid	University of Adelaide, Australia
Hideo Saito	Keio University, Japan
Ming-Hsuan Yang	University of California at Merced, USA

Organizing Chair

Teck Khim Ng	National University of Singapore, Singapore
Junsong Yuan	Nanyang Technological University, Singapore

Workshop Chairs

C.V. Jawahar	IIIT Hyderabad, India
Shiguang Shan	Institute of Computing Technology, Chinese Academy of Sciences, China

Demo Chairs

Bohyung Han	POSTECH, Korea
Koichi Kise	Osaka Prefecture University, Japan

Tutorial Chairs

Chu-Song Chen	Academia Sinica, Tawain
Brendan McCane	University of Otago, New Zealand

Publication Chairs

Terence Sim	National University of Singapore, Singapore
Jianxin Wu	Nanjing University, China

Industry Chairs

Hongcheng Wang	United Technologies Corporation, USA
Brian Price	Adobe, USA
Antonio Robles-Kelly	NITCA, Australia

Steering Committee

In-So Kweon	KAIST, Korea
Yasushi Yagi	Osaka University, Japan
Hongbin Zha	Peking University, China

Honorary Chair

Katsushi Ikeuchi	University of Tokyo, Japan

Area Chairs

Lourdes Agapito	Queen Mary University of London/University College London, UK
Thomas Brox	University of Freiburg, Germany
Tat-Jun Chin	University of Adelaide, Australia
Yung-Yu Chuang	National Taiwan University, Taiwan
Larry Davis	University of Maryland, USA
Yasutaka Furukawa	Washington University in St. Louis, USA
Bastian Goldluecke	University of Konstanz, Germany
Bohyung Han	POSTECH, Korea
Hiroshi Ishikawa	Waseda University, Japan
C.V. Jawahar	IIIT Hyderabad, India
Jana Kosecka	George Mason University, USA
David Kriegman	University of California, San Diego, USA
Shang-Hong Lai	National Tsing-Hua University, Taiwan
Ivan Laptev	Inria Rocquencourt, France
Kyoung Mu Lee	Seoul National University, Korea
Vincent Lepetit	École Polytechnique Fédérale de Lausanne, Switzerland
Jongwoo Lim	Hanyang University, Korea
Simon Lucey	CSIRO/University of Queensland, Australia
Ajmal Mian	University of Western Australia, Australia
Hajime Nagahara	Kyushu University, Japan
Ko Nishino	Drexel University, USA
Shmuel Peleg	The Hebrew University of Jerusalem, Israel
Imari Sato	National Institute of Informatics, Japan
Shin'ichi Satoh	National Institute of Informatics, Japan
Stefano Soatto	University of California, Los Angeles, USA
Jamie Shotton	Microsoft Research, UK
Ping Tan	Simon Fraser University, Canada
Lorenzo Torresani	Dartmouth College, USA
Manik Varma	Microsoft Research, India
Xiaogang Wang	Chinese University of Hong Kong, China
Shuicheng Yan	National University of Singapore, Singapore
Qing-Xiong Yang	City University of Hong Kong, Hong Kong
Jingyi Yu	University of Delaware, USA

Junsong Yuan	Nanyang Technological University, Singapore
Hongbin Zha	Peking University, China
Lei Zhang	Hong Kong Polytechnic University, Hong Kong, China

Program Committee Members

Catherine Achard	Xun Cao	Jen-Hui Cheng
Hanno Ackermann	Gustavo Carneiro	Liang-Tien Chia
Haizhou Ai	Joao Carreira	Chen-Kuo Chiang
Emre Akbas	Umberto Castellani	Shao-Yi Chien
Naveed Akhtar	Carlos Castillo	Minsu Cho
Karteek Alahari	Turgay Celik	Nam Ik Cho
Mitsuru Ambai	Antoni Chan	Jonghyun Choi
Dragomir Anguelov	Kap Luk Chan	Wongun Choi
Yasuo Ariki	Kwok-Ping Chan	Mario Christoudias
Chetan Arora	Bhabatosh Chanda	Wen-Sheng Chu
Shai Avidan	Manmohan Chandraker	Albert C.S. Chung
Alper Ayvaci	Sharat Chandran	Pan Chunhong
Venkatesh Babu	Hong Chang	Arridhana Ciptadi
Xiang Bai	Kuang-Yu Chang	Javier Civera
Vineeth Balasubramanian	Che-Han Chang	Carlo Colombo
Jonathan Balzer	Vincent Charvillat	Yang Cong
Atsuhiko Banno	Santanu Chaudhury	Sanderson Conrad
Yufang Bao	Yi-Ling Chen	Olliver Cossairt
Adrian Barbu	Yi-Lei Chen	Marco Cristani
Nick Barnes	Jieying Chen	Beleznai Csaba
John Bastian	Yen-Lin Chen	Jinshi Cui
Abdessamad Ben Hamza	Kuan-Wen Chen	Fabio Cuzzolin
Chiraz BenAbdelkader	Chia-Ping Chen	Jeremiah D. Deng
Moshe Ben-Ezra	Yi-Ting Chen	Alessio Del Bue
AndrewTeoh Beng-Jin	Tsuhan Chen	Fatih Demirci
Benjamin Berkels	Xiangyu Chen	Xiaoming Deng
Jinbo Bi	Xiaowu Chen	Joachim Denzler
Alberto Del Bimbo	Haifeng Chen	Anthony Dick
Horst Bischof	Hwann-Tzong Chen	Julia Diebold
Konstantinos Blekas	Bing-Yu Chen	Thomas Diego
Adrian Bors	Chu-Song Chen	Csaba Domokos
Nizar Bouguila	Qiang Chen	Qiulei Dong
Edmond Boyer	Jie Chen	Gianfranco Doretto
Steve Branson	Jiun-Hung Chen	Ralf Dragon
Hilton Bristow	MingMing Cheng	Bruce Draper
Asad Butt	Hong Cheng	Tran Du
Ricardo Cabral	Shyi-Chyi Cheng	Lixin Duan
Cesar Cadena	Yuan Cheng	Kun Duan
Francesco Camastra	Wen-Huang Cheng	Fuqing Duan

Zoran Duric
Michael Eckmann
Hazim Ekenel
Naoko Enami
Jakob Engel
Anders Eriksson
Francisco Escolano
Virginia Estellers
Wen-Pinn Fang
Micha Feigin
Jiashi Feng
Francesc Ferri
Katerina Fragkiadaki
Chi-Wing Fu
Yun Fu
Chiou-Shann Fuh
Hironobu Fujiyoshi
Giorgio Fumera
Takuya Funatomi
Juergen Gall
Yongsheng Gao
Ravi Garg
Arkadiusz Gertych
Bernard Ghanem
Guy Godin
Roland Goecke
Vladimir Golkov
Yunchao Gong
Stephen Gould
Josechu Guerrero
Richard Guest
Yanwen Guo
Dong Guo
Huimin Guo
Vu Hai
Lin Hai-Ting
Peter Hall
Onur Hamsici
Tony Han
Hu Han
Zhou Hao
Kenji Hara
Tatsuya Harada
Mehrtash Harandi
Jean-Bernard Hayet
Ran He

Shengfeng He
Shinsaku Hiura
Jeffrey Ho
Christopher Hollitt
Hyunki Hong
Ki Sang Hong
Seunghoon Hong
Takahiro Horiuchi
Timothy Hospedales
Kazuhiro Hotta
Chiou-Ting Candy Hsu
Min-Chun Hu
Zhe Hu
Kai-Lung Hua
Gang Hua
Chunsheng Hua
Chun-Rong Huang
Fay Huang
Kaiqi Huang
Peter Huang
Jia-Bin Huang
Xinyu Huang
Yi-Ping Hung
Mohamed Hussein
Cong Phuoc Huynh
Du Huynh
Sung Ju Hwang
Naoyuki Ichimura
Ichiro Ide
Yoshihisa Ijiri
Sei Ikeda
Nazli Ikizler-Cinbis
Atsushi Imiya
Kohei Inoue
Yani Ioannou
Catalin Ionescu
Go Irie
Rui Ishiyama
Yoshio Iwai
Yumi Iwashita
Arpit Jain
Hueihan Jhuang
Yangqing Jia
Yunde Jia
Kui Jia
Yu-Gang Jiang

Shuqiang Jiang
Xiaoyi Jiang
Jun Jiang
Kang-Hyun Jo
Matjaz Jogan
Manjunath Joshi
Frederic Jurie
Ioannis Kakadiaris
Amit Kale
Prem Kalra
George Kamberov
Kenichi Kanatani
Atul Kanaujla
Mohan Kankanhalli
Abou-Moustafa Karim
Zoltan Kato
Harish Katti
Hiroshi Kawasaki
Christian Kerl
Sang Keun Lee
Aditya Khosla
Hansung Kim
Kyungnam Kim
Seon Joo Kim
Byungsoo Kim
Akisato Kimura
Koichi Kise
Yasuyo Kita
Itaru Kitahara
Reinhard Klette
Georges Koepfler
Iasonas Kokkinos
Kazuaki Kondo
Xiangfei Kong
Sotiris Kotsiantis
Junghyun Kown
Arjan Kuijper
Shiro Kumano
Kashino Kunio
Yoshinori Kuno
Cheng-hao Kuo
Suha Kwak
Iljung Kwak
Junseok Kwon
Alexander Ladikos
Hamid Laga

Antony Lam
Francois Lauze
Duy-Dinh Le
Guee Sang Lee
Jae-Ho Lee
Chan-Su Lee
Yong Jae Lee
Bocchi Leonardo
Marius Leordeanu
Matt Leotta
Wee-Kheng Leow
Bruno Lepri
Frederic Lerasle
Fuxin Li
Hongdong Li
Rui Li
Jia Li
Yufeng Li
Yongmin Li
Yung-Hui Li
Cheng Li
Xin Li
Peihua Li
Xirong Li
Annan Li
Xi Li
Chia-Kai Liang
Shu Liao
T. Warren Liao
Jenn-Jier Lien
Joseph Lim
Ser-Nam Lim
Huei-Yung Lin
Haiting Lin
Weiyao Lin
Wen-Chieh (Steve) Lin
Yen-Yu Lin
RueiSung Lin
Yuanqing Lin
Yen-Liang Lin
Haibin Ling
Hairong Liu
Cheng-Lin Liu
Qingzhong Liu
Miaomiao Liu
Jingchen Liu
Ligang Liu

Haowei Liu
Guangcan Liu
Feng Liu
Shuang Liu
Shuaicheng Liu
Xiaobai Liu
Si Liu
Lingqiao Liu
Chen Change Loy
Feng Lu
Tong Lu
Zhaojin Lu
Le Lu
Huchuan Lu
Ping Luo
Lui Luoqi
Ludovic Macaire
Arif Mahmood
Robert Maier
Yasushi Makihara
Koji Makita
Yoshitsugu Manabe
Rok Mandeljc
Al Mansur
Gian-Luca Marcialis
Stephen Marsland
Takeshi Masuda
Thomas Mauthner
Stephen Maybank
Chris McCool
Xing Mei
Jason Meltzer
David Michael
Anton Milan
Gregor Miller
Dongbo Min
Ikuhisa Mitsugami
Anurag Mittal
Daisuke Miyazaki
Henning Müller
Thomas Moellenhoff
Pascal Monasse
Greg Mori
Bryan Morse
Yadong Mu
Yasuhiro Mukaigawa
Jayanta Mukhopadhyay

Vittorio Murino
Atsushi Nakazawa
Myra Nam
Anoop Namboodiri
Liangliang Nan
Loris Nanni
P.J. Narayanan
Shawn Newsam
Thanh Ngo
Bingbing Ni
Jifeng Ning
Masashi Nishiyama
Mark Nixon
Shohei Nobuhara
Vincent Nozick
Tom O'Donnell
Takeshi Oishi
Takahiro Okabe
Ryuzo Okada
Takayuki Okatani
Gustavo Olague
Martin Oswald
Wanli Ouyang
Yuji Oyamada
Paul Sakrapee
   Paisitkriangkrai
Kalman Palagyi
Hailang Pan
Gang Pan
Sharath Pankanti
Hsing-Kuo Pao
Hyun Soo Park
Jong-Il Park
Ioannis Patras
Nick Pears
Helio Pedrini
Pieter Peers
Yigang Peng
Bo Peng
David Penman
Janez Pers
Wong Ya Ping
Hamed Pirsiavash
Robert Pless
Dilip Prasad
Dipti Prasad Mukherjee
Andrea Prati

Xiao Wu
Yi Wu
Xiaomeng Wu
Rolf Wurtz
Tao Xiang
Yu Xiang
Yang Xiao
Ning Xu
Li Xu
Changsheng Xu
Jianru Xue
Mei Xue
Yasushi Yagi
Koichiro Yamaguchi
Kota Yamaguchi
Osamu Yamaguchi
Toshihiko Yamasaki
Takayoshi Yamashita
Pingkun Yan
Keiji Yanai
Jie Yang
Ruigang Yang
Ming Yang
Hao Yang
Meng Yang
Xiaokang Yang
Yi Yang
Yongliang Yang

Jimei Yang
Chih-Yuan Yang
Bangpeng Yao
Jong Chul Ye
Mao Ye
Sai Kit Yeung
Kwang Moo Yi
Alper Yilmaz
Zhaozheng Yin
Xianghua Ying
Ryo Yonetani
Ju Hong Yoon
Kuk-Jin Yoon
Lap Fai Yu
Gang Yu
Xenophon Zabulis
John Zelek
Zheng-Jun Zha
De-Chuan Zhan
Kaihua Zhang
Tianzhu Zhang
Yu Zhang
Zhong Zhang
Yinda Zhang
Xiaoqin Zhang
Liqing Zhang
Xiaobo Zhang
Changshui Zhang

Cha Zhang
Hong Hui Zhang
Hui Zhang
Guofeng Zhang
Xiao-Wei Zhao
Rui Zhao
Gangqiang Zhao
Shuai Zheng
Yinqiang Zheng
Zhonglong Zheng
Weishi Zheng
Wenming Zheng
Lu Zheng
Baojiang Zhong
Lin Zhong
Bolei Zhou
Jun Zhou
Feng Zhou
Feng Zhu
Ning Zhu
Pengfei Zhu
Cai-Zhi Zhu
Zhigang Zhu
Andrew Ziegler
Danping Zou
Wangmeng Zuo

Best Paper Award Committee

James Rehg   Georgia Institute of Technology, USA
Horst Bischof   Graz University of Technology, Austria
Kyoung Mu Lee   Seoul National University, South Korea

Best Paper Awards

1. Saburo Tsuji Best Paper Award

A Message Passing Algorithm for MRF inference with Unknown Graphs and Its Applications
Zhenhua Wang (University of Adelaide), Zhiyi Zhang (Northwest A&F University), Geng Nan (Northwest A&F University)

2. Sang Uk Lee Best Student Paper Award [Sponsored by Nvidia]

Separation of Reflection Components by Sparse Non-negative Matrix Factorization
Yasuhiro Akashi (Tohoku University), Takayuki Okatani (Tohoku University)

3. Songde Ma Best Application Paper Award [Sponsored by NICTA]

Stereo Fusion using a Refractive Medium on a Binocular Base
Seung-Hwan Baek (KAIST), Min H. Kim (KAIST)

4. Best Paper Honorable Mention

Singly-Bordered Block-Diagonal Form for Minimal Problem Solvers
Zuzana Kukelova (Czech Technical University, Microsoft Research Cambridge),
Martin Bujnak (Capturing Reality), Jan Heller (Czech Technical University),
Tomas Pajdla (Czech Technical University)

5. Best Student Paper Honorable Mention [Sponsored by Nvidia]

On Multiple Image Group Cosegmentation
Fanman Meng (University of Electronic Science and Technology of China),
Jianfei Cai (Nanyang Technological University), Hongliang Li
(University of Electronic Science and Technology of China)

6. Best Application Paper Honorable Mention [Sponsored by NICTA]

Massive City-scale Surface Condition Analysis using Ground and Aerial Imagery
Ken Sakurada (Tohoku University), Takayuki Okatani (Tohoku Univervisty),
Kris Kitani (Carnegie Mellon University)

ACCV 2014 – Outstanding Reviewers

Emre Akbas	Catalin Ionescu	Bernt Schiele
Jonathan Balzer	Suha Kwak	Chunhua Shen
Steve Branson	Junseok Kwon	Sudipta Sinha
Sanderson Conrad	Fuxin Li	Deqing Sun
Marco Cristani	Chen-Change Loy	Yuichi Taguchi
Alessio Del Bue	Scott McCloskey	Toru Tamaki
Anthony Dick	Xing Mei	Dong Wang
Bruce Draper	Yasushi Makihara	Yu-Chiang Frank Wang
Katerina Fragkiadaki	Guy Rosman	Paul Wohlhart
Tatsuya Harada	Mathieu Salzmann	John Wright
Mehrtash Harandi	Pramod Sankar	Bangpeng Yao
Nazli Ikizler-Cinbis	Walter Scheirer	

ACCV 2014 Sponsors

Platnium	Singapore Tourism Board
Gold	Omron Nvidia Garena Samsung
Silver	Adobe ViSenze
Bronze	Lee Foundation Morpx Microsoft Research NICTA

Contents – Part II

3D Vision

Low-Level Vision and Features

Poster Session 2

Poster Session 1

Multi-view Geometry Compression

Siyu Zhu, Tian Fang$^{(\boxtimes)}$, Runze Zhang, and Long Quan

The Hong Kong University of Science and Technology, Hong Kong, China
`tianft@cse.ust.hk`

Abstract. For large-scale and highly redundant photo collections, eliminating statistical redundancy in multi-view geometry is of great importance to efficient 3D reconstruction. Our approach takes the full set of images with initial calibration and recovered sparse 3D points as inputs, and obtains a subset of views that preserve the final reconstruction accuracy and completeness well. We first construct an image quality graph, in which each vertex represents an input image, and the problem is then to determine a connected sub-graph guaranteeing a consistent reconstruction and maximizing the accuracy and completeness of the final reconstruction. Unlike previous works, which only address the problem of efficient structure from motion (SfM), our technique is highly applicable to the whole reconstruction pipeline, and solves the problems of efficient bundle adjustment, multi-view stereo (MVS), and subsequent variational refinement.

1 Introduction

Multi-view geometry represents the intricate geometric relations between multiple views of a 3D scene [1]. Together with the SfM points, it can be optimized as a Maximum Likelihood Estimation, the process of which is called bundle adjustment, and we can also base on multi-view geometry for MVS and subsequent variational refinement. However, for large-scale, irregularly sampled, and highly redundant photo collections, such as Internet photos and video sequences, the statistical redundancy in multi-view geometry severely decreases the reconstruction efficiency and increases the model storage space and transmission capacity.

The overwhelming majority of existing methods generally solve the problem of efficient SfM by eliminating image matching redundancy [2–8], hierarchical decomposition [9–14] and subsampling [15–18]. However, these techniques do not fundamentally reduce the redundancy in multi-view geometry and are difficult to address the problems of efficient MVS and variational refinement. In this paper, we proposed *Multi-View Geometry Compression* (MVGC), which intends to subsample redundant cameras and is highly applicable to the whole reconstruction pipeline, that is it can handle the problems of efficient bundle adjustment, MVS and variational refinement.

Intuitively, our proposed method is based on the observation that a small subset of images is sufficient to guarantee a consistent final reconstruction while preserving its reconstruction accuracy and completeness well. We then formulate

© Springer International Publishing Switzerland 2015
D. Cremers et al. (Eds.): ACCV 2014, Part II, LNCS 9004, pp. 3–18, 2015.
DOI: 10.1007/978-3-319-16808-1_1

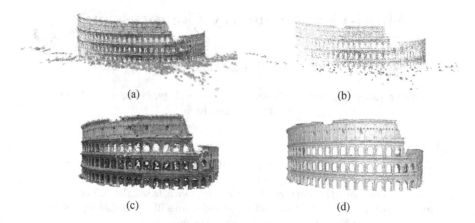

(a)   (b)

(c)   (d)

Fig. 1. Results of our method on the Colosseum data set containing 1789 images. (a) The initial full camera geometry and SfM points which are the inputs of our method. (b) The compressed camera geometry and SfM points that can be used for an efficient bundle adjustment. (c) The accurate and complete stereo reconstruction results based on the compressed multi-view geometry. (d) The variational refinement results from the compressed geometry. Note that it is too computationally expensive for the standard refinement approach to handle the full image collections.

the compression problem as a graph simplification procedure. Based on the full set of images with initial calibration and SfM points, we construct an image quality graph, where each image is a graph vertex and two vertexes are connected if their corresponding image pair can be used for a consistent reconstruction. The problem is then to determine a connected sub-graph with the maximum sum of vertex weight under a certain number of vertexes. A down-sampling algorithm is then introduced as an approximation to solve the problem.

Our work is closely related to research on skeletal graph for efficient SfM [6]. The main difference is that our proposed approach is highly applicable to not only SfM, but also MVS and variational refinement applications. Moreover, the experiment results on both standard and Internet data sets also quantitatively and qualitatively demonstrate that our method increases the efficiency of bundle adjustment, MVS, and variational refinement by approximately a magnitude and better preserves the accuracy and completeness of the final reconstruction than the skeletal graph [6] and other methods.

2   Related Work

During the past few years, many works have been done to reduce redundancy in the 3D reconstruction pipeline. An intuitive idea is to eliminate unnecessary image matching pairs and the vast majority of previous works follow this direction. Rather than matching all image pairs, Agarwal et al. [2] identify a small fraction of candidates by means of vocabulary tree recognition [3]. Frahm et al. [4] utilize approximate GPS tags to capture only nearby image pairs for

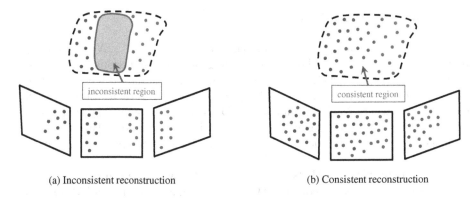

(a) Inconsistent reconstruction   (b) Consistent reconstruction

Fig. 2. The interpretation for a consistent reconstruction. (a) and (b) show that, to preserve a consistent reconstruction, especially for MVS and variational refinement, the intersection of common visible points between the image pair $\{I_i, I_{i+1}\}$ and $\{I_{i+1}, I_{i+2}\}$ cannot be empty.

matching. Wu [5] exploits the characteristic of large-scale matching problem that most of image pairs fail to match, and introduce the preemptive feature matching to filter out superfluous image matching pairs. Since we assume that image matching is given and initial multi-view geometry is also recovered in this paper, all the techniques mentioned are complementary to our work.

The proposed algorithm in this paper is closely related to [2,6–8], which obtain a small skeletal subset of images from a dense scene graphs. However, rather than directly discarding redundant cameras as we do, these works only intend to accelerate the bundle adjustment process by simplifying matching between image pairs and cannot be appropriately applied to other reconstruction steps (e.g. MVS and variational refinement). Moreover, these methods fail to strictly guarantee that the simplified geometry can be used for a consistent reconstruction, which is properly handled in our work by the introduction of quality graph. The hierarchical framework [15] which proposes to resample a dense SfM points still suffers the same problems. Likewise, the approaches above are complementary to our work.

Similar to our method, the authors of [16–18] also propose subsampling approaches to solve SfM problems of video sequences, while they cannot handle diverse and unordered images with complex geometry topology. Canonical view selection methods for robot localization [19] also refer to similar criteria, however, they need different considerations when applied to reconstruction problems.

Instead of reducing input redundancy, divide-and-conquer is also widely used to solve large-scale reconstruction problems. Steedly et al. [9] utilize spectral partitioning to decouple original sequential images into pieces for easier bundle adjustment. Ni et al. [10] split the entire bundle problem into sub-maps with their own coordinate systems for efficient operation, and the authors of [11,12,20] also handle the bundle problem within a relative coordinate system. Rather than recover 3D structure hierarchically at the image level, Farenzena et al. [13] and Gherardi et al. [14] apply divide-and-conquer at the variable level.

3   Problem Formulation

The input to our approach is a set of images $\mathbf{I} = \{I_i \,|\, i = 1, 2, ..., N_\mathbf{I}\}$, where $N_\mathbf{I}$ is the number of cameras. Their corresponding camera calibrations are denoted by $\mathbf{\Pi} = \{\Pi_i | i = 1, 2, ..., N_\mathbf{I}\}$, which are obtained from a standard reconstruction pipeline [21]. A point cloud $\mathbf{P} = \{P_m \,|\, j = 1, 2, ..., N_\mathbf{P}\}$ is then obtained with triangulation, where $N_\mathbf{P}$ is the number of 3D points. It is noteworthy that $\mathbf{P}$ can either be sparse 3D points generated by a general SfM system (e.g. Bundler [22]), or quasi-dense points obtained from a commonly used MVS pipeline (e.g. Quasi-Dense [23]).

Now, the problem of MVGC is defined as follows: given an image set $\mathbf{I}$, its corresponding camera geometry $\mathbf{\Pi}$, and triangulated point cloud $\mathbf{P}$, find an image subset $\mathbf{I}'$ that yields a reconstruction with the least loss of reconstruction accuracy and completeness, which are measured by an increasing function $w(I_i)$ for a given image I_i.

Another issue with our approach is to guarantee that the compressed multi-view geometry can be used for a consistent reconstruction (see Fig. 2), and we therefore introduce the *image quality graph* $G_\mathbf{I}$, where $G_\mathbf{I} = (\mathbf{V}, \mathbf{E})$ is an undirected connected graph, with $\mathbf{V} = \{V_i \,|\, i = 1, 2, ..., n\}$, and each graph vertex V_i corresponds to an image I_i. In order to guarantee that I_i and I_j can be used for a consistent reconstruction, there ought to exist at least one image I_k satisfying that

$$(\mathbf{P}_{I_i} \cap \mathbf{P}_{I_k}) \cap (\mathbf{P}_{I_j} \cap \mathbf{P}_{I_k}) \neq \emptyset, \tag{1}$$

where $\mathbf{P}_{I_i}$ is the set of 3D points visible in camera I_i. And for the graph edge $E_{ij} \in \mathbf{E}$ connecting vertex V_i and V_j, its edge weight $h(E_{ij})$ is defined as the number of cameras $\{I_k\}$ satisfying Eq. (1), that is $h(E_{ij}) = |\{I_k\}|$. Obviously, V_i and V_j is disconnected when $h(E_{ij}) = 0$.

In summary, the problem of MVGC can be mathematically formulated as: given $(\mathbf{I}, \mathbf{\Pi}, \mathbf{P})$ and N_I which is the target number of cameras to be preserved, find $\mathbf{I}' \subset \mathbf{I}$ satisfying

$$\mathbf{I}' = \arg\max_{\mathbf{I}'} \sum_{I_i \in \mathbf{I}'} w(I_i), \tag{2}$$

$$s.t. \quad |\mathbf{I}'| = N_I \text{ and } G_{\mathbf{I}'} \text{ is connected.}$$

4   Approaches

4.1   Graph Construction

Recalling that $G_\mathbf{I} = (\mathbf{V}, \mathbf{E})$, and each graph vertex V_i has a weight scale $w(I_i)$, which is an increasing function denoting the possibility I_i tends to be preserved in the final sub-graph. Obviously, we prefer cameras with high accuracy and completeness measures and we further introduce the regularity measure to avoid irregularly sampled views in the reconstruction scene. Therefore, the weight scale $w(I_i)$ of image I_i is defined as

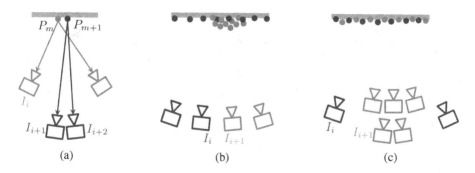

Fig. 3. The illustration of graph vertex measures. (a) 3D points triangulated by cameras with large angles and pixel sampling rate are generally of low covariance (e.g. P_m over P_{m+1}), and cameras with great numbers of such points tend to be remained. (b) Cameras covering 3D points of low density are more inclined to preserve reconstruction completeness (e.g. I_i over I_{i+1}). (c) We prefer under-sampled cameras rather than over-sampled cameras (e.g. I_i over I_{i+1}) to guarantee a uniform distribution of cameras.

$$w(I_i) = w_a(I_i) \cdot w_c(I_i) \cdot w_r(I_i), \tag{3}$$

where $w_a(I_i)$ is the accuracy measure, $w_c(I_i)$ the completeness measure, and $w_r(I_i)$ the regularity measure. Please see Fig. 3 for the visual demonstration.

Accuracy Measure. First, the remained cameras should preserve the final reconstruction accuracy as much as possible. Without ground truth data, camera covariance can be regarded as an alternative to assess the reconstruction accuracy, while even the fast gauge-free covariance estimation method [23] is extremely both space and time consuming for large-scale image collections.

Geometrically, cameras covering more well-qualified 3D points tend to be better constrained and of smaller covariance. For one camera, we utilize the sum of accuracy measure of its visible 3D points as an approximation of camera covariance. Inspired by [24,25], camera pairs with large angles and pixel sampling rate generally triangulate 3D points of high quality (see Fig. 3(a)), and the accuracy measure of a single point P_m observed by the image pair $\{I_i, I_j\}$ is therefore defined as

$$
g_a(P_m, I_i, I_j) = e^{\left(-\frac{(\angle I_i P_m I_j - \sigma_\theta)^2}{2\sigma^2_{\angle I_i P_m I_j}} \right)} \cdot s(P_m, I_i, I_j)
$$
$$
s.t. \quad \sigma_{\angle I_i P_m I_j} = \begin{cases} \theta_1 & \angle I_i P_m I_j \leq \sigma_\theta \\ \theta_2 & \angle I_i P_m I_j > \sigma_\theta \end{cases} \tag{4}
$$

where $s(P_m, I_i, I_j) = \min(1/r(P_m, I_i), 1/r(P_m, I_j))$, $r(P_m, I_i)$ quantifies the diameter of a sphere centered at P_m and its projected diameter equals the pixel spacing in I_i, $\sigma_\theta = 20°$, $\theta_1 = 5°$, and $\theta_2 = 15°$.

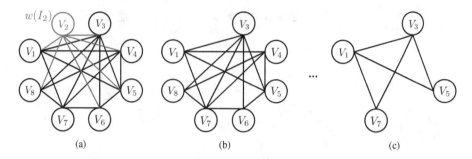

Fig. 4. The graph simplification algorithm. Starting from the initial dense graph shown in (a), we iteratively remove the vertex with the lowest weight and its corresponding adjacent edges until the number of vertexes below a threshold (the final graph is shown in (c)). Meanwhile, the obtained sub-graph is connected so as to guarantee a consistent model.

Therefore, the accuracy measure of one camera I_i is expressed as

$$w_a(I_i) = \sum_{\substack{I_j \in \mathbf{I},\, i \neq j \\ P_m \in \mathbf{P}_{I_i} \cap \mathbf{P}_{I_j}}} g_a(\angle I_i P_m I_j). \tag{5}$$

Completeness Measure. Next, the preserved cameras should cover the whole reconstructed scene, and the completeness in 3D space can be measured by the density of points in 3D. Generally, cameras containing more 3D points of low density better preserve reconstruction completeness (see Fig. 3(b)), and we compute the sum of N_c lowest point density as our camera completeness measure, namely

$$w_c(I_i) = \max_{\mathbf{P}'_{I_i} \subseteq \mathbf{P}_{I_i}, |\mathbf{P}'_{I_i}| = N_c} \sum_{P_m \in \mathbf{P}'_{I_i}} d(P_m), \tag{6}$$

where $d(P_i)$ is the inverse of the density of P_i, and $N_c = 10$.

Regularity Measure. Finally, we should guarantee that the selected cameras are regularly sampled in the reconstruction scene rather than over-sampled in some regions with popular viewpoints and under-sampled in others. Similar to [24], we take the scene content, appearance, and scale into consideration, and introduce the regularity measure $w_r(I_i)$ an increasing function computing the degree the points covered by I_i are also covered by its adjacent cameras. Quantitatively, each point is given a weight counteracting a greater number of visible cameras with a good range of parallax within a neighborhood, and $w_r(I_i)$ is given as the sum of its visible point weights, that is

$$w_r(I_i) = \sum_{\substack{I_j \in \mathbf{I},\, i \neq j \\ P_m \in \mathbf{P}_{I_i} \cap \mathbf{P}_{I_j}}} g_N(P_m) \cdot g_S(P_m). \tag{7}$$

Table 1. Statistics of the SfM data sets and algorithms.

		Sequential			Unstructured		
		Garden	Park	Street	Colosseum	Notre Dame	Trevi
# of images		948	940	684	1789	712	1789
# of images after MVGC		95	94	68	179	71	179
Mean position error [m]	Key frame	0.31	0.24	0.26	–	–	–
	Skeletal graph	0.93	0.82	0.89	0.41	0.34	0.43
	MVGC	0.24	0.19	0.22	0.12	0.11	0.09
Running time [min]	MVGC	0.94	0.88	0.42	2.88	1.57	3.11
	BA with MVGC	0.49	0.66	0.49	0.91	0.45	0.87
	BA without MVGC	6.84	8.14	3.30	10.22	7.23	12.01

Here $g_N(P_m)$ penalizes the trend of greater numbers of features in common with a decreasing angle, and $g_N(P_m)$ is given as

$$g_N(P_m) = \prod_{\substack{I_i, I_j \in \mathbf{I},\ i \neq j \\ P_m \in \mathbf{P}_{I_i} \cap \mathbf{P}_{I_j}}} g_r(P_m, I_i, I_j), \tag{8}$$

where $g_r(P_m, I_i, I_j) = \min((\alpha/\alpha_{\max})^2, 1)$, α is the angle between the rays of I_i and I_j triangulating P_m, and we set $\alpha_{\max} = 60°$, which prefers camera pairs with large angles in all our experiments.

Moreover, $g_S(P_m)$ encourages views with equal or higher resolution than the reference view, and we use

$$g_S(P_m) = \begin{cases} 2/r & 2 \leq r \\ 1 & 1 \leq r < 2 \\ r & r < 1 \end{cases} \tag{9}$$

where $r = r(P_m, I_i)/r(P_m, I_j)$.

4.2 Graph Simplification

Unfortunately, the problem of computing the optimal sub-graph is NP-complete, and we propose an approximation algorithm to obtain it. Starting from an initial dense graph, we first sort the graph vertexes into a priority queue based on their weight and then iteratively delete the vertex with the lowest weight and its adjacent edges until the number of vertexes equals the target number. Meanwhile, there are two issues we should take into consideration. First, the graph edge weight, namely $h(E_{ij})$, changes along with the vertex removal process. When $h(E_{ij}) = 0$, V_i and V_j is disconnected, and we ought to guarantee that the image quality graph is connected until the convergence is met. Second, when the graph is simplified, the graph vertex weight $w(I_i)$ also varies. Obviously, it is computationally unnecessary to update the vertex weight of the entire graph each time a vertex is removed. In our implementation, we update the vertex weight and reallocate the priority queue each time 10 vertexes are removed. Admittedly, the obtained sub-graph is not theoretically optimal, but it still generates satisfactory results.

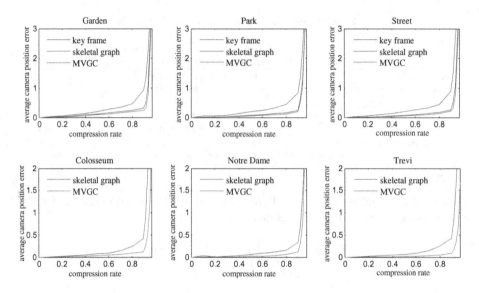

Fig. 5. Average camera position errors after bundle adjustment at different compression rates. We can see that the results of MVGC have lower average camera position errors than those using key frame and skeletal graph on all data sets.

5   Experiments

To demonstrate that the proposed MVGC is highly applicable to the whole pipeline of 3D reconstruction, we present the applications of our method in bundle adjustment, MVS, and variational refinement in the following experiments.

Implementation. Our approach is implemented in C++ and the code is completely CPU-based. All our experiments are tested on a PC with a Quad-core Intel 3.5 GHz processor and 32 GB RAM. We use the publicly available Ceres [26] for bundle adjustment and Quasi-Dense approach [23] for MVS. We also follow the pipeline described in [27] for mesh generation and [28] for variational refinement. The parameters in our implementation are all standard except for N_c, which determines the density of the quality graph and directly effects the running time of MVGC.

Data Set. Three categories of data sets are introduced for testing, and they are respectively video sequences with a resolution of 3M pixels obtained from monochrome video cameras, unstructured high-resolution images from a well-known benchmark [29], and unstructured photo collections from the Internet captured by various cameras with different focal lengths, distortion and sensor noise, under different conditions of lighting, surface reflection and scale.

5.1   Applications in Bundle Adjustment

First, the input images are automatically calibrated using the standard approach [21] and MVGC is then introduced to select a subset of initially calibrated

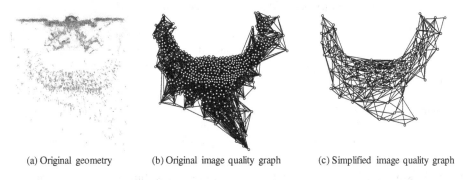

(a) Original geometry   (b) Original image quality graph   (c) Simplified image quality graph

Fig. 6. Graph simplification results of the Trevi data set. Note how the MVGC algorithm preserves the important topology, but significantly reduces the redundancy of the original graph.

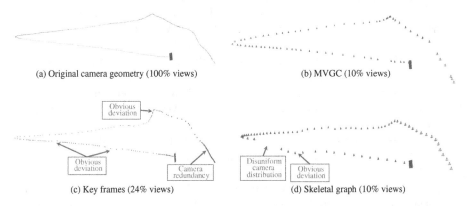

(a) Original camera geometry (100% views)   (b) MVGC (10% views)

(c) Key frames (24% views)   (d) Skeletal graph (10% views)

Fig. 7. Comparisons of video sequence trajectories after bundle adjustment. Compared with the original full sequence, MVGC best preserves the video sequence trajectory after bundle adjustment while the resampled video sequence trajectories using other methods have obvious deviation, redundancy, or disuniform distribution.

views for bundle adjustment. In our implementation, we avoid using multiple full bundle adjustment, which is the main time-consuming part of SfM, before MVGC but divide a large SfM problem into small sub-problems, which are partially bundled, and use the partially bundled geometry as the input geometry for MVGC. After that the full bundle adjustment of each sub-problem and the final bundle adjustment of the global problem are performed. In details, we incrementally add cameras and do partial bundle adjustment for the recently 10 added cameras. When the number of cameras increases relatively by a certain ratio (e.g. 10 %), the geometry of the newly added cameras is regarded as the initially calibrated geometry, and we use MVGC to resample these cameras. Next, the newly resampled cameras together with previously resampled cameras are used for a full bundle adjustment. Then, MVGC is introduced again to resample all the remained cameras and a full bundle adjustment is performed finally.

Table 2. Statistics of the MVS data sets and algorithms.

		Benchmark data sets		Internet data sets		
		Fountain-R25	Herz-Jesu-R23	Square	Notre Dame	Colosseum
# of images		25	23	1907	712	1789
# of images after MVGC		13	12	191	71	179
Running time [min]	MVGC	0.13	0.15	3.26	1.57	2.88
	MVS with MVGC	6.44	6.98	90.14	33.13	85.01
	MVS without MVGC	17.48	16.20	922.23	344.80	835.60

In other words, MVGC do require camera calibrations, but only rough camera calibrations.

The author in [5] shows that partial BA guarantees good camera geometry locally, which can provide satisfactory input geometry for MVGC. The author in [5] also proves that for the majority of large-scale dataset, the time cost of partial BA is much smaller than those of full BA. So the efficiency of SfM improves greatly as we remarkably improve the efficiency of full BA as shown in Table 1. For example, the overall time of full BA of Trevi dataset with and without MVGC are 0.87 and 12.01 min respectively. The partial BA and the other time costs with and without MVGC are 2.73 and 3.96 min respectively. Therefore, the overall time of SfM with and without MVGC are 3.6 and 15.97 min respectively.

Table 1 also shows the statistics of the data sets for bundle adjustment, and about 90 % of cameras are removed using the method of key frame, skeletal graph [6], and MVGC respectively. Here we define compression rate as the percentage of discarding cameras. We can see from Table 1 and Fig. 5 that, on both sequential and unstructured data sets, MVGC obviously outperforms key frame and skeletal graph in average camera position errors after bundle adjustment while improving the efficiency of bundle adjustment by almost a magnitude. Figure 7 gives the qualitative demonstration of the outstanding performance of our method. Figure 6 also provides the visual demonstration of the graph simplification result of the Trevi data set.

5.2 Applications in Multi-view Stereo

Both on the benchmark and Internet data sets, we use full image sets for SfM and MVGC to select a subset of views for dense 3D reconstruction. The general statistics of MVS data sets shown in Table 2 indicate that approximately 50 % of cameras are discarded in the benchmark data sets and 90 % in the Internet data sets. As shown in Figs. 8(a) and (b), the relative error of MVS reconstruction with MVGC is almost the same as that using full image sets on the benchmark data sets. The curves of average relative errors at different compression rates of the Internet data sets are provided in Fig. 8, which further confirms the superiority of MVGC over the skeletal graph and key frame in applications of MVS. Figure 9 provides visual results of MVS of the fountain-R25 and Notre Dame

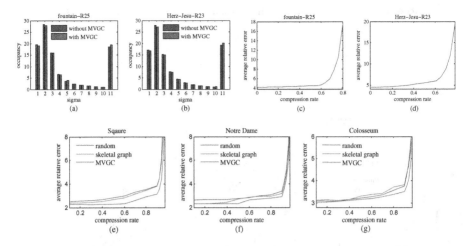

Fig. 8. Average relative errors of benchmark and Internet data sets in the MVS application. (a) and (b) are comparisons of average relative errors of the benchmark data sets between reconstruction using full image sequences and compressed geometry (50 % views). We observe that the absolute reconstruction accuracy using compressed geometry is almost the same as that using complete geometry. (c) and (d) show the average relative errors of the benchmark data sets at different compression rates. (e), (f) and (g) present the average relative errors at different compression rate of the Internet data sets. Likewise, MVGC outperforms the skeletal graph and random image selection methods in any compression rate.

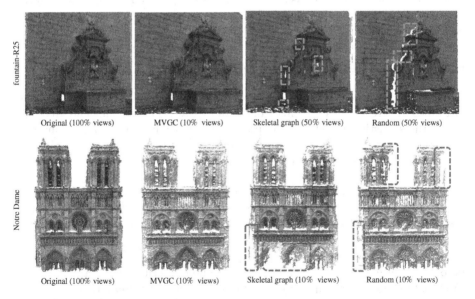

Fig. 9. Comparisons of MVS dense results of the fountain-R25 and Notre Dame data sets in the MVS application. Note the incomplete regions highlighted by dashed rectangles and that the reconstruction from the compressed geometry is complete.

Table 3. Statistics of variational refinement data sets and algorithms.

		Benchmark data sets			Internet data sets		
		Fountain-P11	Entry-P10	Castle-P19	Trevi	Square	Basilica
# of images		11	10	19	1789	1907	1103
# of images after MVGC		6	5	10	54	57	33
Running time [min]	MVGC	0.09	0.07	0.12	3.88	3.67	2.98
	Refinement with MVGC	12.01	8.23	22.61	273.13	324.67	160.00
	Refinement without MVGC	43.36	36.93	86.04	N/A	N/A	N/A

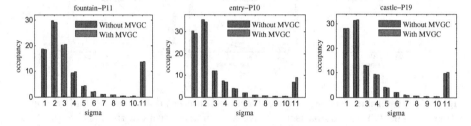

Fig. 10. Relative error histograms of the benchmark data sets in the variational refinement application. It is obvious that the remarkably improved efficiency using MVGC almost compromises no reconstruction accuracy.

data sets. Unlike the MVS results using the skeletal graph and random image selection, which are compromised by incomplete regions, our compressed multiview geometry preserves reconstruction accuracy and completeness best in the final reconstruction.

5.3   Applications in Variational Refinement

In this application, the full image sets are used for SfM and MVS, and we then introduce MVGC to select a subset of views for variational refinement. According to the statistics in Table 3, the proposed algorithm reduces approximately 50 % of the images in the benchmark data sets and 97 % of the images in the Internet data sets for refinement. As demonstrated by the relative error histograms in Fig. 11, the reconstruction accuracy using compressed geometry is almost the same as the one using full image sets on the benchmark data sets but we only spend about 25 % of the running time of the method without compression. Since standard refinement algorithms are generally based on an energy summation traversing all image pairs to compute the cross correlation of photo consistency, as the number of images explodes, the increased time consumption becomes unacceptable, particularly for redundant Internet data sets. Take the Trevi data set as an example, for the full image set approximately 319 k image pairs are needed for pairwise correlation computation, while only 3 % of these image pairs are needed after MVGC. Figures 11 and 12 provide some visual results of variational refinement of the benchmark and Internet data sets.

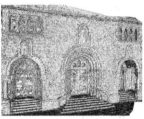 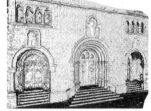 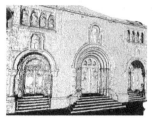

(a) The original triangulated mesh   (b) 100% views for refinement   (c) 32% views for refinement using MVGC

Fig. 11. Comparisons of variational refinement results of the Herz-Jesu-P25 data set in the variational refinement application. The refinement results using compressed geometry still recovers the same details, edges, and topology as the refinement results using full image sets.

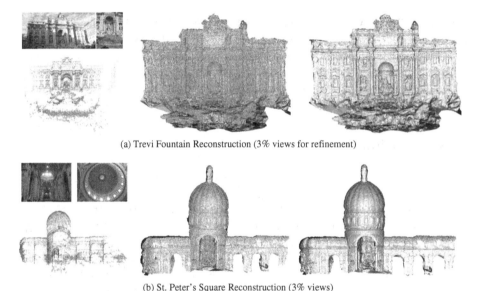

(a) Trevi Fountain Reconstruction (3% views for refinement)

(b) St. Peter's Square Reconstruction (3% views)

Fig. 12. Variational refinement results of the Internet data sets using MVGC. The figures from left to right are samples of Internet image collections, SfM points and corresponding camera geometry, initial triangulated meshes with a decent amount of noise, and finally refined mesh models. We should note that the data sets above cannot be handled by standard refinement methods using full image sets.

5.4 Discussions

Graph Vertex Weight Measures. Another important issue for our experiments is to validate the effectiveness of the accuracy, completeness, and regularity measures in the image quality graph. Table 4 shows the average camera position errors of the sequential and unstructured data sets in SfM for different choices of vertex weight measures. We observe that the MVGC algorithm with accuracy, completeness, and regularity measures performs the best while the absence of anyone of these weight measures will lead to the degeneration of the reconstruction accuracy.

Table 4. Average position errors for different choices of vertex weight measures after bundle adjustment. "A" is the accuracy measure, "C" the completeness measure, and "R" the regularity measure. The MVGC algorithm with accuracy, completeness, and uniformity measures has the lowest average position error after bundle adjustment.

		A + C	A + R	C + R	A + C + R
Sequential data sets	Garden	0.32	0.27	0.30	0.24
	Park	0.26	0.20	0.24	0.19
	Street	0.34	0.31	0.29	0.22
Unstructured data sets	Colosseum	0.19	0.18	0.16	0.12
	Notro Dame	0.22	0.16	0.18	0.11
	Trevi	0.14	0.12	0.12	0.09

Running Time. As indicated in Tables 1, 2, and 3, the running time of MVGC is minor, and the largest is 3.67 min for the Trevi data set. While our proposed method significantly reduces the time and memory consumption of bundle adjustment, MVS, and variational refinement by almost a magnitude, and makes the previously impossible variational refinement using Internet data sets manageable.

6   Conclusions

We propose an approach to compress multi-view geometry by obtaining a subset of views from the original full camera geometry while maximizing the reconstruction accuracy and completeness. The key technical contribution is the introduction of image quality graph, and the problem is then transformed to computing a sub-graph from the original dense graph. MVGC is highly applicable to bundle adjustment, MVS, and variational refinement, and introduces remarkable improvement in efficiency with almost no loss of reconstruction accuracy and completeness. The experiment results on both standard and Internet data sets demonstrate the remarkable improvement in efficiency with almost no loss of reconstruction accuracy and completeness. As for the future work, it is interesting to theoretically explore the optimum subset of multi-view geometry, although our approximation approach has provided satisfactory results. Going forward, hopefully we could extend our method to a hierarchical pipeline so as to validate our pipeline on larger data sets, especially the most prevalent city-scale data sets.

Acknowledgement. We really appreciate the support of RGC-GRF 618711, RGC/NSFC N_HKUST607/11, ITC-PSKL12EG02, and National Basic Research Program of China (2012CB316300).

References

1. Heyden, A., Pollefeys, M.: Tutorial on multiple view geometry. In: Conjunction with ICPR (2000)
2. Agarwal, S., Snavely, N., Simon, I., Seitz, S.M., Szeliski, R.: Building rome in a day. In: ICCV (2009)
3. Nister, D., Stewenius, H.: Scalable recognition with a vocabulary tree. In: CVPR (2006)
4. Frahm, J.-M., Fite-Georgel, P., Gallup, D., Johnson, T., Raguram, R., Wu, C., Jen, Y.-H., Dunn, E., Clipp, B., Lazebnik, S., Pollefeys, M.: Building rome on a cloudless day. In: Daniilidis, K., Maragos, P., Paragios, N. (eds.) ECCV 2010, Part IV. LNCS, vol. 6314, pp. 368–381. Springer, Heidelberg (2010)
5. Wu, C.: Towards linear-time incremental structure from motion. In: 3DTV (2013)
6. Snavely, N., Seitz, S.M., Szeliski, R.: Skeletal sets for efficient structure from motion. In: CVPR (2008)
7. Li, X., Wu, C., Zach, C., Lazebnik, S., Frahm, J.-M.: Modeling and recognition of landmark image collections using iconic scene graphs. In: Forsyth, D., Torr, P., Zisserman, A. (eds.) ECCV 2008, Part I. LNCS, vol. 5302, pp. 427–440. Springer, Heidelberg (2008)
8. Agarwal, S., Snavely, N., Seitz, S.M., Szeliski, R.: Bundle adjustment in the large. In: Daniilidis, K., Maragos, P., Paragios, N. (eds.) ECCV 2010, Part II. LNCS, vol. 6312, pp. 29–42. Springer, Heidelberg (2010)
9. Steedly, D., Essa, I., Dellaert, F.: Spectral partitioning for structure from motion. In: ICCV (2003)
10. Ni, K., Steedly, D., Dellaert, F.: Out-of-core bundle adjustment for large-scale 3D reconstruction. In: ICCV (2007)
11. Mouragnon, E., Lhuillier, M., Dhome, M., Dekeyser, F., Sayd, P.: Real time localization and 3D reconstruction. In: CVPR (2006)
12. Eudes, A., Lhuillier, M.: Error propagations for local bundle adjustment. In: CVPR (2009)
13. Farenzena, M., Fusiello, A., Gherardi, R.: Structure-and-motion pipeline on a hierarchical cluster tree. In: ICCV Workshop on 3D Digital Imaging and Modeling (2009)
14. Gherardi, R., Farenzena, M., Fusiello, A.: Improving the efficiency of hierarchical structure-and-motion. In: CVPR (2010)
15. Fang, T., Quan, L.: Resampling structure from motion. In: Daniilidis, K., Maragos, P., Paragios, N. (eds.) ECCV 2010, Part II. LNCS, vol. 6312, pp. 1–14. Springer, Heidelberg (2010)
16. Fitzgibbon, A.W., Zisserman, A.: Automatic camera recovery for closed or open image sequences. In: Burkhardt, H.-J., Neumann, B. (eds.) ECCV 1998. LNCS, vol. 1406, pp. 311–326. Springer, Heidelberg (1998)
17. Nistér, D.: Reconstruction from uncalibrated sequences with a hierarchy of trifocal tensors. In: Vernon, D. (ed.) ECCV 2000. LNCS, vol. 1842, pp. 649–663. Springer, Heidelberg (2000)
18. Repko, J., Pollefeys, M.: 3D models from extended uncalibrated video sequences. In: Proceeding 3DIM (2005)
19. Booij, O., Zivkovic, Z., Krose, B.: Sparse appearance based modeling for robot localization. In: IROS (2006)
20. Zhu, S., Fang, T., Xiao, J., Quan, L.: Local readjustment for high-resolution 3D reconstruction (2014)

21. Hartley, R., Zisserman, A.: Multiple View Geometry in Computer Vision. Cambridge University Press, Cambridge (2000)
22. Snavely, N., Seitz, S.M., Szeliski, R.: Photo tourism: exploring photo collections in 3D. In: SIGGRAPH (2006)
23. Lhuillier, M., Quan, L.: A quasi-dense approach to surface reconstruction from uncalibrated images. PAMI **27**, 418–433 (2005)
24. Goesele, M., Snavely, N., Curless, B., Hoppe, H., Seitz, S.M.: Multi-view stereo for community photo collections. In: ICCV (2007)
25. Furukawa, Y., Curless, B., Seitz, S.M., Szeliski, R.: Towards internet-scale multi-view stereo. In: CVPR (2010)
26. Agarwal, S., Mierle, K., Others: Ceres solver. https://code.google.com/p/ceres-solver/
27. Kazhdan, M., Bolitho, M., Hoppe, H.: Poisson surface reconstruction. In: Symposium Geometry Proceeding (2006)
28. Delaunoy, A., Prados, E., Gargallo, P., Pons, J.P., Sturm, P.F.: Minimizing the multi-view stereo reprojection error for triangular surface meshes. In: BMVC (2008)
29. Strecha, C., Hansen, W.V., Gool, L.V., Fua, P., Thoennessen, U.: On benchmarking camera calibration and multi-view stereo for high resolution imagery. In: CVPR (2008)

Camera Calibration Based on the Common Self-polar Triangle of Sphere Images

Haifei Huang[1,2], Hui Zhang[2,3(✉)], and Yiu-ming Cheung[1,2]

[1] Department of Computer Science, Hong Kong Baptist University,
Hong Kong, China
[2] United International College, BNU-HKBU, Zhuhai, China
amyzhang@uic.edu.hk
[3] Shenzhen Key Lab of Intelligent Media and Speech,
PKU-HKUST Shenzhen Hong Kong Institution, Shenzhen, China

Abstract. Sphere has been used for camera calibration in recent years. In this paper, a new linear calibration method is proposed by using the common self-polar triangle of sphere images. It is shown that any two of sphere images have a common self-polar triangle. Accordingly, a simple method for locating the vertices of such triangles is presented. An algorithm for recovering the vanishing line of the support plane using these vertices is developed. This allows to find out the imaged circular points, which are used to calibrate the camera. The proposed method starts from an existing theory in projective geometry and recovers five intrinsic parameters without calculating the projected circle center, which is more intuitive and simpler than the previous linear ones. Experiments with simulated data, as well as real images, show that our technique is robust and accurate.

1 Introduction

Camera calibration is a fundamental task in many computer vision applications, such as motion estimation and 3D reconstruction. The main task of camera calibration is to recover the intrinsic and extrinsic parameters. Many calibration methods have been proposed in the past years. They can be classified into two categories: calibration with objects [1–3], and self-calibration [4–6].

In the first category, classical calibration techniques require the use of some highly accurate tailor-made calibration patterns, which are time-consuming and costly. To overcome this drawback, sphere has been introduced into camera calibration in recent years because sphere can be easily found in daily life and its silhouettes can be extracted reliably from image [7]. Besides, it is suitable to calibrate a camera network. As long as the sphere is placed in the common field of view of the cameras, its occluding contours are visible from any position [8].

Sphere, as a calibration target, was first used in [9] to recover the aspect ratio of the two images axes. Later, some nonlinear methods for estimating more camera intrinsic parameters had been presented. In [10], under the assumption of a zero-skew camera, a multi-step nonlinear approach to estimating four intrinsic

© Springer International Publishing Switzerland 2015
D. Cremers et al. (Eds.): ACCV 2014, Part II, LNCS 9004, pp. 19–29, 2015.
DOI: 10.1007/978-3-319-16808-1_2

parameters was presented. In [11], the relation of the image of absolute conic to the image of sphere was well investigated and camera intrinsic parameters were recovered by minimizing the reprojection errors nonlinearly. In [8], a semi-definite programming approach was introduced based on the dual representation of the sphere image. However, there are some problems in nonlinear methods. In [10], error is accumulated seriously in the separated steps. In [11], an appropriate initialization should be given before stating the minimization process. In [8], when noise is large, there could be no solution sometimes. To avoid these deficiencies, from Year 2005, some linear approaches had been introduced. Zhang et al. [12,13], treated two spheres as a surface of revolution [14] and recovered internal parameters by using pole-polar constraints on the image of absolute conic. Ying and Zha [15] interpreted the same constraint presented in [8,11] geometrically, and presented two linear approaches to calibrating the camera by using double contact points and double-contact theorem. Zhao and Liu [16] developed a method by treating a sphere as a revolving stick. Recently, Wong [17] has introduced a stratified approach to recovering extrinsic parameters and intrinsic parameters by finding special point correspondences. Note that the first calibration method presented in [15], as well as methods presented in [8,16], require calculating the projected circle center at the very beginning.

In this paper, we solve the problem of camera calibration using spheres in a new perspective. We investigate the common self-polar triangle of sphere images thoroughly and find that vanishing line of the support plane can be determined by the vertices of such triangles. This allows to find out the imaged circular points, which are used to calibrate the camera. From this perspective, calculating the projected circle center at the very beginning is not necessary and conic homography theory can be interpreted as using the self-dual triangle of sphere images. Note that the proposed method is totally different from the calibration method in [13]. In [13], they investigated the plane formed by the camera center and two sphere centers. They tried to recover the vanishing line of the plane and vanishing point of the plane's normal, while our method is trying to recover the vanishing line of the support plane.

The remainder of this paper is organized as follows. Section 2 briefly introduces some notations and basic equations. Section 3 discusses the common self-polar triangle of two conics. Section 4 presents our novel calibration method. Section 5 shows the experimental results of the proposed method on synthetic and real data sets. Finally, a conclusion is drawn in Sect. 6.

2 Notations and Basic Equations

2.1 The Camera Model

The pinhole camera model is adopted in this paper. In the homogenous coordinate system, let $\mathbf{M} = [X\ Y\ Z\ 1]^\mathbf{T}$ be a world point and $\mathbf{m} = [x\ y\ 1]^\mathbf{T}$ be its image. The imaging process can be represented as

$$u\mathbf{m} = \mathbf{K}[\mathbf{R}|\mathbf{t}]\mathbf{M} \tag{1}$$

where u is a nonzero scale factor, $\mathbf{R}|\mathbf{t}$ denotes a rigid transformation, and $\mathbf{K}$ is the intrinsic parameter matrix with the following format:

$$\mathbf{K} = \begin{bmatrix} \alpha f & s & u_0 \\ 0 & f & v_0 \\ 0 & 0 & 1 \end{bmatrix} \tag{2}$$

In the matrix $\mathbf{K}$, f is the focal length, α is the aspect ratio, (u_0, v_0) is the principal point, and s is the skew.

2.2   The Absolute Conic

The absolute conic was first introduced by Faugeras et al. [4] for camera self-calibration. Let $\mathbf{P} = [X \ Y \ Z \ 0]^{\mathbf{T}}$ be an infinite world point, the absolute conic is formed by the points satisfying $\mathbf{P}^{\mathbf{T}}\mathbf{P} = 0$ in a plane at infinity. The image of the absolute conic ω (IAC) is the conic $\mathbf{K}^{-\mathbf{T}}\mathbf{K}^{-1}$ and its dual ω^* (DIAC) is $\mathbf{K}\mathbf{K}^{\mathbf{T}}$ [18]. Once IAC or DIAC is determined, $\mathbf{K}$ can be easily obtained by Cholesky decomposition [19].

2.3   The Sphere Image

The image of a sphere is a conic because the occluding contour of a sphere is always a circle (see Fig. 1). In [8,13], the algebraic relation between a sphere image and the DIAC is given by

$$\beta_i \mathbf{C}_i^* = \omega^* - \mathbf{o}_i \mathbf{o}_i^{\mathbf{T}} \tag{3}$$

where i is used to indicate the sphere index, β is a nonzero scale factor, $\mathbf{C}^*$ is the dual of the sphere image, and $\mathbf{o}$ is the image of the sphere center (projected circle center). In this paper, when we consider the non-degenerate case, $\mathbf{C}^*$ is equal to $\mathbf{C}^{-1}$.

3   The Common Self-polar Triangle of Sphere Images

In this section, we show that any two disjoint sphere images have a unique common self-polar triangle and present one method to find the vertices of the common self-polar triangle.

3.1   The Pole-polar Relationship

A line l formed by all harmonic conjugates of point $\mathbf{x}$ with respect to a conic $\mathbf{C}$ is called the polar of $\mathbf{x}$, and point $\mathbf{x}$ is called the pole of l. The algebraic relation between pole $\mathbf{x}$ and polar l with respect to a conic $\mathbf{C}$ is given by

$$\mathbf{x} = \mathbf{C}^{-1}\mathbf{l} \tag{4}$$

where $\mathbf{C}^{-1}$ is the dual representation of $\mathbf{C}$ [18].

If the poles of a conic form the vertices of a triangle and their respective polars form its opposite sides, it is called a self-polar triangle(see Fig. 2). If a self-polar triangle is common to two conics, it is called common self-polar triangle (see Fig. 3) [20].

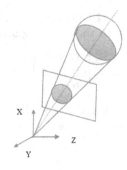

Fig. 1. Projection of a sphere

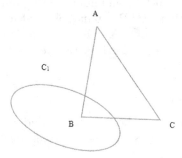

Fig. 2. △**ABC** is a self-polar triangle with respect to conic C_1 when polars of A, B and C are lines BC, AC and AB, respectively.

3.2 The Common Self-polar Triangle of Sphere Images

The relation of two conics to each other has been well studied in [20–22], especially with reference to common self-polar triangle of two conics. By considering two sphere images, we obtain the following proposition.

Proposition 1. *Two disjoint sphere images have a unique common self-polar triangle.*

Proof. In [20], there is one important theorem: If two conics intersect in four distinct points, they have one and only one common self-polar triangle. If they are tangent in two points, they have an infinite number of common self-polar triangles, one vertex of which is at the intersection of the common tangents. In all other cases, two distinct conics have no common self-polar triangle.

Considering two disjoint conics obtained by the image of two spheres, all four intersection points are imaginary and they fall into two conjugate imaginary pairs. Obviously, four intersection points are distinct. According to the theorem mentioned above, we obtain that two disjoint sphere images have a unique common self-polar triangle.   □

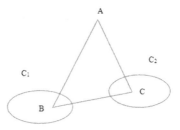

Fig. 3. $\triangle \mathbf{ABC}$ is the common self-polar triangle of two disjoint conics $\mathbf{C}_1$ and $\mathbf{C}_2$ when $\triangle \mathbf{ABC}$ is a self-polar triangle with respect to both $\mathbf{C}_1$ and $\mathbf{C}_2$.

3.3 The Vertices of Common Self-polar Triangle

Let the two sphere images be $\mathbf{C}_1$ and $\mathbf{C}_2$, and if there exists a common pole $\mathbf{x}$ and polar $\mathbf{l}$, the following relationship should be satisfied:

$$\mathbf{l} = \mathbf{C}_1 \mathbf{x}$$
$$\mathbf{l} = \lambda \mathbf{C}_2 \mathbf{x} \tag{5}$$

where λ is a scalar parameter. Subtracting the equations in (5), we get $(\mathbf{C}_1 - \lambda \mathbf{C}_2)x = 0$. By multiplying the inverse of $\mathbf{C}_2$ on both sides, we obtain the following equation:

$$(\mathbf{C}_2^{-1}\mathbf{C}_1 - \lambda \mathbf{I})\mathbf{x} = 0 \tag{6}$$

From the equation of (6), we find the common poles for $\mathbf{C}_1$ and $\mathbf{C}_2$ are the eigenvectors of $\mathbf{C}_2^{-1}\mathbf{C}_1$.

4 Calibration Theory and Method

Based on the above proposition, this section introduces a linear approach to solving the problem of calibration.

4.1 Vanishing Line Recovery

By using the vertices of common self-polar triangle of sphere images, vanishing line of the support plane for the occluding contour can be easily recovered.

Proposition 2. *Let* $\mathbf{C}_1$, $\mathbf{C}_2$ *and* $\mathbf{C}_3$ *be the images of three spheres* $\mathbf{S}_1$, $\mathbf{S}_2$ *and* $\mathbf{S}_3$, $\triangle \mathbf{ABC}$ *be the common self-polar triangle of* $\mathbf{C}_1$, $\mathbf{C}_3$, *and* $\triangle \mathbf{DEF}$ *be the common self-polar triangle of* $\mathbf{C}_1$, $\mathbf{C}_2$, *the vanishing line of the support plane for the occluding contour of* $\mathbf{S}_1$ *is the line* $\mathbf{AD}$.

Proof. In Fig. 4, $\triangle \mathbf{ABC}$ is the common self-polar triangle of $\mathbf{C}_1$, $\mathbf{C}_3$, $\triangle \mathbf{DEF}$ is the common self-polar triangle of $\mathbf{C}_1$, $\mathbf{C}_2$. Let $\mathbf{O}_1, \mathbf{O}_2$ be the imaged sphere centers of $\mathbf{S}_1$, $\mathbf{S}_2$. Multiplying the line $\mathbf{l} = \mathbf{O}_1 \times \mathbf{O}_2$ joining the images of the 2 sphere centers to both sides of (3) gives

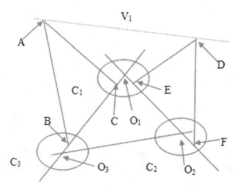

Fig. 4. Vanishing line recovered from vertices of common self-polar triangle of sphere images.

$$\beta_1 \mathbf{C}_1^{-1} \mathbf{l} = \omega^{-1} \mathbf{l}$$
$$\beta_2 \mathbf{C}_2^{-1} \mathbf{l} = \omega^{-1} \mathbf{l} \qquad (7)$$

Let $\beta_1 \mathbf{C}_1^{-1} \mathbf{l} = \beta_2 \mathbf{C}_2^{-1} \mathbf{l} = \mathbf{x}$, we have that $\mathbf{x}$ and $\mathbf{l}$ are the common pole and polar of $\mathbf{C}_1$, $\mathbf{C}_2$. Based on this, in Fig. 4, it is easy to find that line $\mathbf{EF}$ goes through $\mathbf{O}_1, \mathbf{O}_2$. Similarly, line BC goes through $\mathbf{O}_1, \mathbf{O}_3$. Since $\mathbf{A}$ is the pole of BC and $\mathbf{D}$ is the pole of $\mathbf{EF}$, we have that $\mathbf{A}$ and point $\mathbf{D}$ are all harmonic conjugates of $\mathbf{O}_1$ with respect to $\mathbf{C}_1$. According to polar definition described in Subsect. 3.1, point $\mathbf{A}$ and point $\mathbf{D}$ should be on the polar of $\mathbf{O}_1$. Since point $\mathbf{O}_1$ is a projected circle center, its polar should be the vanishing line of the support plane [20]. From those two facts, we obtain that line $\mathbf{AD}$ is the vanishing line. Using the same way, vanishing lines of the support planes for the occluding contours of $\mathbf{S}_2$ and $\mathbf{S}_3$ can be recovered. □

Here, the procedure for recovering the vanishing line of the support plane is briefly summarized below:

1. Obtain sphere images $\mathbf{C}_1$, $\mathbf{C}_2$ and $\mathbf{C}_3$.
2. Calculate vertices of the common self-polar triangle for any two sphere images using (6).
3. Find vertices outside of the sphere images and connect any two of them.

4.2   Calibration Method

As we all know, any circle intersects line at infinity of the support plane in the circular points and circular points lie on the absolute conic. Accordingly, in the image plane, the imaged circular points lie on IAC [18]. If the image of the circle and image of line at infinity are both obtained, we can calculate the images of the two circular points. One pair of imaged circular points provides two independent constraints on IAC. Hence three pairs are needed to fully calibrate. Given three sphere images, we can easily find the self-polar triangle for any two of them. Based on the propositions above, three vanishing lines can be detected

Table 1. Experimental results with 1 pixel noise (50 trials)

Approach	αf	f	s	u_0	v_0
Ground-truth	660	600	0.1	320	240
Semi-definite (nonlinear)	655.3167	595.7662	1.9698	319.6274	238.4794
Orthogonal (linear)	655.2565	595.7586	2.0010	319.8414	238.3899
Our approach (linear)	655.2565	595.7192	2.7449	319.8750	238.6999

and the image of the circular points can be calculated. Consequently, a camera can be calibrated.

The complete calibration algorithm by using the common self-polar triangles of sphere images consists of the following steps:

1. Obtain sphere images $\mathbf{C}_1$, $\mathbf{C}_2$ and $\mathbf{C}_3$.
2. Recover three vanishing lines by using common self-polar triangles.
3. Find the imaged circular points, and then determine ω and obtain $\mathbf{K}$ using the Cholesky factorization.

5 Experiments and Results

5.1 Synthetic Data

In the computer simulations, the synthetic camera has focal length $f = 600$, aspect ratio $\alpha = 1.1$, skew $s = 0.1$, and principal point $(u_0, v_0) = (320, 240)$. The image resolution is: 800×600. An image containing three sphere images is generated. They are uniformly distributed within the image. We choose 500 points on each sphere image, and gaussian noise with zero-mean and σ standard deviation is added to these image points. Ellipses are fitted to these images using a least squares ellipse fitting algorithm. In our experiment, we compare our proposed approach with a nonlinear semi-definite approach presented in [8] and a linear orthogonal approach presented in [13]. To evaluate accuracy and robustness of these methods, we vary the noise level σ from 0 to 6 pixels, and perform 15 independent trials, 30 independent trials as well as 50 independent trials for each noise level. The mean values of these recovered parameters are computed over each run. The average percentage errors of f are shown in Fig. 5. The errors of other parameters, which are not shown here, exhibit similar trend. It can be seen that the errors increase linearly with the the noise level and our method performed as well as others.

Note that the results between our approach and orthogonal approach are very similar. When we calculate the average percentage errors, they are almost the same. That explains why the curves of these two approaches in Fig. 5 are overlapped. In order to show the little difference clearly, estimated parameters under different noise level with 50 trials are shown in Tables 1, 2 and 3.

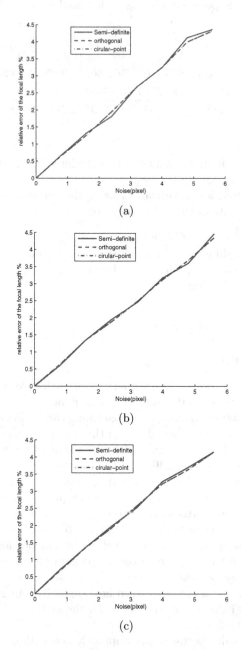

Fig. 5. (a) The estimated results with 15 trials. (b) The estimated results with 30 trials. (c) The estimated results with 50 trials. Due to the results of our approach (Circular-point) and orthogonal approach have little difference, the curves of these two approaches almost overlap.

Table 2. Experimental results with 2 pixels noise (50 trials)

Approach	αf	f	s	u_0	v_0
Ground-truth	660	600	0.1	320	240
Semi-definite (nonlinear)	649.4490	590.3716	3.5963	320.5770	239.1416
Orthogonal (linear)	649.5920	590.5997	3.7439	320.3166	238.6542
Our approach (linear)	649.5920	590.3723	3.9832	320.6633	233.1286

Table 3. Experimental results with 3 pixels noise (50 trials)

Approach	αf	f	s	u_0	v_0
Ground-truth	660	600	0.1	320	240
Semi-definite (nonlinear)	643.8556	585.5044	5.0356	323.2800	236.9793
Orthogonal (linear)	643.8120	585.4920	4.9911	322.3709	237.8458
Our approach (linear)	643.8120	582.6786	3.4279	324.3849	241.1814

Table 4. Real experiment results

Approach	αf	f	s	u_0	v_0
Zhang (ground truth)	1070	1070	0	359	239
Semi-definite (nonlinear)	1107	1108	1.07	352	230
Orthogonal (linear)	1130	1131	1.19	353	232
Our method (linear)	1121	1122	1.05	352	231

5.2   Real Scene

In the real scene experiment, we used 3 plastic balls as calibration objects. Real images were taken with a Canon EOS5D CCD camera. The image resolution is 720×480. The images of spheres were extracted using Canny's edge detector [23], and ellipses are fitted to these images using a least squares ellipse fitting algorithm. The camera is calibrated with the proposed approach, and results are compared with semi-definite approach as well as orthogonal approach. The estimated parameters are listed in Table 4, where the result from the classical method of Zhang [2] is taken as the ground truth. Figure 6b shows the calibration pattern used as ground truth.

5.3   Critical Configuration

Note that in some situations, the calibration process fails. First, when spheres placed near the image centers, the vanishing line of the support plane will be far away from the image center, which will be recovered badly. Second, when any two of the support planes are parallel, less constraints can be obtained and

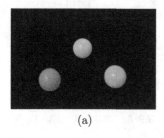
(a)

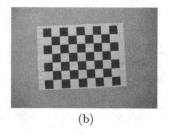
(b)

Fig. 6. (a) Image of three balls. (b) Image of calibration pattern.

the camera can not be calibrated. However, those situations can be avoided by carefully placing spheres.

6   Conclusion

We have proposed a very simple calibration algorithms based on the common self-polar triangles of sphere images, by using a single image of at least three spheres. We have shown how to locate the vertices of the common self-polar triangle and how to recover the vanishing line of the support plane. All computations involved are linear and simple. The experimental results have demonstrated that the proposed method is accurate and robust. Nevertheless, this paper has yet to consider the distortion problem, which will leave for our future studies.

Acknowledgement. The work described in this paper was supported by the National Natural Science Foundation of China (Project no. 61005038 and 61272366) and an internal funding from United International College.

References

1. Tsai, R.Y.: A versatile camera calibration technique for high accuracy 3d machine vision metrology using off-the-shelf tv cameras and lenses. IEEE J. Robot. Autom. **3**, 323–344 (1987)
2. Zhang, Z.: A flexible new technique for camera calibration. IEEE Trans. Pattern Anal. Mach. Intell. **22**, 1330–1334 (2000)
3. Zhang, Z.: Camera calibration with one-dimensional objects. IEEE Trans. Pattern Anal. Mach. Intell. **26**, 892–899 (2004)
4. Faugeras, O.D., Luong, Q.-T., Maybank, S.J.: Camera self-calibration: theory and experiments. In: Sandini, G. (ed.) ECCV 1992. LNCS, vol. 588, pp. 321–334. Springer, Heidelberg (1992)
5. Hartley, R.: An algorithm for self calibration from several views. In: IEEE Conference on Computer Vision and Pattern Recognition, pp. 908–912 (1994)
6. Maybank, S.J., Faugeras, O.D.: A theory of self-calibration of a moving camera. Int. J. Comput. Vis. **8**, 123–151 (1992)
7. Fitzgibbon, A.W., Pilu, M., Fisher, R.B.: Direct least-squares fitting of ellipses. IEEE Trans. Pattern Anal. Mach. Intell. **21**, 476–480 (1999)

8. Agrawal, M., Davis, L.S.: Camera calibration using spheres: a semi-definite programming approach. In: Proceedings of IEEE International Conference on Computer Vision, pp. 782–789 (2003)
9. Penna, M.A.: Camera calibration: a quick and easy way to determine the scale factor. IEEE Trans. Pattern Anal. Mach. Intell. **13**, 1240–1245 (1991)
10. Daucher, D., Dhome, M., Lapreste, J.: Camera calibration from spheres images. In: Eklundh, J.O. (ed.) ECCV 1994. LNCS, vol. 800, pp. 449–454. Springer, Heidelberg (1994)
11. Teramoto, H., Xu, G.: Camera calibration by a single image of balls: from conics to the absolute conic. In: Proceedings of 5th ACCV, pp. 499–506 (2002)
12. Zhang, H., Zhang, G., Wong, K.-Y.K.: Camera calibration with spheres: linear approaches. In: Proceedings of the International Conference on Image Processing, vol. 2, pp. 1150–1153 (2005)
13. Zhang, H., Zhang, G., Wong, K.-Y.K.: Camera calibration from images of spheres. IEEE Trans. Pattern Anal. Mach. Intell. **29**, 499–503 (2007)
14. Wong, K.-Y.K., Mendonça, P.R.S., Cipolla, R.: Camera calibration from surfaces of revolution. IEEE Trans. Pattern Anal. Mach. Intell. **25**, 147–161 (2003)
15. Ying, X., Zha, H.: Geometric interpretations of the relation between the image of the absolute conic and sphere images. IEEE Trans. Pattern Anal. Mach. Intell. **28**, 2031–2036 (2006)
16. Zhao, Z., Liu, Y.: Applications of projected circle centers in camera calibration. Mach. Vis. Appl. **21**, 301–307 (2010)
17. Wong, K.-Y.K., Zhang, G., Chen, Z.: A stratified approach for camera calibration using spheres. IEEE Trans. Image Process. **20**, 305–316 (2011)
18. Hartley, R.I., Zisserman, A.: Multiple View Geometry in Computer Vision. Cambridge University, Cambridge (2000)
19. Gentle, J.E.: Numerical Linear Algebra for Applications in Statistics. Springer, New York (1998)
20. Frederick, S.: Woods: Higher Geometry. Ginn and Company, Boston (1922)
21. Filon, L.N.G.: Introduction to Projective Geometry. Edward Arnold, London (1908)
22. Semple, J., Kneebone, G.: Algebraic Projective Geometry. Oxford Science, Oxford (1952)
23. Canny, J.: A computational approach to edge detection. IEEE Trans. Pattern Anal. Mach. Intell. **8**, 679–698 (1986)

Multi-scale Tetrahedral Fusion of a Similarity Reconstruction and Noisy Positional Measurements

Runze Zhang, Tian Fang[✉], Siyu Zhu, and Long Quan

The Hong Kong University of Science and Technology, Hong Kong, China
tianft@cse.ust.hk

Abstract. The fusion of a 3D reconstruction up to a similarity transformation from monocular videos and the metric positional measurements from GPS usually relies on the alignment of the two coordinate systems. When positional measurements provided by a low-cost GPS are corrupted by high-level noises, this approach becomes problematic. In this paper, we introduce a novel framework that uses similarity invariants to form a tetrahedral network of views for the fusion. Such a tetrahedral network decouples the alignment from the fusion to combat the high-level noises. Then, we update the similarity transformation each time a well-conditioned motion of cameras is successfully identified. Moreover, we develop a multi-scale sampling strategy to reduce the computational overload and to adapt the algorithm to different levels of noises. It is important to note that our optimization framework can be applied in both batch and incremental manners. Experiments on simulations and real datasets demonstrate the robustness and the efficiency of our method.

1 Introduction

Monocular SLAM (Simultaneously Localization And Mapping) is only able to reconstruct camera poses and 3D structures, so called *visual measurements*, up to a similarity transformation due to the gauge freedom [11]. Such a similarity reconstruction is not sufficient for the applications on the navigation, osculation avoidance for robots and unmanned aerial vehicles. Moreover, the noise in feature detections, unbalance features [9], local bundle adjustments [4], and biased depth estimators [17] make the visual measurements contain significant drift in both rotation and translation over a long range movement. Drift-free global positional measurements provided by modern global position system (GPS) can be used to address the aforementioned inherent drawback of monocular SLAM. Some works [3,14] have been done on addressing the scale ambiguity solely. However, the inherent drifting of monocular SLAM makes the error between visual measurements and ground truth no longer follow the normal distribution, which in turn biases the estimation of scale even under maximum likelihood framework. To compensate for the drifting, some other works [6,8,15] directly fuse positional measurements with visual measurements by the metric distances between

© Springer International Publishing Switzerland 2015
D. Cremers et al. (Eds.): ACCV 2014, Part II, LNCS 9004, pp. 30–44, 2015.
DOI: 10.1007/978-3-319-16808-1_3

them, which relies on a good initial similarity transformation to resolve the scale ambiguity and requires aligning both set of data in the same coordinate frame. The estimation of such initial transformation of scales can be problematic when the camera moves under a critical motion such as moving along a straight line, where the rotation around the moving direction is not well constrained. Even worse, low cost GPS sensors on many consumer products give very noisy positional measurement making the estimation of initial similarity transformation less reliable.

In this paper, we propose a novel multi-scale tetrahedral fusion framework. Based on the invariance of the ratios of two distances under a similarity transformation, we define a ratio constraint over a tetrahedral network defined on the cameras that are associated with positional measurements. This configuration is capable of correcting the drift without the knowledge of the global similarity alignment. The global similarity transformation is in turn estimated later on when there is well-conditioned motion. Moreover, we further propagate such positional measurements to the other cameras via relative pose constraints that retain the local camera motion. Geometric constraints based on reprojection error are involved to ensure the consistency between the reconstructed cameras and 3D structures. Finally, a multi-scale scheme that is adapted to different levels of noise of positional measurements is used to sample the tetrahedral and relative pose constraints. All these constraints are formulated as solving a nonlinear least square optimization. After reviewing the related work in Sect. 1.1, we first introduce our key idea on tetrahedral network in Sect. 2.1. Then the formulation is given in Sect. 2.2 along with a discussion on the details of the optimization in Sect. 2.4. In Sect. 3, we finally describe the implementation of our system and present detailed evaluations on our approach.

1.1   Related Work

The work on integrating the positional measurements with a similarity reconstruction can be classified into two categories.

A part of previous research only obtained a metric upgrade by estimating the scale factor between the up-to-scale visual measurement and the metric measurements. Nützi et al. [14] used a spline fitting technique to estimate the scale. Engel et al. [3] proposed a recursive update formula for Maximum likelihood estimation of the scale factor. Their approach takes a metric altitude of a helicopter and the height estimated from a video camera looking downwards to the grounds. In these works, the visual measurement is assumed to be normally distributing around the true estimations. Unfortunately, the assumption is generally not true because the monocular SLAM reconstructs drifted measurements.

Another part of research resolved the drifting problem through the fusion given a good initial similarity alignment. Michot et al. [10] augmented the classic bundle adjustment of reprojection error with a penalty term to minimize the error of the difference of the positional measurements and the similarity reconstruction. Lhuillier [8] proposed a constraint optimization framework on the bundle adjustment that guarantees a small change of reprojection error during the fusion.

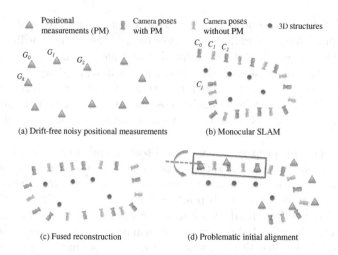

Fig. 1. The illustration of the fusions. (a) and (b) are the positional measurements (PM) and visual measurements that are under an unknown similarity transformation. (c) is an illustration of a successful fusion which successfully estimate the similarity alignment and correct the drift. (d) illustrates the case that the initial similarity alignment is estimated with a critical motion in the red rectangle. Such alignment is unstable because the rotation (the blue arrow) around the moving direction (the green dashed line) is not well constrained (Colour figure online).

Konolige et al. [6] further marginalized the geometric constraint in the bundle adjustment and optimized a pose graph which constraints only the relative pose between the cameras. However, all these works require an initial similarity alignment between the visual measurement and positional measurements. Such an alignment is estimated with a subset of the measurements at the beginning of the fusion, which could be problematic if such subset of measurements is in bad condition, such as forming a straight line. Extended Kalman Filter (EKF) [2,14] has also been used to fuse both the motion and scale simultaneously. In these work, the scale factor is explicitly considered and involved in the state vector of the motion. However, they all required an initial Euclidean registration whose accuracy is very important for the later recursive update.

2   Multi-scale Tetrahedral Fusion

We have two sets of input measurements, a similarity reconstruction generated by monocular SLAM and positional measurements obtained through external sensors such as GPS. The *similarity reconstruction* includes the poses $\mathcal{C} = \{C_j\}$ of the monocular camera at each frame and a set of reconstructed 3D points $\mathcal{P} = \{p_i\}$ as in Fig. 1(b). Each camera is parameterized as $C_j = K_j[R_j|t_j]$. For monocular SLAM, K_j is usually fixed during the capture, so we simply assume K_j is pre-calibrated and drop such terms in the following text. We further denote the extrinsic parameters R_j and t_j as an Euclidean transformation T_j that belongs to $SE(3)$ group. The camera C_j and 3D point p_i are linked by the image feature

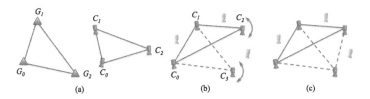

Fig. 2. The illustration of tetrahedral fusion. (a) A toy example of three GPS and visual measurements; (b) Sparse sampling of triangular constraints is not sufficient to constraint the structure; (c) A tetrahedral structure consisting of four triangular constraints can well preserve the shape.

q_{ij} via the projection function $\mathbb{Q}(C_j, p_i)$ if p_i is visible in C_j. The *positional measurement* $\mathcal{G} = \{G_k\}$ are recorded simultaneously when the camera is moving as in Fig. 1(a). Since the temporal sampling rates of vision and positional measurements are usually different, we explicitly align the index set $\{j\}$ and $\{k\}$ to make sure that k denotes the frames with positional measurements while other frames are generally denoted by index j.

Since the coordinate frame of the visual measurement generated by monocular SLAM is unknown, in the alignment-based fusion, a global similarity transformation $S_G = S(G, C, P)$ is first estimated to transform the visual measurement to the coordinate frame of positional measurement as $\hat{C}, \hat{P} = S_G(C, P)$. Then an optimized fused measurement $C', P' = \arg\min_{C', P'} E_{fusion}(C, P, G)$. However, in practice, in the present of noisy positional measurement and the degenerated motions, the estimation of S_G is not always valid and robust. In the following, we introduce a novel framework based on similarity invariants to directly fuse the visual measurement and positional measurement without the knowledge of S_G. The global similarity transformation S_G can then be recovered when there are sufficient measurements and well-conditioned motions. Such decoupling of the alignment from the fusion greatly improves the robustness of the fusion.

2.1 Overview of Tetrahedral Fusion

To fuse a similarity reconstruction with metric positional measurements without alignment, we must make use of similarity invariant properties that are the ratios of distances and the angles. These invariant properties are completely encoded by the ratios of all edge pairs of a triangle. Let $tri = (G_0, G_1, G_2)$ in Fig. 2(a) be a reference triangle. The ratios between its edges, $\|G_0 G_1\|/\|G_1 G_2\|$, $\|G_1 G_2\|/\|G_2 G_0\|$, and $\|G_2 G_0\|/\|G_0 G_1\|$, remain unchanged under a similarity transformation. Let's further denote another triangle as $tri' = (c_0, c_1, c_2)$ whose vertex c_i corresponds to G_i under an unknown similarity transformation. We introduce a ratio constraint on a pair of triangles:

$$E_{ratio}(c_i, c_j, c_k) = \left(\|c_i - c_j\| - \frac{\|G_i G_j\|}{\|G_i G_k\|} \cdot \|c_i - c_k\| \right)^2 \tag{1}$$

For each triangle, three permutations for its vertices give in total three ratio constraints for a triangle.

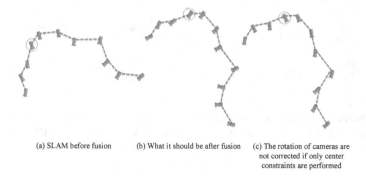

(a) SLAM before fusion   (b) What it should be after fusion   (c) The rotation of cameras are
                                                                      not corrected if only center
                                                                      constraints are performed

Fig. 3. The illustration of the result without rotation constraints. (a) Original SLAM before fusion; (b) Since our fusion result is up to a similarity transformation. The rotation of each camera should remain consistent with original motion. (c) The rotation of each camera cannot be well constrained if only the ratio constraint is applied.

It is theoretically sufficient to exhaustively enumerate all combination of three positional measurements to constraint the fusion. However, such an exhaustive enumeration generates a large number of constraints that overwhelm the computation. A sparse sampling of triangles is thus preferred. Unfortunately, arbitrary sampling does not guarantee a stable fusion. As illustrated in Fig. 2(b), even if the ratio constraints of such two sampled triangles are met with respect to the referenced triangles, such triangles can still rotate arbitrarily around the edge C_0C_1. Hence, to ensure the stabilities of the structure, we introduce tetrahedral constraints, which ensure that all the triangles in four randomly selected vertices must be sampled at the same time as in Fig. 2(c).

Because the ratio constraints in Eq. 1 only maintain the corresponding distance ratio among the position of cameras, the rotation of each camera is not well constrained and is free up to an arbitrary rotation as shown in Fig. 3. We further introduce a term $E_{tertrarot}$ as Eq. 2 to constrain the rotation of cameras with respect to the edges of the sampled tetrahedron:

$$E_{tetrarot}(D_t) = \sum_{i \in D_t} \sum_{j \neq i, j \in D_t} (\frac{(R_i'(c_j' - c_i'))^T (R_i(c_j - c_i))}{||R_i'(c_j' - c_i')|| \cdot ||R_i(c_j - c_i)||} - 1)^2 \quad (2)$$

Actually, the $R_i(c_j - c_i)$ is the projection of translation vector between camera i and j on camera i. And $(R_i'(c_j' - c_i'))^T (R_i(c_j - c_i))/||R_i'(c_j' - c_i')|| \cdot ||R_i(c_j - c_i)||$ is the cosine of angle between such projection before and after fusion. This constraint tries to maintain the consistency between rotation of each camera and the translation between cameras.

Given the tetrahedral constraints, the ratio constraint has a family of trivial solutions that are defined up to a similarity transformation of $\mathcal{G}$. We further introduce two other sets of constraints. One is the relative pose constraint [7], which enforces consistency of the local motion and rotation of the cameras. The other one is the geometric constraints [18], which enforces consistency between the camera poses and 3D points.

2.2 Formulation

Formally, given a reconstruction $\mathcal{C}$ and $\mathcal{P}$ defined up to an arbitrary similarity transformation, and the positional measurement $\mathcal{G}$ in a global geographical reference frame, in the tetrahedral fusion, we are looking for an updated camera poses $\mathcal{C}'$ and 3D points $\mathcal{P}'$, which are still up to a similarity transformation, but associated with $\mathcal{G}$ by minimizing the following energy function.

$$\mathcal{C}', \mathcal{P}' = \arg\min_{\mathcal{C}', \mathcal{P}'} (E_{tetra} + \alpha \cdot E_{pose} + \beta \cdot E_{bundle}), \tag{3}$$

where E_{tetra}, E_{pose}, and E_{bundle} are the energies for tetrahedral constraint, relative pose constraint, and geometric constraint respectively. The tetrahedral constraint is the core of our algorithm, which sets up ratio constraints over a tetrahedral network on the positional measurements. The relative pose constraint embeds the camera poses that do not have corresponding positional measurements into the fusion and makes sure the upgraded camera poses follow the original motion. The last geometric constraint is a classical term that ensures the consistency between camera poses and reconstructed 3D structures. We now present these three terms in details.

Tetrahedral Constraint. The tetrahedral constraint is defined as two parts:

$$E_{tetra} = E_{ratiogps} + E_{rot} \tag{4}$$

The first term is to constrain the ratio relationship between GPS and SLAM as Eq. 5.

$$E_{ratiogps} = \sum_{\{D_t\}} w_t \sum_{i,j,k \in P^3_{(D_t)}} \frac{1}{12} \cdot E_{ratio}(c'_i, c'_j, c'_k), \tag{5}$$

where $P^3_{(D_t)}$ is all the permutations of three cameras in tetrahedron D_t; and the w_t is the weight of the tetrahedral constraint, normalized by the number of tetrahedrons on its sampling level as Sect. 2.3. Because the tetrahedral constraints are relative to both GPS and SLAM data, tetrahedrons $\{D_t\}$ are only sampled in the frames where both GPS and SLAM data are available.

The second part is a tetrahedral constraint for rotation defined in the tetrahedrons D'_t as Eq. 6 to maintain the relative rotation among cameras and tetrahedrons.

$$E_{rot} = \sum_{\{D'_t\}} w'_t E_{tetrarot}(D'_t) \tag{6}$$

Rotation constraints involve only SLAM data, so tetrahedrons $\mathcal{D}' = \{D'_t\}$ are sampled among all the frames.

Relative Pose Constraint. The relative pose constraint [7] penalizes large changes in the relative pose transformation between two connected cameras, C'_i and C'_j. Let the original relative transformation from C_i to C_j be $\Delta T_{ij} = T_i^{-1} T_j$. The relative pose constraint is defined as:

$$E_{pose} = \sum_{\{i,j\}} \| \log_{SE(3)}(T'_i \cdot \Delta T_{ij} \cdot T'^{-1}_j) \|^2_{\Sigma_{ij}}, \tag{7}$$

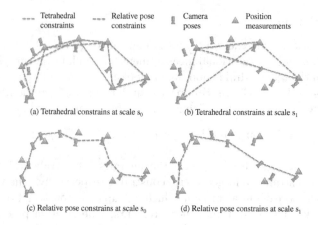

(a) Tetrahedral constrains at scale s_0 (b) Tetrahedral constrains at scale s_1

(c) Relative pose constrains at scale s_0 (d) Relative pose constrains at scale s_1

Fig. 4. The illustration of multi-scale constraints. For clarity, in (a) and (b), tetrahedral constraints are simplified and illustrated as triangular constraints. Please note that the camera poses and positional measurements are roughly aligned in the illustrations for easy understanding, but in the fusion we do not assume any pre-alignment.

where $\log_{SE(3)}(\cdot)$ measures the relative pose error in the tangent space of $SE(3)$ group and Σ_{ij} is the precision matrix of the Mahalanobis distance $\|\cdot\|_{\Sigma_{ij}}$ for 2-tuple camera pose C_i and C_j. We set Σ_{ij} as:

$$\Sigma_{ij} = w_{ij} \begin{bmatrix} \sigma_{trans}^2 I_{3\times3} & 0 \\ 0 & \sigma_{rot}^2 I_{3\times3} \end{bmatrix} \qquad (8)$$

Geometric Constraint. The geometric constraint mimics the bundle adjustment that minimizes the reprojection error in a maximum likelihood estimation manner. It is defined to be

$$E_{bundle} = \sum_{\{q_{ij}\}} \|q_{ij} - \mathbb{Q}(C_j, p_i)\|_{\Sigma}^2, \qquad (9)$$

where Σ is precision matrix for reprojection errors. Conventionally, this term is simply set to identity because the covariance of the reprojection error is hardly known beforehand.

2.3   Multi-scale Constraints

The tetrahedral constraints and relative pose constraints are defined on 4-tuple and 2-tuple relationship respectively. The sampling of such tuples significantly affects the performance of the optimization of Eq. 3. A multi-scale scheme to sample such tuples to fuse different level of details of information is therefore necessary.

The tetrahedral tuples are sampled on the positional measurements $\mathcal{G}$ as in Fig. 4(a) and (b). For each scale $s_l = \lfloor n/2^{L-l} \rfloor$ where $L = \lceil log_2 n \rceil$, $l = 0, \ldots, l_{max}$, we sample the tetrahedron as $(i, i+s_l, i+2s_l, i+3s_l)$ for $i = 0, s_l, 2s_l \ldots \lfloor n/s_l \rfloor s_l$. The sampled tetrahedral tuples for $E_{ratiogps}$ and E_{rot} in Eq. 4 are slightly different. For the first part, the tuples are sampled on overlapped cameras in GPS and

SLAM and l_{max} is set as $L-2$ to constrain ratio on GPS from the smallest scale to the largest. For the second parts, they are sampled on all the cameras in SLAM.

The relative pose constraints are defined on the camera poses $\mathcal{C}$. For each scale $s_l = 2^l$ where $l = 0, 1, \ldots, L_r$, we create the relative pose tuple as $(i, i + s_l)$ for $i = 0, s_l, 2s_l \ldots \lfloor n/s_l \rfloor s_l$ as in Fig. 4(c) and (d).

Instead of setting all the weights w_t, w'_t and w_{ij} of the constraints in every scale uniformly, which makes the fine-scale constraints contribute more than the coarse-scale ones do, we set the sum of the weights of each scale identical to each other.

2.4   Optimization

While the general non-linear least squares problem [13] and its concrete application in bundle adjustment [18] have been well studied in the past decades. We still need carefully decide the weight of the energy terms in Eq. 3, because such terms penalize different objectives are in different sensor systems that cannot be combined directly. In the following, we discuss the strategies of setting the weights. Then we briefly describe how to extend our method to incremental optimization, which is more useful for real-time applications.

Weight Selection. We set the β to be E_{tetra}/E_{bundle} with the initial errors empirically according to the extensive evaluation in [8]. However, the similar strategy does not work for setting α, because the initial error of E_{pose} is 0. Instead, we broke α as $\alpha_{rigid}\alpha_{norm}$. α_{norm} is a normalization factor that ensure the sum of all w_{ij} is the same as the sum of all w_t. α_{rigid} is to control how rigid the original local motion should be. For very noisy positional measurements, α_{rigid} should be increased to avoid overfit to $\mathcal{G}$. In our experiment, α_{rigid} is fixed to 0.1.

Incremental Optimization. For real-time applications, it is unaffordable to setup the tetrahedral network and optimize all the variables globally whenever new measurements arrive. Our framework can be easily modified to support incremental optimization similar to local bundle adjustment [4]. Let's call the last n frames that are involved in the incremental optimization as active frames. Only the constraints in Eq. 3 that overlap the active frames are kept. Moreover, the parameters that lay in the non-active frames are fixed during the optimization.

3   Implementation and Experiments

We implemented a standard visual SLAM system to generate the visual measurement from a video taken by a monocular camera. We first detect and track features with Harris corners and KLT tracker. Only the tracks spanning more than five frames are kept for camera pose estimation. Visual keyframes are inserted whenever less than 70 % of tracks are kept from last keyframes. To initialize the reconstruction, a sliding window containing the last three consecutive keyframes is used to scan the tracked frames until a 5-point triplet reconstruction [12] is succeeded with a sufficient baseline and enough inlier tracks. Then the camera poses of

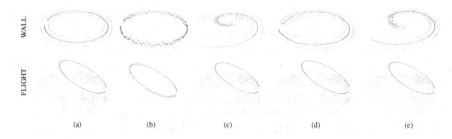

Fig. 5. Simulation datasets and results. Top row: WALL; bottom row: FLIGHT. (a) Ground-truth; (b) Perturbed GPS; (c) Visual SLAM; (d) Results by our method; (e) Results by IBA [8].

consecutive frames are resectioned using 3-point pose estimation algorithm. A new 3D point is triangulated and verified whenever the baseline among its visible cameras is large enough. Local bundle adjustment [4] is used to improve the local consistency of the estimated 3D points and cameras. The implementation of our tetrahedral fusion according to Eq. 3 is quite straight forward. Ceres Solver [1] is used to solve the non-linear least square optimization. All our implementation is written in C++ without any GPU optimization. The experiments are carried out on a PC equipped with Intel Core i7-930 CPU and 16GB ram. All parameters are set to the default value introduced in the paper, while the weight in Eq. 3 are set by the strategy described in Sect. 2.4. The fusion process now runs on our test platform at about 9 fps.

3.1   Simulation Experiments

Because of the lack of ground-truth for the experiment data, we generate two simulation datasets, named as WALL and FLIGHT. WALL is to simulate a common forward moving motion for humans and ground vehicles. It is generated by constructing two concentric circular walls and making the camera move along the corridor between the two walls. The camera is kept looking forward during the whole simulation. FLIGHT is to simulate a typical flight of an UAV that takes video using a camera looking downwards vertically at the ground. The simulated camera takes off and lands, moving in circle and shooting at a flat ground. Random 3D points are sampled on the synthetic scenes and projected back to the moving cameras to construct the simulated feature tracks for SLAM. Each projection in feature tracks is perturbed by a random noise at 0.5 pixels. The predefined camera moving trajectories are considered as the ground truth GPS measurement $\{G_k^*\}$. The ground truth are shown in Fig. 5(a). Random perturbation σ_{gps} is added to $\{G_k^*\}$ to generate the perturbed GPS measurements $\{G_k\}$ as shown in Fig. 5(b). The reconstructed trajectories by SLAM as shown in Fig. 5(c) are used as the visual measurement $\{C_j\}$. In the following, we first evaluate our fusion result via visual inspection and then carefully study how the fusion works with respect to different parameter settings and noise levels comparing with the state-of-the-art positional fusion IBA [8]. The following experiments are performed by batch version of our method and IBA [8].

Table 1. Mean (m), standard deviation (σ) and maximum value (∞) of absolute position error of camera locations with respect to perturbed GPS (gps) and ground-truth GPS (gt). SLAM is the result of visual SLAM. Tetra is our method. IBA is method in [8].

		m^{gps}	σ^{gps}	∞^{gps}	m^{gt}	σ^{gt}	∞^{gt}
WALL	SLAM	123.5	67.39	212.1	123.5	67.42	212.0
	Tetra	**12.33**	**5.603**	**19.53**	**12.53**	**5.475**	**20.17**
	IBA	103.0	56.08	176.2	103.0	56.05	176.2
FLIGHT	SLAM	6.317	1.909	12.76	6.317	2.797	10.40
	Tetra	3.386	**1.833**	9.885	**1.481**	**0.7583**	**3.051**
	IBA	**3.299**	1.900	**9.771**	1.608	1.011	3.261

Qualitative Evaluation. The visual SLAM result of dataset WALL, as shown in Fig. 5(c), suffers from serious drift, because the forward moving motion gives very narrow baseline between consecutive frames and makes the reconstruction with large bias. However, after the tetrahedral fusion with the noisy GPS data as shown in Fig. 5(b), we get a visually plausible trajectory as shown in Fig. 5(d) that almost close the loop perfectly. In contrast, as shown in the top row of Fig. 5(e), IBA [8] cannot deal with drift because the initial similarity alignment is biased due to the drifted visual measurement and noisy positional measurements. In the dataset FLIGHT, Fig. 5(d) and (e) do not show too much difference visually between our method and IBA, since the result of visual SLAM has very small error.

Quantitative Evalution. Here we quantitatively evaluate our method using the absolute camera position error with respect to the ground truth GPS. Since our fusion framework yields only an up-to-scale reconstruction, an optimal similarity transform is computed to align the SLAM result and GPS before the computation of the absolute error. First, Table 1 illustrates the absolute position error of our method compared with original visual SLAM and IBA when the perturbation added to the ground-truth GPS is $\sigma_{gps} = 4$, where the size of the simulation scene is roughly 100. Then to evaluate the effectiveness of the energy terms in Eq. 3, we carry out the fusion without the relative pose constraint E_{pose} and geometry constraint E_{bundle}. Moreover, we study the performance of our framework with uniform weights for each piece of constraint in Eq. 3. In these experiments, we vary the perturbation of GPS to $\sigma_{gpsz} = 2, 4, 8$. The results are plotted and listed in Fig. 6 and Table 2. We can easily find that our fusion method with adaptive weighting gives best results in terms of absolute position error in most cases. However, an exception is the case when the noise level is low. Such result is reasonable, because given the GPS measurements with very little noise, any good algorithm should rely on GPS measurement directly. Therefore, our fusion without relative pose gives better results than the fusion with all constrains. The uniform weighting also performs better because the uniform weighting strategy essentially weights less the relative pose term since the number of the relative pose constraints is far less than the tetrahedral constraints.

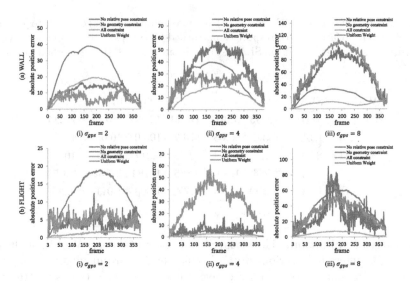

Fig. 6. Absolute position error of each frame with respect to the ground-truth GPS for the fusion using different configurations of energy terms and weights.

Table 2. Mean (m), standard deviation (σ) and maximum value (∞) of absolute position error with respect to the ground-truth GPS (gt) on simulation datasets by the fusion using different configurations of energy terms and weights.

		$\sigma_{gps} = 2$			$\sigma_{gps} = 4$			$\sigma_{gps} = 8$		
		m^{gt}	σ^{gt}	∞^{gt}	m^{gt}	σ^{gt}	∞^{gt}	m^{gt}	σ^{gt}	∞^{gt}
WALL	No relative pose	11.63	3.518	17.7	36.63	14.77	57.17	58.84	26.28	102.1
	No geometry	24.98	12.47	38.95	25.54	12.71	39.70	22.32	8.927	32.64
	All constraint	12.83	5.581	19.53	**12.63**	**5.600**	**20.04**	**8.979**	**3.169**	**16.78**
	Uniform weight	**6.105**	**2.700**	**14.71**	21.43	6.407	32.34	68.40	32.26	114.0
FLIGHT	No relative pose	3.810	1.853	12.37	4.878	2.904	19.09	26.96	18.64	91.22
	No geometry	12.06	5.175	18.90	3.447	1.807	6.245	38.16	18.48	61.34
	All constraint	**0.614**	**0.696**	**1.908**	**1.481**	**0.7583**	**3.051**	**3.971**	**2.297**	**7.750**
	Uniform weight	4.001	1.626	9.326	29.32	13.50	60.85	30.90	13.53	56.05

3.2   Real-Video Experiments

In this section, we test our fusion with six real videos divided in two groups. The first group includes five real videos with noisy or incomplete GPS data. The first video is part of part 1 in New College Dataset [16], which is called "NEW" in the following. The next three video "GARDEN", "HOUSE", "PARK" are taken by a monocular camera mounted on an unmanned aerial vehicle, the GPS measurement is output by the on-board flight controller. These videos are taken at 10 Hz with the resolution 686 × 452 pixels, while the positional measurements are recorded at about 3 Hz. The last video "CAMPUS" is captured on a ground vehicle with the resolution 640 × 480 pixels at 15 Hz, while the GPS measurements are recorded at about 10 Hz. The second group contains one real video "2011_09_26_drive_0117" in the raw data in KITTI vision benchmark [5], which is one of the longest videos of raw data. In the following, this video is called "KITTI". The GPS in this data

Table 3. Statistics on the running time of batch fusion for the real video datasets.

	# of iterations	# of visual frames	# of GPS frames	# of tracks	# of projections	Total time
NEW	163	2552	324	74717	1087035	21348.6s
GARDEN	158	881	288	47088	454655	172.5s
HOUSE	154	826	322	52904	453929	132.8s
PARK	186	632	247	30597	379133	250.9s
CAMPUS	167	2395	2395	149725	1011778	15996.9s
KITTI	171	666	564	162509	990748	13657.3s

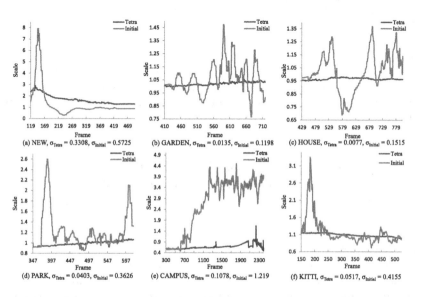

Fig. 7. The scale estimation on the real video datasets. Green line: the initial scale estimated by aligning the SLAM measurements of the latest 20 frames with the corresponding GPS. Red line: the scale estimated by aligning our fused measurements with the corresponding GPS measurements. $\sigma_{initial}$ and σ_{tetra} are the standard deviation of the initial scales and the scale estimated by our fusion respectively.

is enough accurate and regarded as ground-truth on the benchmark. We regard the original GPS as ground-truth in our experiment and add Gaussian noise to the original GPS data to generate noised GPS. The scale of datasets in our experiment and running time of batch fusion is listed in Table 3.

Group Without Ground-Truth. Since we do not have the access to the specification of the GPS sensors, we have little knowledge on the accuracy of the GPS measurement. To quantize the magnitude of the noise of GPS, we compute the standard deviation of the magnitude of angular acceleration, listed as σ_a at the top row of Table 4. Figure 8(ii) shows the noisy GPS measurement of NEW, GARDEN and CAMPUS visually. Though the σ_a of NEW is not large, Fig. 8 shows that its GPS

Table 4. Mean (m) and standard deviation (σ) of absolute position error of camera locations with respect to GPS measurement (gps) for real data. m^{2d} is the mean value of the ratio between the reprojection error after fusion and the reprojection error of SLAM [8]. Tetra is our method. IBA is method in [8].

	NEW, $\sigma_a = 15.66°$			GARDEN, $\sigma_a = 25.80°$			HOUSE, $\sigma_a = 24.44°$		
	m^{gps}	σ^{gps}	m^{2d}	m^{gps}	σ^{gps}	m^{2d}	m^{gps}	σ^{gps}	m^{2d}
SLAM	6.12037	3.60924	(1)	2.833	1.000	(1)	4.040	1.365	(1)
Tetra	**0.03089**	**0.5483**	1.004	0.115	**0.566**	1.624	**0.2857**	**0.6410**	3.713
IBA	2.38272	1.56625	24.82	**0.0729**	0.5662	1.64673	1.500	0.7680	4.47081
	PARK, $\sigma_a = 24.68°$			CAMPUS, $\sigma_a = 31.04°$					
	m^{gps}	σ^{gps}	m^{2d}	m^{gps}	σ^{gps}	m^{2d}			
SLAM	3.170	2.223	(1)	157.1	80.97	(1)			
Tetra	**0.2713**	**0.6276**	9.752	**2.520**	2.698	**1.582**			
IBA	0.4737	0.6376	26.2039	7.319	**1.360**	2.8881			

Table 5. Mean (m^{gt}) and standard deviation (σ^{gt}) of absolute position error of camera locations with respect to original GPS measurement for "KITTI".m^{gps} and σ^{gps} is with respect to noised GPS measurement.m^{2d} is the mean value of the ratio between the reprojection error after fusion and the reprojection error of SLAM [8]. Tetra is our method. IBA is method in [8].

	m^{gt}	σ^{gt}	∞^{gt}	m^{gps}	σ^{gps}	∞^{gps}	m^{2d}
SLAM	5.456	2.174	8.731	5.863	2.151	9.436	(1)
Tetra	**0.5621**	**0.6313**	**1.928**	**0.9096**	**0.7564**	**3.335**	**0.9969**
IBA	0.6365	0.8466	2.495	0.9273	0.8843	3.417	7.340

data is incomplete, which corresponds to the situation where GPS information cannot be obtained in urban valley environment. With such noisy GPS measurements, we estimate the scale factor between GPS and visual measurements by finding the best similarity transformation to align the latest 20 GPS measurements with the corresponding SLAM measurements. The green plots in Fig. 7 show that the estimated scale is very noisy, which makes the fusion with positional measurement not stable using alignment-based method. Even worse, the SLAM measurements contain very large drifting as shown in Figs. 8(c.i) and 7(e). In contrast, even without the initial alignment, our method successful fuses the GPS and SLAM measurements, which in turn makes the estimation of scales very robust as shown in the red plots of Fig. 7.

To compare the absolute position errors with IBA, we take all SLAM measurements and corresponding GPS measurements to estimate a robust similarity transformation, so that IBA can successfully fuse the GPS and SLAM measurements. We also compute the ratio between the reprojection error of fusion results and the reprojection error of SLAM for a comparison. The statistic of the comparison listed in Table 4 shows that our fusion method gives the best results in most cases. Although sometimes IBA gives comparable results, it is noted that IBA requires a robust alignment before fusion, while ours can fuse the positional measurements even such alignment is not valid.

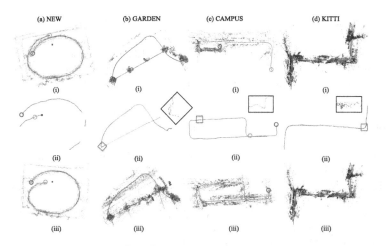

Fig. 8. The results of batch version of our method on NEW, GARDEN, CAMPUS and KITTI. (i) The results of SLAM; (ii) GPS measurements(noised GPS for KITTI), the region in the blue rectangle is zoomed in and shown in the black rectangle; (iii) Our fusion results. The orange and red circles indicate the corresponding visual and GPS measurements to show the large drift in visual SLAM.

Group with Ground-Truth. Since the GPS data of "KITTI" is enough accurate and regarded as ground-truth, we add Gaussian noise with $\sigma = 0.2$ in three directions to the original GPS data and the original GPS data is used as ground-truth to give quantitative evaluation in our experiment. The detail of noised GPS is shown as Fig. 8(d.ii). As shown in Table 5, our method generates better results than the-state-of-art method IBA [8]. We also estimate the scale factor between GPS and visual measurements as above experiment on dataset without ground-truth and Fig. 7(f) shows that the result is robust.

4   Conclusions

In this paper, we propose a multi-scale tetrahedral fusion framework. The key insight of our method is the usage of the ratio of distances that is invariant under similarity transformation, which decouples the task of fusion from the task of similarity alignment. The tetrahedral network ensures a sparse sampling of the ratio constraints, while the multi-scale scheme further adapts the fusion to different level of noisy positional measurements. Our framework is capable of fusing a similarity reconstruction with positional data even when the similarity alignment is not valid. The fused results can help to resolve the scale ambiguity robustly.

Acknowledgement. Real-time videos Garden, House, Park are provided by DJI and CAMPUS is provided by Key Laboratory of Machine Perception (Ministry of Education) in Peking University. This work is supported by RGC-GRF 618711, RGC/NSFC N_HKUST607/11, ITC-PSKL12EG02, and National Basic Research Program of China (2012CB316300).

References

1. Agarwal, S., Mierle, K.: Ceres Solver: Tutorial & Reference. Google Inc
2. Dusha, D., Mejias, L.: Error analysis and attitude observability of a monocular gps/visual odometry integrated navigation filter. Int. J. Robot. Res. **31**, 714–737 (2012)
3. Engel, J., Sturm, J., Cremers, D.: Camera-based navigation of a low-cost quadro-copter. In: 2012 IEEE/RSJ International Conference on Intelligent Robots and Systems (IROS), pp. 2815–2821. IEEE (2012)
4. Eudes, A., Lhuillier, M.: Error propagations for local bundle adjustment. In: CVPR, pp. 2411–2418 (2009)
5. Geiger, A., Lenz, P., Stiller, C., Urtasun, R.: Vision meets robotics: the kitti dataset. Int. J. Rob. Res. (IJRR) **32**, 1231–1237 (2013)
6. Konolige, K., Agrawal, M.: FrameSLAM: from bundle adjustment to real-time visual mapping. IEEE Trans. Robt. **24**, 1066–1077 (2008)
7. Kummerle, R., Grisetti, G., Strasdat, H., Konolige, K., Burgard, W.: g^2o: A general framework for graph optimization. In: ICRA, pp. 3607–3613 (2011)
8. Lhuillier, M.: Incremental fusion of structure-from-motion and gps using constrained bundle adjustments. IEEE Trans. Pattern Anal. Mach. Intell. **34**, 2489–2495 (2012)
9. Mei, C., Sibley, G., Cummins, M., Newman, P., Reid, I.: Rslam: a system for large-scale mapping in constant-time using stereo. Int. J. Comput. Vis. **94**, 198–214 (2011)
10. Michot, J., Bartoli, A., Gaspard, F.: Bi-objective bundle adjustment with application to multi-sensor slam. In: 3DPVT, p. 3025 (2010)
11. Morris, D.D.: Gauge Freedoms and uncertainty modeling for three-dimensional computer vision. Ph.D. thesis, Carnegie Mellon University (2001)
12. Nistér, D.: An efficient solution to the five-point relative pose problem. IEEE Trans. Pattern Anal. Mach. Intell. **26**, 756–777 (2004)
13. Nocedal, J., Wright, S.: Numerical Optimization. Springer, New York (2000)
14. Nützi, G., Weiss, S., Scaramuzza, D., Siegwart, R.: Fusion of imu and vision for absolute scale estimation in monocular slam. J. Intell. Robt. Syst. **61**, 287–299 (2011)
15. Rehder, J., Gupta, K., Nuske, S., Singh, S.: Global pose estimation with limited gps and long range visual odometry. In: 2012 IEEE International Conference on Robotics and Automation (ICRA), pp. 627–633. IEEE (2012)
16. Smith, M., Baldwin, I., Churchill, W., Paul, R., Newman, P.: The new college vision and laser data set. Int. J. Robot. Res. **28**, 595–599 (2009)
17. Sibley, G., Sukhatme, G., Matthies, L.: The iterated sigma point kalman filter with applications to longrange stereo. In: Proceedings of Robotics: Science and Systems, pp. 263–270 (2006)
18. Triggs, B., McLauchlan, P.F., Hartley, R.I., Fitzgibbon, A.W.: Bundle adjustment – a modern synthesis. In: Triggs, B., Zisserman, A., Szeliski, R. (eds.) ICCV-WS 1999. LNCS, vol. 1883, pp. 298–372. Springer, Heidelberg (2000)

DEPT: Depth Estimation by Parameter Transfer for Single Still Images

Xiu Li[1,2], Hongwei Qin[1,2]([✉]), Yangang Wang[3], Yongbing Zhang[1,2], and Qionghai Dai[1]

[1] Department of Automation, Tsinghua University, Beijing, China
{li.xiu,zhang.yongbing}@sz.tsinghua.edu.cn,
qionghaidai@tsinghua.edu.cn
[2] Graduate School at Shenzhen, Tsinghua University, Beijing, China
qhw12@mails.tsinghua.edu.cn
[3] Microsoft Research Asia, Beijing, China
yangangw@microsoft.com

Abstract. In this paper, we propose a new method for automatic depth estimation from color images using parameter transfer. By modeling the correlation between color images and their depth maps with a set of parameters, we get a database of parameter sets. Given an input image, we compute the high-level features to find the best matched image sets from the database. Then the set of parameters corresponding to the best match are used to estimate the depth of the input image. Compared to the past learning-based methods, our trained database only consists of trained features and parameter sets, which occupy little space. We evaluate our depth estimation method on the benchmark RGB-D (RGB + depth) datasets. The experimental results are comparable to the state-of-the-art, demonstrating the promising performance of our proposed method.

1 Introduction

Images captured with conventional cameras lose the depth information of the scene. However, scene depth is of great importance for many computer vision tasks. 3D applications like 3D reconstruction for scenes (*e.g.*, Street View on Google Map), robot navigation, 3D videos, and free view video(FVV) [1] all rely on scene depth. Depth information can also be useful for 2D applications like image enhancing [2] and scene recognition [3]. Recent RGB-D imaging devices like Kinect are greatly limited on the perceptive range and depth resolution. Neither can they extract depth for the existing 2D images. Therefore, depth estimation from color images has been a useful research subject.

In this paper, we propose a novel depth estimation method to generate depth maps from single still images. Our method applies to arbitrary color images.

Electronic supplementary material The online version of this chapter (doi:10. 1007/978-3-319-16808-1_4) contains supplementary material, which is available to authorized users.

D. Cremers et al. (Eds.): ACCV 2014, Part II, LNCS 9004, pp. 45–58, 2015.
DOI: 10.1007/978-3-319-16808-1_4

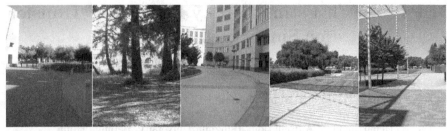

(a) Test images

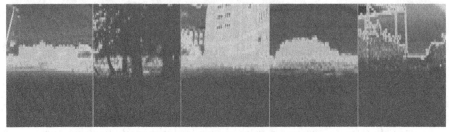

(b) Estimated depth maps by DEPT

Fig. 1. Selected images and corresponding depth maps estimated by DEPT. The darker the red is, the further (from the imaging device) the objects are. The darker the blue is, the closer the objects are.

We build the connection between image and depth with a set of parameters. A parameter sets database is constructed, and the parameter sets are transferred to input images to get the corresponding depth maps. Some estimation results are shown in Fig. 1.

As a reminder, the paper is organized as follows. In Sect. 2, the related techniques are surveyed. In Sect. 3, we introduce our proposed DEPT (depth estimation by parameter transfer) method in details. We demonstrate our method on the RGB-D benchmark datasets in Sect. 4. Finally, we conclude our work in Sect. 5.

2   Related Works

In this section, we introduce the techniques related to this paper, which are respectively depth estimation from a single image, and parameter transfer.

2.1   Depth Estimation from Single Images

The reason Depth estimation from a single image is possible lies in that there are some monocular depth cues in a 2D image. Some of these cues are inferred from local properties like color, shading, haze, defocus, texture variations and gradients, occlusions and so on. Global cues are also crucial to inferring depth, as the ability humans have. So, integrating local and global cues of a single image to estimate depth is reasonable.

There are semi-automatic and automatic methods for depth estimation from single images. Horry et al. [4] propose *tour into the picture*, where the user interactively adds planes to an image to make animation. The work of Zhang et al. [5] requires the user to add constrains manually to images to estimate depth.

Automatic methods for single image depth estimation come up in recent years. Hoiem et al. [6] propose *automatic photo pop-up*, which reconstructs an outdoor image using assumed planar surfaces of it. Delage et al. [7] develop a Bayesian framework applied to indoor scenes. Saxena et al. [8] propose a supervised learning approach, using a discriminatively-trained Markov Random Field (MRF) that incorporates multi-scale local and global image features. Then, they improve this method in [9]. After that, depth estimation from predicted semantic labels is proposed by Liu et al. [10]. A more sophisticated model called Feedback Enabled Cascaded Classification Models (FE-CCM) is proposed by Li et al. [11]. One typical depth estimation method is Depth Transfer, developed by Karsch et al. [12]. This method first builds a large scale RGB-D images and features database, then acquires the depth of the input image by transferring the depth of several similar images after warping and optimizing procedures.

Under specific conditions, there are other depth extract methods, such as dark channel prior proposed by He et al. [13], proved effective for hazed images.

The method closest to ours is the parametric model developed by Wang et al. [14] for describing the correlation between single color images and depth maps. This work treats the color image as a set of patches and derives the correlation with a kernel function in a non-linear mapping space. They get convincing depth map through patch sampling. However, this work only demonstrates the effectiveness of the model, and can't estimate depth with an arbitrary input image. Our improvements are two-fold: we extend this model from one image to many, and we transfer parameter set to an arbitrary input image according to best image set match.

2.2   Parameter Transfer

We carry out a survey on transfer methods in the field of depth estimation. The non-parametric scene parsing by Liu et al. [15] avoids explicitly defining a parametric model and scales better with respect to the training data size. The Depth Transfer method by Karsch et al. [12] leverages this work and assumes that scenes with similar semantics should have similar depth distributions after densely aligned. Their method has three stages. First, given an input image, they find K best matched images in RGB space. Then, the K images are warped to be densely aligned with the input. Finally, they use an optimization scheme to interpolate and smooth the warped depth values to get the depth of the input.

Our work is different in three aspects. First, instead of depth, we transfer parameter set to the input image, so we don't need post process like warping. Second, our database is composed of parameter sets instead of RGB-D images, so the database occupies little space. Third, the depth values are computed with the transferred parameter set directly, so we don't need an optimization procedure after transfer.

3   DEPT: Depth Estimation by Parameter Transfer

In this section, we first introduce the modeling procedure for inferring the correlation between color images and depth maps. Then, we introduce the parameter transfer method in detail.

3.1   The Parametric Model

The prior work of Wang *et al.* [14] proposes a model to build the correlation between a single image I and its corresponding depth map D with a set of parameters. We extend this by using a set of similar images IS and their corresponding depth map DS. So the parameters contain information of all the images in the set.

We regard each color image as a set of overlapped fixed-size color patches. We will discuss the patch size later. For each image, we sample the patches $x_1, x_2, ..., x_p$ and their corresponding depth values from RGB-D image set. To avoid over-fitting, we only sample p patches from each image. In our experiment, we set p as 1000, and the samples account for 0.026 % of the total patches in one image. We use a uniform sampling method, *i.e.*, we separate the image into grids and select samples uniformly from all the grids. By denoting N as the number of images in an image set, totally we sample $N \times p$ patches. Specially, for single image, $N = 1$.

Modeling the Correlation Between Image and Depth. After the sampling procedure, we model the correlation by measuring the sum squared error between the depth $\hat{\mathbf{d}}$ mapped with the sampled color patches and the ground truth depth $\mathbf{d}$. The model is written as

$$E = \sum_{i=1}^{p \times N} |tr(W^T \sum_{j=1}^{n} \gamma_j \phi(x_i * f_j)) - d_i|^2, \tag{1}$$

where E is the sum squared estimation error, p is the number of sample patches per image, N is the number of images in the image set, f_j is the filters, n is the number of filters, ϕ is the kernel function to map the convoluted patches and sum them up to *one patch*, γ_j is the weight of each convoluted patch, W is the weight matrix, whose size is the same of the *one patch*, aiming at integrating the overall information from each patch.

Equation 1 can be rewritten as

$$E = \sum_{i=1}^{p \times N} |\mathbf{w}^T \phi(X_i F) \gamma - d_i|^2, \tag{2}$$

where X_i is a matrix reshaped from patch x_i. The row size of X_i is the same as f_i, while $F = [f_1, f_2, ..., f_n]$, $\gamma = [\gamma_1, \gamma_2, ..., \gamma_n]^T$. $\mathbf{w}$ is the result of concatenating all the entries of W.

At the image level, F describes the texture gradient cues of the RGB image by extracting the frequency information. γ describes the variance of filters. We use Principle Component Analysis (PCA) to initialize F, and optimize it afterwards. As for the size of filter, we need to balance between efficiency and effect. However, we use W to integrate the global information, so we can choose smaller sized filters to reduce time consuming. $\phi(\cdot)$ is set as $\phi(x) = \log(1 + x^2)$, as it has been proven effective in [14].

Estimating Model Parameters. First, we rewrite Eq. 2 as

$$E = \|M\phi(XF)\gamma - \mathbf{d}\|_2^2, \tag{3}$$

and

$$E = \|\mathbf{\Gamma}\phi(F^T\hat{X})\mathbf{w} - \mathbf{d}\|_2^2, \tag{4}$$

where X is got by concatenating all the X_i in Eq. 2. $\hat{X}$ is got by concatenating all the X_i^T. Each row of M is $\mathbf{w}^T$, and each row of $\mathbf{\Gamma}$ is γ^T. So Eq. 3 is a least square problem of γ, and Eq. 4 is a least square problem of $\mathbf{w}$. Then we minimize E by optimizing the filters F. Finally we get a set of parameters, consisting of F, γ, and $\mathbf{w}$.

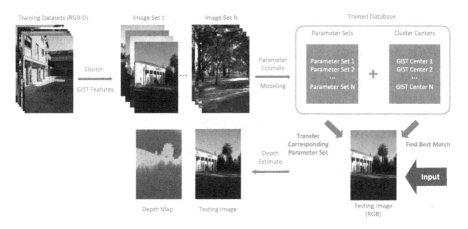

Fig. 2. Our pipeline for estimating depth. First we build a parameter set database, then the parameter set is transferred to the input image according to the best matched GIST feature. Finally, the parameter set is used to estimate the depth.

3.2 Parameter Transfer

Our parameter transfer procedure, outlined in Fig. 2, has three stages. First, we build a parameter set database using training RGB-D images. Second, given an input image, we find the most similar image sets using high-level image features, and transfer the parameter set to the input image. Third, we compute the depth of the input image.

Parameter Set Database Building. Given a RGB-D training dataset, we compute high-level image features for each image. Here, we use GIST [16] features, which can be used to measure similarities of images. Then, we category the training images to N sets, using KNN (K Nearest Neighbors) cluster method. And we get the central GIST feature for each image set. For each image set, the corresponding parameter set is obtained using our parameter estimate model. The central GIST features and corresponding parameter sets compose our parameter set database. Actually, this database is so small as to occupy much less space compared to the RGB-D datasets.

Image Set Matching. Given an input image, we compute its GIST feature and find the best matched central GIST feature from our trained database. Then the parameter set corresponding to the best matched central GIST feature (*i.e.* the central GIST feature of the most similar image set) is transferred to the input image. We define the best match as

$$G_{best} = \min_{i=1,2,...,N} \|G_{input} - G_i\|, \tag{5}$$

where G_{input} denotes the GIST feature of the input image, and G_i denotes the central GIST feature of each image set.

As the most similar image set match the input closely in feature space, the overall semantics of the scenes are similar. At the low level, the cues such as the texture gradient, texture variation, and color are expected to be roughly similar to some extend. With the model above, the parameters connecting the images and depth maps should be similar. So, it is reasonable to transfer the parameter set to the input image.

Depth Estimation. We use the color patches of the input image and the transferred parameter set to map the estimation depth. The computational formula is:

$$\hat{\mathbf{d}} = M\phi(XF)\gamma, \tag{6}$$

where X is the patches, F is the filters, γ is the weight to balance the filters. M is the weight matrix. These parameters are all from the parameter set.

4   Experiment

In this section, we evaluate the effectiveness of our DEPT method on single image RGB-D datasets.

4.1   RGB-D Datasets

We use the Make3D Range Image Dataset [17]. The dataset is collected using 3D scanner and the corresponding depth maps using lasers. There are totally 534 images separated into two parts, which are the training part containing 400 images and the testing part containing 134 images, respectively. The color image resolution is 2272×1704, and the ground truth depth map resolution is 55×305.

4.2 Image Cluster

We compute the GIST features for each image in the training dataset. Then we use KNN algorithm to cluster the images into N sets, here we set N as 30. The images are well separated according to the scene semantics. The silhouette plot in Fig. 3 measures how well-separated the resulting image sets are. Lines on the right side of 0 measure how distant that image is from neighboring image sets. Lines on the left of 0 indicate that image is probably assigned to the wrong set. The vertical axis indicates different clusters (image sets). As we can see, most of the images are well clustered. As for the choosing of N, we test a series of values with a step of 10. The results around 30 are close, and 30 is the best. The cluster number can also be accurately set according to existing pattern classification methods (*e.g.* methods to find best k in k-means algorithm).

An example image set is shown in Fig. 5. It can be seen that the clustered images have roughly similar semantic scene. The depth distributions also seem similar, as are shown in the color images as well as the depth maps.

4.3 Parameter Sets Estimation

For each image set, we estimate the corresponding model parameters. The overlapped patch size is set 15×15. The filter size is set as 3×3. We separate each image into grids and uniformly sample 1000 patches per image. So for an N

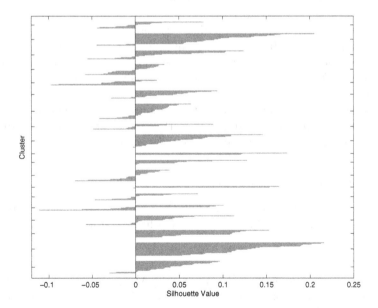

Fig. 3. Silhouette plot of the KNN cluster result. Each line represents an image. Lines on the right side of 0 measure how distant that image is from neighboring image sets. Lines on the left of 0 indicate that image is probably assigned to the wrong set. The vertical axis indicates different clusters (image sets).

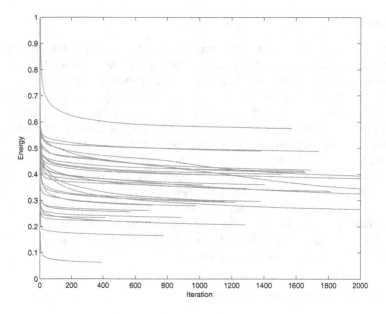

Fig. 4. Energy decline curves of the 30 image sets. E is on a ln scale.

sized image set, totally $1000 \times N$ patches are sampled, which occupy $0.026\,\%$ of the whole image set. We initialize the filters with PCA method, and optimize all the parameters using warm-start gradient descent method. The iteration stop condition is $E < 10^{-6}$. In our experiment, the energy (i.e., the sum squared errors E) declines as Fig. 4 shows. As can be seen, most of the curves come to a steady state after about 1000 iterations. The smaller the steady energy is, the more similar the images in that set are.

For each image set, we obtain one optimized parameter set. The 30 parameter sets and the corresponding cluster centers (the center of the GIST features in each image set) make up the parameter sets database.

4.4 Depth Estimation by Parameter Transfer

For each of the testing 134 images, we find the best matched image set from the parameter sets database and compute the depth maps using the computational formula of Eq. 6.

Quantitative Comparison with Previous Methods. We calculate three common error metrics for the estimated depth. Denoting $\hat{\mathbf{D}}$ as the estimated depth and $\mathbf{D}$ as the ground truth depth, we calculate **RE** (*relative error*):

$$\mathbf{RE} = \frac{|\hat{\mathbf{D}} - \mathbf{D}|}{\mathbf{D}}, \qquad (7)$$

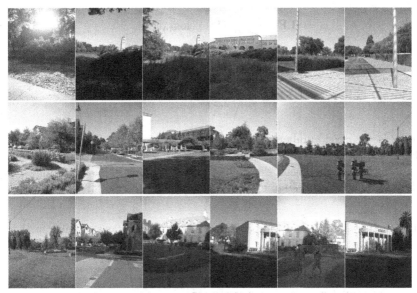

(a) One clustered image set

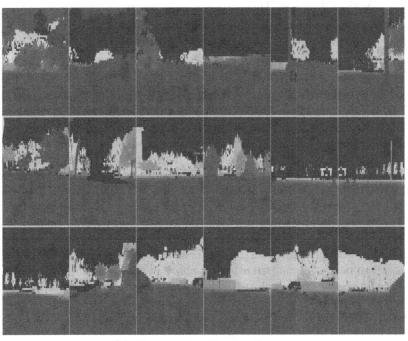

(b) The corresponding depth maps

Fig. 5. One example image set after image cluster procedure. (a) is a clustered image set, containing 18 semantic similar images, (b) are their corresponding depth maps. The depth distributions in the images are roughly similar.

LE ($\log_{10}$ *error*):
$$\mathbf{LE} = |\log_{10}(\hat{\mathbf{D}}) - \log_{10}(\mathbf{D})|, \tag{8}$$

and **RMSE** (*root mean squared error*):

$$\mathbf{RMSE} = \sqrt{\sum_{i=1}^{P}(\hat{\mathbf{D}}_i - \mathbf{D}_i)^2/P}, \tag{9}$$

where P is the pixel number of a depth map.

Error measure for each image is the average value of all the pixels on the ground truth resolution scale (55×305). Then the measures are averaged over all the 134 images to get final error metrics, which are listed in Table 1.

Table 1. Average error and database size comparison of various estimate methods.

Method	RE	LE	RMSE	Trained Database
Depth MRF [8]	0.530	0.198	16.7	-
Make3D [17]	0.370	0.187	-	-
Feedback Cascades [11]	-	-	15.2	-
Depth Transfer [12]	0.361	0.148	15.1	2.44 GB
DEPT(ours)	0.489	0.182	16.9	188 KB

As can be seen, our results are better than Depth MRF [8] in view of **RE** and **LE**, better than Make3D [17] in view of **LE**. Totally speaking, the results of DEPT are comparable with the state-of-the-art learning based automatic methods. Especially, DEPT only requires a very small sized database, and once the database is built, we can compute the depth directly. Built from the 400 training RGB-D images that occupy 628 MB space, our database size is only 188 KB (0.03 %). As a contrast, the trained database of Depth Transfer [12] occupies 2.44 GB[1] (about 4 times of the original dataset size). Though our method has *disadvantage* in average errors over the Depth Transfer [12], we have large *advantages* in database space consuming and computer performance requirement(in [12], the authors claim Depth Transfer requires a great deal of data (GB scale) to be stored concurrently in memory in the optimization procedure), which are especially crucial when the database grows in real applications.

Further more, our method also has advantages in some of the estimation effects, as is detailed in the following qualitative evaluation.

Qualitative Evaluation. A qualitative comparison of our estimated depth maps, depth maps estimated by Depth Transfer [12] and the ground truth depth

---

[1] Implemented with the authors' public codes at http://research.microsoft.com/en-us/downloads/29d28301-1079-4435-9810-74709376bce1/.

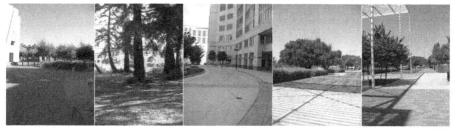

(a) Test images

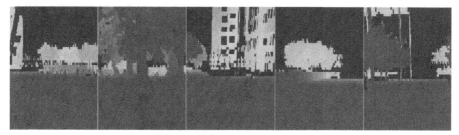

(b) Ground truth depth maps

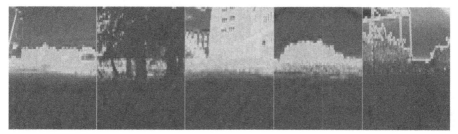

(c) Estimated depth maps by DEPT (our method)

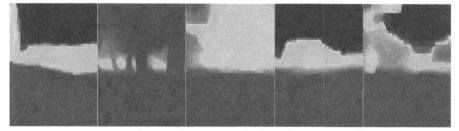

(d) Estimated depth maps by Depth Transfer [12]

Fig. 6. Performance comparison: scenes of streets, squares and trees. (a) show some test images containing streets, squares or trees, (b) are corresponding ground truth depth maps, (c) are estimated depth maps by DEPT (our method), (d) are estimated depth maps by Depth Transfer [12]

maps are demonstrated in Figs. 6 and 7. As can be seen, our estimated depth maps are visually reasonable and convincing, especially in the details like texture variations (e.g., the tree in the second column of Fig. 6) and relative depth

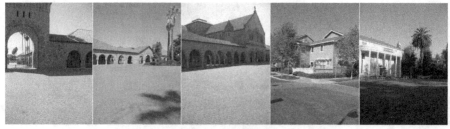

(a) Test images

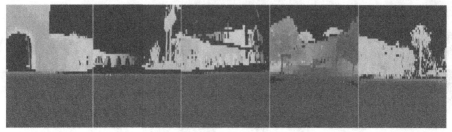

(b) Ground truth depth maps

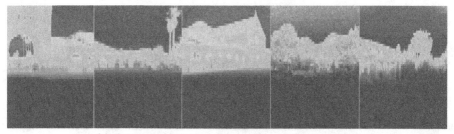

(c) Estimated depth maps by DEPT (our method)

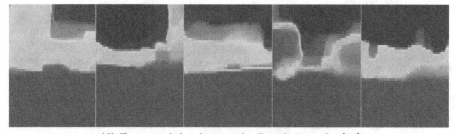

(d) Estimated depth maps by Depth Transfer [12]

Fig. 7. Performance comparison: scenes of buildings. (a) show some test images containing buildings, (b) are corresponding ground truth depth maps, (c) are estimated depth maps by DEPT (our method), (d) are estimated depth maps by Depth Transfer [12]

(e.g., the pillars' depth in the last column of Fig. 6 is well estimated by our DEPT method, while Depth Transfer [12] estimates wrong). Actually, some of our results are even more accurate than the ground truth (e.g., in the third column in Fig. 7, there is a large part of wrong depth in the building area of the ground truth depth map). The ground truth maps have some scattered noises, which may result from the capturing device. While the noises in our depth maps are less because of the using of overall information in the image set. But we must point out that the sky areas in our depth maps are not as pleasing, which may result from the variation of sky color and texture among various images in a set, especially when the cluster result is biased. This may result in the increase of average error in the previous metrics. However, as the increasing of RGB-D images acquired by depth imaging devices, our database can expand easily due to the extremely small space consuming, which means we may get more and more accurate matched parameter sets for existing RGB images and video frames.

5   Conclusion and Future Works

In this paper, we propose an effective and fully automatic technique to restore depth information from single still images. Our depth estimation by parameter transfer (DEPT) method is novel in that we use clustered scene semantics similar image sets to model the correlation between RGB information and D (depth) information, obtaining a database of parameter sets and cluster centers. DEPT only requires the trained parameter sets database which occupies much less space compared with previous learning based methods. Experiments on RGB-D benchmark datasets show quantitatively comparable to the state-of-the-art and qualitatively good results. The estimated depth maps are visually reasonable and convincing, especially in the details like texture variations and relative depth. Further more, as the increasing of RGB-D images acquired by depth imaging devices, our database can expand easily due to the extremely small space consuming. In the future work, we would like to improve the cluster accuracy by exploring more accurate similarity metrics that are applicable to our image and depth correlation model. And we suppose it is also meaningful to improve the depth estimation performance for video frames by using optical flow features or other features related to time coherence.

Acknowledgement. This work is supported by National Natural Science Foundation of China (Grant No. 71171121/61033005) and National 863 High Technology Research and Development Program of China (Grant No. 2012AA09A408).

References

1. Liu, Q., Yang, Y., Ji, R., Gao, Y., Yu, L.: Cross-view down/up-sampling method for multiview depth video coding. IEEE Sig. Process. Lett. **19**, 295–298 (2012)
2. Li, F., Yu, J., Chai, J.: A hybrid camera for motion deblurring and depth map super-resolution. In: 2008 IEEE Conference on Computer Vision and Pattern Recognition CVPR 2008, pp. 1–8. IEEE (2008)
3. Torralba, A., Oliva, A.: Depth estimation from image structure. IEEE Trans. Pattern Anal. Mach. Intell. **24**, 1226–1238 (2002)

4. Horry, Y., Anjyo, K.I., Arai, K.: Tour into the picture: using a spidery mesh interface to make animation from a single image. In: Proceedings of the 24th Annual Conference on Computer Graphics and Interactive Techniques, pp. 225–232. ACM Press/Addison-Wesley Publishing Co. (1997)

5. Zhang, L., Dugas-Phocion, G., Samson, J.S., Seitz, S.M.: Single-view modelling of free-form scenes. J. Vis. Comput. Animation **13**, 225–235 (2002)

6. Hoiem, D., Efros, A.A., Hebert, M.: Automatic photo pop-up. ACM Trans. Graph. (TOG) **24**, 577–584 (2005). ACM

7. Delage, E., Lee, H., Ng, A.Y.: A dynamic bayesian network model for autonomous 3d reconstruction from a single indoor image. In: 2006 IEEE Computer Society Conference on Computer Vision and Pattern Recognition, vol. 2, pp. 2418–2428. IEEE (2006)

8. Saxena, A., Chung, S.H., Ng, A.Y.: Learning depth from single monocular images. In: Advances in Neural Information Processing Systems, pp. 1161–1168 (2005)

9. Saxena, A., Chung, S.H., Ng, A.Y.: 3-d depth reconstruction from a single still image. Int. J. Comput. Vis. **76**, 53–69 (2008)

10. Liu, B., Gould, S., Koller, D.: Single image depth estimation from predicted semantic labels. In: 2010 IEEE Conference on Computer Vision and Pattern Recognition (CVPR), pp. 1253–1260. IEEE (2010)

11. Li, C., Kowdle, A., Saxena, A., Chen, T.: Towards holistic scene understanding: feedback enabled cascaded classification models. In: Advances in Neural Information Processing Systems, pp. 1351–1359 (2010)

12. Karsch, K., Liu, C., Kang, S.B.: Depthtransfer: depth extraction from video using non-parametric sampling. IEEE Transactions on Pattern Analysis and Machine Intelligence (2014)

13. He, K., Sun, J., Tang, X.: Single image haze removal using dark channel prior. IEEE Trans. Pattern Anal. Mach. Intell. **33**, 2341–2353 (2011)

14. Wang, Y., Wang, R., Dai, Q.: A parametric model for describing the correlation between single color images and depth maps. Signal Processing Letters **21** (2014)

15. Liu, C., Yuen, J., Torralba, A.: Nonparametric scene parsing via label transfer. IEEE Trans. Pattern Anal. Mach. Intell. **33**, 2368–2382 (2011)

16. Oliva, A., Torralba, A.: Modeling the shape of the scene: a holistic representation of the spatial envelope. Int. J. Comput. Vis. **42**, 145–175 (2001)

17. Saxena, A., Sun, M., Ng, A.Y.: Make3d: learning 3d scene structure from a single still image. IEEE Trans. Pattern Anal. Mach. Intell. **31**, 824–840 (2009)

Object Ranking on Deformable Part Models with Bagged LambdaMART

Chaobo Sun[(⊠)], Xiaojie Wang, and Peng Lu

School of Computer, Beijing University of Posts and Telecommunications,
Beijing, China
{cbsun,xjwang,lupeng}@bupt.edu.cn

Abstract. Object detection methods based on sliding windows has long been considered a binary classification problem, but this formulation ignores order of examples. Deformable part models, which achieves great success in object detection, have the same problem.This paper aims to give better order to detections given by deformable part models. We use a bagged LambdaMART to model both pair-wise and list-wise relationships between detections. Experiments show our ranking models not only significantly improve detection rates compared to basic deformable part model detectors, but also outperform classification methods with same features.

1 Introduction

Detection of objects in natural images has always been a difficult problem in computer vision, due to the complexity of backgrounds and the large variances of objects in the same category. Data-driven methods in recent years [12,18] have achieved reasonable results. In these methods, object detection is formulated into a binary classification problem: to distinguish the object patches and non-object ones from a set of candidates. The candidates can be generated using either sliding windows [12] or objectness based methods [2,9].

Deformable Part Models(DPM) have achieved great success in object detection. Though DPMs generate solid sets of candidates with hierarchical templates [12] to model the deformation inside categories, they also suffer from the shortcoming of binary classification formulation. Our experiments show that with an enlarged set of detections and the correct order of the detections, the performance of DPMs may be significantly prompted. This observation reveals the role of order in object detection, and make it a natural way that developing a learning to rank framework to improve DPMs.

With ranking perspective on object detection, we can remodel object detection as object ranking, which aims to recover the ground truth order given a set of candidate detections. The set, can contain all possible windows in a spatial pyramid, or the output of previous detection system.

When comparing object ranking to classical object detection methods, we find that the classical methods fail to capture the relationships between detections. The relationships, contains both pair-wise and list-wise information, plays

© Springer International Publishing Switzerland 2015
D. Cremers et al. (Eds.): ACCV 2014, Part II, LNCS 9004, pp. 59–71, 2015.
DOI: 10.1007/978-3-319-16808-1_5

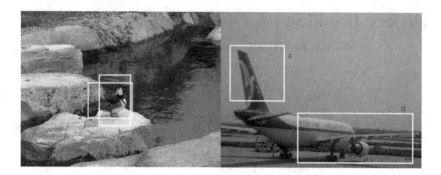

Fig. 1. In the image on the left-hand side, detection a and b are both true detections, but a is definitely a better detection than b; In the image on the right-hand side, c and d are both false detections whose overlap ratios with ground truth objects are below 0.5, but still we can tell d is better than c.

a central role in ranking. As Fig. 1 shows, A ranking model focuses on "Why is a detection better than another" rather than "Why is a detection true".

We have a discussion on background works in Sect. 2. Section 3.1 makes a review of LambdaMART. Section 3.2 discusses why object ranking is useful. Section 3.3 describes our ranking model based on ensemble of decision trees, which uses bagged [5] LambdaMART [19], with a training procedure with increasing dataset. Experiments in Sect. 4 discuss the features we use, the potential of DPM, show the comparison between ranking and classification. We then make analysis on the errors before and after ranking, and discuss the impact factors of our ranking model.

2   Related Work

Research on generic object detection is originating from person detection [10]. From then on sliding-window methods with HOG pyramids have been a main stream on object detection. For every category of objects, sliding-window build a set of templates to represent all its poses. During training, cropped objects and backgrounds are extracted to train the template. During detecting, a matching score is computed at every position in the feature space, then the position with scores above a threshold is considered to be an object position [10].

Deformable part models [12] have greatly pushed the research on object detection. As a variation of sliding windows, DPMs establish a set of hierarchical templates for every category of objects. Each template is organized into a root and its parts. Not only the appearance(vision features) of roots and parts, but also the parts' relative positions(structural features) to the root are taken into consider, so that DPMs can tolerate a certain degree of deformation.

Our work is basically based on DPM. But different from the way using strong supervised information [3,4], we aim to improve DPM by using extra image information beyond HOG, which is relatively simple.

Many excellent works have shown that object detection can benefit from objectness models [2,9,18]. Objectness models aim to provide a small set of detection candidates with high recall. Then classifiers are applied on the candidates. Our work is similar to this approach in the way that we both use two-stage modeling, but we use deformable part models rather than objectness models to generate more reliable, and smaller sets of candidates, also we use ranking rather than classification as the post procedure.

Gradient Boosted Decision Trees(GBDT) based methods have achieved great success in learning to rank problems [6]. They use a pair-wise loss from ranknet models [7]. GBDTs are then extended to LambdaMART [19] by introducing list-wise information [8]. We use a bagged LambdaMART to rank detections, this method is similar with [13], but differs in the way how bagging samples are generated, our generating scheme is based on pairs rather than examples, and is a more natural way in the task of object detection.

There are many types of useful image features for object detection, among which Histograms of gradient(HOG) features [10] have long been a primal one, Local Binary Patterns(LBP) [1] are proved to be a good supplement for HOG, Color SIFT has also been a standard feature using in methods based on selective search [18], local contrast information and saliency are also useful [2].

In recent years features from deep convolutional neural networks(CNN) [15] achieved very high performance [14]. Features learned by well-structured deep CNNs are good descriptors for images, and are powerful tools for object detection.

3 Ranking Model for Object Detection

3.1 Why Ranking?

Classical learning to rank systems focus on selecting relevant items from a set of candidates. Object detection is similar to these models, if we interpret the searching space of object detection as a set of candidates. Following the way of Pascal VOC evaluation [11], the set of candidates are all positions of all images in a dataset. The aim of object detection is then selecting candidates that have more overlap ratios with ground truth objects.

In information retrieval systems, when modeling the relationship of some samples $\{x_i\}_{i=1}^n$ and their corresponding labels $\{y_i\}_{i=1}^n$, there are three types of information:

- item-wise information, direct relationships between every x_i and y_i.
- pair-wise information, relationships between a paired (x_i, x_j).
- list-wise information, information retrieval metrics of a list $x_1, x_2, \ldots, x_n$, such as mean average precision(MAP).

On the other hand, the standard evaluation metric for object detection is MAP, so it is natural that taking MAP of detections into account during training. While it is quite difficult for classification which focuses on item-wise labels, adding list-wise information to a ranking model is straight-forward [8].

The key difficulty for applying ranking models on object detection is its large space of candidates. All rectangles in images are candidates to rank. Sliding window methods largely reduce the number of candidates by making the constraint that all candidates should be in certain sizes [10], while in recent years there are several useful technologies directly aiming at shrinking the space of candidates [2,9].

3.2 LambdaMART

Cross Entropy Loss. Suppose that we have a list of detections, labeled with their overlap ratios with ground truth objects. We first generate a set of pairs based on the list, let the set be J, each pair (i, j) in the set J means that detection x_i has a higher overlap ratio than x_j with some ground truth objects. We then define a cross entropy loss function on pairs in J.

To begin the definition, we define a simple empirical distribution on every pair (i, j) in J:

$$\bar{P}_{ij} \equiv \begin{cases} 1, (i, j) \in J \\ 0, (j, i) \in J \end{cases} \tag{1}$$

The empirical probability is a statistical measure of the pair-wise information in training datasets. During the train stage of our model, the score function is applied on each detection, and the score outputted would also generate a model distribution. We define it in a form of sigmoid function:

$$P_{ij} \equiv \frac{1}{1 + e^{-\sigma(f_i - f_j)}} \tag{2}$$

For simplicity, we use f_i to denote a score function for sample x_i.

The two distributions should be as close as possible. We use cross entropy to measure the divergence of them:

$$C_{ij} = -\bar{P}_{ij} log(P_{ij}) - (1 - \bar{P}_{ij}) log(1 - P_{ij}) \tag{3}$$

Combining Eqs. (1) ,(2) and (3), we got:

$$C_{ij} = log(1 + e^{-\sigma(f_i - f_j)}) \tag{4}$$

MART. A MART model is an ensemble of regression decision trees, the score for a feature x is defined as:

$$f^m(x) = \sum_{k=1}^{m} \eta^k t^k(x) \tag{5}$$

where $t^k(x)$ is the score of kth regression decision tree, η is the learning rate.

Suppose that $m - 1$ trees are trained, and the mth tree is now to be trained. Note that in MART model, a new regression tree tries to capture the gradient of total cost, that is, let the gradient for a single example x_i be λ_i^m, the mth tree trained to fit the dataset $\{(x_i, \lambda_i^m)\}_{i=1}^k$. We have:

$$\lambda_i^m \equiv \sum_{j:(i,j)\in J or (j,i)\in J} \frac{\partial C_{ij}^{m-1}}{\partial f_i^{m-1}} \tag{6}$$

Recall the derivative of C_{ij}, which is defined in Eq. 4, has following feature:

$$\frac{\partial C_{ij}}{\partial f_i} = \frac{-\sigma}{1 + e^{-\sigma(f_i - f_j)}} = -\frac{\partial C_{ij}}{\partial f_j} \tag{7}$$

let $\dfrac{\partial C_{ij}^{m-1}}{\partial f_i^{m-1}}$ be λ_{ij}^m, we can re-write λ_i^m as:

$$\lambda_i^m = \sum_{j:(i,j) \in J} \lambda_{ij}^m - \sum_{j:(j,i) \in J} \lambda_{ij}^m \tag{8}$$

LamdbaMART. While the above formulation well models pair-wise information, weights of λs are introduced to capture list-wise information.

$$\lambda_{ij} = \frac{-\sigma}{1 + e^{-\sigma(f_i - f_j)}} \|\Delta MAP_{ij}\| \tag{9}$$

where ΔMAP_{ij} is the change of mean average precision if positions of x_i and x_j are exchanged.

3.3 Bagged LambdaMART with an Increasing Training Set

We have discussed in Sect. 3.1 why object detection is more a ranking problem instead of classification, but there are still significant differences between object detection and classical ranking problems. The first difference is that the list of candidates in object detection is much larger. In classical ranking tasks, candidates are divided into different groups, because only candidates in the same group have relationships, comparison between groups are meaningless. While in object detection, a candidate is comparable with all other candidates in the dataset, not only from the same image, so an ideal list for object detection is a list contains all candidates detected on all images in the dataset.

Suppose there are m images in the dataset, and we generate n detection candidates per image, then the ranking list has length $m * n$, and when applying LambdaMART in which pairs are needed to be generated, that is, $O((m * n)^2)$ pairs(if the relationships between candidates are not sparse, they are usually not), computing the loss of all pairs are both time consuming and memory consuming.

The second difference is that there are too many low-ranking candidates relative to high-ranking ones. This is a main difficulty for nearly all object detection systems [12,18,20]. DPM results have largely reduced the difficulty by providing a credible candidate sets, but we still have a ratio of 25 : 1 between high-ranking detections with low-ranking ones.

Based on above observations, we use an ensemble of ranking models with increasing training set for detection. The framework of training is shown in Fig. 2.

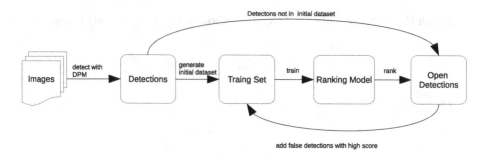

Fig. 2. The training procedure

Increasing Training Set. We generate the training set in an increasing way. The training set is initialized with good candidates whose overlap ratios are above a threshold, others are stored in a set of **open detections**, trained models are applied on this set and detections with high scores are added into the training set and removed from the set of open detections. Operating like this iteratively, we are supposed to get final model after a certain number of iterations.

Increasing training datasets, which are widely used in object detection systems, aim to solve the unbalance problem of true and false examples. Our implementation is similar to previous methods based on classification, but the motivation is quite different.

It is notable that in the ranking perspective on object detection, there is no unbalance problem for training data, as we focus mainly on pair-wise and list-wise information, rather than item-wise labels. So it is possible to include all examples in training set, and train a model in a single round, our iterative setting is aiming to reduce the difficulty in computing.

Bagging. At each iteration, once training set is prepared, the training set forms a single list for ranking. To reduce computational complexity, we use bagging methods to randomly split the whole set into smaller subsets. A splittings is a bagging [5] set of samples, in the way that splitting on examples are equivalent to sampling on pairs.

To ensure pairs are sampled uniformly, suppose we have K subsets, and the probability of sample x_i be grouped into subset $k(1 \leq k \leq K)$ is p_i^k, then the probability of pair (i,j) be sampled in this splitting is $\dfrac{\sum\limits_{k=1}^{K} p_i^k \cdot p_i^k}{K}$. We can then make probability a constraint by simply setting $p_i^k = \frac{1}{K}$. That means if each example is assigned into subsets uniformly, then the pairs are sampled uniformly.

We then train a LambdaMART model for every splitting, then the ensemble of LambdaMART models are obtained as the final model at this iteration.

Bagged LambdaMART can be interpreted as a matrix of decision trees, as Fig. 3 shows, trees in the model are ensembled in both gradient boosted scheme, and bagging scheme.

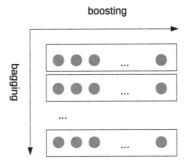

Fig. 3. Ensemble of decision trees as a matrix

4   Experiments

4.1   Deep Features

We use Caffe [16] to extract deep features. The network is the pretrained model in Caffe. The architecture of the neural network, is defined in [17]. For each detection windows, the image patch bounded by it are feed into the network, and the output of penultimate layer are taken as features. These features have been proved to be powerful in object-based image recognition problems [14], and it would be more powerful after fine-tuning on Pascal VOC datasets, but as our focusing are the ranking procedure, we just use the original features.

4.2   Potential of DPM

Deformable Part Models, which learn certain number of templates for objects, suffer from the large variance of objects in a category, but we argue that by enlarging the detection set on each image, and giving them the correct order, deformable part models can achieve much better performance.

We enlarge the detection set by selecting k-best detections per image, instead of using a static threshold. Figure 4 shows that under k-best scheme, recall is an increasing function on k.

To illustrate the importance of correct order, we evaluate detections in both orders: the order given by DPM detectors, and the order given by their overlap ratios.

Table 1 shows the results of comparison on Pascal VOC2007 datasets [11], which is also the potential of DPM.

4.3   Model Comparison on Pascal VOC Benchmarks

While correct order can significantly improve the performance of DPM, how to recover the correct order is a main challenging. As discussed above, ranking is a straight-forward way. We also implement a binary classification re-scoring procedure based on SVM for comparison.

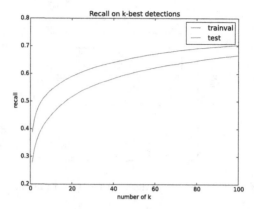

Fig. 4. recalls are growing by increasing k on both trainval and test dataset of Pascal VOC 2007, but the growth would be very slow when k is large.

Table 1. DPM order is the order according to DPM scores, and GT order is the order according to overlap ratios with ground truth objects. When detections are given, DPM results in GT order are the upper bound of DPM.

	plane	bike	bird	boat	bottle	bus	car	cat	chair	cow
DPM order	0.310	0.597	0.040	0.121	0.235	0.506	0.546	0.171	0.177	0.228
GT order	0.748	0.875	0.700	0.609	0.602	0.879	0.710	0.912	0.755	0.698

	table	dog	horse	mbike	person	plant	sheep	sofa	train	tv	AVG
DPM order	0.221	0.046	0.583	0.479	0.418	0.085	0.188	0.359	0.454	0.408	0.309
GT order	0.898	0.893	0.876	0.845	0.691	0.662	0.641	0.960	0.868	0.785	0.780

Table 2 shows that our ranking model outperforms classification model based on SVM. The results proved our guess: by modeling more information, ranking models are more powerful than classification models in object detection.

In Table 2 we make an extra comparison between our results and [14], which uses the same features, much larger candidate sets(1000–2000 detections per image, giving higher recall than DPM), and svm classifiers. With a smaller set of candidates, our models plays better on 9 categories, and average rate on all categories are very close (only a difference of 0.3).

The implementation in [14] uses training and testing set of detections generated by selective search, which contains 1000–2000 detections per image. We obtain close performance to them with a smaller set of candidates.

Figure 5 shows top detections from negatives of DPM. The ranking model are more strong at detecting truncated objects or objects in complex backgrounds.

4.4 Analysis of Ranking Model

Following [18], we initialize the training set with detections whose overlap ratios are above 0.2. At each iteration, 5000 detections with highest score in the set of open detections are added into the training set.

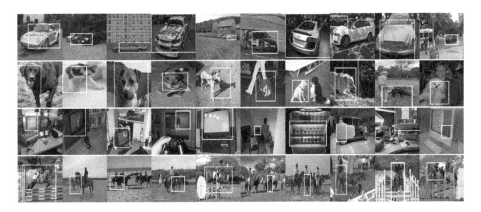

Fig. 5. Top detections of car, dog, tvmonitor and horse, which are considered negative by original DPM, but judged positive by our ranking model.

Table 2. DPM is the original results, DPM+svm is the results, DPM+rank is results form our ranking model, DeepF is the result reported in [14].

	plane	bike	bird	boat	bottle	bus	car	cat	chair	cow
DPM	0.310	0.597	0.040	0.121	0.235	0.506	0.546	0.171	0.177	0.228
DPM+svm	0.421	0.555	0.341	0.194	0.261	0.519	0.545	0.428	**0.327**	0.291
DeepF	**0.531**	0.589	**0.354**	**0.296**	0.223	0.5	**0.577**	**0.524**	0.191	**0.435**
DPM+rank	0.467	**0.668**	0.259	0.194	**0.307**	**0.594**	0.570	0.392	0.291	0.365
	table	dog	horse	mbike	person	plant	sheep	sofa	train	tv	AVG
DPM	0.221	0.046	0.583	0.479	0.418	0.085	0.188	0.359	0.454	0.408	0.309
DPM+svm	0.391	0.337	0.501	0.591	0.417	0.192	0.313	0.329	0.451	0.477	0.394
DeepF	**0.408**	**0.436**	0.476	0.54	0.391	**0.23**	**0.423**	0.336	0.514	**0.552**	0.426
DPM+rank	0.335	0.240	**0.651**	**0.629**	**0.445**	0.167	0.309	**0.449**	**0.586**	0.541	0.423

Figure 6 shows detection rates at different iterations. The first three rounds of training is useful, but training after 3 rounds makes little contribution. At the beginning iterations of training, MAP grows significantly, but after 3 rounds, there is no significant promotion when increasing the number of iterations.

4.5 Analysis of Errors

Under the standard evaluation metric of MAP, true detections are the detections which have overlap ratios below 0.5, and false detections just the opposite. When focusing on false detections, it is a natural idea that these errors are caused by different reasons, so that a fine-grained analysis is reasonable.

We divide detection errors into 3 types: location errors; confusion with other categories; background errors. We argue that only background errors are *real* errors. Location errors at least provides the correct information about the existence of objects, while confusion errors may suggest visual similarities of different categories.

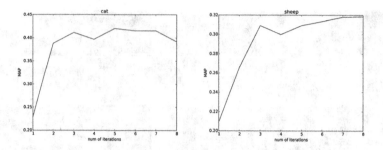

Fig. 6. We use two categories to select a best number of iterations. We train ranking models on trainval dataset of Pascal VOC 2007, and test them on the a subset of the test dataset.

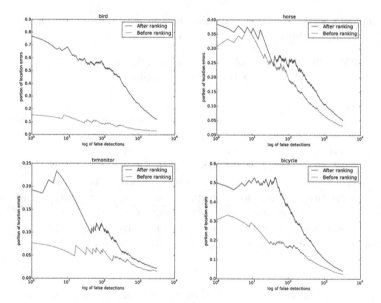

Fig. 7. We select 4 representative classes: bird, on which the performance of DPM is very poor; horse, on which the performance of DPM is very good; tvmonitor and bicycle are artificial objects with middle level performance.

We define location errors as the false detections with relatively high overlap ratios(above 0.2). As Fig.7 shows, giving the same number of total errors, the proportion of location errors after ranking are much higher than that before ranking.

The result means that false detections with higher overlap ratios are given higher ranking, and the our ranking model has a strong ability of distinguishing a not so bad example from totally bad ones. Then, by introducing pair-wise and list-wise information, the ranking model meets the expectation that learning "why a detection is better than another".

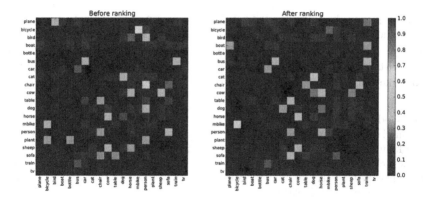

Fig. 8. Confusion matrices before and after ranking. These matrices are not standard confusion matrices, only errors are shown in them so that the diagonals are all zero. Each row in the matrices represents distribution of mis-recognition errors for a specific detector.

Another important type of errors is confusion with other categories. Figure 8 shows the confusion matrices on top 100 errors before and after ranking.

Overall distribution of confusions before and after ranking are similar. There are some common pairs in both matrices, like **bicycle** and **motorbike**; **car** and **bus**; **horse** and **cow**; **train** and **bus**. These pairs are all similar categories in vision, it is difficult to distinguish even by human visually, human may distinguish them by other information.

Besides similar pairs discussed above, it is interesting that there are two significant confusion in the matrix before ranking: recognizing bird as aeroplane, and recognizing person as chair. They are both dismissed in the matrix after ranking. It shows that when HoG features focus on the shape and structure of images, deep features are more complex and more powerful to distinguish images by appearance.

5 Conclusion and Future Work

Our whole work in this paper is motivated by the ignorance of order information by classical object detection methods. Under the guidance of this idea, we propose a bagged LambdaMART for object detection. We evaluate the models on k-best results generated by deformable part models, with deep features from convolutional neural network. Experiments show an improvement by ranking not only compared to original DPM, but also svm-based re-scoring method applied on DPM. Our model also achieves close result with state of the art methods which use the same feature. We also implement several fine-grained evaluations on detection errors, which also provides solid evidence for the role of ranking in object detection.

But it is also notable that the combination of ranking model and deep features does not explore total potential of DPM, there is still a long way to go to recover the ground truth order.

Our object ranking framework can be used as a post-processing stage of any object candidates generating system. Although the k-best results of DPM are small and reliable, there are many objectness based methods which generate results with much higher recall. It would be also useful to run the ranking model on that methods.

Acknowledgments. This work was partially supported by National Natural Science Foundation of China(Project No.61273365 and No. 61100120), the Fundamental Research Funds for the Central Universities (No. 2013RC0304), National High Technology Research and Development Program of China(No. 2012AA011104) and discipline building plan in 111 base(No. B08004) and Engineering Research Center of Information Networks, Ministry of Education.

References

1. Ahonen, T., Hadid, A., Pietikäinen, M.: Face recognition with local binary patterns. In: Pajdla, T., Matas, J.G. (eds.) ECCV 2004. LNCS, vol. 3021, pp. 469–481. Springer, Heidelberg (2004)
2. Alexe, B., Deselaers, T., Ferrari, V.: What is an object? In: 2010 IEEE Computer Society Conference on Computer Vision and Pattern Recognition, pp. 73–80. IEEE, June 2010
3. Azizpour, H., Laptev, I.: Object detection using strongly-supervised deformable part models. In: Fitzgibbon, A., Lazebnik, S., Perona, P., Sato, Y., Schmid, C. (eds.) ECCV 2012, Part I. LNCS, vol. 7572, pp. 836–849. Springer, Heidelberg (2012)
4. Branson, S., Perona, P., Belongie, S.: Strong supervision from weak annotation: Interactive training of deformable part models. In: 2011 IEEE International Conference on Computer Vision (ICCV), pp. 1832–1839, November 2011
5. Breiman, L.: Bagging predictors. Mach. Learn. **24**(2), 123–140 (1996)
6. Burges, C.: From ranknet to lambdarank to lambdamart: an overview. Learning **11**, 23–581 (2010)
7. Burges, C., Shaked, T., Renshaw, E., Lazier, A., Deeds, M., Hamilton, N., Hullender, C.: Learning to rank using gradient descent. In: Proceedings of the 22nd International Conference on Machine Learning, pp. 89–96. ACM (2005)
8. Burges, C.J.C., Ragno, R., Le, Q.V.: Learning to rank with nonsmooth cost functions. In: NIPS, vol. 6, pp. 193–200 (2006)
9. Cheng, M.-M., Zhang, Z., Lin, W.-Y., Torr, P.H.S.: BING: Binarized normed gradients for objectness estimation at 300fps. In: IEEE CVPR (2014)
10. Dalal, N., Triggs, B.: Histograms of oriented gradients for human detection. In: IEEE Computer Society Conference on Computer Vision and Pattern Recognition, CVPR 2005, vol. 1, pp. 886–893. IEEE (2005). De Europe
11. Everingham, M., Van Gool, L., Williams, C.K.I., Winn, J., Zisserman, A.: The PASCAL Visual Object Classes Challenge, (VOC2007) Results 92007). http://www.pascal-network.org/challenges/VOC/voc2007/workshop/index.html
12. Felzenszwalb, P.F., Girshick, R.B., McAllester, D., Ramanan, D.: Object detection with discriminatively trained part-based models. IEEE Trans. Pattern Anal. Mach. Intell. **32**(9), 1627–1645 (2010)

13. Ganjisaffar, Y., Caruana, R., Lopes, C.V.: Bagging gradient-boosted trees for high precision, low variance ranking models. In: Proceedings of the 34th International ACM SIGIR Conference on Research and Development in Information Retrieval, pp. 85–94. ACM (2011)
14. Girshick, R., Donahue, J., Darrell, T., Malik, J.: Rich feature hierarchies for accurate object detection and semantic segmentation (2013). arXiv preprint arXiv:1311.2524
15. Jarrett, K., Kavukcuoglu, K., Ranzato, M., LeCun, Y.: What is the best multi-stage architecture for object recognition? In: IEEE 12th International Conference on Computer Vision, pp. 2146–2153. IEEE (2009)
16. Jia, Y.: Caffe: An open source convolutional architecture for fast feature embedding (2013). http://caffe.berkeleyvision.org/
17. Krizhevsky, A., Sutskever, I., Hinton, G.E.: Imagenet classification with deep convolutional neural networks. In: Pereira, F., Burges, C.J.C., Bottou, L., Weinberger, K.Q. (eds.) Advances in Neural Information Processing Systems 25, pp. 1097–1105. Curran Associates Inc (2012)
18. van de Sande, K.E.A., Uijlings, J.R.R., Gevers, T., Smeulders. Segmentation as selective search for object recognition. In: 2011 IEEE International Conference on Computer Vision (ICCV), pp. 1879–1886. IEEE (2011)
19. Wu, Q., Burges, C.J.C., Svore, K.M., Gao, J.: Ranking, boosting, and model adaptation. Tecnical report, MSR-TR-2008-109 (2008)
20. Zhu, L., Chen, Y., Yuille, A., Freeman, W.: Latent hierarchical structural learning for object detection. In: 2010 IEEE Conference on Computer Vision and Pattern Recognition (CVPR), pp. 1062–1069. IEEE (2010)

Representation Learning with Smooth Autoencoder

Kongming Liang, Hong Chang[✉], Zhen Cui, Shiguang Shan, and Xilin Chen

Key Lab of Intelligent Information Processing of Chinese
Academy of Sciences (CAS), Institute of Computing Technology,
CAS, Beijing 100190, China
{kongming.liang,hong.chang,zhen.cui,shiguang.shan,
xilin.chen}@vipl.ict.ac.cn

Abstract. In this paper, we propose a novel autoencoder variant, smooth autoencoder (SmAE), to learn robust and discriminative feature representations. Different from conventional autoencoders which reconstruct each sample from its encoding, we use the encoding of each sample to reconstruct its local neighbors. In this way, the learned representations are consistent among local neighbors and robust to small variations of the inputs. When trained with supervisory information, our approach forces samples from the same class to become more compact in the vicinity of data manifolds in the new representation space, where the samples are easier to be discriminated. Experimental results verify the effectiveness of the representations learned by our approach in image classification and face recognition tasks.

1 Introduction

How to represent images and videos has been an important and fundamental problem in computer vision, as the performance of various computer vision approaches relies on the choice of feature representations. Traditional hand-crafted low level image features, such as Scale Invariant Feature Transform (SIFT), Histogram of Oriented Gradients (HOG), Local Binary Patterns (LBP), have shown their effectiveness for many specific vision problems. However, these features are sub-optimal shallow representations, which require domain knowledge and have limited generalization ability. Instead of designing features manually, a more promising approach is to learn effective feature representations automatically from vision data, through *representation learning*. For various computer vision tasks, an ideal feature representation should be *robust* for small variations, *smooth* for preserving data structures and *discriminative* for classification related tasks.

Recently, representation learning in deep learning context has aroused a great deal of interests in machine learning and computer vision community. Deep models learn multi-layer nonlinear transformations from the input data to the output representations, which is more powerful in feature extraction than hand-crafted shallow models. Moreover, deep models can progressively capture more abstract

© Springer International Publishing Switzerland 2015
D. Cremers et al. (Eds.): ACCV 2014, Part II, LNCS 9004, pp. 72–86, 2015.
DOI: 10.1007/978-3-319-16808-1_6

features at higher layers, corresponding to the hierarchical human vision system. Representative deep learning methods such as convolutional neural networks (CNN), deep belief networks (DBN) and stacked autoencoders (SAE) have achieved great successes in image classification [1], action recognition [2], object tracking [3], etc. Among the building blocks of these models, autoencoders directly learn a parametric feature mapping function by minimizing the reconstruction error between input and its encoding (i.e., representation). In addition, various regularization terms are proposed to improve the basic autoencoders. Sparse autoencoders penalize the hidden unit to be sparse by L1 penalty [4,5] or Kullback–Leibler divergence [6] with respect to the binomial distribution. Denoising autoencoders (DAE) [7,8] learn a representation which is robust to small random perturbations. Contractive autoencoders (CAE) [9] reduce the number of effective freedom degrees of the representation by adding an analytic contractive penalty. Both DAE and CAE are robust to small changes of the inputs among the training examples. Moreover, CAE is capable of representing nonlinear manifolds, as its output encodings contract in the directions orthogonal to the underlying data manifold. This paper focuses on parametric representation learning along the direction of autoencoder variants.

It is always preferred to preserve the manifold structure at the same time of representation learning. As proved in [10], preserving the consistence in representation of similarity between local neighbors is essential for nonlinear feature learning. Classical manifold learning methods [11–13] learn embedding coordinates instead of explicit feature mappings, thus limit their usage as feature extractors. Local sparse coding methods [14,15] are capable of revealing the manifold structure, but their iterative coding process is far from efficient. Recent works incorporate manifold regularization into deep learning models and obtain parametric feedforward encoders on nonlinear manifolds, e.g., deep learning via semi-supervised embedding [16] and CAE [9]. However, it is not natural to incorporate supervisory information into these models during layerwise pretraining, so they can seldom learn discriminative representations.

In this paper, we propose a novel parametric representation learning method, smooth autoencoder (SmAE), which possesses more advantages than previous related methods mentioned above. Specifically, our approach explicitly characterizes the similarity between input samples by minimizing the weighted reconstruction error of each sample from its local neighbors, instead of itself as previous autoencoders do. Therefore, the resultant feature mappings vary smoothly on manifolds. In addition, since SmAE constrains adjacent samples to have similar feature representations, the learned feature representations are robust to small variations as the input changes on the manifold. Moreover, SmAE can learn discriminative representations by making use of supervisory information. When trained in (semi-)supervised learning setting, SmAE can increase the within-class compactness in the learned representation space. Figure 1 illustrates the classwise contractive process of our method. Experiments on image classification and face recognition show the effectiveness of the proposed method. The good performance of our method relies on its advantages briefly summarized as follows: (1) smooth representations on data manifold, (2) robust to small variations and (3) discriminative ability due to classwise contraction.

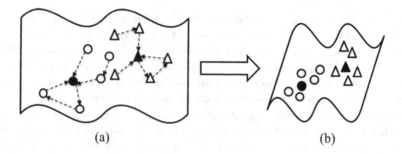

(a)   (b)

Fig. 1. Illustration of within-class contraction. The learned function maps the samples from original space (a) to feature space (b). Circles and triangles represent samples with different labels. The solid circles and triangles denote the sample correspondences between the original space and feature space. The dashed arrows between samples indicate the neighborhood relations.

The rest of this paper is organized as follows. In Sect. 2, we first review some popular autoencoder variants. Our method is then presented in Sect. 3 in detail. The relationship between SmAE and other relevant methods is discussed in Sect. 4. Experimental results on image classification and face recognition are reported in Sect. 5. Finally, we conclude this paper in Sect. 6.

2   Autoencoders and Its Variants

Autoencoders [17], as the name suggests, consist of two stages: encoding and decoding. It was first used to reduce dimensionality by setting the number of encoder output units less than the input. The model is usually trained using back-propagation in an unsupervised manner, by minimizing the reconstruction error of the decoding results from the original inputs. With the activation function chosen to be nonlinear, an autoencoder can exact more useful features than some common linear transformation methods such as PCA. If the dimension of encoding output is set higher than the input dimension, the encoding result will be enriched and more expressive. By stacking multiple pretrained autoencoders followed by a supervised classifier, the deep autoencoders will generate more abstract and high-level semantic features which are beneficial for image classification.

Basic Autoencoder (AE). The encoder is a function that maps the input data $x \in \mathbb{R}^{d_x}$ to d_h hidden units to get the feature representation or code as:

$$h = f(x) = s_f(Wx + b_h), \tag{1}$$

where s_f is a nonlinear activation function, typically a sigmoid function $s_f(z) = \frac{1}{1+e^{-z}}$, or a hyperbolic tangent function $s_f(z) = tanh(z) = \frac{e^z - e^{-z}}{e^z + e^{-z}}$. The parameters of the encoder are a $d_h \times d_x$ weight matrix W and a bias vector $b_h \in \mathbb{R}^{d_h}$.

The decoder function g maps the outputs of hidden units back to the original input space as:

$$y = g(h) = s_g(W' h + b_o),\tag{2}$$

where s_g is the activation function which usually has the same form as that in the encoder. The parameters of the decoder are a $d_x \times d_h$ weight matrix W' and a bias vector $b_o \in \mathbb{R}^{d_x}$. In this paper, we choose both the encoding and decoding activation function to be sigmoid function and only consider the tied weights case, in which $W' = W^T$.

To find the model parameters $\theta = \{W, b_h, W', b_o\}$, autoencoders are trained by minimizing the reconstruction error on a set of training data $x_i \in \mathbb{R}^{d_x}, i = 1, ..., n$. The objective function optimized by AE is:

$$J_{AE}(\theta) = \sum_{i=1}^{n} L(x_i, g(f(x_i))),\tag{3}$$

where L is a loss function which is usually decided according to the input range. If the input is in $[0,1]$, cross-entropy loss $L(\mathbf{x}, \mathbf{y}) = \sum_{i=1}^{d_x} x_i log(y_i) + (1-x_i)log(1-y_i)$ is usually used. In the other cases, square error $L(x, y) = \|x - y\|^2$ is typically chosen.

Sparse Autoencoders (SpAE). Sparse autoencoder [6] is an basic autoencoder regularized by a weight decay term and a sparsity constraints on the hidden units. The objective function of SpAE is:

$$J_{SpAE}(\theta) = \sum_{i=1}^{n} L(x_i, g(f(x_i))) + \lambda \sum_{ij} W_{ij}^2 + \beta \sum_{j=1}^{d_h} KL(\rho \| \widetilde{\rho}_j),\tag{4}$$

where $\widetilde{\rho}_j = \frac{1}{n}\sum_{i=1}^{n} h_j(x_i)$ is the average activation of hidden unit j and the $KL(\rho \| \widetilde{\rho}_j) = \rho log\frac{\rho}{\widetilde{\rho}_j} + (1-\rho)log\frac{1-\rho}{1-\widetilde{\rho}_j}$ is the KL divergence between Bernoulli random variables with mean ρ and $\widetilde{\rho}_j$. The second term tends to decrease the magnitude of the weights and prevent over-fitting. β and λ control the tradeoff among the loss and two penalty terms.

Denoising Autoencoders (DAE). To make the representations robust to partial corruption of the input patterns, Vincent et al. [7,8] present an alternative form to train autoencoders. Instead of directly reconstructing the original input samples, denoising autoencoders learn to reconstruct the clean input x_i from the artificially corrupted counterpart $\widetilde{x}_i$. DAE is trained by optimizing the following objective function:

$$J_{DAE}(\theta) = \sum_{i=1}^{n} \mathbb{E}_{\widetilde{x}_i \sim q(\widetilde{x}_i | x_i)}[L(x_i, g(f(\widetilde{x}_i)))].\tag{5}$$

Typically, two common corruptions are additive isotropic Gaussian noise, $\widetilde{x} = x + \epsilon, \epsilon \sim \mathcal{N}(0, \sigma^2 I)$, and binary masking noise, where a random fraction of inputs are set to zero.

Contractive Autoencoders (CAE). To robustness to small perturbations around the training points, [9] proposes a regularization that measures the sensitivity of the encodings with respect to the input. The contractive auto-encoder(CAE) has the following objective function:

$$J_{CAE}(\theta) = \sum_{i=1}^{n} \left(L(\boldsymbol{x_i}, g(f(\boldsymbol{x_i}))) + \lambda \left\| \mathcal{J}_f(\boldsymbol{x_i}) \right\|_F^2 \right), \tag{6}$$

where $\mathcal{J}_f(\boldsymbol{x_i}) = \sum_{jk}(\frac{\partial h_j(\boldsymbol{x_i})}{\partial x_{ik}})^2$ is the Jacobian matrix which encourages the mapping to the feature space to be contractive in the neighborhood of the training data.

3   Smooth Autoencoders

In this paper, we propose a novel autoencoder variant, smooth autoencoders (SmAE), to learn nonlinear feature representations. For each input, SmAE aims to reconstruct its *target neighbors*, instead of reconstructing itself as traditional autoencoder variants do. Formally, the objective function of SmAE is defined as:

$$J_{SmAE}(\theta) = \sum_{i=1}^{n} \sum_{j=1}^{k} w(\boldsymbol{x_j}, \boldsymbol{x_i}) L(\boldsymbol{x_j}, g(f(\boldsymbol{x_i}))) + \beta \sum_{j=1}^{d_h} KL(\rho \| \tilde{\rho}_j), \tag{7}$$

where $w(\cdot, \cdot)$ is a weight function defined through a smoothing kernel $w(\boldsymbol{x_j}, \boldsymbol{x_i}) = \frac{1}{Z}\mathcal{K}(d(\boldsymbol{x_j}, \boldsymbol{x_i}))$, and the item Z is used to guarantee $\sum_{j=1}^{k} w(\boldsymbol{x_j}, \boldsymbol{x_i}) = 1$ for all i. k is the number of target neighbors of $\boldsymbol{x_i}$(see Sect. 3.1 for detail discussions). $d(\cdot, \cdot)$ is a distance function which measures the feature distance/similarity in the original space. The first term in Eq. (7) forces neighboring input samples to have similar representations. In this way, the resultant feature representations are not only robust to local variations but also smooth as the input samples vary on the manifold. The second term in the objective function regularizes on model complexity by using KL sparsity.

Besides the advantages of robustness and smoothness, SmAE can learn discriminative representations under (semi-)supervised learning settings, with proper selection of target neighbors. In the following subsections, we discuss on the choice of target neighbors and the reconstruction loss term in more details, and then describe the model training process.

There are different ways to define the weight function by using arbitrary kernel functions $\mathcal{K}(\cdot)$ and distance functions $d(\cdot, \cdot)$. Some common choices of kernel functions include Gaussian kernel, as well as triangular, uniform and tricube kernels. The distance function can be chosen as any standard distance functions based on L_p norm or learned through metric learning methods designed by domain experts. In this paper we choose Gaussian kernel which is widely used for manifold learning:

$$w(\boldsymbol{x_j}, \boldsymbol{x_i}) = \begin{cases} \frac{1}{Z} exp(-\frac{\|\boldsymbol{x_i} - \boldsymbol{x_j}\|^2}{\sigma}) & \boldsymbol{x_j} \in \mathcal{N}_i \\ 0 & \text{otherwise} \end{cases} \tag{8}$$

$\mathcal{N}_i$ denotes the target neighborhood of sample x_i. The bandwidth of kernel σ is selected by cross-validation in our experiments. In this setting, the normalization item is $Z = \sum_{j=1}^{k} exp(-\frac{\|x_i - x_j\|^2}{\sigma})$.

3.1 Target Neighbors

Target neighbors can have different definitions, depending on the learning tasks and domain knowledge. Concretely speaking, we may decide the target neighbors according to unsupervised, supervised and semi-supervised learning settings, as well as the characteristics of learning tasks and training data.

Unsupervised Target Neighbors. For each x_i from the training data, we may choose k nearest neighbors based on an appropriate metric, such as Euclidian, Mahalanobis and cosine. In this paper, we use Euclidian distance to define the neighbourhood. The k nearest neighbors are considered as the k target neighbors and the corresponding distances are used to compute the weight function.

Supervised Target Neighbors. Under this setting, target neighbours are defined as k nearest neighbors with the same label of x_i. Besides the traditional global metrics, some local metrics can also be used to compute the weight function.

Beyond label information and original distance, smooth autoencoders can also utilize other forms of information, such as pairwise constraints, artificial deformation and temporal/spatial coherence to define or generate target neighbours. When we make use of supervisory information to decide the supervised target neighbors, SmAE can increase the within-class compactness in the learned representation space, as illustrated in Fig. 1. In this way, SmAE can learn discriminative representations in supervised and semi-supervised learning settings.

3.2 The Loss Function

Two typical loss functions commonly adopted in training autoencoders are squared error $L_{se}(x, y) = \|x - y\|^2$ and cross-entropy loss $L_{ce}(x, y) = -x \cdot log(y) - (1 - x) \cdot log(1 - y)$, where $\cdot$ denotes the element-wise product operator. When the input data and feature representation are normalized in [0,1], the cross-entropy loss function is usually applied.

If the cross-entropy loss function is chosen, the weighted reconstruction error of SmAE for sample x_i can be simplified into the form $-\sum_{j=1}^{k} w(x_j, x_i)x_j \cdot log(g(f(x_i))) - (1 - \sum_{j=1}^{k} w(x_j, x_i)x_j) \cdot log(1 - g(f(x_i)))$. Let us consider

$$\widetilde{x}_i = \sum_{j=1}^{k} w(x_j, x_i)x_j \tag{9}$$

as a transformed version of x_i. Then, the objective function of SmAE can be rewritten as:

$$J_{SmAE}(\theta) = \sum_{i=1}^{n} L_{ce}(\widetilde{x}_i, g(f(x_i))) + \beta \sum_{j=1}^{d_h} KL(\rho\|\widetilde{\rho}_j). \tag{10}$$

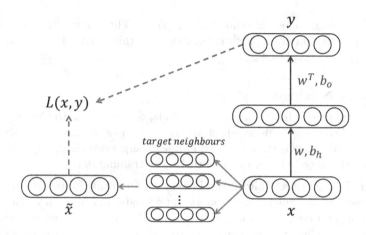

Fig. 2. Smooth autoencoder with cross-entropy loss

Therefore, SmAE can be considered as an ordinary sparse autoencoder, with new deformation samples constructed according to Eq. (9) as the reconstruction targets. Figure 2 shows the actual model architecture of SmAE with cross-entropy loss. In all experiments in this paper, cross-entropy loss is adopted as the loss function.

3.3   Model Pretraining and Stacking

Similar with previous autoencoder variants, smooth autoencoder can be used to build a deep network. For the first layer in the deep model, we choose the target neighbors defined in 3.1 and calculate the transformed version according to (9) for each training sample. The objective function (10) is minimized using standard back-propagation algorithm. The optimization procedure in layer-wise pretraining for smooth autoencoder based on cross-entropy loss function is shown in Algorithm 1. The representations learned by the first layer are then used as the input of the second layer, and so on so forth. After layer-wise pretraining, the network parameters are further fine-tuned using label information provided on top of the network in the supervised case.

4   Discussions

The smooth autoencoders possess close relationship with popular methods including sparse coding and other autoencoder variants.

4.1   Relationship with Sparse Coding

Standard sparse coding solves the following optimization problem:

$$\min_{\substack{D \in \mathbb{R}^{d_x \times K} \\ \alpha_i \in \mathbb{R}^{K}, i=1,\dots,n}} \sum_{i=1}^{n} (\|\boldsymbol{x_i} - D\boldsymbol{\alpha_i}\|_2^2 + \gamma |\boldsymbol{\alpha_i}|_1), \tag{11}$$

Algorithm 1. Layer-wise pretraining of Smooth Autoencoder with Cross Entropy loss

---

Input: The training data set $\{x_i\}_{i=1}^n$
Output: learned weight W, bias b_h, b_o

1: Compute the transformed versions $\{\tilde{x}_i\}_{i=1}^n$ for each training data, and initialize W, b_h, b_o
2: **while** not stopping criterion **do**
3:     Set $\Delta W = 0, \Delta b_h = 0, \Delta b_o = 0$
4:     Perform the feedforward pass, compute the activation of the hidden layer $z_i^h = W x_i + b_h$ and output layer $z_i^o = W^T s_f(z_i^h) + b_o$
5:     Compute the error term:
$$\delta_i^o = \frac{\partial L_{ce}((\tilde{x}_i, g(f(x_i))))}{\partial z_i^o} = -\left(\frac{\tilde{x}_i}{s_g(z_i^o)} + \frac{1-\tilde{x}_i}{1-s_g(z_i^o)}\right) \cdot s_g'(z_i^o)$$
$$\delta_i^h = \left(W\delta_i^o + \beta\left(\frac{\rho}{\hat{\rho}_i} + \frac{1-\rho}{1-\hat{\rho}_i}\right)\right) \cdot s_f'(z_i^h)$$
6:     Compute the partial derivatives:
$$\Delta W = \sum_{i=1}^n \frac{J_{SmAE}(W,b_h,b_o;x_i)}{\partial W} = \sum_{i=1}^n s_f(x_i)\delta_i^{oT} + \delta_i^h x_i^T;$$
$$\Delta b_h = \sum_{i=1}^n \frac{J_{SmAE}(W,b_h,b_o;x_i)}{\partial b_h} = \sum_{i=1}^n \delta_i^o;$$
$$\Delta b_o = \sum_{i=1}^n \frac{J_{SmAE}(W,b_h,b_o;x_i)}{\partial b_o} = \sum_{i=1}^n \delta_i^h;$$
7:     Update W, b_h, b_o by gradient descent
8: **end while**

---

where $D = [d_1, d_2, ..., d_K] \in \mathbb{R}^{d_x \times K}$ is the dictionary to be learned, with d_i being the ith atom. α_i is the encoding of sample x_i with respect to dictionary D. The factor γ is used to balance the reconstruction error and sparsity penalty. An autoencoder can be viewed as sparse coding with explicit encoding function (i.e., an forward inference process) if the decoder is linear. Therefore, the direct encoding of autoencoders may be used to approximately replace the computation-expensive sparse coding by our intuition.

Some variants of sparse coding methods also attempt to use the local property from a manifold perspective. Local coordinate coding(LCC) [14] approximately represents each data point by a linear combination of its nearby anchor points from the view of reconstruction. More Recently, Smooth sparse coding(SSC) [15] is proposed to incorporate local feature similarities into the sparse coding framework. Different from them, our proposed method can learn an explicit encoding process with better robustness in small variations as well as discriminative ability due to within-class compactness. Besides, the proposed SmAE can further be easily stacked into a deep framework, which also makes the whole model optimized globally with back-propagation.

4.2 Relationship with Other Autoencoder Variants

Both smooth autoencoders and sparse autoencoders use the sparsity constraints to push the majority of representations close to zero. Sparse autoencoders encode the samples individually and ignore the mutual dependence. Therefore, small variances in the input space may result in distinct changes on the learned representations. Different from sparse autoencoders, smooth autoencoders can capture

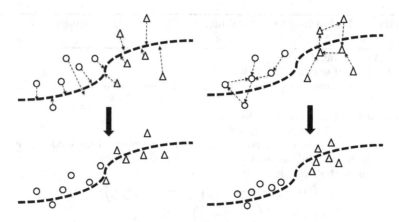

Fig. 3. Comparison between contractive autoencoder (the left) and smooth autoencoder (the right). The dashed curve refers the manifold that data rely on.

the local similarity by explicitly considering manifold structures, and thus the learned representations are less sensitive to variational inputs.

When the cross entropy loss function is adopted, the weighted reconstruction error of smooth autoencoders has similar form with denoising autoencoders, as expressed in Eq. (10). However, the robustness of denoising autoencoders is stochastic which is determined by the corruption progress. Smooth autoencoder uses transformed samples generated by target neighbors to model local variance. Therefore, the learning processing is analytic rather than stochastic, and the learned representations are more effective for classification tasks.

Smooth autoencoders are closely related to contractive autoencoders, as both of them learn robust representations along data manifolds. CAE penalizes on the Frobenius of the Jacobian matrix of the encoding function. As illustrated in Fig. 3, this penalty makes the representations contractive in the direction of noise which is orthogonal to the manifold. SmAE penalizes weighted reconstruction errors on target neighbors to guarantee robust and smooth representations. However, contractive autoencoders do have limitations: it is robust only to infinitesimal input variations and it cannot learn discriminative representations. Smooth autoencoders alleviate these limitations as they consider relaxed variations within local neighborhoods and increase within-class compactness using supervisory information.

5   Experiments

We evaluate smooth autoencoders as a representation learner in handwritten digit recognition on MNIST dataset [18] and its variations [19], and in face recognition on the Extended YaleB [20] and AR face [21] datasets. In our method, the main model parameters are chosen by cross-validating on the training set or using the available validation set.

5.1   Hand Digital Recognition

We first verify the effectiveness of SmAE on the widely used MNIST dataset, which consists of handwritten digit images with 28×28 pixels. The original MNIST dataset and MNIST variations are used in the following experiments.

Classification on MNIST. Following the standard protocol of MNIST, 60,000 images from MNIST dataset are used for training and 10,000 for testing. To intrinsically validate the effectiveness of the proposed method, here we compare several baselines, including AE, SpAE, DAE and CAE. In the proposed SmAE, the network is constrained with tied weights and the sigmoid activation function. The number of hidden nodes is set to 1000. To verify the effectiveness of preservation of neighbor structures, here we only consider unsupervised SmAE by choosing $k = 5$ target neighbors in the unsupervised way (see Sect. 3.1). The comparison results are reported in Table 1. As shown in this table, unsupervised smooth autoencoder has lower classification error than AE, SpAE and DAE, and is even comparable to the state-of-the-art method CAE. Furthermore, if we stack two SmAEs into a deep framework, the proposed method can sharply reduce the error rate to **1.06 %**.

Table 1. Classification Results of different autoencoders on MNIST dataset

Method	AE	SpAE	DAE [7]	CAE [9]	SmAE
Test error(%)	1.68	1.19	1.18	1.14	1.15

Classification on MNIST Variation. As a benchmark, MNIST variation [19] is usually used to evaluate deep learning algorithms recently. It contains various classification tasks. Here, we choose three tasks: "mnist-basic", "mnist-rot" and "rect" to test our method. "mnist-basic" is a subset dataset of MNIST. Images in "mnist-rot" are rotated by an angle generated uniformly between 0 and 2π radians. The above two datasets both contain 10000 samples for training, 2000 samples for validating and 50000 samples for testing. "rect" is a binary classification task to discriminate between wide and long rectangles. It has 1000, 200 and 50000 samples as training, validating and testing sets respectively.

As the deep learning algorithms have reached the state-of-the-art performance, here we compare those classic deep learning methods with properly stacked layers, including stacked AE (SAE), DAE, CAE and Restricted Boltzman Machine (RBM). In our method, we use the unsupervised target neighbor to define the weight function. After layerwise pretraining, the network is further finetuned with a softmax classifier. The hyper-parameters such as layer sizes, sparsity penalty and kernel bandwidth are obtained by using the validation set. In Fig. 4, we report the classification accuracy of all comparison methods, in the above three classification tasks, where the digit after the method name marks the number of layers in its deep network, e.g., "SmAE-2" means the proposed model network is constructed by stacking two SmAEs. The other comparison results

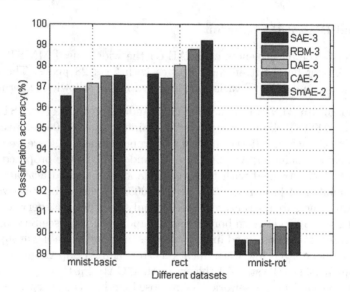

Fig. 4. Classification accuracy on MNIST variations (Color figure online).

are quoted from the related published literatures [7] and [9], whose reported best results are shown in this table. In most cases, smooth autoencoders achieve comparable and even better results than the other current state-of-the-art methods.

To explicitly show the good property of smooth autoencoder, we do the 2D visualization on the mnist-basic dataset. In Fig. 5, different colors represent the images from 0~9 digits. Principal Component Analysis is used to reduce the dimensions of the representations learned by conventional autoencoder, unsupervised smooth autoencoder and supervised smooth autoencoder. All the three methods are respectively abbreviated as AE-2, SmAE-2.unsup and SmAE-2.sup, since the number of hidden layers is two. We use all the 10000 training data and randomly choose 10000 test data for comparison. As shown in the figure, the unsupervised SmAE-2 can capture locality property which makes the data more separable than the conventional autoencoder. By further using the label information, the supervised SmAE-2 can learn representations which distinctly increase the within-class compactness. In addition, we randomly choose 5 samples of each digit from test data and construct the affinity matrix as shown in Fig. 6. As we can see, samples from the same digit are highly compacted in SmAE-2.sup.

5.2   Face Recognition

In this section, we conduct extensive experiments on two standard face datasets, extended YaleB [20] and AR face [21], to evaluate the proposed method. Extended YaleB dataset consists of 2,414 frontal-face images of 38 persons under 64 illumination conditions. The original images are cropped to 50×50 pixels. For each person, we randomly sample 32 images for training and the rest for testing. AR dataset contains the frontal images of 126 persons, which are collected across two

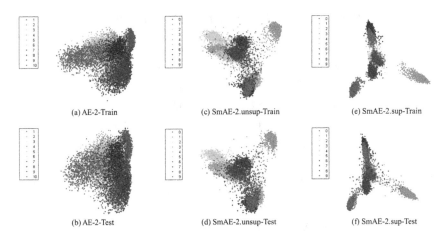

Fig. 5. 2D visualization of within-class compactness

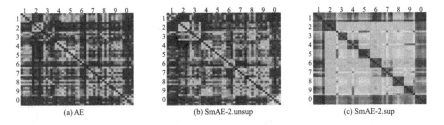

Fig. 6. Affinity Matrix of mnist-basic

separate sessions with different facial expressions, lighting and occlusion variations. Following the standard evaluation protocol, we random choose 50 males and 50 females with 2,600 images to verify the proposed methods. Among them, 20 images per person are randomly selected for training and the rest six of each person for testing. All the images are cropped into 80×64 pixels gray images.

First, we perform single layer smooth autoencoder and compare it with different autoencoder variants. Besides unsupervised SmAE, here we also consider the supervised case by using manual labels in the construction neighbor weights to further enhance the discriminative feature learning. Both methods are respectively abbreviated as SmAE.unsup and SmAE.sup. In our methods, the nearest neighbors $k = 5$ and $k = 10$ are respectively set for the unsupervised and supervised cases. The number of the hidden units is set to be 600. A softmax classifier is connected to the output layer to check the performance on face recognition. The parameter σ is set to be 0.05, β and ρ are set to 0.1. For other methods, we try to tune their referred parameters and reported the best results. As shown in Table 2, under both unsupervised and supervised setting, smooth autoencoder can still improve the recognition performance by using the preservation of manifold structures in our proposed SmAE.

Table 2. Single Layer Face Recognition Rate(%)

Method	Extended YaleB	AR face	Mean
SpAE	94.07	93.50	93.79
DAE	93.57	93.17	93.37
CAE	93.82	93.83	93.83
SmAE.unsup	94.17	94.00	94.09
SmAE.sup	95.16	95.00	95.08

Table 3. Face recognition rates (%) on Extended YaleB and AR face database

Method	Extended YaleB	AR face
K-SVD	90.5	90.0
SRC	88.6	74.5
LC-KSVD	95.0	93.7
DDL-PC2	95.3	96.6
MMDL	97.3	97.3
SmAE-2	**98.2**	**98.4**

Next, we further compare our method with several related face feature representation methods by using the solider sparse coding theory, including K-SVD [22], SRC [23], LC-KSVD [24], DDL-PC2 [25] and MMDL [26]. All these comparison methods have demonstrated their robust representation ability in the description of images. To learn more abstract and robust representation, in our method we stack two-layer smooth autoencoders by using supervised target neighbor definition. The number of units in both hidden layers are set to 1000. k is set to 5 and the parameters σ, β and ρ are simply set to be 0.1 without further tuning. We conduct 10-round random experiments, and then report average recognition rate in Table 3. As we can see, smooth autoencoders achieve the highest accuracies on both datasets. This further demonstrates that the representation learned by our method is more effective for image classification.

6   Conclusions and Future Work

In this paper, we present a novel neural network method: Smooth Autoencoder. By using the encoding of a sample to reconstruct its target neighbors instead of itself, the relationship between similar local features can be captured. We further show the representations learned by our method are robust to small variations. By making use of supervisory information, smooth autoencoder can enhance within-class compactness which is beneficial for classification tasks. Experimental results show that our approach improves the conventional autoencoder and achieve comparable or better performance on handwritten digit recognition and face recognition. For future work, we can extend the target neighbor definition to different applications, such as action recognition in spatial-temporal videos.

Acknowledgement. This work is partially supported by the National Natural Science Foundation of China under contract No. 61390515, 61272319, and 61202297 and Natural Science Foundation of Fujian Province under contract No.2013J01239.

References

1. Krizhevsky, A., Sutskever, I., Hinton, G.E.: Imagenet classification with deep convolutional neural networks. In: NIPS (2012)
2. Ji, S., Xu, W., Yang, M., Yu, K.: 3d convolutional neural networks for human action recognition. IEEE Trans. Pattern Anal. Mach. Intell. **35**, 221–231 (2013)
3. Wang, N., Yeung, D.Y.: Learning a deep compact image representation for visual tracking. In: NIPS (2013)
4. Ngiam, J., Coates, A., Lahiri, A., Prochnow, B., Le, Q.V., Ng, A.Y.: On optimization methods for deep learning. In: ICML (2011)
5. Ranzato, M., Boureau, Y.L., LeCun, Y.: Sparse feature learning for deep belief networks. In: NIPS (2007)
6. Xie, J., Xu, L., Chen, E.: Image denoising and inpainting with deep neural networks. In: NIPS (2012)
7. Vincent, P., Larochelle, H., Bengio, Y., Manzagol, P.A.: Extracting and composing robust features with denoising autoencoders. In: ICML (2008)
8. Vincent, P., Larochelle, H., Lajoie, I., Bengio, Y., Manzagol, P.A.: Stacked denoising autoencoders: learning useful representations in a deep network with a local denoising criterion. J. Mach. Learn. Res. **11**, 3371–3408 (2010)
9. Rifai, S., Vincent, P., Muller, X., Glorot, X., Bengio, Y.: Contractive auto-encoders: explicit invariance during feature extraction. In: ICML (2011)
10. Bengio, Y., Courville, A., Vincent, P.: Representation learning: a review and new perspectives. IEEE Trans. Pattern Anal. Mach. Intell. **35**, 1798–1828 (2013)
11. Roweis, S.T., Saul, L.K.: Nonlinear dimensionality reduction by locally linear embedding. Science **290**, 2323–2326 (2000)
12. Tenenbaum, J.B., De Silva, V., Langford, J.C.: A global geometric framework for nonlinear dimensionality reduction. Science **290**, 2319–2323 (2000)
13. Belkin, M., Niyogi, P.: Laplacian eigenmaps for dimensionality reduction and data representation. Neural Comput. **15**, 1373–1396 (2003)
14. Yu, K., Zhang, T., Gong, Y.: Nonlinear learning using local coordinate coding. In: NIPS (2009)
15. Balasubramanian, K., Yu, K., Lebanon, G.: Smooth sparse coding via marginal regression for learning sparse representations. In: ICML (2013)
16. Weston, J., Ratle, F., Mobahi, H., Collobert, R.: Deep learning via semi-supervised embedding. In: Montavon, G., Orr, G.B., Müller, K.-R. (eds.) Neural Networks: Tricks of the Trade, 2nd edn. LNCS, vol. 7700, pp. 639–655. Springer, Heidelberg (2012)
17. Hinton, G.E., Zemel, R.S.: Autoencoders, minimum description length, and helmholtz free energy. In: NIPS (1994)
18. LeCun, Y., Bottou, L., Bengio, Y., Haffner, P.: Gradient-based learning applied to document recognition. Proc. IEEE **86**, 2278–2324 (1998)

19. Larochelle, H., Erhan, D., Courville, A., Bergstra, J., Bengio, Y.: An empirical evaluation of deep architectures on problems with many factors of variation. In: ICML (2007)
20. Georghiades, A.S., Belhumeur, P.N., Kriegman, D.: From few to many: Illumination cone models for face recognition under variable lighting and pose. IEEE Trans. Pattern Anal. Mach. Intell. **23**, 643–660 (2001)
21. Martinez, A.M.: The ar face database. Technical report 24 (1998)
22. Aharon, M., Elad, M., Bruckstein, A.: K-svd: an algorithm for designing overcomplete dictionaries for sparse representation. IEEE Trans. Signal Process. **54**, 4311–4322 (2006)
23. Wright, J., Yang, A.Y., Ganesh, A., Sastry, S.S., Ma, Y.: Robust face recognition via sparse representation. IEEE Trans. Pattern Anal. Mach. Intell. **31**, 210–227 (2009)
24. Jiang, Z., Lin, Z., Davis, L.S.: Learning a discriminative dictionary for sparse coding via label consistent k-svd. In: CVPR (2011)
25. Guo, H., Jiang, Z., Davis, L.S.: Discriminative dictionary learning with pairwise constraints. In: Lee, K.M., Matsushita, Y., Rehg, J.M., Hu, Z. (eds.) ACCV 2012, Part I. LNCS, vol. 7724, pp. 328–342. Springer, Heidelberg (2013)
26. Wang, Z., Yang, J., Nasrabadi, N., Huang, T.: A max-margin perspective on sparse representation-based classification. In: CVPR (2013)

Single Image Smoke Detection

Hongda Tian$^{(\boxtimes)}$, Wanqing Li, Philip Ogunbona, and Lei Wang

Advanced Multimedia Research Lab, ICT Research Institute,
School of Computer Science and Software Engineering,
University of Wollongong, Wollongong, Australia
{ht615,wanqing,philipo,leiw}@uow.edu.au

Abstract. Despite the recent advances in smoke detection from video, detection of smoke from single images is still a challenging problem with both practical and theoretical implications. However, there is hardly any reported research on this topic in the literature. This paper addresses this problem by proposing a novel feature to detect smoke in a single image. An image formation model that expresses an image as a linear combination of smoke and non-smoke (background) components is derived based on the atmospheric scattering models. The separation of the smoke and non-smoke components is formulated as convex optimization that solves a sparse representation problem. Using the separated quasi-smoke and quasi-background components, the feature is constructed as a concatenation of the respective sparse coefficients. Extensive experiments were conducted and the results have shown that the proposed feature significantly outperforms the existing features for smoke detection.

1 Introduction

Vision-based smoke detection has many advantages over the traditional photo-electric or ionization-based smoke detectors, including being suitable for both closed and open spaces and providing early detection with information on the location and intensity [1–5]. Despite the recent advances [4,5], almost all existing detection algorithms are video-based and the video is assumed to be captured by stationary cameras in order to facilitate the motion detection and feature extraction involved in these algorithms. However, such requirement can be hardly met in an open space where cameras are inevitably jittering under severe and dynamic environment, such as wind. Our experiments (see Sect. 5.7) have shown that camera jittering can significantly degrade the performance of video-based smoke detection. If the surveillance is based on battery-powered sensor network, the available power supply, computing resource, or bandwidth is hardly sufficient for video processing and smoke detection. In this case, surveillance images rather than videos are available. Furthermore, when a pan-tilt-zoom (PTZ) camera is used in video-based smoke detection, the unreliable background modeling will cause the failure of most systems. In such circumstances, detection of smoke from single images becomes highly desirable. This desirability comes at a price because image-based detection is much more challenging than video-based systems as it

© Springer International Publishing Switzerland 2015
D. Cremers et al. (Eds.): ACCV 2014, Part II, LNCS 9004, pp. 87–101, 2015.
DOI: 10.1007/978-3-319-16808-1_7

is no longer possible to estimate the background required for the separation of the smoke component in the state-of-the-art methods recently proposed in [4,5]. To the best of our knowledge, there is little study reported on single image-based smoke detection. This paper presents a novel method to address this problem.

The main contributions of the paper are three-fold: (i) Based on the atmospheric scattering (attenuation and airlight) models [6], an image formation model for smoke is derived. This model explains how smoke scatters the light reflected from the background of the scene and also serves as a source of light through scattering. The model suggests that an image patch covered by smoke can be approximated as a linear combination of two components; one component is contributed by smoke while the other is contributed by the background. The weight of the composition is a function of the thickness and the scattering coefficient of the smoke. (ii) Guided by the image model, dictionary-based sparse representation for the two components is used to separate an image into quasi-smoke and quasi-background components through a convex optimization process. The coefficients of both components are concatenated as a novel feature for detection. The experimental results verified that the proposed feature is reliable and highly discriminative. (iii) A method to differentiate light smoke and heavy smoke and a method to differentiate smoke and fog/haze are presented. Preliminary results on these are reported in the paper.

The remainder of the paper is organized as follows: a brief review of existing video-based smoke detection methods is provided in Sect. 2. Based on the atmospheric scattering models, an image formation model for smoke is derived in Sect. 3. The proposed method based on the image formation model is presented in Sect. 4. Experimental results are shown in Sect. 5 along with discussions. Finally, the paper is concluded with some perspectives on future work in Sect. 6.

2   Related Work

The success of existing video-based smoke detection methods lies in identifying robust visual features to characterize smoke. To motivate the rationale for the proposed feature some representative video-based smoke detection methods are reviewed with respect to the features they used. The features have been based on the characteristics of smoke including motion, color, edge and texture.

From motion point of view, an accumulative motion model has been proposed to capture the motion characteristics of smoke in [7]. Other research efforts have extracted motion features of smoke using optical flow [8,9]. However, no motion information is available from a single image. The fact that the color of smoke is usually grayish provides a clue for the extraction of color features [1–3,10–13]. However, this paper focuses on detection of smoke from single gray-scale images.

Given the video of a scene, blurred edges could be observed in smoke-covered areas and the consequent decrease in high frequency has been used as cue to perform smoke detection [1,2,11]. However, this decrease in high frequency is not unique to smoke coverage and is hard to measure its extent from a single image due to the lack of background information. Owing to the dispersive distribution

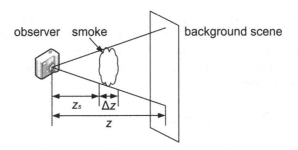

Fig. 1. Smoke usually appears at a certain distance from the observer with limited thickness along the line of sight.

of smoke, texture features have been extracted for smoke detection [3,10,13,14]. Additionally, it is also noted that the transmission [15], fractal [16] and histograms of oriented gradient (HOG) [9] have been employed to detect smoke.

Recently, to reduce the level of noise introduced into the extracted features by the background, an image separation approach has been proposed for smoke detection [4,5]. It actively separates the smoke component, if any, from the background. Texture features are then extracted from the separated smoke component for detection.

In summary these methods require a video sequence captured by a stationary camera and in the case of color feature, a color camera. Hence in general, they cannot deal with smoke detection from a single gray-scale image. The proposed feature for single image smoke detection is based on the physics of smoke formation and is able to encode reliable information for detection.

3   Physics-Based Image Formation Model

To develop computer vision systems that are able to operate in adverse weather conditions (e.g. fog/haze), the dichromatic atmospheric scattering model was proposed in [6]. The model accounts for the presence of scattering medium (e.g. fog/haze) in the entire space and expresses the final spectral irradiance $\mathbf{F}(z, \lambda)$ received by the observer (e.g. camera) as the sum of the irradiance $\mathbf{T}(z, \lambda)$ of directly transmitted light and the irradiance $\mathbf{A}(z, \lambda)$ of airlight:

$$\mathbf{F}(z, \lambda) = \mathbf{T}(z, \lambda) + \mathbf{A}(z, \lambda), \tag{1}$$

where z is the distance between the scene and observer, and λ refers to the wavelength of light. Specifically, $\mathbf{T}(z, \lambda)$ is related to the attenuation of a beam of light as it travels through the scattering medium. $\mathbf{A}(z, \lambda)$ is related to the phenomenon whereby the medium behaves like a source of light, which is caused by the scattering of environmental illumination by particles of the medium.

In the case of smoke, the smoke will act as the scattering medium like fog/haze. However, unlike fog/haze, smoke usually does not occupy the entire space of the scene. Assume that smoke appears at distance z_s from a camera and its thickness along the line of sight is Δz, as shown in Fig. 1. There are no point sources of light, that the irradiance at each background scene point is dominated by the ambient radiance, and the irradiance due to other scene points is not significant. By ignoring the multiple scattering, a formation model for smoke can be derived using the reasoning similar to that in [6] as follows:

$$\mathbf{T}(z,\lambda) = g\frac{e^{-\beta(\lambda)\Delta z}}{z^2}\mathbf{L}_\infty(\lambda)\rho(\lambda); \tag{2}$$

$$\mathbf{A}(z,\lambda) = g\int_{z_s}^{z_s+\Delta z}\mathbf{L}_\infty(\lambda)\beta(\lambda)e^{-\beta(\lambda)z}dz$$
$$= ge^{-\beta(\lambda)z_s}(1 - e^{-\beta(\lambda)\Delta z})\mathbf{L}_\infty(\lambda), \tag{3}$$

where g is a constant that accounts for the optical settings of the imaging system, $\beta(\lambda)$ is the scattering coefficient, $\mathbf{L}_\infty(\lambda)$ is the radiance of the horizon ($z = \infty$) at wavelength λ, and $\rho(\lambda)$ represents the reflectance properties and aperture of the scene point. Substituting Eqs. (2) and (3) into Eq. (1) yields

$$\mathbf{F}(z,\lambda) = (1 - \Omega(\Delta z,\lambda))\mathbf{B}(z,\lambda) + \Omega(\Delta z,\lambda)\mathbf{S}(z_s,\lambda), \tag{4}$$

where

$$\Omega(\Delta z,\lambda) = 1 - e^{-\beta(\lambda)\Delta z};$$
$$\mathbf{B}(z,\lambda) = \frac{g}{z^2}\mathbf{L}_\infty(\lambda)\rho(\lambda); \tag{5}$$
$$\mathbf{S}(z_s,\lambda) = ge^{-\beta(\lambda)z_s}\mathbf{L}_\infty(\lambda).$$

Equation (4) is the image formation model for smoke. $\mathbf{B}(z,\lambda)$ accounts for the background under clear air when there is no smoke. In the rest of the paper, it is referred to as the background component or non-smoke component interchangeably. $\mathbf{S}(z_s,\lambda)$ represents the pure smoke at distance z_s from the observer, which is referred to as the smoke component. The parameter $\Omega(\Delta z,\lambda) \in [0,1]$ depends on the thickness Δz of the smoke. It can be assumed constant within a small area where Δz would not vary much. In the rest of the paper it is referred to as the blending parameter. Note the derived model Eq. (4) indicates an additive relationship between smoke and non-smoke components.

4   Proposed Method

This paper adopts block-based detection scheme in order to achieve early detection (smoke will usually cover a very small area at the early stage) and localization of the smoke.

4.1   Smoke Detection on Block Level

Let $\mathbf{f} \in \mathbb{R}^N$ be a given image block with N pixels, $\mathbf{b} \in \mathbb{R}^N$ and $\mathbf{s} \in \mathbb{R}^N$ be the corresponding background and smoke components. Then the image formation model described by Eq. (4) can be written as

$$\mathbf{f} = (1 - \omega)\mathbf{b} + \omega\mathbf{s} + \mathbf{n}, \tag{6}$$

where $\mathbf{n} \in \mathbb{R}^N$ represents modeling noise. From Eq. (5), it is apparent that the blending parameter $\Omega(\Delta z, \lambda)$ depends on the scattering coefficient $\beta(\lambda)$ of smoke and the thickness Δz of the smoke along the line of sight. Assuming that the scattering coefficient of smoke does not change appreciably within the visible wavelength and the thickness of smoke is constant within a small image block, $\Omega(\Delta z, \lambda)$ is a constant within the image block, and the quantity is referred to as the blending parameter, ω, on block level. Guided by the image formation model and in order to extract reliable features for smoke detection from a single image block $\mathbf{f}$, the background component $\mathbf{b}$ should be separated from the smoke component $\mathbf{s}$. Intuitively, the problem can be formulated as the minimization of the power of the residual noise:

$$\min_{\omega, \mathbf{b}, \mathbf{s}} \|\mathbf{f} - \omega\mathbf{s} - (1 - \omega)\mathbf{b}\|_2^2 \quad s.t. \quad \omega \in [0, 1]. \tag{7}$$

Given only a single input image block $\mathbf{f}$, further constraints are required to obtain an unique and reliable solution to Eq. (7). A good estimation of $\mathbf{b}$, $\mathbf{s}$, and ω is expected if both $\mathbf{b}$ and $\mathbf{s}$ could be well modeled according to the visual property of non-smoke and pure smoke. If each image block is considered as a point in an N-dimensional space, pure smoke images are likely to lie in multiple low-dimensional subspaces. Driven by the progress of sparse representation [17] in recent years, if sample smoke images can be collected or generated to capture the distribution of pure smoke in the space, it is expected that any specific pure smoke image would have a sparse representation with respect to the samples. Similar argument can be made for samples of non-smoke images. Such a collection of samples represents a dictionary and each sample in the dictionary is typically referred to as a basis. Both dictionaries, one for pure smoke and the other for non-smoke, are designed such that they lead to sparse representations over only one type of image content (either pure smoke or non-smoke). To fix these ideas let $\mathbf{D_s} \in \mathbb{R}^{N \times J}(N \ll J)$ be a dictionary for pure smoke and each column of $\mathbf{D_s}$ be a basis. Then a pure smoke image $\mathbf{s}$ is expected to be sparse in $\mathbf{D_s}$:

$$\mathbf{s} = \mathbf{D_s x_s} \quad s.t. \quad \|\mathbf{x_s}\|_0 \leq M_s, \tag{8}$$

where $\|\mathbf{x_s}\|_0$ counts the number of non-zero entries in $\mathbf{x_s}$. Similarly a non-smoke image $\mathbf{b}$ is expected to be sparse in a dictionary $\mathbf{D_b} \in \mathbb{R}^{N \times L}(N \ll L)$ for non-smoke:

$$\mathbf{b} = \mathbf{D_b x_b} \quad s.t. \quad \|\mathbf{x_b}\|_0 \leq M_b. \tag{9}$$

Here M_s and M_b are the upper bounds for the number of non-zero entries in the sparse coefficients $\mathbf{x_s}$ and $\mathbf{x_b}$ respectively. Considering Eqs. (8) and (9) as the models for pure smoke and non-smoke respectively, Eq. (7) can be rewritten as follows:

$$\min_{\omega, \mathbf{x_b}, \mathbf{x_s}} \{\|\mathbf{f} - \omega\mathbf{D_s x_s} - (1 - \omega)\mathbf{D_b x_b}\|_2^2 + \eta\|\mathbf{x_b}\|_0 + \gamma\|\mathbf{x_s}\|_0\} \quad s.t. \quad \omega \in [0, 1],$$
$$\tag{10}$$

where η and γ are regularization parameters. Due to the non-convexity of the ℓ_0-norm, it is replaced with the ℓ_1-norm, which is the common practice in the literature:

$$\min_{\omega, \mathbf{x_b}, \mathbf{x_s}} \{\|\mathbf{f} - \omega \mathbf{D_s x_s} - (1 - \omega)\mathbf{D_b x_b}\|_2^2 + \eta\|\mathbf{x_b}\|_1 + \gamma\|\mathbf{x_s}\|_1\} \quad s.t. \quad \omega \in [0,1].$$
$$(11)$$

The optimization problem expressed by Eq. (11) is convex with respect to one of $\mathbf{x_b}$, $\mathbf{x_s}$, and ω when fixing the other two. One may propose to optimize the three terms alternately. However, ω and $(1 - \omega)$ are coupled with $\mathbf{x_s}$ and $\mathbf{x_b}$ respectively by multiplication, which indicates that $\mathbf{x_b}$, $\mathbf{x_s}$, and ω may not be well estimated to reflect their true values, if no other constraints are imposed. Noting that the optimal ω is a scalar, we can always absorb ω into $\mathbf{x_s}$ and $(1-\omega)$ into $\mathbf{x_b}$ in Eq. (11), and solve for $\omega \mathbf{x_s}$ and $(1 - \omega)\mathbf{x_b}$. The only changes are to scale down γ and η by ω and $(1 - \omega)$ respectively. This does not significantly change the essence of optimization, but helps to reduce one unknown ω. Based on this consideration, the following variables are defined

$$\mathbf{y_b} = (1 - \omega)\mathbf{x_b}; \qquad \mathbf{y_s} = \omega \mathbf{x_s}. \tag{12}$$

Then Eq. (11) can be written as

$$\min_{\mathbf{y_b}, \mathbf{y_s}} \|\mathbf{f} - \mathbf{D_s y_s} - \mathbf{D_b y_b}\|_2^2 + \eta'\|\mathbf{y_b}\|_1 + \gamma'\|\mathbf{y_s}\|_1. \tag{13}$$

In this case, $\mathbf{D_b y_b}$ and $\mathbf{D_s y_s}$ can be regarded as the scaled version of the background and smoke component respectively; and they will be referred to as quasi-background and quasi-smoke component respectively in the rest of the paper. Given $\mathbf{f}$, $\mathbf{D_b}$, and $\mathbf{D_s}$, Eq. (13) can be solved through alternate optimization with regard to $\mathbf{y_b}$ and $\mathbf{y_s}$ respectively by using sparse coding algorithms such as the feature-sign search algorithm [18]. Each is a convex problem and the convergence of the optimization is guaranteed [19]. Once the difference between the objective function (Eq. (13)) values in two consecutive iterations is less than a predefined threshold, the optimal $\mathbf{y_b}$ and $\mathbf{y_s}$ can be obtained. For any input image block $\mathbf{f}$ and irrespective of whether it contains smoke, $\mathbf{y_b}$ and $\mathbf{y_s}$ are estimated to model the quasi-background and quasi-smoke component respectively. Both $\mathbf{y_b}$ and $\mathbf{y_s}$ are expected to encode useful information of the input image block $\mathbf{f}$. As a result, they are concatenated as a novel feature to characterize $\mathbf{f}$. The extracted feature is input to a support vector machine (SVM) classifier. A decision is made on whether there is smoke or not in $\mathbf{f}$.

4.2   Discussions

It is noted that an image formation model similar to Eq. (6) was also used for video-based smoke detection in [4,5], image matting in [20,21], and single image haze removal in [22]. In [4,5], background modeling based on the information of previous video frames is a strict prerequisite for image separation. In this paper a different separation method is proposed for single image smoke detection. User interactions are usually required for image matting. Our image model was derived from the atmospheric scattering models and the proposed method for smoke detection is fully automatic. A dark channel prior was assumed for outdoor haze-free images for restoring high quality haze-free images in [22]. The removal of haze does not require a good separation of haze and the input image in [22] must be a color image to employ the dark channel prior. In this paper, given a single gray-scale image, quasi-smoke is separated from quasi-background to extract reliable features for smoke detection. A somewhat related work was reported in [23] but our work differs from it in two key aspects. First, the separation problem in [23] was for a mixture of texture and piece-wise smooth components. Second, the dictionaries used in that work were restricted from well known transforms such as the curvelet and discrete cosine transforms. As shown later in the paper, the dictionaries $\mathbf{D_b}$ and $\mathbf{D_s}$ are learned from real samples so as to adapt to the smoke and non-smoke classes.

5   Experimental Results

In this section, some preparations for the experiments including the data sets used are described in Sect. 5.1. Some separated quasi-smoke and quasi-background components are shown in Sect. 5.2. To explore the separability between smoke and general non-smoke classes based on the proposed feature, experiments with a binary classification task are performed in Sect. 5.3. To explore the separability among the classes of heavy smoke, light smoke, and general non-smoke based on the proposed feature, results of a ternary classification task are reported in Sect. 5.4. As fog/haze share similar visual appearance with smoke, they may pose a challenge for single image smoke detection. Thus, it is instructive to test whether smoke and fog/haze could be differentiated using the proposed feature; and this is studied in Sect. 5.5. The effectiveness of the proposed feature for smoke detection in real applications is validated in Sect. 5.5 as well. Furthermore, the computational complexity of the proposed algorithm is analyzed in Sect. 5.6. Finally, to make a comparison between video-based smoke detection and image-based smoke detection under the situation that cameras are jittering, experiments are conducted in Sect. 5.7.

5.1   Data Sets and Experimental Setup

Smoke and non-smoke images with the size of 16×16 pixels were collected. These block images were then divided into two parts, one for training the smoke and non-smoke dictionaries and the other for training and testing the classifiers for smoke detection. Notice that the images for learning dictionaries were strictly excluded for classifier training/testing.

Given an input image block $\mathbf{f}$, two over-complete dictionaries $\mathbf{D_b}$ and $\mathbf{D_s}$ are required to solve Eq. (13). To adapt smoke and non-smoke classes, K-SVD [24] was adopted to train $\mathbf{D_b}$ and $\mathbf{D_s}$ from the training samples. Specifically,

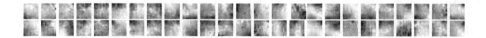

Fig. 2. Examples of the bases from the learnt dictionary $\mathbf{D_s}$ for smoke.

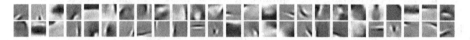

Fig. 3. Examples of the bases from the learnt dictionary $\mathbf{D_b}$ for non-smoke.

1000 pure smoke images with the size of 16×16 pixels were used to learn $\mathbf{D_s}$. To make $\mathbf{D_b}$ have good generalization ability, 60000 non-smoke images with the size of 16×16 pixels that were randomly cropped from the images in the CIFAR-100 data set [25], were used to learn $\mathbf{D_b}$. In the experiments, both $\mathbf{D_b}$ and $\mathbf{D_s}$ have the size of 256×500. Some basis samples from $\mathbf{D_s}$ and $\mathbf{D_b}$ are shown in Figs. 2 and 3 respectively.

To construct a data set of smoke for training and testing the classifier, 5000 images with the size of 16×16 pixels were manually cropped based on visual observation from 25 publicly available video clips of smoke. These video clips [1–3], cover indoor and outdoor, short and long distance surveillance scenes with different illuminations. Furthermore, half of the 5000 block images are heavy smoke and the rest are light smoke.

To construct a data set of general non-smoke for training and testing the classifier, which cover a large variety of real life image patches, 5000 images with the size of 16×16 pixels were randomly cropped from the images in the 15-scene data set [26].

To construct a data set of fog/haze image patches for training and testing the classifier, 10 fog/haze images were collected from [22,27–29]. 2500 images with the size of 16×16 pixels were cropped from the fog/haze regions in those images; there are 250 block images in each collected image.

In addition, four video clips that were captured by unstable cameras were chosen. 1000 images with the size of 16×16 pixels were manually cropped from the videos. Half of these block images are smoke (either heavy or light) and the rest are non-smoke foreground objects. Notice the 1000 cropped block images are associated with 1000 background block images that were estimated through video-based background modeling [30].

5.2 Separation of Quasi-smoke and Quasi-background

Given a test image block $\mathbf{f}$ and the trained dictionaries $\mathbf{D_b}$ and $\mathbf{D_s}$, the corresponding sparse coefficients $\mathbf{y_b}$ and $\mathbf{y_s}$ are estimated by solving Eq. (13). Then quasi-background component $\mathbf{D_b y_b}$ and quasi-smoke component $\mathbf{D_s y_s}$ are calculated. For an image which includes many blocks, the separation can be performed on every block in a sliding window manner. To validate the separation performance, the collage in Fig. 4 shows some separated quasi-smoke and quasi-background components.

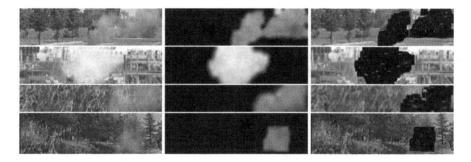

Fig. 4. Quasi-smoke and quasi-background separation (column 1: the test images, column 2: the separated quasi-smoke components, column 3: the separated quasi-background components).

5.3 Binary Classification with the Proposed Feature

Given 5000 smoke image blocks and 5000 general non-smoke image blocks, the separability between them based on the proposed feature was studied. Specifically, each of the 10000 block images was considered as f. Given the trained dictionaries D_b and D_s, the corresponding sparse coefficients y_b and y_s were estimated by solving Eq. (13). The concatenated y_b and y_s was considered as a novel feature to characterize the test image block and as input to SVM classifier to determine whether it contains smoke. In the rest of the paper, the proposed feature will be referred to as SC.

The visual features based on motion, color, and edge are not suitable for smoke detection from a single gray-scale image. Thus texture feature was adopted in this paper. As local binary pattern (LBP) [31] has been successfully used in texture classification tasks and was applied to video-based smoke detection in [3–5], it was adopted for comparison in our experiments. As shown in [4,5], the texture feature extracted from the separated smoke component is more reliable than that extracted from the original video frame. In our experiments LBP was extracted from the separated components as well. After y_b and y_s were obtained, quasi-background component $D_b y_b$ and quasi-smoke component $D_s y_s$ could be estimated. Similar to the trick used in [4,5], LBP simply extracted from $D_s y_s$ was considered as a feature for smoke detection, and will be referred to as LBP_S in the rest of the paper. Additionally, the concatenated LBP extracted respectively from $D_b y_b$ and $D_s y_s$ may encode discriminative information and was tested as well; and this will be referred to as LBP_C in the rest of the paper. For completeness, LBP that was extracted from the original image block f without performing separation was also tested; and this will be referred to as LBP in the rest of the paper.

Both linear and radial basis function (RBF) kernel SVM were tested and 5-fold cross validation was performed in our experiments in the rest of the paper, unless otherwise specified. The classification accuracies are reported in Table 1. As shown in the table, among the four features tested, the proposed feature SC achieves the highest accuracy in the binary classification of smoke and general

Table 1. Accuracies for binary classification of smoke and general non-smoke (*LBP*: extracted from the original image block **f**; *LBP$_S$*: extracted from the quasi-smoke component $\mathbf{D_s y_s}$ only; *LBP$_C$*: extracted from both the quasi-smoke component $\mathbf{D_s y_s}$ and the quasi-background component $\mathbf{D_b y_b}$ and then concatenated).

Feature	*LBP*	*LBP$_S$*	*LBP$_C$*	*SC (Proposed)*
Accuracy (%)	68.96	80.49	85.58	**94.9**

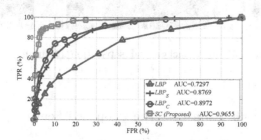

Fig. 5. ROC curves for binary classification of smoke and general non-smoke (*LBP*: extracted from the original image block **f**; *LBP$_S$*: extracted from the quasi-smoke component $\mathbf{D_s y_s}$ only; *LBP$_C$*: extracted from both the quasi-smoke component $\mathbf{D_s y_s}$ and the quasi-background component $\mathbf{D_b y_b}$ and then concatenated).

non-smoke. As expected, the texture feature *LBP* extracted without component separation has the worst performance. With the texture information of both quasi-background and quasi-smoke components considered, *LBP$_C$* is more discriminative than *LBP$_S$*, which only represents the texture feature of quasi-smoke component. Furthermore, the receiver operating characteristics (ROC) curves are adopted as performance measurement. They are shown in Fig. 5 along with area under the curve (AUC) values. It is evident that the proposed feature *SC* outperforms all the other three features.

The optimum SVM parameters obtained after tuning (5-fold cross validation on 10000 image blocks) were used to train a SVM classifier using the proposed feature. Some classification results based on the SVM are shown in Fig. 6. In each scene shown in Fig. 6, one smoke region and one non-smoke region were selected manually for illustration purpose; these are indicated using blue rectangle. Then some block images were randomly selected from the two regions as test samples. The smoke and non-smoke blocks classified by using the proposed feature are indicated by red block and green block respectively. Although there are a few classification errors on block level, the selected regions indicated by blue rectangle will not be misclassified if simple majority voting is employed.

5.4   Ternary Classification with the Proposed Feature

Generally at the onset, smoke starts out lightly colored in a video surveillance scene. In order to be useful for early smoke detection, the algorithm should be able to differentiate amongst heavy smoke, light smoke, and non-smoke. Furthermore,

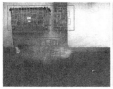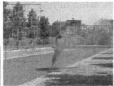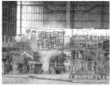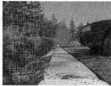

Fig. 6. Illustrative classification results (blue rectangle: the selected region; red block: classified as smoke; green block: classified as non-smoke) (Color figure online).

the algorithm should not be sensitive to false alarm caused by some objects with high homogeneous appearance such as clothes and vehicle body. This consideration motivates us to explore the separability among the classes of heavy smoke, light smoke, and general non-smoke based on the proposed feature. For this, a ternary classification task was conducted, which has not been reported in the literature.

Specifically, 2500 block images were randomly selected from the data set of general non-smoke. Given these 2500 general non-smoke, 2500 heavy smoke, and 2500 light smoke image blocks, separation experiments were performed and the proposed feature SC was extracted. For our comparative evaluation, LBP, LBP_S and LBP_C were also extracted as texture feature. The classification accuracies are reported in Table 2. Similar to the binary classification case, among all the four features the highest accuracy is observed when using the proposed feature SC. It is also noted that, for ternary classification of heavy smoke, light smoke, and general non-smoke, the features LBP_S, LBP_C and SC extracted based on the separated components still outperform LBP. For clarity, the confusion matrix for ternary classification based on SC is shown in Table 3. As can be noticed, most non-smoke can be differentiated from heavy smoke and light smoke. The main misclassification occurs between heavy smoke and light smoke.

5.5 Smoke Detection: Real Application Considerations

The separability between smoke and general non-smoke classes based on the proposed feature has been validated in Sect. 5.3 and 5.4. As mentioned before, fog/haze may pose a challenge for single image smoke detection. To better understand this challenging case, the separability between smoke and fog/haze classes was explored. Note this is the first time it is being reported in the literature. This consideration is also useful when specifying the classifiers to be used in a real smoke detection application.

Table 2. Accuracies for ternary classification of heavy smoke, light smoke, and general non-smoke (LBP: extracted from the original image block $\mathbf{f}$; LBP_S: extracted from the quasi-smoke component $\mathbf{D_s y_s}$ only; LBP_C: extracted from both the quasi-smoke component $\mathbf{D_s y_s}$ and the quasi-background component $\mathbf{D_b y_b}$ and then concatenated).

Feature	LBP	LBP_S	LBP_C	SC *(Proposed)*
Accuracy (%)	51.92	62.77	73.61	**84.47**

Table 3. Confusion matrix for ternary classification of heavy smoke, light smoke, and general non-smoke based on the proposed feature SC.

		Detected		
		Heavy	Light	Non-smoke
Truth	Heavy	81.4%	18.2%	0.4%
	Light	13.6%	76.2%	10.2%
	Non-smoke	1.2%	3%	95.8%

2500 block images were randomly selected from the smoke data set. Given these 2500 smoke (including both heavy and light) and 2500 fog/haze block images, separation experiments were conducted and the proposed feature SC was extracted. To make a comparison, LBP_C which has been proved to be the best among LBP features was extracted from quasi-smoke and quasi-background components as texture feature.

A binary classification task on these image blocks yielded classification accuracies of 76.6% and 77.5% when using LBP_C and SC respectively. Note that the study on the differentiation of smoke from fog/haze is preliminary. It can be expected from the above experiments that the proposed feature SC will outperform LBP-based features in a realistic case where smoke, fog/haze and non-smoke (excluding fog/haze) coexist.

Based on the results so far obtained, the proposed feature SC, has been validated to effectively separate between the classes of smoke and general non-smoke; and the classes of smoke and fog/haze. In a smoke detection system application it will be preferable to filter out general non-smoke at a first stage of smoke detection. Then smoke and fog/haze are further differentiated at a second stage. Based on this consideration, a tree-structured classifier may have good generalization ability in terms of classification between smoke and non-smoke. To validate this hypothesis, such a classifier was constructed and tested for its effectiveness in detecting smoke. Using the data sets described in Sect. 5.1, two partitions (training and test data) were created. In the training set, there are 1500 block images including either heavy or light smoke, 1500 general non-smoke block images selected randomly, and 1500 fog/haze block images. The test set comprises 3500 smoke block images, 3500 general non-smoke block images, and 1000 fog/haze block images. A SVM was trained using SC on the 1500 smoke block images and 1500 general non-smoke block images; and this classifier is referred to as *Classifier1*. Another SVM was trained using SC on the 1500 smoke block images and 1500 fog/haze block images; and this is referred to as *Classifier2*. For comparison, a SVM was also trained using SC on the 1500 smoke block images and 3000 non-smoke (including both general and fog/haze) block images; and this is referred to as *Classifier3*. *Classifier1* and *Classifier2* were simply concatenated as a tree-structured classifier; and this is referred to as *Classifier4*. Given the 3500 smoke block images and 4500 non-smoke (including 3500 general and 1000 fog/haze) block images in the test set, image separation

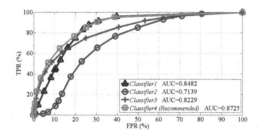

Fig. 7. ROC curves for single image smoke detection based on the four classifiers.

was performed and SC was extracted. The ROC curves for smoke detection based on the four classifiers are shown in Fig. 7, where AUC values are also provided. Overall *Classifier4* outperforms all the other three classifiers. Trained on smoke and fog/haze images only, *Classifier2* gives the worst performance among all the classifiers. The ROC curve based on *Classifier4* also indicates the effectiveness of the proposed feature SC for single image smoke detection.

5.6 Computational Complexity

In the proposed method, most computation time is spent in the step of feature extraction, that is, obtaining the sparse coefficients to represent the quasi-smoke and quasi-background components by solving Eq. (13). In this step, the sparse coefficients $\mathbf{y_b}$ and $\mathbf{y_s}$ are alternately calculated using the feature-sign search algorithm. The complexity of this step is $O(K_1 K_2 (K_3^3 + K_4^3))$, where K_1 is the number of iterations within the feature-sign search algorithm, K_2 is the number of alternations, K_3 is the number of non-zero entries in $\mathbf{y_b}$, and K_4 is the number of non-zero entries in $\mathbf{y_s}$. Typical values of K_1, K_2, K_3 and K_4 for our experiments are 5, 15, 30 and 20 respectively.

5.7 Smoke Detection with Jittering Cameras

When cameras jitter, video-based smoke detection algorithms could lead to poor performance due to the unreliable background modeling and feature extraction. However, single image smoke detection, which does not rely on the information of previous video frames, should perform well. To validate this, experiments using real video data were conducted. Given 1000 block images cropped from the video clips captured by jittering cameras, the proposed single image smoke detection method yielded a classification accuracy of 95.5 %. The state-of-the-art video-based smoke detection algorithm presented in [5] achieved only 54.5 %.

6 Conclusion and Future Work

In this paper, a novel feature, namely the sparse coefficients associated with an over-complete dictionary representation, has been proposed to detect smoke from a single image. The proposed feature arises from two parts; one representing the smoke component of the input image and the other representing the non-smoke component. We derived a component-based image formation model for smoke using the atmospheric scattering models and formulated an optimization scheme that allowed the separation of quasi-smoke and quasi-background components. The effectiveness of the proposed feature for single image smoke detection was validated by the experimental results. Furthermore, practical consideration for the design of a smoke detection system that could be useful in specifying required classifiers was presented. As an indicator for successful smoke separation, a good estimation of ω is meaningful from the perspective of both theoretical and practical consideration and this will be pursued in our continuing work.

Acknowledgement. This work was partly supported by SNS Unicorp Pty Ltd.

References

1. Calderara, S., Piccinini, P., Cucchiara, R.: Vision based smoke detection system using image energy and color information. Mach. Vis. Appl. **22**, 705–719 (2011)
2. Toreyin, B.U., Dedeoglu, Y., Cetin, A.E.: Wavelet based real-time smoke detection in video. In: EUSIPCO (2005)
3. Yuan, F.: A double mapping framework for extraction of shape-invariant features based on multi-scale partitions with adaboost for video smoke detection. Pattern Recogn. **45**, 4326–4336 (2012)
4. Tian, H., Li, W., Wang, L., Ogunbona, P.: A novel video-based smoke detection method using image separation. In: ICME, pp. 532–537 (2012)
5. Tian, H., Li, W., Wang, L., Ogunbona, P.: Smoke detection in video: an image separation approach. IJCV **106**, 192–209 (2014)
6. Narasimhan, S.G., Nayar, S.K.: Vision and the atmosphere. IJCV **48**, 233–254 (2002)
7. Yuan, F.: A fast accumulative motion orientation model based on integral image for video smoke detection. Pattern Recogn. Lett. **29**, 925–932 (2008)
8. Kolesov, I., Karasev, P., Tannenbaum, A., Haber, E.: Fire and smoke detection in video with optimal mass transport based optical flow and neural networks. In: ICIP (2010)
9. Park, J., Ko, B., Nam, J.Y., Kwak, S.: Wildfire smoke detection using spatiotemporal bag-of-features of smoke. In: WACV, pp. 200–205 (2013)
10. Jakovcevic, T., Stipanicev, D., Krstinic, D.: Visual spatial-context based wildfire smoke sensor. Mach. Vis. Appl. **24**, 707–719 (2013)
11. Labati, R.D., Genovese, A., Piuri, V., Scotti, F.: Wildfire smoke detection using computational intelligence techniques enhanced with synthetic smoke plume generation. IEEE Trans. Syst. Man Cybern.: Syst. **43**, 1003–1012 (2013)
12. Morerio, P., Marcenaro, L., Regazzoni, C.S., Gera, G.: Early fire and smoke detection based on colour features and motion analysis. In: ICIP, pp. 1041–1044 (2012)
13. Wang, Y., Chua, T.W., Chang, R., Pham, N.T.: Real-time smoke detection using texture and color features. In: ICPR, pp. 1727–1730 (2012)
14. Tian, H., Li, W., Ogunbona, P., Nguyen, D.T., Zhan, C.: Smoke detection in videos using non-redundant local binary pattern-based features. In: MMSP, pp. 1–4 (2011)

15. Long, C., et al.: Transmission: a new feature for computer vision based smoke detection. In: Wang, F.L., Deng, H., Gao, Y., Lei, J. (eds.) Artificial Intelligence and Computational Intelligence. LNCS, vol. 6319, pp. 389–396. Springer, Heidelberg (2010)

16. Maruta, H., Nakamura, A., Yamamichi, T., Kurokawa, F.: Image based smoke detection with local hurst exponent. In: ICIP, pp. 4653–4656 (2010)

17. Wright, J., Ma, Y., Mairal, J., Sapiro, G., Huang, T.S., Yan, S.: Sparse representation for computer vision and pattern recognition. Proc. IEEE **98**, 1031–1044 (2010)

18. Lee, H., Battle, A., Raina, R., Ng, A.Y.: Efficient sparse coding algorithms. In: NIPS (2007)

19. Bezdek, J.C., Hathaway, R.J.: Convergence of alternating optimization. Neural Parallel Sci. Computations **11**, 351–368 (2003)

20. Bai, X., Sapiro, G.: Geodesic matting: a framework for fast interactive image and video segmentation and matting. IJCV **82**, 113–132 (2009)

21. Levin, A., Lischinski, D., Weiss, Y.: A closed-form solution to natural image matting. IEEE TPAMI **30**, 228–242 (2008)

22. He, K., Sun, J., Tang, X.: Single image haze removal using dark channel prior. IEEE TPAMI **33**, 2341–2353 (2011)

23. Starck, J.L., Elad, M., Donoho, D.L.: Image decomposition via the combination of sparse representations and a variational approach. IEEE TIP **14**, 1570–1582 (2005)

24. Aharon, M., Elad, M., Bruckstein, A.: K-SVD: an algorithm for designing overcomplete dictionaries for sparse representation. IEEE Trans. Sig. Process. **54**, 4311–4322 (2006)

25. Krizhevsky, A.: Learning multiple layers of features from tiny images. Technical report (2009)

26. Lazebnik, S., Schmid, C., Ponce, J.: Beyond bags of features: spatial pyramid matching for recognizing natural scene categories. In: CVPR, pp. 2169–2178 (2006)

27. Fattal, R.: Single image dehazing. ACM Trans. Graph. **27**, 1–9 (2008)

28. Kopf, J., Neubert, B., Chen, B., Cohen, M., Cohen-Or, D., Deussen, O., Uyttendaele, M., Lischinski, D.: Deep photo: model-based photograph enhancement and viewing. ACM Trans. Graph. **27** (2008)

29. Tan, R.T.: Visibility in bad weather from a single image. In: CVPR (2008)

30. Stauffer, C., Grimson, W.E.L.: Learning patterns of activity using real-time tracking. IEEE Trans. Pattern Anal. Mach. Intell. **22**, 747–757 (2000)

31. Ojala, T., Pietikainen, M., Maenpaa, T.: Multiresolution gray-scale and rotation invariant texture classification with local binary patterns. IEEE TPAMI **24**, 971–987 (2002)

Adaptive Sparse Coding for Painting Style Analysis

Zhi Gao[1][✉], Mo Shan[2], Loong-Fah Cheong[3], and Qingquan Li[4,5]

[1] Interactive and Digital Media Institute, National University of Singapore,
Singapore, Singapore
gaozhinus@gmail.com

[2] Temasek Laboratories, National University of Singapore, Singapore, Singapore
sholmes9091@gmail.com

[3] Electrical and Computer Engineering Department,
National University of Singapore, Singapore, Singapore
eleclf@nus.edu.sg

[4] The State Key Laboratory of Information Engineering in Surveying,
Mapping, and Remote Sensing, Wuhan University, Wuhan, China
qqli@whu.edu.cn

[5] Shenzhen Key Laboratory of Spatial Smart Sensing and Services,
Shenzhen University, Shenzhen, China

Abstract. Inspired by the outstanding performance of sparse coding in applications of image denoising, restoration, classification, etc., we propose an adaptive sparse coding method for painting style analysis that is traditionally carried out by art connoisseurs and experts. Significantly improved over previous sparse coding methods, which heavily rely on the comparison of query paintings, our method is able to determine the authenticity of a single query painting based on estimated decision boundary. Firstly, discriminative patches containing the most representative characteristics of the given authentic samples are extracted via exploiting the statistical information of their representation on the DCT basis. Subsequently, the strategy of adaptive sparsity constraint which assigns higher sparsity weight to the patch with higher discriminative level is enforced to make the dictionary trained on such patches more exclusively adaptive to the authentic samples than via previous sparse coding algorithms. Relying on the learnt dictionary, the query painting can be authenticated if both better denoising performance and higher sparse representation are obtained, otherwise it should be denied. Extensive experiments on impressionist style paintings demonstrate efficiency and effectiveness of our method.

1 Introduction

Painting analysis has been carried out by art connoisseurs and experts traditionally, and the procedure could be fairly costly and subjective. Even worse, the conclusions made in this way could be changed over time due to the emergence of new historical evidence. Therefore, assisting the authentication by less biased

---

Zhi Gao and Mo Shan—denotes joint first author.

© Springer International Publishing Switzerland 2015
D. Cremers et al. (Eds.): ACCV 2014, Part II, LNCS 9004, pp. 102–117, 2015.
DOI: 10.1007/978-3-319-16808-1_8

automatic method has been attracting increased attention from the communities of art, mathematics and engineering, etc. Although appealing, and much cross-disciplinary interaction of image analysis researcher and art historians has been reported, a survey of the representative literature [1, 9, 11, 14, 19–21] reveals that the research of painting authentication using computer vision techniques is still in its early stage.

Currently, most published research of computerized painting analysis focuses on two tasks: to distinguish authentic painting from its forgery, given a set of authentic samples; to classify the query authentic one for dating challenge or stylometry comparison, given multiple sets of authentic samples. Intuitively, such identification and classification like tasks can be easily solved by exploiting the latest achievements in pattern classification. However, due on one hand to the requirement of sophisticated high-level art knowledge which should be conveyed and applied mathematically, on the other hand to the lack of sufficient well-prepared positive and negative samples[1], a classifier with satisfactory performance still demands extensive efforts.

Inspired by the outstanding performance of sparse coding which has achieved the state-of-the-art performance in a variety of applications including image denoising and restoration, action classification and recognition, face recognition and abnormal (or irregularity) detection, etc., it has been applied for painting analysis as well in recent years [9, 15, 16]. In the widely celebrated paper published on Nature [18], sparse coding is demonstrated with the capability of capturing well the localized orientation and spatial frequency information existed in the training images. Nevertheless, when applied to artistic analysis, sparse coding exploits very little artistic knowledge, perhaps due to the difficulty of incorporating the stylistic information into the standard training procedure. Moreover, such methods make the final decision based on the comparison of pertinent statistic, either among multiple query samples or among multiple sets of given authentic samples, for the authentication and dating challenge tasks respectively. However, it is not always the case to distinguish the authentic one from its imitations, and the more realistic problems is to determine authenticity for one query sample given a set of authentic samples. Consequently, several questions of practical importance could be raised: firstly, is it possible to import any artistic knowledge appropriately into the sparse coding model to capture more characteristics of the painting? Secondly, how to estimate a decision boundary to determine how much a query painting can deviate from the training data before it could be categoried as being too different to be authentic or consistent?

In this paper, we propose an adaptive sparse representation algorithm in which the DCT baseline is leveraged to overcome the aforementioned drawbacks of most available methods in some extent. Firstly, instead of brushstrokes or features, discriminative patches containing the most representative characteristics of the given authentic samples are extracted via exploiting the statistical

---

[1] Due on one hand to the copyright issue, the high quality reproductions of the paintings in the museums are rarely publicly available even for research purpose, on the other hand to the fact that museums usually have no interests to acquire and keep paintings that are known as forgeries.

information of their representation on the DCT basis. Moreover, such patches are sorted according to their distinctiveness. Subsequently, the strategy of adaptive sparsity constraint which assigns higher sparsity regularization weight to the patch with higher discriminative level is enforced to make the dictionary trained on such patches more exclusively adaptive to the authentic samples than dictionary trained via previous sparse coding algorithms. Relying on the learnt dictionary, the query painting can be authenticated if both better denoising performance and more sparse representation are obtained than the results obtained on the baseline DCT basis, otherwise it should be denied. Herein the DCT basis is chosen to represent the general style to some extent, which is used to set a baseline for comparison purpose. In this way, a decision boundary can be built. Besides the sparsity measure, here we further exploit a well proved conclusion in sparse coding community that the dictionaries learned from the data itself significantly outperform predefined dictionaries, such as DCT, curvelets, wedgelets and various sorts of wavelets in the generative tasks including denoising, restoration, etc., since the learnt dictionary is more suitably adapted to the given data [5,8]. We apply such conclusion from another direction, namely, if the testing image can be better denoised by using the learnt dictionary than DCT, it can be determined as more consistent with the dictionary (basis) learned from the authentic samples. Extensive experiments including classification of van Gogh's paintings from different periods, dating challenge and stylometry measure demonstrate the efficiency and effectiveness of our method. In particular, to our knowledge, the experiment of painting classification based on decision boundary is conducted in a computerized artistic analysis fashion for the first time.

The main contributions of our work may be summarized as follows. Firstly, a novel patch extraction method is developed based on the statistics on the DCT basis. Secondly, an improved sparse coding algorithm is proposed for stylistic assessment of the paintings, incorporating the prior statistics of extracted patches Thirdly, a decision boundary is estimated based on a baseline measure leveraging the DCT basis, enabling the attribution of a single query painting. Last but not the least, insightful observations are drawn for the analysis of the paintings by van Gogh produced in different periods.

2   Related Work

Research efforts based on computational techniques to study art and cultural heritages have emerged in the recent years, interested readers can refer to such surveys [19–21] for a comprehensive introduction. Here, we focus on the most relevant works. Currently, according to the characteristics extracted from digital paintings and on which the following process performs, the main approaches of computerized painting analysis can be roughly divided into three categories: feature based, brushstroke based and sparse coding based.

In order to perform the high-level analysis on paintings, various methods have been proposed to capture their perceivable characteristics based on the features of color and texture [23], fractal dimension [22], etc. Without attempting to be exhaustive, other features include HOG2 × 2, local binary pattern (LBP), dense

SIFT (scale-invariant feature transform) have also been tested [4]. However, such feature based methods can hardly be generalized to deal with paintings of different artists, since they reply heavily on the prior knowledge of different artists to select proper features to represent their artworks, and the challenge of this regard has been pointed out in [11].

As suggested by art connoisseurs and experts that the pattern of brushwork is an important indicator of styles, methods have been developed tailored to the brushstroke analysis. The work [14] published on PAMI applied the brushwork traits to authenticate and date the paintings of van Gogh. However, brushstrokes are too difficult to be crisply segmented out using off-the-shelf detector. Several brushstroke extraction methods have been proposed [2,14], but codes of such methods are not publicly available. Based on brushstroke detection, a variety of mathematic tools, such as neural network [17], hidden Markov Models (HMM) [10], multiresolution HMM [13], have been applied to represent and model the information of brushstroke width, length, curvature, shapes, etc. Subsequently, SVM classifier is trained on the given data to perform a specific task. In summary, researchers in this study identified several challenges deserving more efforts. Firstly, it is very difficult to automatically extract the strokes and art theory required to be exploited. Secondly, there is an urgent demand for more sophisticated mathematical models which are capable of capturing the subtle visual characteristics in paintings. Thirdly, it is difficult to train a satisfactory classifier without sufficient well-prepared positive and negative samples.

Motivated by its outstanding performance in various applications in computer vision and signal processing, sparse coding has been applied to the recognition of authentic paintings as well. In 2010, the work [9] applied the sparse coding model for the first time on quantification of artistic style to determine authentication of drawings of Pieter Bruegel the Elder and received a lot of attention in the media. Therein, the dictionary is firstly learned based on the given authentic paintings according to the sparse coding model, and the authentication is performed on the sparsity measure of representations on the learnt dictionary. The one whose representation coefficients are more sparse will be determined as authentic. In [15], sparse coding is applied to perform stylometry measure on van Gogh's paintings of different periods. Instead of measuring the sparsity of the representation coefficient, the similarity measure is performed on the dictionary itself. The strength of the sparse coding algorithm is that it can capture the visual features in the painting through the overlapping patches extracted. However, the standard dictionary training adopted previously does not integrate the discriminative features that are indicative of styles, such as brushstrokes, possibly because the extraction of brushstrokes and the modeling involves extensive domain knowledge.

3   Our Adaptive Sparse Coding Algorithm

3.1   Notation

To facilitate the description, we first introduce the notation adopted in this paper. Matrices and vectors are in bold capital, bold lower-cased fronts respectively.

We define for $q \geq 1$, the ℓ_q-norm of a vector $\boldsymbol{x}$ in $\mathbb{R}^m$ as $||\boldsymbol{x}||_q \triangleq \left(\sum_{i=1}^{m} |\boldsymbol{x}[i]|^q\right)^{1/q}$, where $\boldsymbol{x}[i]$ denotes the i-th entry of $\boldsymbol{x}$. The ℓ_0-pseudo-norm is defined as the number of nonzero elements in a vector. We consider the Frobenius norm of a matrix $\boldsymbol{X}$ in $\mathbb{R}^{m \times n}$: $||\boldsymbol{X}||_F \triangleq \left(\sum_{i=1}^{m} \sum_{j=1}^{n} |\boldsymbol{X}[i,j]|^2\right)^{1/2}$. $\boldsymbol{x}_i$ or $\boldsymbol{X}(:,i)$ represents the i-th column of $\boldsymbol{X}$, $\boldsymbol{X}(j,:)$ is the j-th row of $\boldsymbol{X}$.

3.2 Previous Sparse Coding Algorithm for Painting Analysis

Mathematically, the basic sparse coding algorithm amounts to solve the following optimization problem (as Eq. (1)) or its tightest convex surrogate (as Eq. (2)):

$$\min_{D,X} ||\boldsymbol{Y} - \boldsymbol{DX}||_2 \quad \text{s.t.} \ \forall \ 1 \leqslant i \leqslant N, \ ||\boldsymbol{x}_i||_0 \leqslant k \tag{1}$$

$$\min_{D,X} ||\boldsymbol{Y} - \boldsymbol{DX}||_2 + \lambda ||\boldsymbol{X}||_1 \tag{2}$$

where $\boldsymbol{Y} \in \mathbb{R}^{d \times N}$ contains all the available image patches $\{\boldsymbol{y}\}_{i=1}^{N}$ as columns, and similarly, $\boldsymbol{X} \in \mathbb{R}^{n \times N}$ contains all the sparse representation vectors $\{\boldsymbol{x}\}_{i=1}^{N}$. Sparse representation aims to find both the dictionary $\boldsymbol{D} \in \mathbb{R}^{d \times n}$ and the representations $\boldsymbol{X}$. In Eq. (1), k is a given constant controlling the sparsity, usually $k \ll d$ to keep $\boldsymbol{X}$ sparse and $d < n$ to ensure the over-completeness of $\boldsymbol{D}$. In Eq. (2), λ is the regularization parameter to balance the ℓ_2 representation fidelity term and the ℓ_1 sparsity penalty term. In fact, extensive efforts have been devoted to the algorithms to find the global optimal solution of $\boldsymbol{D}$ and $\boldsymbol{X}$ efficiently, and lots of methods have been proposed. For more knowledge in this regard, readers are advised to refer to such monograph [7] and references therein.

The typical framework of using sparse coding for artistic authentication can be summarized briefly as this: $\boldsymbol{D}_{tr}$ is firstly trained on the given authentic paintings, then the representation matrices of two testing samples, the authentic one and a forgery, are computed based on $\boldsymbol{D}_{tr}$. As [9,16] did, kurtosis is applied to measure the sparseness of matrix. The one whose representation matrix is more sparse, namely the kurtosis value is larger, is determined as authentic. Obviously, such methods rely on the comparison of kurtosis of multiple query paintings without taking their difference of content complexity into account. The limitation of [9] will be demonstrated in the experiment part, Sect. 4.1.

3.3 Discriminative Patches Extraction

To facilitate more perceivable characteristics of the authentic paintings being learned by sparse coding model, here we propose to extract discriminative patches according to the statistics of their representation on the DCT basis.

Given a painting, we firstly estimate its representation coefficient matrix on the predefined DCT basis by replacing $\boldsymbol{D}$ in Eq. (2) with $\boldsymbol{D}_{dct}$, as below:

$$\min_{X_{dct}} ||\boldsymbol{Y} - \boldsymbol{D_{dct}X_{dct}}||_2 + \lambda ||\boldsymbol{X}_{dct}||_1 \tag{3}$$

where the image patches $\{y\}_{i=1}^{N}$ are of size 12×12 pixels, extracted from the whole image with half size sliding; the number of DCT atoms is 512, namely D_{dct} is of dimensions 144×512; and the recommended value of λ is 0.6. As D_{dct} is predefined and known, we apply the ℓ_1-ls algorithm [12] to estimate X_{dct}. Here, we clarify that the default patch size is 12×12 pixels extracted with half size sliding, the default atom number of dictionary, either predefined DCT or learned on training data, is 512. Such default parameters are used in this paper, except where indicated.

As well known that the DCT basis is usually used for image compression, an image patch with more complex content requires more DCT basis functions to represent, and vice versa. To measure the content complexity of an image patch of size n $\times$ n pixels, the activity measure is proposed in [7], a higher value indicating the presence of more complex content, as below:

$$Activity\,(I) = \sum_{i=2}^{n}\sum_{j=1}^{n}|I\,[i,j] - I\,[i-1,j]| + \sum_{i=1}^{n}\sum_{j=2}^{n}|I\,[i,j] - I\,[i,j-1]| \quad (4)$$

It is worth mentioning that the outline in the painting is mainly decided by the object itself, and includes little characteristics of the artist. Therefore we eliminate such pixels first based on the segmentation results of K-means segmentation. In our work, the DCT basis (or say dictionary) which is popularly applied as initialization for dictionary learning in sparse coding is applied as a baseline to represent a general painting style. Therefore, patches which do not conform to such criteria are defined as discriminative, which contain representative characteristics of specific artist. Mathematically, discriminative patches are those patches with lower kurtosis (namely, more atoms used for representation) and relatively lower activity (namely, content is simpler). Instead of using the values directly, we perform discriminative patches extraction based on the sorting of values of both kurtosis and activity, as summarized in Algorithm 1.

In Fig. 1, the result of discriminative patches extraction is shown. Moreover, the intermediate result of outline detection of K-means segmentation is also included. Through careful observation, we find that such extracted patches cover most of the area with obvious brushstrokes, especially, areas with impasto are extracted successfully, which are supposed to be the most representative characteristics of the artist [25]. In contrast to those brushstroke detection methods which are limited for oil painting, our discriminative patch extraction method is more general, and can be easily applied on other kinds of artworks. In fact, we have tried other bases including wavelet and coutourlet for this part, and find that the DCT basis works well to meets our requirement.

3.4   Adaptive Sparse Coding Algorithm

With discriminative patches P_i^d $(i = 1, \ldots, K)$ in hand, whose discriminative level (represented as dl_i) is the descending order, we propose the following adaptive sparse coding model, as below:

Algorithm 1. Discriminative Patches Extraction.

Input: A painting image IM;

Output: Discriminative patches: P_i^d, $i = 1, \ldots, K$;

1: Get patches of size 12×12 pixels from IM with half-size sliding: P_i, $i = 1, \ldots, N$;

2: Get the boundary map IM_e by performing the K-means segmentation on IM;

3: Based on IM_e, obtain patches without boundary pixels: P_i, $i = 1, \ldots, M$;

4: Set $K = M \times 0.2$; //20 % of the patches will be extracted.

5: Using Eq.(3), compute coefficient vector $\boldsymbol{x}_i$ for patch P_i, $i = 1, \ldots, M$, compute the kurtosis for each coefficient vector and sort in ascending order, get kurArray;

6: Compute activities for the patches P_i, $i = 1, \ldots, M$, and sort the values in ascending order, get actArray;

7: Set $nCounter = 0$; //to count how many discriminative patches have been found.

8: **for** j=1; $j <= 20$; j++

9:     **for** k=1; $k <= j$; k++

10:        **if** $nCounter < K$

11:            Find patches whose kurtosis value is the begining $j \times 5\%$ in the kurArray;

12:            Find patches whose activity value is the begining $k \times 5\%$ in the actArray;

13:            Find intersection of patches found in step 11, 12, save to the discriminative patches, P_i^d, $i = 1, \ldots, p$;

14:            $nCounter = nCounter + p$;

15:        **end for**

16: **end for**

17: In the discriminative patches list, the first K patches are exported.

$$\min_{D,X} \|\boldsymbol{Y} - \boldsymbol{D}\boldsymbol{X}\|_1 + \sum_{i=1}^{K} \lambda_i \|\boldsymbol{x}_i\|_1, \; \lambda_i = \lambda_{min} + \frac{dl_i - dl_{min}}{dl_{max} - dl_{min}}(\lambda_{max} - \lambda_{min})$$

$$(5)$$

where the adaptive regularization parameter λ_i, instead of a constant, is applied to balance the representation fidelity term and the sparsity penalty term, and $\lambda_{max} = 2.5$, $\lambda_{min} = 0.5$. Obviously, patch with higher dl value will be assigned with larger λ value. In other words, if the patch with more discriminative information is enforced to be represented with less dictionary atoms. Crafted in this way, the dictionary can better represent the stylistic features. Compared with

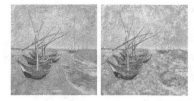

Fig. 1. Result of discriminative patches extraction. Left: edge detected by K-means. Right: extracted discriminative patches.

Fig. 2. Authentication on query samples from van Gogh (left) and Monet (right).

Eq. (2), another significant difference is that the ℓ_1-norm based representation fidelity is applied, since it is less vulnerable to outliers, as proved in [6,24]. In this way, our learnt dictionary is robust to the outliers generated from the flaws of previous operations.

To tackle the optimization problem of Eq. (5), we separate it into two sub-problems, sparse coding for training samples and dictionary updating. Briefly, the objective function of each sub-problem is defined as below:

$$\min_{\boldsymbol{x}_i} \sum_{i=1}^{K} ||\boldsymbol{y}_i - \boldsymbol{D}\boldsymbol{x}_i||_1 + \lambda_i\,||\boldsymbol{x}_i||_1\,,\ i = 1,\ldots,K \tag{6}$$

Eq. (6) is to estimate the sparse coefficients of each training patch, when $\boldsymbol{D}$ is given. We can rewrite Eq. (6) into an equivalent ℓ_1 approximation problem:

$$\min_{\boldsymbol{x}_i} \sum_{i=1}^{K} \left\lVert \begin{pmatrix} \boldsymbol{y}_i \\ \boldsymbol{0} \end{pmatrix} - \begin{pmatrix} \boldsymbol{D} \\ \lambda_i \boldsymbol{I} \end{pmatrix} \boldsymbol{x}_i \right\rVert_1,\ i = 1,\ldots,K \tag{7}$$

With $\boldsymbol{X}$ fixed, the dictionary $\boldsymbol{D}$ can be updated as follows:

$$\min_{\boldsymbol{D}}\ ||\boldsymbol{Y} - \boldsymbol{D}\boldsymbol{X}||_1 \tag{8}$$

All the sub-problems in Eqs. (7) and (8) are standard ℓ_1-regression problems. We resort to the iterative reweighted least squares (IRLS) [3] for solutions, and the algorithm is summarized as below:

In Algorithm 2, δ is a small positive value ($\delta = 0.001$ in our experiments). Each iteration of IRLS involves minimizing a quadratic objective function. The global optimum can be reached by taking derivatives and setting them to zeros.

An intuitive yet important question on adaptive sparse coding model is that why not apply much larger λ value to make the dictionary more adaptive to the patches. However, this is not the case. If λ is out of certain range, although the solution of $\boldsymbol{D}, \boldsymbol{X}$ still can be obtained, but results in a poor representation fidelity measure. This observation again justifies that besides kurtosis, the representation fidelity measure must be taken into account to evaluate how well a dictionary is learned, or how well the signal is consistent with the dictionary. Here, we further exploit a well proved conclusion in sparse coding that the dictionary learned from the data itself is more adapted to the data, resulting in significantly better denoising performance than applying predefined dictionaries [8], therefore, the denoising performance, namely the PSNR (peak signal-noise ratio) value is also incorporated to indicate the reconstructive power of the dictionary. In summary, on the same testing sample, if the learnt dictionary can achieve higher PSNR and higher kurtosis than that of applying DCT, the testing is deemed as much consistent with the dictionary. Here, the importance of estimating a reasonable range for the dynamic λ must be highlighted. The value of $\lambda_{max} = 2.5$, $\lambda_{min} = 0.5$ applied in our work is based on extensive experiments.

Algorithm 2. Adaptive Sparse Coding Algorithm.

Input:

Image patches matrix $Y \in \mathbb{R}^{d \times K}$, λ_{max}, λ_{min}, and the atom numbers of D is n;

Output:

Solution $D \in \mathbb{R}^{d \times n}$, $X \in \mathbb{R}^{n \times K}$ of Eq.(5);

1: Initialization: set D as overcomplete DCT dictionary;

2: **while** not converged **do**

3:    //**Lines 4 is the sparse coding stage to solve Eq. 7.**

4:    apply the IRLS method to solve X :

     the key objective function for IRLS is:

     $min_{x_i} \sum_{j=1} \omega_i^j (y_i[j] - D(j,:)x_i)^2 + \sum_{j=1}^n \eta^j (\lambda_i x_i[j])^2$;

     $\omega_i^j = \frac{1}{\sqrt{(y_i[j] - D(j,:)x_i)^2 + \delta}}$, $\eta^j = \frac{1}{\sqrt{(0 - I(j,:)x_i)^2 + \delta}}$

5:    //**Lines 6 is the dictionary update stage to solve Eq. 8.**

6:    apply the IRLS method to update D:

     $min_{D(i,:)} \left\| (Y(i,:))^T - (D(i,:)X)^T \right\|_1$, $i = 1, \ldots, d$;

     the key objective function for IRLS is:

     $min_{D(i,:)} \sum_{j=1}^N \phi_i^j (Y[i,j] - D(i,:)x_j)^2$;

     $\phi_i^j = \frac{1}{\sqrt{(Y[i,j] - D(i,:)x_j)^2 + \delta}}$

     normalize each column of D after all rows are updated;

7: **end while**

8: Output D, X.

---

4   Experiments and Analysis

4.1   Authentication Experiment

The direct comparison strategy of [9] is questionable, since the decision relying on the single statistic of sparse representation could be unfair (or biased). The bias arises because the difference between query samples in terms of the content complexity has not been taken into account.

To demonstrate the effect of content complexity, let us take an authentication example shown in Fig. 2, in which the given set of authentic paintings are from van Gogh, and the objective is to determine the authenticity of two query paintings, from van Gogh and Monet respectively. A dictionary is trained from van Gogh's painting, and then the kurtosis values of the sparse coefficients of the two query paintings associated with the van Gogh dictionary are computed. As a result, the kurtosis of van Gogh's painting is 43.00, whereas that of the Monet's painting is 61.24. This clearly contradicts the assumption drawn in [9] that the painting from the same style has a higher kurtosis.

Previous method fails in this case where the content of the authentic van Gogh's painting is more complex than Monet's, thus resulting in dense coefficients, which will lead to the wrong conclusion that Monet's painting is authentic to a van Gogh's dictionary.

In our method, we estimate the decision boundary of a single query sample via leveraging the DCT basis as baseline, where the margin is obtained by the original kurtosis subtracting off that associated with the DCT basis. The motivation behind the introduction of a baseline is because the DCT basis, being unbiased and often used for dictionary initialization, can represent the general style. It then follows that a decision boundary can be estimated by comparing the sparse representation of a test painting to this baseline. Instead of using the original kurtosis values, the margin is perceived as a more suitable measure. Consequently, for the same paintings used previously, the margin for van Gogh's painting is 29.56, while that for Monet's is 29.72. The effect of content complexity is thus mitigated to certain extent.

Besides kurtosis, which shows the representativeness of the dictionary, the denoising performance is another important measure indicative of the reconstructive power of the dictionary. Here the denoising performance is also compared against the DCT basis. Using the dictionary trained from the same space, the PSNR margin for van Gogh's painting is 1.46 dB compared with -1.72 dB for Monet's. The positive PSNR margin for van Gogh's painting demonstrates that the dictionary trained from the same image space is indeed better than DCT basis in terms of the reconstruction ability. On the contrary, DCT basis denoises Monet's painting better than the dictionary trained from van Gogh.

In summary, the lack of a decision boundary in the previous methods can be addressed by introducing DCT basis as a baseline, and then the sparse representation and denoising performance can be compared against it. Sparser representation and better denoising performance indicate that the query painting is authentic, belonging to the same image space with the dictionary.

4.2   Style Diversity Experiment

To analyze the style diversity in the context of decision boundary, we follow the experimental settings in [15]. The objective of this experiment is to determine the similarity of van Gogh's paintings in different periods.

As mentioned before, the collection of data set for painting analysis is quite challenging, since the high quality reproductions owned by the museums are rarely publicly available. Hence we employ an alternative way to acquire the large amount of paintings needed for the experiments, by using a python script to collect paintings from the web, following the same strategy of [4]. The paintings collected are mainly from WIKIART, which provides artworks in public domain.

The given training set comprises of paintings by van Gogh produced in four periods, namely Paris Period, Arles Period, Saint-Remy Period and Auvers-sur-Oise Period. 20 paintings are chosen from each period, thus totally 80. Among these paintings, 5 in each period are randomly selected to form a group of 20 paintings to represent the overall style of van Gogh, which is used for training the dictionary. 20 paintings by Monet are also included as a group of outliers.

The sparsity and denoising performance are plotted in Fig. 3. The horizontal axis shows the PSNR margin between the van Gogh dictionary and DCT basis, whereas the vertical axis reveals the kurtosis margin. These values are normalized such that their magnitudes are smaller than 1. The hollow markers represent the original data and the filled markers indicate the position of the mean values.

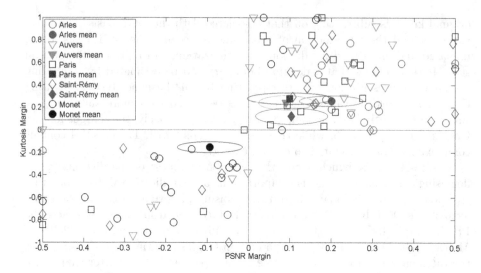

Fig. 3. Style similarity for van Goghs painting from four periods and Monets painting. Hollow marker is for each painting, filled marker is for the mean values of each group (Color figure online).

The plot demonstrates that as outliers, most of Monet's paintings lie in the third quadrant and have negative kurtosis and PSNR margin on average, suggesting that they are from a different image space. For the majority of van Gogh's paintings located in the first quadrant, those from Paris Period have a higher mean kurtosis, which indicates that this period is more similar to overall van Gogh style than other three periods, meaning that van Gogh's paintings can be represented better by the Paris Period. These observations are consistent with the conclusion drawn in [15].

In addition to the similarity analysis in [15], we also measure the spread of the paintings in each period. This is achieved by computing the variation of the kurtosis margin and PSNR margin, which are set to be the minor and major axis of the ellipses centered at the mean. It could be observed that the Paris Period has the longest major axis, revealing that the stylistic variation of this period is the greatest among the four periods. This observation agrees with the fact that the painter constantly varies his style and technique during his stay in Paris.

To summarize, the Paris Period is the most similar one to van Gogh's overall style. The consistency of our finding with the previous paper demonstrates the efficiency of our method. Furthermore, our algorithm finds that his painting techniques vary most frequently during Paris Period as well, which shed some new lights on style diversity analysis. The experiment also shows that the DCT basis is capable of providing a decision boundary for authentication, and successfully identifying the outliers.

4.3   Classification of van Gogh's Painting from Four Periods

To illustrate the usefulness and accuracy of the painting authentication based on a decision boundary, a novel experiment is designed to classify van Gogh's paintings produced in the four periods. The dataset is the same with the experiment in Sect. 4.2, except that only 10 paintings are chosen from each period to reduce computational time. The details of these paintings are listed in the supplementary material.

The experimental procedure is as follows. Firstly, a dictionary is trained from the 10 paintings randomly selected from each of the four periods. Secondly, the kurtosis margin and the PSNR margin of each painting associated with the four dictionaries are computed and then plotted respectively. Under the scenario where all the paintings are painted by the same painter, the 'authentic' paintings are defined as those produced in the same period with the dictionary. For instance, the paintings in the Arles Period are 'authentic' to the dictionary of this period, and the paintings in other three periods are regarded as 'forgeries'. Having a sparser representation and better denoising performance by the trained dictionary in a specific period than the DCT, the paintings located in the first quadrant are deemed to be from the same image space of that dictionary and are authentic. Therefore, the first quadrant is the decision boundary to determine authenticity for each query painting.

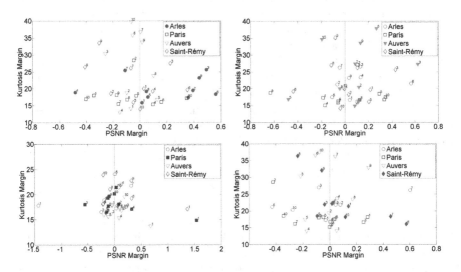

Fig. 4. Classification plots of the four periods. Filled markers: paintings in the same period with the dictionary used for testing. Hollow markers: paintings in other periods (Color figure online).

The classification results are plotted in Fig. 4. The results demonstrate that our method classifies the paintings with acceptable accuracy. For instance, most of the paintings in the Arles Period, Saint-Remy Period and Auvers-sur-Oise

Period are correctly identified. This has corroborated the usefulness of the decision boundary since most of the authentic paintings indeed lie in the first quadrant. Nevertheless, there are some paintings from other periods misclassified as authentic. This may be explained by the high similarity of these paintings observed from the similarity experiment. After all they are all painted by the same artist.

As for Paris Period, only 5 authentic paintings are correctly identified. However, the low accuracy does not necessarily undermine the effectiveness of the decision boundary. From the experiment in Sect. 4.2, it is observed that the paintings in the Paris Period vary most significantly in styles. Hence it is not surprising to find that the dictionary trained from these paintings cannot represent each painting well. From this perspective, this result is consistent with our findings in the previous experiment.

To sum up, the decision boundary built upon kurtosis and PSNR margin is able to classify paintings with high accuracy even in the extremely challenging case where both the positive and negative samples are paintings of van Gogh. Furthermore, the classification accuracy can be increased by selecting the paintings with high stylistic consistency.

4.4 Dating Challenge

While the paintings used in the experiment in Sect. 4.3 can be easily dated by the connoisseurs as to which period they belong, the attribution for other paintings by van Gogh are more ambiguous. To address the real dating problems raised by experts, which has also been explored extensively in [1,14], we examine three paintings which seem to share the traits of varied periods.

The paintings under examination are Still Life: Potatoes in a Yellow Dish (f386), Willows at Sunset (f572), and Crab on its Back (f605), as shown in Fig. 5. The decisions for these paintings are still under debate among connoisseurs because some insist that they belong to Paris Period while others argue that they belong to Provence Period, corresponding to the Arles and Saint-Remy Period in the similarity and period classification experiments.

For the ground truth, two groups of artworks, each containing eight paintings produced in Paris Period and Provence Period respectively, are selected and we train two dictionaries from each group. Then the kurtosis margin and PSNR margin associated with the dictionaries are plotted. From Fig. 5, it is clear that f386 should be dated to the Provence Period since it is located in the first quadrant when using the Provence dictionary. Similarly, f572 is dated to the Paris Period. One may wonder how to date f605 since both locations are in the second quadrant. In fact, this painting can be dated to the Provence Period because both kurtosis and PSNR margin are higher for the Provence dictionary. Moreover, in the previous works it is highlighted that compared with f386, f605 is less similar to the paintings in the Provence Period. This is also reflected in our results since the PSNR margin for f605 is negative when using the Provence dictionary, meaning that the reconstructive power of the Provence dictionary is less significant for f605 in comparison to f386. In short, the effectiveness of

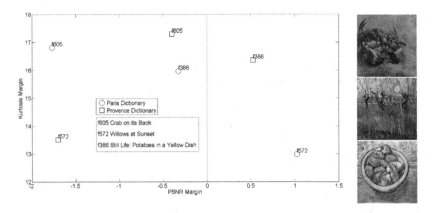

Fig. 5. Dating results (left) of three test paintings (right).

the painting classification based on decision boundary can also be demonstrated when applied to address the dating question. Which period a painting belongs to not only depends on the quadrant but also relates to the comparison of the margins. Although the correct attribution of the three paintings investigated is controversial in the art historical literature, the conclusion reached in our experiment is consistent with the examinations conducted by other state-of-the-art computerized painting analysis methods. Hence it may be concluded that the performance of our method is also superior.

5   Conclusion

In this paper we have developed a groundbreaking method for painting style analysis. Leveraging the proposed DCT baseline, both the discriminative patches extraction in the early stage and the decision making in the final stage are performed efficiently and successfully. In between, an adaptive sparse coding algorithm is proposed to learn the perceivable characteristics of the artist, provided a set of authentic data is given. A promising aspect of our method is that the authenticity of a single query painting can be determined based on a decision boundary. With this procedure we have performed extensive authentication and classification experiments where consistent conclusions are drawn. We have also shown that our novel approach of authentication based on a decision boundary sheds some new lights on style diversity analysis. Furthermore, our method can classify paintings with high stylistic similarity fairly accurately. We believe that with the advances in vision and machine learning, more art related questions can be addressed from a computational point of view.

Acknowledgement. This work is supported by these Grants: theory and methods of digital conservation for cultural heritage (2012CB725300), PSF Grant 1321202075, and the Singapore NRF under its IRC@SG Funding Initiative and administered by the IDMPO at the SeSaMe centre.

References

1. Abry, P., Wendt, H., Jaffard, S.: When Van Gogh meets Mandelbrot: multifractal classification of painting's texture. Sig. Process. **93**, 554–572 (2013)
2. Berezhnoy, I.E., Postma, E.O., van den Herik, H.J.: Automatic extraction of brush-stroke orientation from paintings. Mach. Vis. Appl. **20**, 1–9 (2009)
3. Bissantz, N., Dmbgen, L., Munk, A., Stratmann, B.: Convergence analysis of generalized iteratively reweighted least squares algorithms on convex function spaces. SIAM J. Optim. **19**, 1828–1845 (2009)
4. Blessing, A., Wen, K.: Using machine learning for identification of art paintings. Technical report, Stanford University, Stanford (2010)
5. Castrodad, A., Sapiro, G.: Sparse modeling of human actions from motion imagery. IJCV **100**, 1–15 (2012)
6. Cong, Z., Xiaogang, W., Wai-Kuen, C.: Background subtraction via robust dictionary learning. EURASIP J. Image Video Process. **2011** (2011)
7. Elad, M.: Sparse and Redundant Representations: From Theory to Applications in Signal and Image Processing. Springer, New York (2010)
8. Elad, M., Aharon, M.: Image denoising via sparse and redundant representations over learned dictionaries. IEEE Trans. Image Process. **15**, 3736–3745 (2006)
9. Hughes, J.M., Graham, D.J., Rockmore, D.N.: Quantification of artistic style through sparse coding analysis in the drawings of pieter bruegel the elder. In: Proceedings of the National Academy of Sciences, vol. 107, pp. 1279–1283 (2010)
10. Jacobsen, R.: Digital painting analysis: authentication and artistic style from digital reproductions. Ph.D. thesis, Aalborg University, Aalborg (2012)
11. Johnson, C.R., Hendriks, E., Berezhnoy, I.J., Brevdo, E., Hughes, S.M., Daubechies, I., Li, J., Postma, E., Wang, J.Z.: Image processing for artist identification. IEEE Sig. Process. Mag. **25**, 37–48 (2008)
12. Koh, K., Kim, S.J., Boyd, S.P.: An interior-point method for large-scale l1-regularized logistic regression. J. Mach. Learn. Res. **8**, 1519–1555 (2007)
13. Li, J., Wang, J.Z.: Studying digital imagery of ancient paintings by mixtures of stochastic models. IEEE Trans. Image Process. **13**, 340–353 (2004)
14. Li, J., Yao, L., Hendriks, E., Wang, J.Z.: Rhythmic brushstrokes distinguish van gogh from his contemporaries: findings via automated brushstroke extraction. IEEE Trans. PAMI **34**, 1159–1176 (2012)
15. Liu, Y., Pu, Y., Xu, D.: Computer analysis for visual art style. SIGGRAPH Asia 2013 Technical Briefs, p. 9. ACM (2013)
16. Mairal, J., Bach, F., Ponce, J.: Task-driven dictionary learning. IEEE Trans. PAMI **34**, 791–804 (2012)
17. Melzer, T., Kammerer, P., Zolda, E.: Stroke detection of brush strokes in portrait miniatures using a semi-parametric and a model based approach. In: International Conference on Pattern Recognition, vol. 1, pp. 474–476 (1998)
18. Olshausen, B.A., Field, D.J.: Emergence of simple-cell receptive field properties by learning a sparse code for natural images. Nature **381**, 607–609 (1996)
19. Stork, D.G.: Computer vision and computer graphics analysis of paintings and drawings: an introduction to the literature. In: Jiang, X., Petkov, N. (eds.) CAIP 2009. LNCS, vol. 5702, pp. 9–24. Springer, Heidelberg (2009)
20. Stork, D.G., Coddington, J.: Computer image analysis in the study of art. In: Proceeding of SPIE, vol. 6810 (2008)
21. Stork, D.G., Coddington, J., Bentkowska-Kafel, A.: Computer vision and image analysis of art II. In: Proceeding of SPIE, vol. 7869 (2011)

22. Taylor, R.P., Micolich, A.P., Jonas, D.: Fractal analysis of pollock's drip paintings. Nature **399**, 422–422 (1999)
23. van den Herik, H.J., Postma, E.O.: Discovering the visual signature of painters. In: Kasabov, N. (ed.) Future Directions for Intelligent Systems and Information Sciences. STUDFUZZ, vol. 45, pp. 129–147. Springer, Heidelberg (2000)
24. Wagner, A., Wright, J., Ganesh, A., Zhou, Z., Mobahi, H., Ma, Y.: Toward a practical face recognition system: robust alignment and illumination by sparse representation. IEEE Trans. PAMI **34**, 372–386 (2012)
25. Yelizaveta, M., Tat-Seng, C., Ramesh, J.: Semi-supervised annotation of brushwork in paintings domain using serial combinations of multiple experts. In: Proceedings of the 14th Annual ACM International Conference on Multimedia, pp. 529–538. ACM (2006)

Efficient Image Detail Mining

Andrej Mikulík, Filip Radenović[⊠], Ondřej Chum, and Jiří Matas

Center for Machine Perception, Department of Cybernetics, Faculty of EE,
Czech Technical University in Prague, Prague, Czech Republic
filip.radenovic@cmp.felk.cvut.cz

Abstract. Two novel problems straddling the boundary between image retrieval and data mining are formulated: for every pixel in the query image, (i) find the database image with the maximum resolution depicting the pixel and (ii) find the frequency with which it is photographed in detail.

An efficient and reliable solution for both problems is proposed based on two novel techniques, the hierarchical query expansion that exploits the document at a time (DAAT) inverted file and a geometric consistency verification sufficiently robust to prevent topic drift within a zooming search.

Experiments show that the proposed method finds surprisingly fine details on landmarks, even those that are hardly noticeable for humans.

1 Introduction

Visual image and specific object search engines have gone through a rapid development in the past decade. Methods that evolved from the bag of visual words [26] show considerable diversity and differ significantly from the original, e.g. those aggregating local descriptors like Fischer kernel [23] or VLAD [12]. But all the approaches attempt to rank images according to the similarity to the query image or region.

Finding and displaying the most similar images in a large dataset, however, may neither be the most exciting user experience nor useful for solving a particular search task since near duplicates or very similar images are retrieved, see Fig. 9. This was recently pointed out by Mikulik *et al.* [18] who propose a different search task: given a user-specified region in the query image, find the most detailed images in the database, or more precisely, images having the largest number of pixels within the query region.

In this work, we generalize the approach to the following formulation: given a query image, automatically, without any user specified hint, *find all "interesting" parts within the spatial extent of the query*. Two definitions of "interesting" lead to different tasks. The first is to find, for all pixels in the query, the highest resolution images depicting it, Fig. 1. The second is to find regions of interest that are the most often photographed, Fig. 2 (right). For more examples and comparison of the two tasks, see also Figs. 10 and 11.

In order to solve those tasks efficiently in a large, unordered image collection, a number of issues has to be tackled. Namely, an efficient retrieval of matching

© Springer International Publishing Switzerland 2015
D. Cremers et al. (Eds.): ACCV 2014, Part II, LNCS 9004, pp. 118–132, 2015.
DOI: 10.1007/978-3-319-16808-1_9

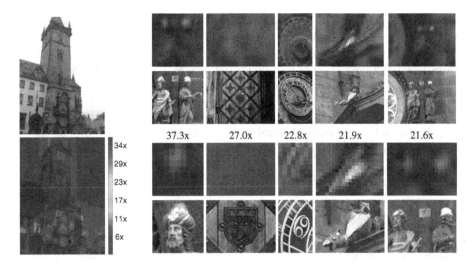

Fig. 1. Top five ranked images (right, 2nd row) automatically retrieved by the highest resolution transform. Compare the resolution of the corresponding parts (right, 1st row) of the query image (left, top). The difference in resolution is best appreciated in the visualization on selected details (right, 3rd and 4th row). The scaling factor achieved at each pixel is shown below the query image.

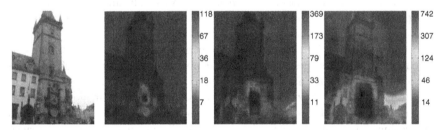

Fig. 2. The number of images showing a pixel (three images on the right) of the Astronomical clock query (left) only covering a small percentage of the original query: 0–1 %, 1–3 %, 3–10 %, from left to right respectively. The percentage is related to the size of the detail photographed.

sub-images with significantly different resolution has to be addressed, together with an effective rejection of false matches to prevent topic drifts. Towards this end, we introduce a novel concept of detail mining called hierarchical query expansion.

The results of the method are illustrated in Figs. 1 and 2, which show the query image, a sample of the discovered images of details from the dataset and two visualizations of localized interesting parts of the query image. The color in Fig. 1 (left, bottom) codes the maximal resolution found in the dataset. In Fig. 2 (right) the color codes the number of images found and backprojected into the query image.

The outputs show what the most interesting details for the crowds visiting the landmark are and which details are worth seeing (taking a picture of). It helps the user to find or focus on interesting details or suggests additional queries. Annotations (such as Flickr tags) of the discovered images can be used for describing parts of the image as in [4]. The output of the proposed detail mining can be also used as a initial step for finding iconic view of the details [28].

The rest of the paper is structured as follows: the components of the search engine based on bag-of-words retrieval are reviewed in Sect. 2. The novel method is introduced in Sect. 3 and experiments are given in Sect. 4. Section 5 concludes the paper.

2   Related Work

This section reviews relevant approaches to specific object search. Currently, methods based on aggregation of local features, such as [12,23], have become popular. Despite recent results on approximate localization using VLAD descriptor [2], these methods perform poorly when geometric constraints are to be enforced. Thus, these methods are not suitable for sub-image search with large scale change.

This paper builds on the bag-of-words image representation which was first adopted in the domain of visual search in [26]. Virtually all aspects of BoW-type representation have been studied in great detail: feature detectors and descriptors [3,15–17,29], vocabulary construction [10,19,21,24,26], spatial verification and re-ranking [10,24], document metric learning [5,11,13], dimensionality reduction [9], burstiness and feature dependency detection [5,11,14], and query expansion and automatic failure recovery [7,8,11,22,25].

The proposed method exploits a recent variant of the BoW image representation using an inverted file augmented with geometric information [27] for efficient image scoring. The closest approach to ours is [18] which attempts to retrieve a single user-specified sub-window with the highest resolution. Unlike Mikulík et al., no supervision by the user is provided in this work, and all possible locations are considered simultaneously. To avoid severe contamination by irrelevant images, a novel geometric consistency verification method is introduced.

Compared to other methods that efficiently find clusters of related images, such as [4], this paper focuses on extreme geometric changes, especially towards large changes of scale in order to obtain images with the greatest details.

The application domain of this paper is similar to the recent work of Weyand and Leibe [28] on hierarchical iconoid shift, which, given a landmark, provides iconic views of objects at different scales on that landmark. In [28], images are obtained separately for each landmark, using textual ques and GPS tags, and each collection of such images is indexed separately. In contrary, our approach has only one large collection of images without any further annotation, and the landmark (or any image with details to be discovered) is not defined beforehand. In [28], the images are exhaustively matched, which is a time demanding offline process. Our method works online and takes only several seconds to find the details of a given image. Note that compared to [28], this paper deals with a more difficult task, as linking details to full views in the exhaustive matching is easier than the other way round, see Fig. 3.

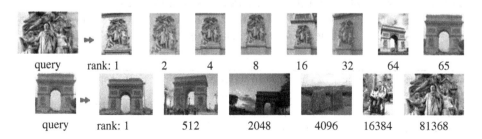

Fig. 3. Reaching the full view from a detail and vice versa by conventional image retrieval. When querying with an image of a detail, the full view is returned in the top few images. When querying with the full view, the detailed images are ranked low, typically even below a large number of false positives.

2.1 What Is This?

The proposed method builds upon the ideas introduced by Mikulik *et al.* in [18]. We review this work in detail as the zoom-in queries are used. The method [18] is based on the bag-of-words image search engine. In the first step, features are detected and described in the given query image. Posting lists (rows of inverted files) of the query visual words are fetched and images in the dataset scored according to the weighted bag-of-words. The standard tf-idf weighting scheme is used but in addition, visual words scores to the separate bins according to the logarithm of the scale change. A score in a bin is re-weighted linearly to prefer scaling-up (zoom-in) and to suppress scaling-down.

In our experiments, we compressed the scale information of each feature into 4 bits. This allows to separate features into 16 bins. Edges of the bins are learned on the subset of images to equalize the histogram of log scales.

In standard systems the score is evaluated in one go for each document when scalar products are computed between whole posting lists and a query BoW vector. To enable taking into account the scale change, the score of a document is computed during traversing of the inverted file in a *document at a time* (DAAT) manner [27]. A heap of the top S scored images is kept, where S is a chosen length of the shortlist.

Images in the shortlist are spatially verified using RANSAC [6] and incremental spatial verification (iSP) [7], and re-ordered according to the scale of found geometric transformation. This ranking is prone to false positives more than standard ranking – according to number of model inliers. The problem was already mentioned in [18].

3 Efficient Image Detail Mining

This section describes the proposed method in detail. The goal of this paper is to find the finest details for every location in the image and to find regions that are commonly photographed by the crowds. Two issues prevent a simple solution of applying the method described in the previous section to every location in the image: computational efficiency and the risk of high false positive rate.

Algorithm 1. Overview of the zooming algorithm. Note that step 5 represents a trade-off between the query time and output quality.

Input: Bag-of-words of the query image Q
Output: Ranked list of images R

---

1. Fetch posting list of query visual words from inverted file.
2. Score with tf-idf weights and re-weight according to scale change of the features. Create the shortlist.
3. Spatially verify images in the shortlist estimating affine transformation A with RANSAC.
4. Rank images according to $\det(A)$ (descend order).
5. Group images.
6. Return the result or form the expanded query with context learning and goto 1.

3.1 Hierarchical Query Expansion

It has been demonstrated many times that the query expansion technique [1,8] significantly improves the quality of retrieval performance, especially on the recall. We introduce a novel method for detail mining called hierarchical query expansion. After the initial query, the image is divided into sub-regions and a new, expanded, query is issued for each of the sub-regions. The partitioning of the image is driven by the density of the photographed details – the focus of the crowds. Since people tend to take pictures of individual and well aligned objects, regions depicted in a number of overlapping images are good candidates for detail mining. There are three issues that need to be addressed in order to efficiently deliver qualitatively appealing results: image coverage, low redundancy, and consistency.

Image Coverage and Low Redundancy. Typically, on well-known landmarks, certain details are photographed significantly more often than others. Considering only the top results without considering their spatial layout, as most of the query expansion approaches do, would result in neglecting details that are still available in the image collection, but are depicted on a lower number of photographs. In order to obtain details in all parts of the image, lower ranked images that are not overlapping with higher ranked images are considered.

For efficiency, the retrieved images are spatially clustered and large clusters are sub-sampled. Each such cluster provides a simple generative model of a certain part of the image on a higher resolution level than the original query. The clusters are used to issue an expanded zoom-in query, to obtain further details. The procedure can be iterated, however our experiments suggest that a single application of hierarchical query expansion is sufficient to obtain most of the details present in the database.

Consistency. Since in our approach the user does not provide a region of interest, a number of seemingly harmless and uninteresting regions, such as railings in the corner of the image, can expand into enormous number of false positive images. To eliminate such a topic drift, we introduce a novel mechanism to detect and eliminate inconsistencies in the retrieved results. A test is performed as an additional spatial verification between result images to ensure that no false positive will be introduced into any expanded query. In the test, an affine transformation $A_{j,i}$ mapping features from result image i to result image j is obtained. In addition, the mappings $A_{q,i}$ and $A_{q,j}$ to the query image q estimated in the initial retrieval phase are used. For a consistent pair of result images i and j, it holds $A_{q,i} \approx A_{q,j} A_{j,i}$. However, for false positive results caused by repeated patterns or bursty features, the three mappings are typically inconsistent, see Fig. 4.

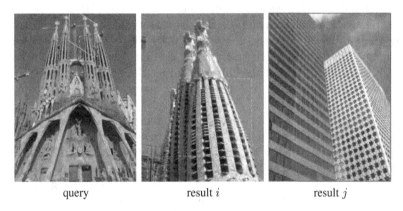

query   result i result j

Fig. 4. The geometric consistency test. The solid parallelogram in the query image denotes the projected image border of result j through the transformation estimated between the query and result j. The dashed parallelogram in the query image is again the border of result j, now transformed by composition of transformations through result image i. The dashed parallelogram in result i is the transformed image boundary from result j.

3.2   Expansion Regions Selection

Images obtained by the zoom-in query (with a minimal scale change of 2) are first filtered by geometric verification against the query image. Only images with at least t_1 inliers are considered. The estimated mapping of the result images to the query is then used to backproject the images. Consequently, the result images are grouped based on location and scale in the query image. Finally, on each group a geometric consistency test is performed, before the expanded queries are issued.

Choice of t_1 Parameter. The number of matching features as a level of confidence of match correctness has been previously used in query expansion techniques [8]. In our case, when a significant change of scale is required, the parameter t_1 can be set much lower than in standard query expansion. It stems from the fact that the number of features exponentially decreases with the scale of the feature – this is caused by the scale dependent non-maxima suppression in the feature detectors. Therefore, the probability of random geometric match is substantially decreased by the requirement of zooming-in. Experimentally, we have found that as little as two consistent features with a query image ($t_1 = 2$) provides acceptable results. Note that this result is in combination with a large vocabulary (16M visual words) and the novel geometric consistency test among the result images. In our experiments, we set $t_1 = 4$.

Result Grouping. A simple greedy algorithm is used to group the result images for the hierarchical query expansion. First, a place (a pixel) in the query image covered by the largest number of images is found. The image with the highest estimated scale change covering that pixel is selected as a cluster seed. Images with at least 50 % overlap with the seed image are included in the cluster. The cluster is removed and the whole procedure is repeated.

Note that unlike in [28], the goal is not to produce an iconic view of the detail, but to group images relevant to that certain detail for the purpose of query expansion. If the size of the cluster is larger than 6 images, the 6 images with the largest scale change are used for the query expansion for efficiency reasons.

Each cluster is subject to a geometric consistency test. First, inliers to the geometric transformation $A_{j,i}$ between image pairs in a cluster are detected. For geometric consistency, at least 50 % of those matches need to be consistent with the composite transformation $A_{j,q}A_{q,i}$.

If a cluster contains only a single image and the consistency test cannot be evaluated, such a cluster is discarded, unless it has at least t_2 geometrically consistent features with the query image and thus small probability of being a false match. In the presented experiments $t_2 = 8$. An example of clusters of geometrically consistent images is shown in Fig. 5.

3.3 Discussion

The proposed method can be seen as a special type of image clustering. In image clustering, false links can be introduced by users inserting visual tags into their images, as depicted in Fig. 6. These links are difficult to detect and complex heuristics are often used. Our approach naturally eliminates such issue, as a large scale change is required, while the tags, no matter how complex, typically have a fixed scale.

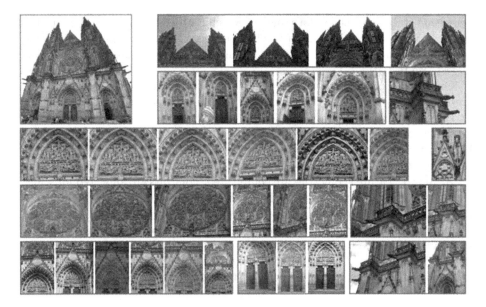

Fig. 5. Groups of spatially verified images selected for further query expansion. The original query is shown in the top-left corner with a blue border (Colour figure online).

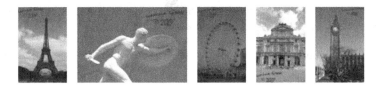

Fig. 6. A common issue for image clustering methods. Totally unrelated scenes linked via a graphical tag superimposed over the images.

4   Experiments

A search engine was built on a dataset of 620,000 images downloaded from Flickr, searching for tags of famous landmarks, European countries and cities, and architectonic keywords.

4.1   Dataset Preparation

Following the common practice in the recent work on image retrieval, multi-scale Hessian-affine features [17] were detected and described by the SIFT descriptor [15].

The hierarchical two level k-means algorithm with approximate nearest neighbor [20] is used to learn a balanced vocabulary with 16 millions visual words [19]. The vocabulary is learned on all 620,000 images (nearly 1.3×10^9 SIFT descriptors). Mikulik *et al.* [19] studied the effect of vocabulary size and showed that increasing it boosts the performance of specific object retrieval and that the speed of tf-idf scoring is increased. The speed is significantly increasing up to 16 million visual words with a negligible increase up to 64 million words (the largest size tested).

One disadvantage of the large vocabularies – that the resulting search trees are unbalanced – has been addressed by the shallow hierarchical tree proposed in [19]. The second disadvantage is the higher computational complexity of building the large vocabulary. The 16 million visual word dictionary is a compromise between the time required for the offline vocabulary building and performance. According to [19], even larger vocabularies would lead to higher performance.

As in [22], feature geometries are compressed. Four bits are allocated for scale and 12 bits for shape compression. The compressed geometries are stored in the inverted file along with the visual words for fast access during DAAT scoring [27].

We have manually annotated results for six different landmarks. As an example of very difficult false positives even for humans, we show a selection of high ranked false positives (Fig. 7) for the Arc de Triomphe query. The false positive images come from the same landmark, just from a different side.

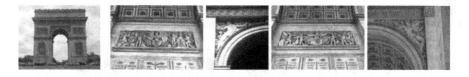

Fig. 7. Some highly ranked false positives for the Arc de Triomphe query (left).

4.2   Scale Change

This experiment shows scale change in the highest ranked images for two different settings. The standard retrieval system and our new method with query expansion, designed for discovering as many details as possible, are compared. As it can be seen from Fig. 8, our method retrieves a large portion of detailed images. Figure 9 shows that retrieved images from our system are more informative than images from standard retrieval.

In case of the Astronomical clock from Fig. 1, the displayed images – local maxima in the resolution, are in our method ranked in the first five in comparison to ranks usually above 5000 in standard retrieval. As the length of the shortlist is limited because of efficiency, these images are not even considered for verification and thus are surrounded by false positives.

4.3   Maximum Scale

Figures 10 and 11 show further examples of very fine details. The maximum scale is typically achieved by images of some interesting detail or eventually by a false match, as shown in Figs. 10 and 11. The false matches are rare and are results of

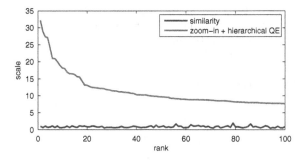

Fig. 8. Scale change for the 100 top scored images. Comparison of the standard nearest neighbor (most similar) and zoom-in with hierarchical query expansion (QE) methods. The query and the first few results are shown in Fig. 9.

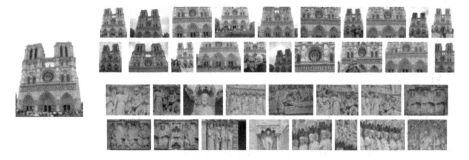

Fig. 9. A comparison of the highest ranked images for two different settings. The query image on the left is used in both cases. The first two rows on the right show top 20 results of the standard nearest neighbor (NN) system optimizing average precision (i.e. similarity). The last two rows show the top 16 images after query expansion of chosen groups of images. Note that while the NN search retrieves many very similar results, the result of our approach is much more informative.

the query expansion. The spatial consistency test is not performed on the final results to reduce the response time.

On the other hand, the frequency distribution is dominated by a relatively small (and thus not interesting) scale change from the query image. Most of such images show people in front of the landmark with a part of the building in the background. The biggest difference between the location of the details and frequently photographed spots is in the Arc de Triomphe, where many people have their photo taken upwards with the arc above them.

Quantitative results are given in Table 1. We summarize results over six different landmark queries. The number of images that were retrieved as details of the landmark showing scale change larger than 3, the value of largest zoom, and the number of false positive images in top 10, 50, and 100 images with largest zoom were recorded. On all landmarks, very fine details were detected with reasonable false positive rates. The three tables compare results for different types of result verification. The most conservative method based on standard spatial verification [24] combined with the proposed geometric consistency of

Table 1. Performance on the six annotated queries with different verification methods. From left to right: query name, the number of retrieved images with zoom larger than 3, the maximum zoom achieved, the number of false positives in top ten, fifty and hundred retrieved images respectively.

Standard spatial verification with the proposed geometric consistency test on groups

Query	NumImgs	MaxZoom	FP@10	FP@50	FP@100
Astronomical clock	2297	37.33	0	1	3
Sacre Cœur	174	16.47	0	6	16
St. Vitus Cathedral	398	32.64	0	3	8
Sagrada Familia	305	20.27	0	0	0
Notre Dame	510	34.84	0	0	0
Arc de Triomphe	444	27.46	1	9	19

iSP [7] with the geometric consistency test on groups

Query	NumImgs	MaxZoom	FP@10	FP@50	FP@100
Astronomical clock	2564	29.25	3	8	18
Sacre Cœur	335	21.85	1	8	20
St. Vitus Cathedral	599	31.16	0	7	14
Sagrada Familia	348	22.92	0	4	6
Notre Dame	625	41.47	0	3	11
Arc de Triomphe	717	28.16	0	18	30

iSP [7] without the geometric consistency test on groups

Query	NumImgs	MaxZoom	FP@10	FP@50	FP@100
Astronomical clock	3210	40.29	2	8	14
Sacre Cœur	623	26.71	1	7	20
St. Vitus Cathedral	651	31.16	0	5	17
Sagrada Familia	474	22.92	0	1	4
Notre Dame	777	41.47	6	22	33
Arc de Triomphe	912	28.17	1	??	45

result groups produces very low false positive rates and the lowest number of retrieved images. With the incremental spatial verification (iSP) [7], the number of false positive images has the tendency to increase. This trend is further pronounced when skipping the group geometric consistency test.

Speed performance of every stage of the proposed algorithm is recorded in Table 2. Importance of the group consistency test stage is additionally amplified looking at these results. Skipping this stage will not significantly decrease total duration of the query but it will noticeably increase the number of false positives in several queries, i.e. in the Notre Dame and the Arc de Triomphe query (as shown in Table 1).

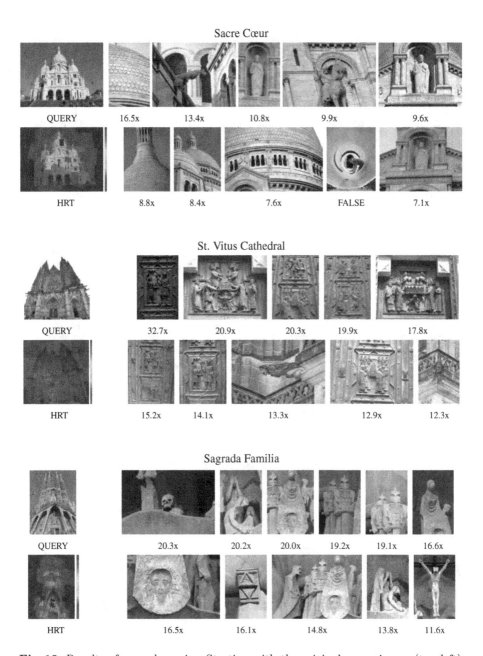

Fig. 10. Results of several queries. Starting with the original query image (top left), the high resolution transform (HRT) (bottom left) is obtained and details are found automatically. The retrieved images (right) with the largest relative scale change (after removal of multiple examples of the same detail).

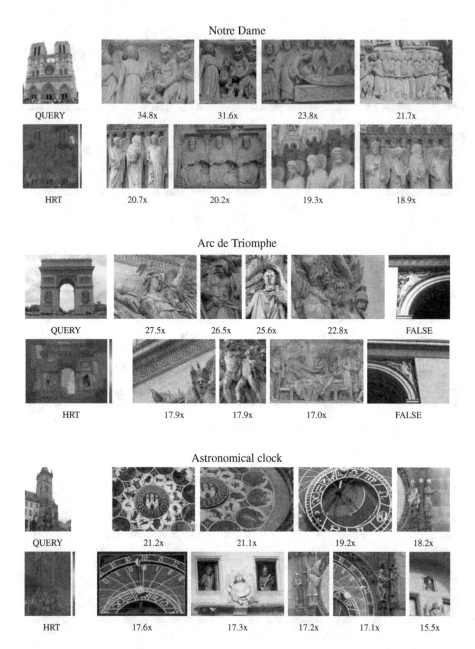

Fig. 11. Results of several queries. Starting with the original query image (top left), the high resolution transform (HRT) (bottom left) is obtained and details are found automatically. The retrieved images (right) with the largest relative scale change (after removal of multiple examples of the same detail). For the Astronomical clock query five images with the largest relative scale change are shown in Fig. 1 (right).

Table 2. Duration of the highest resolution transform (HRT) as a whole and of all the stages on a single 2.6 GHz machine. From left to right: query name, duration of the initial zoom-in query, duration of the grouping stage, duration of the geometric consistency test performed on each group, duration of QE query performed on each group, total duration of the query.

Query	Zoom-in	Grouping	Group SP	hierQE	Total
Astronomical clock	8.2 s	4.8 s	0.6 s	25.0 s	38.5 s
Sacre Cœur	2.9 s	1.1 s	0.2 s	5.1 s	9.3 s
St. Vitus Cathedral	8.3 s	5.5 s	0.7 s	16.7 s	31.2 s
Sagrada Familia	1.6 s	0.5 s	0.1 s	2.8 s	5.0 s
Notre Dame	10.3 s	11.3 s	0.8 s	14.9 s	37.3 s
Arc de Triomphe	4.3 s	2.8 s	0.8 s	13.4 s	21.3 s

5   Conclusions

A pair of novel problems has been formulated: given a query image, for every pixel, find an image with the maximum resolution depicting it and find the most photographed parts of the image. The solution to the problems relies on a hierarchical query expansion that exploits the DAAT inverted files and a new geometric consistency verification step that is sufficiently robust to prevent topic drift.

Experiments show that the false positive rate of the proposed method is well below the level needed for user acceptability and that surprising details on the tested landmarks are found, even those that are hardly noticeable by inspection in the query image. On a single 2.6 GHz machine, the computation of the highest resolution transform takes 5–40 s depending mainly on the number of relevant images.

Acknowledgement. The authors were supported by the MSMT LL1303 ERC-CZ, GACR P103/12/G084, and SGS13/142/OHK3/2T/13 grants.

References

1. Arandjelovic, R., Zisserman, A.: Three things everyone should know to improve object retrieval. In: Proceedings of CVPR, pp. 2911–2918 (2012)
2. Arandjelović, R., Zisserman, A.: All about VLAD. In: Proceedings of CVPR (2013)
3. Bay, H., Tuytelaars, T., Van Gool, L.: SURF: speeded up robust features. In: Leonardis, A., Bischof, H., Pinz, A. (eds.) ECCV 2006, Part I. LNCS, vol. 3951, pp. 404–417. Springer, Heidelberg (2006)
4. Chum, O., Matas, J.: Large-scale discovery of spatially related images. IEEE PAMI **32**(2), 371–377 (2010)
5. Chum, O., Matas, J.: Unsupervised discovery of co-occurrence in sparse high dimensional data. In: Proceedings of CVPR (2010)
6. Chum, O., Matas, J., Kittler, J.: Locally optimized RANSAC. In: Michaelis, B., Krell, G. (eds.) DAGM 2003. LNCS, vol. 2781, pp. 236–243. Springer, Heidelberg (2003)
7. Chum, O., Mikulik, A., Perdoch, M., Matas, J.: Total recall II: query expansion revisited. In: Proceedings of CVPR, pp. 889–896. IEEE Computer Society (2011)

8. Chum, O., Philbin, J., Sivic, J., Isard, M., Zisserman, A.: Total recall: automatic query expansion with a generative feature model for object retrieval. In: Proceedings of ICCV (2007)
9. Jégou, H., Chum, O.: Negative evidences and co-occurences in image retrieval: the benefit of PCA and whitening. In: Fitzgibbon, A., Lazebnik, S., Perona, P., Sato, Y., Schmid, C. (eds.) ECCV 2012. LNCS, pp. 774–787. Springer, Heidelberg (2012)
10. Jégou, H., Douze, M., Schmid, C.: Hamming embedding and weak geometric consistency for large scale image search. In: Forsyth, D., Torr, P., Zisserman, A. (eds.) ECCV 2008. LNCS, vol. 5302, pp. 304–317. Springer, Heidelberg (2008)
11. Jégou, H., Douze, M., Schmid, C.: On the burstiness of visual elements. In: Proceedings of CVPR (2009)
12. Jégou, H., Douze, M., Schmid, C., Pérez, P.: Aggregating local descriptors into a compact image representation. In: Proceedings of CVPR (2010)
13. Jégou, H., Harzallah, H., Schmid, C.: A contextual dissimilarity measure for accurate and efficient image search. In: Proceedings of CVPR (2007)
14. Knopp, J., Sivic, J., Pajdla, T.: Avoiding confusing features in place recognition. In: Daniilidis, K., Maragos, P., Paragios, N. (eds.) ECCV 2010, Part I. LNCS, vol. 6311, pp. 748–761. Springer, Heidelberg (2010)
15. Lowe, D.G.: Distinctive image features from scale-invariant keypoints. Int. J. Comput. Vis. 60(2), 91–110 (2004)
16. Mikolajczyk, K., Schmid, C.: Scale and affine invariant interest point detectors. Int. J. Comput. Vis. 1(60), 63–86 (2004)
17. Mikolajczyk, K., Tuytelaars, T., Schmid, C., Zisserman, A., Matas, J., Schaffalitzky, F., Kadir, T., Van Gool, L.: A comparison of affine region detectors. Int. J. Comput. Vis. 65, 43–72 (2005)
18. Mikulík, A., Chum, O., Matas, J.: Image retrieval for online browsing in large image collections. In: Brisaboa, N., Pedreira, O., Zezula, P. (eds.) SISAP 2013. LNCS, vol. 8199, pp. 3–15. Springer, Heidelberg (2013)
19. Mikulík, A., Perdoch, M., Chum, O., Matas, J.: Learning vocabularies over a fine quantization. Int. J. Comput. Vis. 103(1), 163–175 (2013)
20. Muja, M., Lowe, D.G.: Fast approximate nearest neighbors with automatic algorithm configuration. In: VISSAPP (2009)
21. Nister, D., Stewenius, H.: Scalable recognition with a vocabulary tree. In: Proceedings of CVPR (2006)
22. Perdoch, M., Chum, O., Matas, J.: Efficient representation of local geometry for large scale object retrieval. In: Proceedings of CVPR (2009)
23. Perronnin, F., Liu, Y., Sanchez, J., Poirier, H.: Large-scale image retrieval with compressed fisher vectors. In: Proceedings of CVPR (2010)
24. Philbin, J., Chum, O., Isard, M., Sivic, J., Zisserman, A.: Object retrieval with large vocabularies and fast spatial matching. In: Proceedings of CVPR (2007)
25. Philbin, J., Chum, O., Isard, M., Sivic, J., Zisserman, A.: Lost in quantization: improving particular object retrieval in largescale image databases. In: Proceedings of CVPR (2008)
26. Sivic, J., Zisserman, A.: Video google: a text retrieval approach to object matching in videos. In: Proceedings of ICCV, pp. 1470–1477 (2003)
27. Stewénius, H., Gunderson, S.H., Pilet, J.: Size matters: exhaustive geometric verification for image retrieval. In: Fitzgibbon, A., Lazebnik, S., Perona, P., Sato, Y., Schmid, C. (eds.) ECCV 2012, Part III. LNCS, pp. 693–706. Springer, Heidelberg (2012)
28. Weyand, T., Leibe, B.: Discovering details and scene structure with hierarchical iconoid shift. In: Proceedings of ICCV, IEEE (2013)
29. Winder, S., Hua, G., Brown, M.: Picking the best daisy. In: Proceedings of CVPR (2009)

Accuracy and Specificity Trade-off in k-nearest Neighbors Classification

Luis Herranz$^{(\boxtimes)}$ and Shuqiang Jiang

Key Laboratory of Intelligent Information Processing, Institute of Computing
Technology, Chinese Academy of Sciences, Beijing, China
luis.herranz@vipl.ict.ac.cn

Abstract. The k-NN rule is a simple, flexible and widely used non-parametric decision method, also connected to many problems in image classification and retrieval such as annotation and content-based search. As the number of classes increases and finer classification is considered (e.g. specific dog breed), high accuracy is often not possible in such challenging conditions, resulting in a system that will often suggest a wrong label. However, predicting a broader concept (e.g. dog) is much more reliable, and still useful in practice. Thus, sacrificing certain specificity for a more secure prediction is often desirable. This problem has been recently posed in terms of accuracy-specificity trade-off. In this paper we study the accuracy-specificity trade-off in k-NN classification, evaluating the impact of related techniques (posterior probability estimation and metric learning). Experimental results show that a proper combination of k-NN and metric learning can be very effective and obtain good performance.

1 Introduction

Visual recognition is a basic problem in computer vision, and is a key component in image retrieval and automatic annotation systems. User generated annotations tend to be ambiguous and noisy, and often not representative of the content. In addition, the tagging process is tedious and time consuming, so often users just do not annotate their own content. Automatically classifying and annotating images is thus highly desirable.

Exploiting hierarchical semantic relations between related classes can improve the classification accuracy [1] and can be used to speed up classification [2]. However, the goal of these methods is still to predict a label among the original set of training labels (leaf nodes in the hierarchy).

In practice, when the number of categories becomes larger and the differences between them are more subtle (fine-grained classification), the accuracy is not high, and the suggested label is often not accurate. Recently, Deng et al. [3] proposed a different approach with the objective of trading off accuracy and specificity. When the confidence in a particular SVM prediction is not high enough, hierarchical semantic relations are leveraged to suggest less specific tags,

© Springer International Publishing Switzerland 2015
D. Cremers et al. (Eds.): ACCV 2014, Part II, LNCS 9004, pp. 133–146, 2015.
DOI: 10.1007/978-3-319-16808-1_10

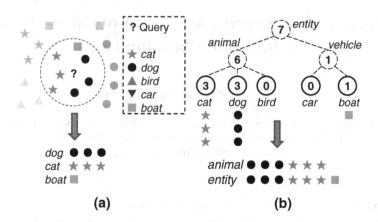

Fig. 1. k-NN classification with semantic hierarchy: (a) votes in flat classification, (b) vote aggregation in broader concepts.

but with higher confidence. Thus, if the prediction of a dog breed is not reliable, perhaps just simply suggest *dog*.

The k-nearest neighbors (k-NN) rule is a widely used non-parametric classification method despite its simplicity. It has the advantage of not requiring training and the capability to easily incorporate new information. The idea is to find the k nearest neighbors training samples to a query feature vector and select the most frequent class. However, this may be difficult in practice when the number of classes increases and becomes more difficult to discriminate between closely related classes, leading to high uncertainty in the prediction (see Fig. 1a). Recently, semantic hierarchies have been used in k-NN classification, in particular to learn tree structured metrics [4], but accuracy-specificity trade-offs in k-NN have not been studied.

In this paper we study the accuracity-specificity trade-off in k-NN classification, by considering voting in internal nodes of the hierarchy (see Fig. 1b). We focus on related techniques, such as metric learning [3,5–7] and posterior probability estimation [8,9]. We include specific analysis and evaluation metrics (semantic similarity, accuracy-specificity F score) to evaluate the performance of the method in the accuracy-specificity framework. The rest of the paper is organized as follows. Section 2 describes the accuracy-specificity framework. In Sect. 3 we describe its extension to k-NN classification. Sections 4 and 5 present the experimental evaluation and the conclusions.

2   The Accuracy-Specificity Framework

In this section we briefly review the specificity-accuracy framework and the Dual Accuracy Reward Trade-off Search (DARTS) algorithm proposed by Deng et al. [3].

2.1 Accuracy and Specificity

In flat classification, only one class is considered correct, so the prediction is either right or wrong. However, in hierarchical classification not only the leaf concept is correct but also the ancestors. The main difference is that broader concepts are easier to predict correctly but at the same time provide less useful information. This can be modeled as a trade-off between accuracy and specificity. We can describe a hierarchy of concepts as a graph $H = (V, E)$, with each node $v \in V$ representing a concept. The leaf nodes $Y \subset V$ are mutually exclusive concepts and form the classes for flat classification. Let $x \in X$ represent a training feature vector and $y \in Y$ the corresponding label. A classifier $\tilde{y} = f(\tilde{x})$ predicts a label $\tilde{y} \in V$ for the test feature vector $\tilde{x}$. Now, evaluating the classifier on a test set, we can obtain the average accuracy as $A(f) = \frac{1}{|S|} \sum_{x \in S} [f(x) \in \pi(y)]$ where $\pi(y)$ represents the set of correct predictions (i.e. those in the path from the correct leaf node to the root node, including y), and $[P]$ is 1 if the statement P is true, otherwise is 0.

In a hierarchy of concepts, several nodes are correct classifications, however we should choose the most informative one, which in our case is the most specific one. Thus, we would prefer *cat* to *entity*, and *Siamese* to *cat*, provided that all of them are correct predictions. A suitable measure is the information gain with respect to predicting the root node [3], measured as $g_v = log_2 |Y| - log_2 \sum_{y \in Y} [v \in \pi(y)]$ which increases from the root node (zero gain) to leaf nodes (maximum gain). We assumed all leaf nodes are equally probable (i.e. uniform prior). Figure 2a shows the corresponding information gain of the semantic hierarchy in Fig. 1b. We can compute the average information gain (of correct predictions) in the classifier f as $G(f) = \frac{1}{|S|} \sum_{x \in S} g_{f(x)} [f(x) \in \pi(Y)]$.

2.2 Making Conservative Predictions

A typical flat classifier does not consider other option than venturing a (fine grained) prediction, no matter whether it is right or wrong. However, sometimes

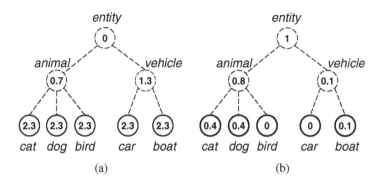

(a)   (b)

Fig. 2. Example of k-NN classification with hierarchical concepts: (a) information gain at each node, (b) estimation of the likelihood in the example in Fig. 1a ($k = 7$).

it is possible to estimate the confidence of the classifier in its prediction, which enables a way to reject the prediction. In the accuracy-specificity framework this can be seen as predicting the root node, when the classifier estimates that the prediction is highly probable to be wrong

$$f(x) = \begin{cases} f(x) & \text{if } p(v|x) \geq \alpha \\ \tilde{v} & \text{otherwise} \end{cases}$$

where $\tilde{v} \in V$, and $0 < \alpha \leq 1$ is an arbitrary minimum accuracy to accept a prediction.

When a full hierarchy is available, intermediate nodes can also be selected, allowing a finer trade-off between accuracy and specificity. In particular, the objective of the DARTS algorithm [3] is to maximize the information gain given a certain accuracy guarantee α

$$\begin{aligned} \text{maximize} \quad & G(f) \\ \text{s.t.} \quad & A(f) \geq \alpha \end{aligned} \tag{1}$$

Using Lagrange multipliers, the constrained optimization problem (1) can be expressed as

$$L(f) = G(f) + \lambda(A(f) - \alpha) \tag{2}$$

and then find the value of λ maximizing the Lagrange function $L(f)$. In the DARTS algorithm, this value is found by estimating posterior probabilities and selecting the node with the maximum expected information gain. For SVMs, Platt scaling [10] is used to estimate probabilities at each node, and the value of λ is found via binary search.

3   Application to k-nearest Neighbors Classification

Including the internal nodes of a hierarchy in k-NN can be done by simply aggregating votes from children nodes (see Fig. 1b). Then the only parameter to be set is k. However, good performance depends on the metric used to measure the distance. To include rejection and trading off accuracy and specificity, we also need to estimate posterior probabilities.

3.1   Estimating Class Probabilities

For a given k and a test image x, we can define its k-nearest neighborhood $\mathcal{N}_k(x)$ as a set with the points in the training set with lower distance to x. For convenience we assume they are ordered by increasing distance. The simplest estimator of the posterior probability k-NN is the fraction of neighbors that belong to that class [8]

$$p(v|x) = \frac{k^{(v)}}{k} = \frac{1}{k} \sum_{u \in \mathcal{N}_k(x)} [u \in v] \tag{3}$$

where $k^{(v)}$ indicates the number of the k-nearest neighbors belonging to the class represented by the node v. Note that this estimator is also valid for internal nodes.

The probability estimator in (3) ignores the distance and the order of the neighbors. We can include weights in (3) to emphasize closer neighbors and estimate the probability as

$$p\left(v|x\right) = \frac{1}{k} \sum_{\substack{i=1 \\ u_i \in \mathcal{N}_k\left(x\right)}}^{k} w_i \left[u_i \in v\right] \tag{4}$$

where u_i represents the i-th nearest neighbor and $w_i \geq 0$ the corresponding weight. The weights are learned using the method proposed by Atiya [9], which uses a softmax representation to model weights and then maximizes the likelihood. We enforce decreasing weights with distance $w_1 \geq \ldots \geq w_i \geq \ldots \geq w_k$ to avoid randomness.

3.2 Metring Learning

The selection of the nearest neighbors depends essentially on the particular metric $d\left(x_i, x_j\right)$ used to evaluate distances. Common used metrics (e.g., such as the Euclidean distance, may not be the most suitable in general. If training data is available, an appropriate metric can be learned to capture the specific characteristics of the feature space.

During the last ten years, automatic metric learning has been intensively studied, resulting in large number of learning methods (see [7] for a recent survey). There is no clear algorithm performing better than others, and sometimes the Euclidean distance still has better performance than a learned metric. Due to the complexity of visual feature spaces, the performance of different methods usually varies significantly from problem to problem, and from dataset to dataset. For that reason, we will consider three widely used metric learning approaches and evaluate them in our case.

Most metric learning methods learn a distance of the form $d_M\left(x_i, x_j\right) = \sqrt{\left(x_i - x_j\right)^T M \left(x_i - x_j\right)}$. The metric is parametrized by the positive semi-definite matrix M, which is usually learned from a regularized convex optimization problem, with constraints representing the relations between pairs of samples. In such pairwise relations, pairs can be reduced to two classes: similar (same label) and dissimilar (different label). In particular the ITML [11] algorithm enforces constants of the type $d_M^2\left(x_i, x_j\right) \leq t_{similar}$ if $y_i = y_j$ for similar pairs (and $d_M^2\left(x_i, x_j\right) \geq t_{dissimilar}$ if $y_i \neq y_j$ for dissimilar pairs). The cost function is the Bregman divergence between M and a target matrix (typically the identity).

In the large margin metric learning (LMNN) framework, the goal is to pull target neighbors (same label) into the k-neighborhood, and push impostors (different label) away. Here, the constraints are relative and local to the neighborhood. Given triplets (x_i, x_j, x_k), the distance to impostors must be larger (with a safety margin) than the distance to target neighbors $(d^2_M (x_i, x_j) \leq d^2_M (x_i, x_k) + 1$, where x_j represents a genuine neighbor of x_i and x_k an impostor. We considered the original LMNN algorithm [5] and BoostMetric [6] which decomposes M in a combination of rank-one matrices which enables fast learning using boosting.

To satisfy the constraints, in practice slack variables are included in the constraints and in the objective function. One problem with these formulations is the polynomial complexity, as the number of constraints grows as $O(n^2)$ in the case of pairwise constraints and as $O(n^3)$ in the case of triplets. In practice, a small subset of these constraints is subsampled to keep a reasonable complexity.

4   Experimental Evaluation

4.1   Dataset and Settings

We evaluated the performance of k-NN classification over the ILSVCR65 dataset and the corresponding semantic hierarchy [3][1]. The dataset contains images of *animals* and *vehicles* further classified in *birds*, *cats* and *dogs*, and *boats* and *cars*, respectively (see Fig. 1b). Note that there is no *mammal* category in this taxonomy, so *birds* are as similar to *cats* and *dogs* as *cats* are to *dogs*. Finally these categories are further classified in 7, 5, 31, 5 and 9 fine-grain categories (57 leaf nodes), respectively. Although leaf nodes are balanced (each flat classifier is trained with the same number of images) the semantic hierarchy is not, resulting in a strong bias towards some parent nodes, such as *animal*, and particularly *dog*. Labels are assigned only at leaf nodes, represented each with 100/50/150 images in the training/validation/test sets.

To represent the images we used the LLC [12] features provided with the dataset. The original features include two spatial pyramid levels (1×1 and 3×3), for a total of 100 K dimensions. As k-NN is not practical in such high dimensional space, we only kept the first level of the spatial pyramid (10K dimensions) and reduced the features to 50 dimensions using PCA.

4.2   Results

In our experiments we study the performance of different accuracy-specificity strategies, including flat k-NN classification (FLAT), flat with rejection (FLAT-REJ) and the DARTS method, evaluated for different values of α. We learned metrics using the LMNN, BoostMetric and ITML algorithms using the implementations provided by their authors[2,3,4]. Due to the large number of samples,

---

[1] The ILSVCR65 dataset, hierarchy and the DARTS source code are available at http://www.image-net.org/projects/hedging/.
[2] http://www.cse.wustl.edu/~kilian/code/lmnn/lmnn.html.
[3] http://code.google.com/p/boosting/.
[4] http://www.cs.utexas.edu/~pjain/itml/.

considering all the possible pairs/triplets constraints is extremely costly, so we sampled a significant number (i.e. still millions of constraints). We used grid search to adjust the corresponding parameters, measuring the k-NN classification accuracy ($k = 20$) in the validation set to prevent overfitting.

The average classification accuracy in the test set is shown in Table 1. We see that, unfortunately, using the metrics learned with LMNN and BoostMetric lead to worse performance than simply using the Euclidean distance. In contrast, the metric learned with ITML improves significantly the accuracy. This may suggest that the large margin framework is not suitable for this particular problem, due to the huge number of triplet constraints, of which only a small fraction are considered in practice. This small fraction (still millions of constraints) may not be large enough to learn a metric properly. Typically, these algorithms are evaluated with very successful results for smaller datasets with relative low dimensional feature spaces and few classes, when all or a significant fraction of triplet constraints can be considered. Our case is more challenging and in practice we had to discard a large amount of triplet constraints to keep the training time reasonable. In contrast, ITML considers pairwise constraints, which scale better with the number of samples and classes, and results in an improved accuracy.

We also measured the semantic similarity between the prediction and the ground truth (leaf node) as [13]

$$s\left(v,y\right) = \frac{\left|\pi'\left(v\right) \bigcap \pi'\left(y\right)\right|}{\max\left(\left|\pi'\left(v\right)\right|, \left|\pi'\left(y\right)\right|\right)}$$

where v is the predicted node, y is the ground truth leaf node and $\pi'\left(v\right)$ indicates the path from v to the root node (excluding v) and $\left|\pi'\left(v\right)\right|$ indicates the length of that path. In contrast to accuracy, that only considers a binary outcome for a test sample (either correct or wrong classification), the semantic similarity gives a graded score which may be a more suitable measure when including internal nodes as predictions (e.g. a *dog* should be more similar to a *cat* than to a *boat*, because both are *animals*). In fact, the flat classification accuracy of SVM[5] is higher than k-NN with ITML, but the semantic similarity is lower, and as we will see this is related with a poorer accuracy-specificity performance. This suggest that, after metric learning, the feature space is structured in a more semantically meaningful way, in which leaf node misclassifications are likely to be predicted as a still relatively similar leaf node class. In contrast, SVM does not change the structure of the feature space but finds nonlinear decision boundaries. Thus the accuracy may be higher, but misclassifications tend to be less related semantically to the true class than in k-NN with metric learning.

The corresponding accuracy-specificity curves were obtained varying the value of α, from 0 to 0.99 (note that FLAT-REJ with $\alpha = 0$ corresponds to the flat classifier). Specificity is measured as normalized information gain. Figure 3

---

[5] In [3] SVM achieves higher classification accuracy using spatial pyramid and 100K-dim features, in contrast to the 50-dim features (no spatial pyramid) used in our experiments.

Table 1. Flat classification results.

Evaluation metric	k-NN				SVM
	Euclidean	LMNN	BoostMetric	ITML	
Accuracy (%)	18.02	16.34	9.87	21.19	**24.01**
Semantic similarity(%)	60.94	59.79	54.15	**64.16**	62.01

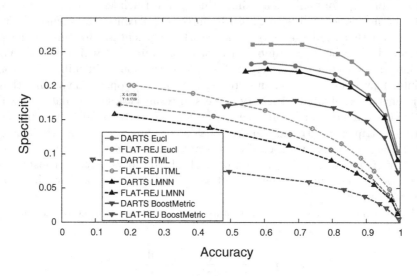

Fig. 3. Effect of metric learning over the accuracy-specificity curve ($k = 30$).

shows the curves for different decision, metric learning methods and $k = 30$. We can observe that, in terms of accuracy-specificity trade-off, DARTS consistently outperforms FLAT-REJ, increasing the accuracy and still keeping a higher average specificity. In addition, an appropriate metric improves significantly the performance, not only in flat k-NN classification (compare Table 1) but also in accuracy-specificity curves.

As shown in Fig. 4, the choice of the method used to estimate posterior probabilities is not so critical. We also compare the curves for several values of k, with larger neighborhoods performing better (we show more results later). Interestingly, Atiya's method [9] improves slightly the performance for large neighborhoods, while not being useful in smaller ones.

In order to further study the effect of the parameter k in the performance, we also use a variation of the F-score to evaluate the accuracy-specificity performance

$$F(f) = \max_{\lambda \in [0,1)} \left(\frac{2\,A\,(f_\lambda)\,G\,(f_\lambda)}{A\,(f_\lambda) + G\,(f_\lambda)} \right)$$

where f_λ is the classifier that maximizes (2) for λ. As mentioned earlier, small neighborhoods are not suitable in this problem. The size of the neighborhood

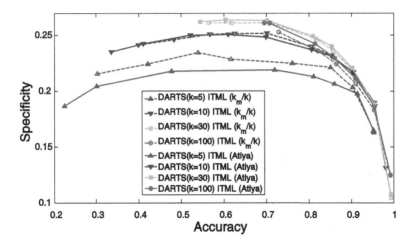

Fig. 4. Effect of the probability estimation method over the accuracy-specificity curve.

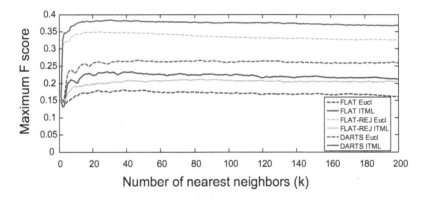

Fig. 5. Best accuracy-specificity F score for different k.

trades off accuracy in the estimation and locality. A more accurate estimation of the posterior probability requires more neighbors, but then the neighborhood in the feature space is more spread, leading to less localized prediction. The accuracy-specificity F score is a compact way to compare different methods (see Fig. 5, using Atiya's estimator) and their dependency with k. First, we can see that the performance gain of both DARTS and metric learning over the flat classifiers and the Euclidean distance is consistent and very robust to the particular choice of k. Actually, for neighborhoods large enough (say $k \geq 20$) F scores are almost constant. For smaller values the performance decreases significantly. We can also observe a slow but steady decay in the performance due to a less localized prediction. For that reason we set $k = 30$ in the remaining experiments.

Finally, Fig. 6 compares the performance of DARTS with SVM classification and DARTS with k-NN. The performance of SVM is comparable to k-NN with Euclidean distance. Note that in this variation there is no training at all if we

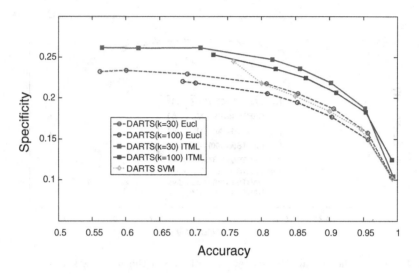

Fig. 6. Comparison of k-NN and SVM approaches.

use (3) to estimate posterior probabilities. Using ITML k-NN outperforms SVM for this feature space. As we mentioned earlier, a better metric not only helps to increase the flat accuracy, but also helps to structure the feature space in such a way that semantic relations are better preserved. The resulting nearest neighbors are also more semantically related, which provides a better way to estimate the posterior probability at different levels of the hierarchy, so the DARTS method can make better decisions. As we discussed earlier, the average semantic similarity of predictions in the flat classifier is a good indicator of how suitable the feature space is for this framework.

Figure 7 shows the fraction of predictions and their associated information gain (or predicted incorrectly). The flat classifier always ventures a prediction so the amount of both correct and incorrect is relatively high. With a rejection option, many wrong predictions are rejected and labeled as *entity* (root node) but also some correct predictions. DARTS further reduces the amount of very specific correct predictions, and keeps a similar rate of wrong predictions as FLAT-REJ. However, the amount of predictions assigned to the root node is reduced considerably, and they are assigned to more specific intermediate nodes, which is more useful. Higher values of α reduce the number of wrong predictions but also increase the number of uncertain predictions (i.e. *entity*) and also reduce the number of correct predictions with highest specificity.

Figure 8 shows some examples of how wrong predictions in the flat classifier can be recovered as less specific labels, but still more useful than a wrong prediction. FLAT-REJ can sometimes anticipate a wrong prediction but predicts it as *entity*. In contrast, DARTS provides more specific labels. Some examples of the k-nearest neighbors for specific images are shown in Fig. 9. Although neighbors of the same class are not as many as desirable, the selected neighbors often

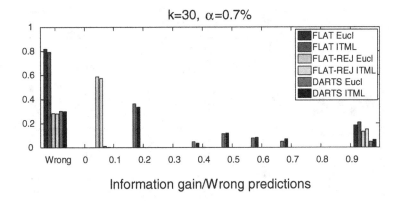

Fig. 7. Information gain and wrong predictions.

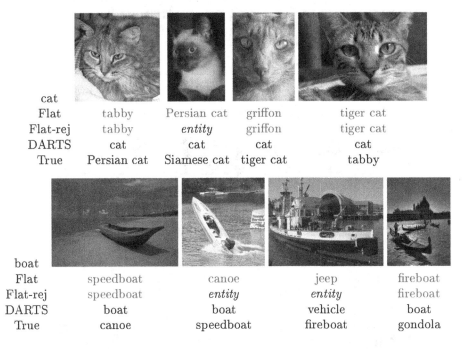

Fig. 8. Examples of wrong predictions in flat classification recovered to less specific but correct predictions ($k = 30$, $\alpha = 0.7$). Rejected cases in FLAT-REJ are labeled as *entity* (non-informative).

belong to related superclasses (e.g. *dog*, *car*), so it seems reasonable to use them to infer a useful label.

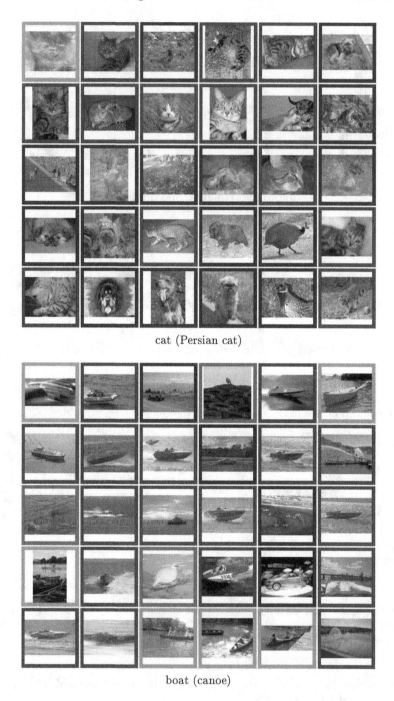

cat (Persian cat)

boat (canoe)

Fig. 9. Nearest neighbors (by increasing distance) to the first image of each broad category in Fig. 8. Green (red) frames indicate the level of semantic similarity (dissimilarity) (Color figure online).

5   Conclusion

The k-NN framework is simple but powerful. It can achieve very competitive performance, and even outperform SVM using the same features. As a non-parametric method, it can incorporate new samples to the model without need for retraining (other than metric learning and/or weights in (4) if desired to update them, but not strictly necessary).

We observed that the structure of the feature space after metric learning reflects a more suitable structure to deal with flat misclassifications, which is exploited in k-NN classification to effectively trade off accuracy and specificity. This results in even better accuracity-specificity trade-off than classifiers with higher flat classification accuracy, such as SVM. In this case, semantic similarity is more suitable than flat accuracy to measure the performance. We also noticed that a wrong choice of metric learning method may result in disappointing results, particularly in the experiments performed with methods using triplet constraints.

Experiments show promising results with relatively low dimensionality (50 dimensions). SVM can still achieve better performance resorting to very high dimensional features (100 K dimensions) [3]. In future work we would like to target larger scale datasets and also higher dimensional features. However, scalability in k-NN classification is the main obstacle, so approximate search methods and structures may be necessary. Search in very high dimensional features spaces is also very demanding. Moreover, current metric learning methods do not scale well either, due to the use of paiwise and triplet constraints. Thus, further fundamental research in k-NN classification tools and metric learning methods seems necessary to make it practical for larger datasets and higher dimensional spaces.

Acknowledgement. This work was supported in part by the National Natural Science Foundation of China: 61322212, 61035001 and 61350110237, in part by the Key Technologies R&D Program of China: 2012BAH18B02, in part by National Hi-Tech Development Program (863 Program) of China: 2014AA015202, and in part by the Chinese Academy of Sciences Fellowships for Young International Scientists: 2011Y1GB05.

References

1. Fergus, R., Bernal, H., Weiss, Y., Torralba, A.: Semantic label sharing for learning with many categories. In: Daniilidis, K., Maragos, P., Paragios, N. (eds.) ECCV 2010, Part I. LNCS, vol. 6311, pp. 762–775. Springer, Heidelberg (2010)
2. Griffin, G., Perona, P.: Learning and using taxonomies for fast visual categorization. In: CVPR (2008)
3. Deng, J., Krause, J., Berg, A.C., Li, F.F.: Hedging your bets: optimizing accuracy-specificity trade-offs in large scale visual recognition. In: CVPR, pp. 3450–3457 (2012)
4. Hwang, S.J., Grauman, K., Sha, F.: Learning a tree of metrics with disjoint visual features. In: NIPS, pp. 621–629 (2011)

5. Weinberger, K.Q., Saul, L.K.: Distance metric learning for large margin nearest neighbor classification. JMLR **10**, 207–244 (2009)
6. Shen, C., Kim, J., Wang, L., van den Hengel, A.: Positive semidefinite metric learning using boosting-like algorithms. JMLR **13**, 1007–1036 (2012)
7. Kulis, B.: Metric learning: a survey. Found. Trends Mach. Learn. **5**, 287–364 (2013)
8. Fukunaga, K., Hostetler, L.: k-nearest-neighbor bayes-risk estimation. IEEE Trans. Inform. Theory **21**, 285–293 (1975)
9. Atiya, A.F.: Estimating the posterior probabilities using the k-nearest neighbor rule. Neural Comput. **17**, 731–740 (2005)
10. Platt, J.: Probabilistic outputs for support vector machines and comparison to regularized likelihood methods. In: Smola, A.J., Bartlett, P., Scholkopf, B., Schuurmans, D. (eds.) Advances in Large Margin Classifiers, pp. 61–74. MIT Press, Cambridge (1999)
11. Davis, J.V., Kulis, B., Jain, P., Sra, S., Dhillon, I.S.: Information-theoretic metric learning. In: ITML, pp. 209–216 (2007)
12. Wang, J., Yang, J., Yu, K., Lv, F., Huang, T.S., Gong, Y.: Locality-constrained linear coding for image classification. In: CVPR, pp. 3360–3367 (2010)
13. Budanitsky, A., Hirst, G.: Evaluating wordnet-based measures of lexical semantic relatedness. Comput. Linguist. **32**, 13–47 (2006)

Multi-view Point Cloud Registration Using Affine Shape Distributions

Jia Du$^{(\boxtimes)}$, Wei Xiong, Wenyu Chen, Jierong Cheng, Yue Wang,
Ying Gu, and Shue-Ching Chia

Visual Computing Department, Institute for Infocomm Research,
Singapore, Singapore
{duj,wxiong,chenw,chengjr,ywang,guy,scchia}@i2r.a-star.edu.sg

Abstract. Registration is crucial for the reconstruction of multi-view single plane illumination microscopy. By using fluorescent beads as fiduciary markers, this registration problem can be reduced to the problem of point clouds registration. We present a novel method for registering point clouds across views. This is based on a new local geometric descriptor - affine shape distribution - to represent the random spatial pattern of each point and its neighbourhood. To enhance its robustness and discriminative power against the missing data and outliers, a permutation and voting scheme based on affine shape distributions is developed to establish putative correspondence pairs across views. The underlying affine transformations are estimated based on the putative correspondence pairs via the random sample consensus. The proposed method is evaluated on three types of datasets including 3D random points, benchmark datasets and datasets from multi-view microscopy. Experiments show that the proposed method outperforms the state-of-the-arts when both point sets are contaminated by extremely large amount of outliers. Its robustness against the anisotropic z-stretching is also demonstrated in the registration of multi-view microscopy data.

1 Introduction

With recent advances in multi-view single plane illumination microscopy (multi-view SPIM) [1–5], high resolution in vivo volume images for relatively large biological specimens can be obtained by fusing the volume images from multiple views into a single volume. Registration is an essential step to align the volume images across views into one common coordinate system before information fusion. The state-of-the-arts, the bead-based registration [3,6], use fluorescent beads embedded in the mounting medium around the sample, which allows for accurate and sample-independent reconstruction. By considering the beads as fiduciary markers, the registration for multi-view SPIM can be reduced to the problem of point cloud registration.

The bead-based registration for multi-view SPIM brings new challenges to the field of point cloud registration. We use a simple example to illustrate the main challenges of this ill-posed problem, as shown in Fig. 1. Firstly, no presuming geometries or distinctive image features can be used to establish the

© Springer International Publishing Switzerland 2015
D. Cremers et al. (Eds.): ACCV 2014, Part II, LNCS 9004, pp. 147–161, 2015.
DOI: 10.1007/978-3-319-16808-1_11

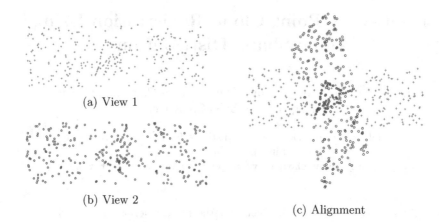

(a) View 1

(b) View 2

(c) Alignment

Fig. 1. Point cloud registration for multi-view SPIM. For the point clouds from two views, there exists a common but unknown spatial point patterns (the contour of a fish) as shown in Panels (a) and (b). The underlying spatial transformation between views is affine. As shown in Panel (c), the proposed method aims to detect the points of correspondence and solve for the underlying transformation in the present of an extremely large amount of outliers and missing data in both point clouds.

correspondence pairs of points between views since beads are randomly distributed in the medium without texture information. In addition, there exist optical distortions such as the anisotropic z-stretching of each view introduced by the differential refraction index mismatch between water and the mounting medium [3]. Thus, the underlying spatial transformation between views is affine, rather than rigid. Most importantly, the common point patterns across views are contaminated by an extremely large amount of outliers (up to 90 % of thousands of points) due to the imaging setting of the SPIM: beads can be observed only in the illuminated region under each view, and the overlaps between illuminated regions across views are small. The opacity of samples and light scattering also give rise to missing correspondence in the overlapping region.

Our method tries to overcome the above challenges. We first propose a local geometric descriptor: affine shape distribution. The descriptor represents the affine invariant shapes for local point patterns between views and also takes into account the positional uncertainty of each point. To address the outliers or missing data within the local constellation of each point, a permutation and voting scheme based on affine shape distributions is introduced to enhance its robustness and discriminative power against the missing data and outliers. The common patterns preserved across views are identified by matching the entries of affine shape distribution among all possible combinations of neighbouring points. Next, the difference between affine shape distributions is measured by the Fréchet distance, which allows us to represent each distribution as a high-dimensional vector in Euclidean space. Therefore, a hierarchical tree-based algorithm with logarithmic complexity is used to efficiently search for the putative matching pairs across views among hundreds of thousands of entries due to the highly combinatorial nature of this problem. The underlying affine transformation is estimated based on the putative correspondence pairs via the random sample consensus [7]. Finally, the proposed method is evaluated under different parameter settings and compared against the state-of-the-arts on both the benchmark datasets for point cloud matching and real datasets from multi-view SPIM.

2   Related Works

Point cloud registration is a fundamental yet challenging task in many areas such as computer vision, robotics and autonomous systems and medical image analysis to name but a few (see e.g., [8–10] for comprehensive reviews). Based on the optimization strategies, they can be separated into two main categories.

The methods in the first category employ an objective function, a closed form expression to measure the dissimilarity between the aligned point sets under the tentative transformation. The correspondence detection and transformation estimation is conducted iteratively during the minimization of the objective function. The iterative closest point (ICP) [11] method is one of most well-known algorithm to iteratively find point correspondence based on the nearest neighbour relationship and update the transformations. However, ICP is prone to being trapped in local minima, especially under bad initial alignments. To address this problem, the robust point matching (RPM) [12] relaxes point correspondence to be continuously valued and employs deterministic annealing for optimization. The coherent point draft (CPD) [13] method uses one point set to represent the Gaussian mixture model and converts point matching into the problem of fitting the model to another point set. Similarly, the robust point set matching uses Gaussian mixture model (RPM-GMM) [14] to minimize the distance between two mixtures of Gaussian representing two point sets. Despite their success in many applications, those approaches tend to degrade badly if the proportion of outliers in the point sets become large [15].

Another popular strategy is to use a two-stage process. In the first stage, a set of putative correspondences are computed by using a feature-descriptor distance to reduce the set of possible matches. The second stage is designed to remove the outliers in the correspondence set and estimate the transformation, where a standard procedure to enforce the global geometric consistency of the correspondence is RANSAC [7]. Notably, the first stage is crucial to the success of those methods. If discriminative features (e.g., SIFT [16]) are used, the correspondence detection problem can be greatly alleviated. For problems where the features are non-discriminative, it is pairwise geometric information that helps in finding the right correspondence. The 4-points congruent sets method (4PCs) [17] matches the pairs of widely separated 4 points within the same plane. Spin images [18] compute 2D histograms of points falling within a cylindrical volume by means of a plane spins around the normal of its underlying surface. 3D shape context [19] generalizes the basic idea of spin images by accumulating

3D histograms of points within a sphere centered at the feature point. However, the needs to find the particular geometry such as coplanar four points for 4PCs or the normal of their underlying surface for 3D shape context make them unsuitable for our problem. The most related to our work is the bead-based registration in Fiji-Plugin [3], where the author introduces a translation and rotation invariant local geometric descriptor by representing each point as a vector in the six-dimensional descriptor space. The vector was determined by the unique constellation of its four neighbouring points and similar descriptors in different views had a small Euclidean distance. The drawback of this descriptor is its sensitivity to selection of the neighbourhood of individual points under different local spatial density of the points. To address this problem, a rotation invariant local feature is proposed using group integration [6]. However, neither descriptors takes into account outliers or missing data within the local constellation of individual constituent points and their descriptors are not affine-invariant.

Belonging to the second category, our approach addresses the limitations of the state-of-the-arts, the bead-based registration in Fiji-Plugin [3] and can achieve good results in difficult data. The contributions of the proposed method include:

1. a novel local geometric descriptor, i.e., affine shape distribution, which represents the affine invariant shape for local point patterns together with its positional uncertainty;
2. a permutation and voting scheme, which enhances robustness and discriminative power of affine shape distributions against the outliers or missing data within the local constellation of each point;
3. an efficient search scheme for the putative matching pairs using a hierarchical tree-based algorithm allowing for fast and precise point cloud registration.

3   Methodology

In this section, we first define an representation for the local spatial pattern of one point together with its neighbours, named as affine shape. Next, the probability distributions of the affine shape are derived from their positional uncertainty. Finally, we introduce a complete algorithm to establish the putative correspondence based on affine shape distributions and estimate the underlying spatial transformation between the random point sets of two views.

3.1   Affine Shape for Local Point Patterns

Let's have one point $\mathbf{p} \in \mathbb{R}^d$ and its k neighbours, $\mathbf{p}_1, \mathbf{p}_2, ..., \mathbf{p}_k$, where k is the minimum number of points required to define a canonical frame that is invariant to affine transformations. In other word, k points form a simplex to define an affine basis. (e.g., $k = 3$ in two dimensional case and $k = 4$ in three dimensional case).

Given a point $\mathbf{p}$ and its k neighbours with an arbitrary order, an affine invariant labelling for its k neighbours can first be performed based on their affine invariant coefficients. Assume $\mathbf{p}_1, \mathbf{p}_2, ..., \mathbf{p}_k$ is not degenerate, point $\mathbf{p}$ can be represented by a weighted linear combination of its k neighbours. Here $\mathbf{p} = \sum_{i=1}^{k} w_i \mathbf{p}_i = [\mathbf{p}_1, \mathbf{p}_2, ..., \mathbf{p}_k]\mathbf{w}$, with $\sum_{i=1}^{k} w_i = 1$. The coefficients, w_i, are known to be invariant to any affine transformation applied to the point set. We can rearrange the order of those points by sorting their corresponding $|w_i|$ in ascending order. Given any selected point $\mathbf{p}$, this rearrangement allows for an affine invariant labelling for its neighbours and thus avoids the need for the calculation of all the possible permutations of its k neighbours. In the rest of this paper, we consider the points $\mathbf{p}_1, \mathbf{p}_2, ..., \mathbf{p}_k$ arranged in such a way, with $\mathbf{p}_k$ according to the point with the largest $|w_i|$.

Given one point $\mathbf{p}$ with its k neighbours, $\mathbf{p}_1, \mathbf{p}_2, ..., \mathbf{p}_k$, as labelled above, we show that the shape of the $k + 1$ points can be represented as a point at standardized Euclidean shape space [20], Ω, which is a subspace of $\mathbb{R}^d$. Let's take the three dimensional case ($k = 4$) for instance. We first choose one point, say $\mathbf{p}_4$, as the local frame origin. Then, a matrix, $A = [\mathbf{p}_1 - \mathbf{p}_4, \mathbf{p}_2 - \mathbf{p}_4, \mathbf{p}_3 - \mathbf{p}_4]$, can be defined by subtracting the origin, $\mathbf{p}_4$, from the other points. Similarly, we subtract the selected point, $\mathbf{p}$, by the origin and denote $\mathbf{p}_t = \mathbf{p} - \mathbf{p}_4$. We now consider the inverse mapping of A, A^{-1}, which transforms the three points, $\mathbf{p}_1$, $\mathbf{p}_2$, $\mathbf{p}_3$, to the points with unit length on x, y and z axes respectively. By applying the mapping to the selected point in the local frame, $\mathbf{p}_t$, we get a vector, $\mathbf{q} \in \Omega$, at standardized Euclidean shape space as

$$\mathbf{q} = [\mathbf{p}_1 - \mathbf{p}_4, \mathbf{p}_2 - \mathbf{p}_4, \mathbf{p}_3 - \mathbf{p}_4]^{-1} \cdot (\mathbf{p} - \mathbf{p}_4) = A^{-1}\mathbf{p}_t. \tag{1}$$

Note that the vector, $\mathbf{q}$, encodes the affine invariant spatial patterns of those five points ($\mathbf{p}$ and $\mathbf{p}_{1,2,3,4}$) and serves as a descriptor for the local point pattern. Thus, we refer to $\mathbf{q}$ as the affine shape of these $(k + 1)$ points.

3.2 Affine Shape Distribution

We now address the problem of inherent uncertainty of observed points. There are two sources of uncertainty in the resulting affine shape representations. One comes from the uncertainty of the observed point $\mathbf{p}$ itself, while another stems from the variability of the affine basis.

Let's consider that the position of each point $\mathbf{p}$ is a random variable following a Gaussian distribution function with mean $\bar{\mathbf{p}}$ and covariance matrix $\Sigma_\mathbf{p} \in \mathbb{R}^{d \times d}$. If we assume the affine basis have no variability, the affine shape, $\mathbf{q}$, also follows a Gaussian distribution function with mean $\bar{\mathbf{q}} = A^{-1}\bar{\mathbf{p}}$ and covariance matrix $\Sigma_\mathbf{q} = A^{-1}\Sigma_\mathbf{p}A^{-\top}$.

To consider the uncertainty of the points used to define the affine basis, we make use of the following classic theorem [21].

Proposition 1 (Uncertainty Propagation). *Let v be a random vector in $\mathbb{R}^d$ with mean $\bar{v}$ and covariance matrix Σ, and $f : \mathbb{R}^d \to \mathbb{R}^{d'}$ be an affine map. Then $f(v)$ is a random vector in $\mathbb{R}^{d'}$ with mean $f(\bar{v})$ and covariance matrix $J\Sigma J^\top$, where J is the Jocabian matrix of f at point $\bar{v}$.*

For the three dimensional case, given 4 points as a simplex, we can calculate its affine matrix, A, from Eq. (1). The Jacobian matrix of A for each entry of the 4 points is equal to

$$\frac{\partial vec(A)}{\partial vec(\mathbf{p}_{1,2,3,4})} = \begin{bmatrix} I_3 & 0 & 0 & -I_3 \\ 0 & I_3 & 0 & -I_3 \\ 0 & 0 & I_3 & -I_3 \end{bmatrix}, \tag{2}$$

where 0 is a 3×3 all-zero matrix and I_3 is a 3×3 identity matrix. Differentiating $AA^{-1} = I_3$, we obtain that $d(A^{-1}) = -A^{-1}dAA^{-1}$. Using the Kronecker product $\otimes$, it can be rewritten as $vec(d(A^{-1})) = -(A^{-\top} \otimes A^{-1})vec(dA)$. Thus, we can calculate the Jacobian of A^{-1} at A with respect to the 4 points, as follows

$$J = \frac{\partial vec(A^{-1})}{\partial vec(\mathbf{p}_{1,2,3,4})} = -(A^{-\top} \otimes A^{-1}) \frac{\partial vec(A)}{\partial vec(\mathbf{p}_{1,2,3,4})}. \tag{3}$$

Following the Proposition 1, we get

$$\Sigma_{A^{-1}} = J \cdot \text{diag}\left(\Sigma_{\mathbf{p}_1}, \Sigma_{\mathbf{p}_2}, \Sigma_{\mathbf{p}_3}, \Sigma_{\mathbf{p}_4}\right) \cdot J^\top, \tag{4}$$

where $\text{diag}\left(\Sigma_{\mathbf{p}_1}, \Sigma_{\mathbf{p}_2}, \Sigma_{\mathbf{p}_3}, \Sigma_{\mathbf{p}_4}\right)$ denotes the block-diagonal matrix of size 12×12 with block matrices $\Sigma_{\mathbf{p}_1}, \Sigma_{\mathbf{p}_2}, \Sigma_{\mathbf{p}_3}, \Sigma_{\mathbf{p}_4}$ on its diagonal. Note that we consider the position variation of each point is independent on each other.

Based on Eq. (1), we can naturally get $\Sigma_{\mathbf{p}_t} = \Sigma_{\mathbf{p}} + \Sigma_{\mathbf{p}_4}$ for $\mathbf{p}_t$. Again, by using the Proposition 1, the complete $\Sigma_{\mathbf{q}}$ considering the variation in all the points can be given as

$$\Sigma_{\mathbf{q}} = L\Sigma_{A^{-1}}L^\top + A^{-1}\Sigma_{\mathbf{p}_t}A^{-\top}, \tag{5}$$

where $L = [\text{diag}(\mathbf{p}_t) \ \text{diag}(\mathbf{p}_t) \ \text{diag}(\mathbf{p}_t)]$ is a 3×9 block matrix with 3 identical 3×3 blocks.

It is worth noting that the probabilistic distribution of affine shape is invariant to rotation and translation. In addition, its mean, $\bar{\mathbf{q}}$, is equal to the affine invariant coefficients, while its covariance matrix, $\Sigma_{\mathbf{q}}$, encodes the information related to the affine bases and uncertainties of the points. In the rest of this paper, we refer this probabilistic distribution of affine shape as affine shape distribution.

3.3   Fréchet Distance for Affine Shape Distributions

To measure the difference between two affine shape distributions, we adopt Fréchet distance between multivariate normal distributions [22] as

$$\text{dist}\left(\mathcal{N}(\bar{\mathbf{q}}_1, \Sigma_{\mathbf{q}_1}), \mathcal{N}(\bar{\mathbf{q}}_2, \Sigma_{\mathbf{q}_2})\right) = |\bar{\mathbf{q}}_1 - \bar{\mathbf{q}}_2|^2 + \text{tr}\left[\Sigma_{\mathbf{q}_1} + \Sigma_{\mathbf{q}_2} - 2(\Sigma_{\mathbf{q}_1}\Sigma_{\mathbf{q}_2})^{\frac{1}{2}}\right], \tag{6}$$

where $\text{tr}(\cdot)$ stands for the trace of a matrix and $|\cdot|$ is L^2 norm in vector space. Noting that the first term measures the Euclidean distance between two affine-invariant coefficients in the space of Ω. The second term accounts for the difference between the non-rigid parts (skewing and anisotropic scaling) of two underlying affine transformations and the positional uncertainties of all the points.

3.4   Point Cloud Matching Using Affine Shape Distributions

A robust point matching has to satisfy two requirements: the stability and the discrimination power. The stability means, given the constellation of a point and its m neighbours in one view, the corresponding pattern of one point together with its m neighbours can also be found in another view. However, it is not easy to find such correspondent pairs of patterns. Affine transformation may change the Euclidean distance between points, and thus changes the members of neighbourhood of one point selected by nearest neighbours searching. The constellation of local point patterns can also be contaminated by the unexpected occlusion and outliers occurred in the local neighbourhood for the given point. Therefore, given any point, we need to consider a larger neighbourhood by including its nearest n neighbours, where $n > m$. Then, all possible combinations of m points from n nearest points should be examined. As long as at least one combination of m points is common, a stable feature for matching of point patterns can be established.

The discrimination power ensures that different point patterns in one view should match their respective patterns in another view. However, it is often not the case since similar affine shape distributions can be obtained from other different spatial pattern of points. To increase the discrimination power, we have to consider the case when $m > k$ and assume there exist at least $\binom{m}{k}$ common combinations of k points out of $\binom{n}{k}$ possible combinations from the n nearest points. To enforce this constraint, a voting system is introduced to establish a matching between two point patterns in different views only when there exist at least $\binom{m}{k}$ pairs of similar entries of affine shape distributions between their corresponding local neighbourhoods.

Algorithm 1. affine shape distribution generation for point matching

---

Input   : a random point set P with N number of points
Output: affine shape distributions with $\binom{n}{k} \cdot N$ number of entries
1 **for** *each point* **p** *in P* **do**
2   **for** *each combination of its k points out its n nearest neighbours* **do**
3   Calculate the mean $\bar{\mathbf{q}}$ via Eq. (1)
4   Estimate the covariance matrix $\Sigma_{\mathbf{q}}$ via Eq. (5)

Given a random point set, all the entries of its affine shape distributions can be calculated as detailed in Algorithm 1. The next step is to establish the putative correspondence pairs between those entries of two point sets. Due to the highly combinatorial nature of this problem, there is a need for speeding up the search for potential matching pairs among the huge amount of entries for affine shape distributions. Inspired by the ideas in [22], we transform the covariance matrix of each affine shape distributions into a diagonal matrix. As discussed in the work [23], under the commutative case, the calculation of the Fréchet distance between two affine shape distributions in Eq. (6) can be simplified as

$$\text{dist}\left(\mathcal{N}(\bar{\mathbf{q}}_1, \Sigma_{\mathbf{q}_1}), \mathcal{N}(\bar{\mathbf{q}}_2, \Sigma_{\mathbf{q}_2})\right) = |\bar{\mathbf{q}}_1 - \bar{\mathbf{q}}_2|^2 + \left| vec(\Sigma_{\mathbf{q}_1}^{\frac{1}{2}}) - vec(\Sigma_{\mathbf{q}_2}^{\frac{1}{2}}) \right|^2. \quad (7)$$

Note that each affine shape distribution can be represented by a vector in a feature space with L^2 norm. Therefore, for each entry of affine shape distribution, we employ a KD-tree to search for its nearest neighbours as potential matching pairs in this high dimensional vector space. The complete algorithm for random point matching based on affine shape distributions is summarized in Algorithm 2.

Algorithm 2. robust point matching based on affine shape distributions

---

    Input   : two random point sets X and Y related by an underlying affine
             transformation
    Output: a set of putative correspondence pairs and an estimated affine
             transformation
1 Calculate the affine shape distributions for X and Y using Algorithm 1
2 **for** *each entries of the distributions of X* **do**
3   Search for its nearest neighbour in the entries of Y based on Eq. (7)
4   Add one vote for the pair of points based on the matching of their entries
5 **for** *each pairs of points* **do**
6   Keep the pairs of points with the number of votes greater or equal than $\binom{m}{k}$
        as putative correspondence between X and Y
7 Estimate the underlying affine transformation based on the putative
  correspondence via RANSAC [7]

---

4 Results

4.1 Experiments on Synthetic 3D Random Points

In this experiment, we evaluate the performance of the proposed method under different parameter settings. To generate data sets of 3D random points, we first generate 100 points randomly distributed in a $100 \times 100 \times 100$ space as inliers of one view. We obtain the corresponding inliers in another view by transforming those points using an random affine transformation and independently adding Gaussian positional jitter, $\mathcal{N}(0, \sigma^2 I_3)$, to each point. Next, we add outliers randomly into the surrendering regions of the inliers for both views. For each trial, we compare the ground truth with the putative correspondences detected by the proposed method before further refinement via RANSAC. Their precision and recall ratios are recorded for 100 random trials. Three types of experiments are conducted under different parameter settings.

For the first type of experiment, we fix the number of nearest neighbours, $n = 8$, and vary the number of common neighbours, m, under different amounts of outliers with $\sigma = 0.1$. As shown in Fig. 2(a), when $m = 5$, it achieves a good balance between the discriminative power and robustness against outliers. Similarly, given $m = 5$ as fixed, the second type of experiments varies n under the different number of outliers with $\sigma = 0.1$. According to Fig. 2(b), a trade-off between precision and recall ratios for the choice of n is obtained when $n = 8$. Therefore, we can fix the parameters ($m = 5, n = 8$) for the rest of experiments. Finally, to investigate the influence of positional jitter for the proposed method, we evaluate its performance under four levels of Gaussian positional jitter ($\sigma = 0.01, 0.1, 0.5, 1$) respectively. Theoretically, the expected relative distance between points, r, is equal to $1/\rho^{1/3}$, where ρ is the density of the point cloud. In our case, the range of r are from 15 to 22 depending on total number of points including both inliers and outliers. Compared to the relative distance between local neighbors, the registration problem under the high levels of Gaussian positional jitter ($\sigma \geq 0.5$) is considered quite challenging. As shown in Fig. 2(c), when the level is high ($\sigma \geq 0.5$), both precision and recall ratios for true correspondent pairs drop rapidly. Similar results were also reported in [6]. It is a well-known limitation that such descriptors derived from local point pattern are relatively sensitive to the positional jitter due to their dependence on local spatial constellation of points [24]. Despite their limitations, this type of local descriptors are widely used in many applications such as camera-based document image retrieval [25] and pose estimation using a projected dense dot pattern [26], for its robustness against large number of outliers.

4.2 Experiments on Benchmark Datasets

In this experiment, we focus on investigating the robustness of the proposed methods against the large number of outlier. Two types of point patterns ('fish' and 'character') from the benchmark synthesized datasets [12] are used to evaluate the performance of our method against the state-of-the-arts. Those methods include iterative closest point (ICP) [11], coherent point drift (CPD) [13] and robust point set matching using Gaussian mixture model (RPM-GMM) [14], whose source codes are publicly available. We also compare our method with the algorithm described in [3] noted as Fiji. We implement our method using Matlab and all the methods are run on a laptop with 2.2GHz CPU and 8G RAM. Rigid transformation between two point sets is applied for a fair comparison since the available version of RPM-GMM only supports the estimation of rigid transformation.

In each trial, we generate a random rigid transformation and apply it to the prototype patterns to obtain a pair of point patterns related by the transformation. Both patterns are located within an area of size 10×10. We also add a Gaussian positional jitter with $\sigma = 0.001$ to each point of the transformed prototype patterns. To evaluate the performances of the methods under heavy outliers or occlusions, two types of tests are designed: (1) Outlier test. Random outliers following an uniform spatial distribution are added to both sides of the point patterns respectively; (2) Occlusion test. We remove a portion of true correspondence from both point patterns and add same numbers of random outliers

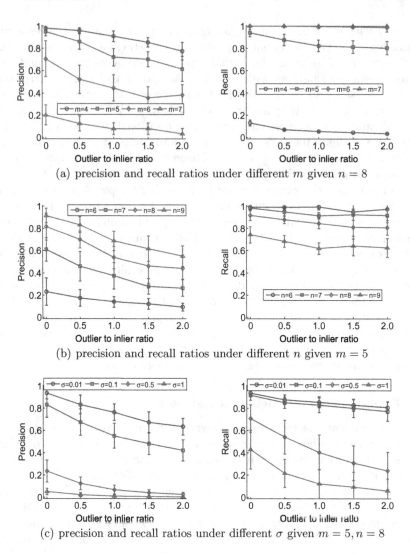

(a) precision and recall ratios under different m given $n = 8$

(b) precision and recall ratios under different n given $m = 5$

(c) precision and recall ratios under different σ given $m = 5, n = 8$

Fig. 2. The mean and standard deviation of precision and recall ratios over 100 random trials under different parameter settings against different numbers of outliers.

as those of the removed inliers to both sides of the point patterns. The examples of the synthesized point sets of both types are shown in Fig. 3. One point set is considered as the moving point set while the other is taken as the fixed point set. The matching error is defined as the mean of Euclidean distances between the inliers in the fixed point set and their correspondences in the transformed moving point set obtained by each method. The average matching errors over 100 random trials by all the methods for two types of tests are shown in Fig. 4. Obviously, the performances of our method are much better than others especially under heavy outliers and occlusions. For ICP, the large mean and standard deviation of registration error arise under all the cases due to local minima and bad initial alignments. CPD, RPM-GMM and Fiji perform well in the cases with a few outliers or occlusions, but they yield far less robust alignments than our method under the cases with large amount of outliers or occlusions. The average running times of different methods are listed in Table 1. Our method is slower than others as we need to consider combinatorial optimizations.

Table 1. Average running times of different methods against the total number of points N (in seconds).

	$N = 100$	$N = 200$	$N = 500$	$N = 1000$
ICP	0.2640	0.428	1.109	3.414
CPD	0.0169	0.086	0.196	0.896
RPM-GMM	0.0554	0.061	0.093	0.162
Fiji	0.517	1.162	2.615	12.581
Ours	1.524	3.210	9.480	25.020

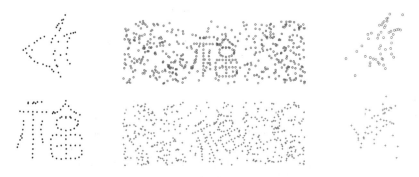

Fig. 3. Left column shows the prototype shapes for fish and character. The middle column shows an example of character case with outliers, where the points in one view are plotted as blue circles while those in another view are red crosses. The right column shows an example of fish case with occlusion.

4.3 Experiments on Dataset from Multiview SPIM

The data set of multi-view SPIM is obtained from [27] associated with [3]. A live Drosophila egg was recorded from seven views with angles of 45°. Each view contains approximately two thousands of fluorescent beads of 0.5 μm diameter. The resulting images have a size of $(1040 \times 1388 \times 90)$ with voxels of size $(0.731\,\mu m \times 0.731\,\mu m \times 2\,\mu m)$.

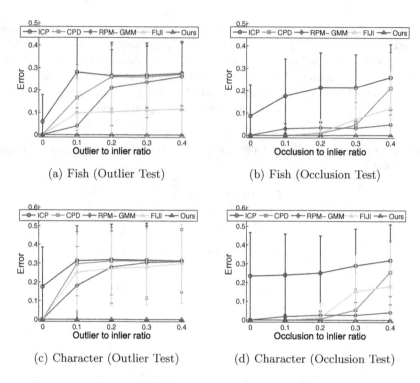

(a) Fish (Outlier Test)   (b) Fish (Occlusion Test)

(c) Character (Outlier Test)   (d) Character (Occlusion Test)

Fig. 4. The mean and standard deviation of matching errors over 100 random trials by different methods for the two types of tests.

The beads of all the views are first extracted with subpixel accuracy using a difference of Gaussian filter [28]. We set $\sigma = 1$ for this experiments. An example of the result by the proposed method is shown in Fig. 5. To conduct quantitative comparisons against the state-of-the-arts (CPD and the bead-based registration in Fiji-Plugin [3]), the ground truth of corresponding beads across views is required. Since the Fiji-Plugin is a well-established method in this field, we first register each image to the image of first view using the Fiji-Plugin and consider the detected corresponding beads as ground truth. Then, we apply all the methods to estimate the underlying transformations across views. The registration error is defined by the average Euclidean distance between beads of ground truth in the first view and their correspondences of another view warped by the estimated transformations using each method. As listed in Table 2, the proposed method achieves comparable registration accuracies for all the views as the Fiji-Plugin, while the CPD yields large registration errors. The average execution times for the CPD, Fiji-Plugin and our method are around 35, 37 and 76 seconds respectively.

It is well-known that there exists the anisotropic z-stretching of each view introduced by the differential refraction index mismatch between water and agarose since the sample is never perfectly centered in the agarose column [3].

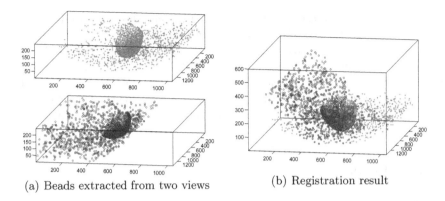

(a) Beads extracted from two views

(b) Registration result

Fig. 5. Illustration of the bead-based registration result between two views using the proposed method. Panel (a) shows the extracted bead from two views. Noting that the contours of samples in both views are mistakenly identified as beads. Later, they are automatically treated as outliers by the proposed method. The result of registration between two views with a rotation around 45° are illustrated in Panel (b). The yellow circles indict the correspondence pairs detected by the proposed method.

Table 2. Comparison of the average registration errors between the reference beads in view 1 and those in the rest of views.

	View 2	View 3	View 4	View 5	View 6	View 7
CPD	135.91	238.00	313.29	306.70	300.06	161.68
Fiji	0.6326	0.8373	0.8763	1.0952	1.2159	1.1177
Ours	0.5701	0.8567	1.1384	1.9056	1.5877	1.8183

To evaluate the effect of anisotropic z-stretching on registration accuracy, an affine transformation, $\mathrm{diag}(1, 1, s_z)$, is created, where s_z is a scaling factor on z-axis. We apply those additional affine transformations to the images of the first two views to simulate anisotropic z-stretching. We simulate four levels of anisotropic scaling with $s_z = 0.6, 0.7, 0.8, 0.9$, where the level with $s_z = 0.6$

Table 3. Comparison of the average registration errors and the number of true correspondent pairs under different levels of anisotropic scaling in z-axis (s_z). Note that the total number of pairs of true correspondence as inliers is 219 and the total number of extracted beads in two views are 2736 and 2538 respectively.

		$s_z = 0.9$	$s_z = 0.8$	$s_z = 0.7$	$s_z = 0.6$
Fiji	average error	0.6223	0.8534	63.56	160.2
	corresp. pairs	62	12	0	0
Ours	average error	0.5690	0.5917	0.5857	0.6394
	corresp. pairs	71	42	27	14

is the one with the largest anisotropic scaling among all of the levels. Table 3 shows the average registration error and the numbers of true correspondence pairs detected by each method under different scaling factors s_z. Note that the local descriptor used by the Fiji-Plugin is not affine-invariant as we discussed in the related work section. Therefore, for the case with large anisotropic scaling ($s_z = 0.6, 0.7$), the proposed method can register well, while the Fiji-Plugin fails due to the inadequate number of true correspondence pairs detected by its local descriptor.

5   Conclusion

We have presented a point cloud registration using affine shape distributions for multi-view SPIM. The proposed method detects the points of correspondence and solves for the underlying transformation in the presence of an extremely large amount of outliers and missing data in both point clouds. Experiments show this method is more reliable against the large amount of outliers and the anisotropic scaling of the underlying affine transformation, even in cases when the well-established methods fail. However, our method is sensitive to positional jitter. Hence, our future work is to explore descriptors which are robust to potential positional jitter and non-linear deformations.

References

1. Swoger, J., Verveer, P., Greger, K., Huisken, J., Stelzer, E.H.: Multi-view image fusion improves resolution in three-dimensional microscopy. Opt. Express **15**, 8029–8042 (2007)
2. Keller, P.J., Schmidt, A.D., Santella, A., Khairy, K., Bao, Z., Wittbrodt, J., Stelzer, E.H.: Fast, high-contrast imaging of animal development with scanned light sheet-based structured-illumination microscopy. Nat. Meth. **7**, 637–642 (2010)
3. Preibisch, S., Saalfeld, S., Schindelin, J., Tomancak, P.: Software for bead-based registration of selective plane illumination microscopy data. Nat. Meth. **7**, 418–419 (2010)
4. Krzic, U., Gunther, S., Saunders, T.E., Streichan, S.J., Hufnagel, L.: Multiview light-sheet microscope for rapid in toto imaging. Nat. Meth. **9**, 730–733 (2012)
5. Schmid, B., Shah, G., Scherf, N., Weber, M., Thierbach, K., Campos, C.P., Roeder, I., Aanstad, P., Huisken, J.: High-speed panoramic light-sheet microscopy reveals global endodermal cell dynamics. Nat. Commun. **4**, 2207 (2013)
6. Temerinac-Ott, M., Keuper, M., Burkhardt, H.: Evaluation of a new point clouds registration method based on group averaging features. In: 2010 20th International Conference on Pattern Recognition (ICPR), pp. 2452–2455. IEEE (2010)
7. Fischler, M.A., Bolles, R.C.: Random sample consensus: a paradigm for model fitting with applications to image analysis and automated cartography. Commun. ACM **24**, 381–395 (1981)
8. Salvi, J., Matabosch, C., Fofi, D., Forest, J.: A review of recent range image registration methods with accuracy evaluation. Image Vis. Comput. **25**, 578–596 (2007)
9. Zhang, D., Lu, G.: Review of shape representation and description techniques. Pattern Recogn. **37**, 1–19 (2004)

10. Aldoma, A., Marton, Z.C., Tombari, F., Wohlkinger, W., Potthast, C., Zeisl, B., Rusu, R., Gedikli, S., Vincze, M.: Tutorial: point cloud library: three-dimensional object recognition and 6 DOF pose estimation. IEEE Robot. Autom. Mag. **19**, 80–91 (2012)
11. Besl, P., McKay, N.D.: A method for registration of 3-D shapes. IEEE Trans. Pattern Anal. Mach. Intell. **14**, 239–256 (1992)
12. Chui, H., Rangarajan, A.: A new point matching algorithm for non-rigid registration. Comput. Vis. Image Underst. **89**, 114–141 (2003)
13. Myronenko, A., Song, X.: Point set registration: coherent point drift. IEEE Trans. Pattern Anal. Mach. Intell. **32**, 2262–2275 (2010)
14. Jian, B., Vemuri, B.C.: Robust point set registration using gaussian mixture models. IEEE Trans. Pattern Anal. Mach. Intell. **33**, 1633–1645 (2011)
15. Lian, W., Zhang, L.: Robust point matching revisited: a concave optimization approach. In: Fitzgibbon, A., Lazebnik, S., Perona, P., Sato, Y., Schmid, C. (eds.) ECCV 2012, Part II. LNCS, vol. 7573, pp. 259–272. Springer, Heidelberg (2012)
16. Lowe, D.G.: Distinctive image features from scale-invariant keypoints. Int. J. Comput. Vis. **60**, 91–110 (2004)
17. Aiger, D., Cohen-Or, N.J.: 4-points congruent sets for robust pairwise surface registration. ACM Trans. Graph. (TOG) **27**, 85 (2008)
18. Johnson, A.E., Hebert, M.: Using spin images for efficient object recognition in cluttered 3D scenes. IEEE Trans. Pattern Anal. Mach. Intell. **21**, 433–449 (1999)
19. Frome, A., Huber, D., Kolluri, R., Bülow, T., Malik, J.: Recognizing objects in range data using regional point descriptors. In: Pajdla, T., Matas, J.G. (eds.) ECCV 2004. LNCS, vol. 3023, pp. 224–237. Springer, Heidelberg (2004)
20. Leung, T.K., Burl, M.C., Perona, P.: Probabilistic affine invariants for recognition. In: Proceedings of the 1998 IEEE Computer Society Conference on Computer Vision and Pattern Recognition, pp. 678–684. IEEE (1998)
21. Sur, F.: Robust matching in an uncertain world. In: 2010 20th International Conference on Pattern Recognition (ICPR), pp. 2350–2353. IEEE (2010)
22. Dowson, D., Landau, B.: The frechet distance between multivariate normal distributions. J. Multiv. Anal. **12**, 450–455 (1982)
23. Givens, C.R., Shortt, R.M., et al.: A class of wasserstein metrics for probability distributions. Mich. Math. J. **31**, 231–240 (1984)
24. Grimson, W.E.L., Huttenlocher, D.P., Jacobs, D.W.: A study of affine matching with bounded sensor error. In: Sandini, G. (ed.) ECCV 1992. LNCS, vol. 588, pp. 291–306. Springer, Heidelberg (1992)
25. Nakai, T., Kise, K., Iwamura, M.: Use of affine invariants in locally likely arrangement hashing for camera-based document image retrieval. In: Bunke, H., Spitz, A.L. (eds.) DAS 2006. LNCS, vol. 3872, pp. 541–552. Springer, Heidelberg (2006)
26. McIlroy, P., Izadi, S., Fitzgibbon, A.: 3D pose estimation using a projected dense dot pattern. IEEE Transactions on Visualization and Computer Graphics **20**, 839–851 (2014)
27. Preibisch, S.: The 7-angle spim dataset of drosophila. http://fly.mpi-cbg.de/preibisch/nm/HisYFP-SPIM.zip. Accessed Mar 2014
28. Lindeberg, T.: Scale-space Theory in Computer Vision. Springer, Heidelberg (1993)

Part Detector Discovery in Deep Convolutional Neural Networks

Marcel Simon[✉], Erik Rodner, and Joachim Denzler

Computer Vision Group, Friedrich Schiller University of Jena, Jena, Germany
marcel.simon@uni-jena.de
http://www.inf-cv.uni-jena.de

Abstract. Current fine-grained classification approaches often rely on a robust localization of object parts to extract localized feature representations suitable for discrimination. However, part localization is a challenging task due to the large variation of appearance and pose. In this paper, we show how pre-trained convolutional neural networks can be used for robust and efficient object part discovery and localization without the necessity to actually train the network on the current dataset. Our approach called "part detector discovery" (PDD) is based on analyzing the gradient maps of the network outputs and finding activation centers spatially related to annotated semantic parts or bounding boxes. This allows us not just to obtain excellent performance on the CUB200-2011 dataset, but in contrast to previous approaches also to perform detection and bird classification jointly without requiring a given bounding box annotation during testing and ground-truth parts during training.

1 Introduction

In recent years, the concept of *deep learning* has gained tremendous interest in the vision community. One of the key ideas is to jointly learn a model for the whole classification pipeline from an input image to the final outputs. A successful model especially for classification are deep convolutional neural networks (CNN) [1]. A CNN model can be seen as the concatenation of several processing steps similar to algorithmic steps in previous "non-deep" recognition models. The steps sequentially transform the given input into a likely more abstract representation [2–4] and finally to the expected output.

Due to the large number of free parameters, deep models usually need to be learned from large-scale data, such as the ImageNet dataset used in [1], and learning is a computationally demanding step. The very recent work of [5–7] shows that pre-trained deep models can also be exploited for datasets which they have not been trained on. In particular, efficient and very powerful feature representations can be obtained that lead to a significant performance improvement on several vision benchmarks. Our work follows a similar line of thought and

Electronic supplementary material The online version of this chapter (doi:10.1007/978-3-319-16808-1_12) contains supplementary material, which is available to authorized users.

This work was supported by Nvidia with a hardware donation.

D. Cremers et al. (Eds.): ACCV 2014, Part II, LNCS 9004, pp. 162–177, 2015.
DOI: 10.1007/978-3-319-16808-1_12

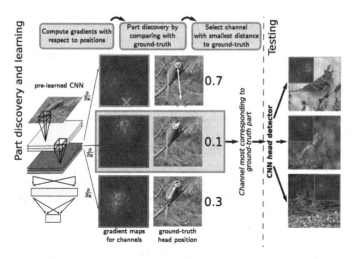

Fig. 1. Outline of our approach during learning using the *part strategy*: (1) compute gradients of CNN channels with respect to image positions, (2) estimate activation centers, (3) find spatially related semantic parts to select useful channels that act as part detectors later on.

in particular the question we were interested in is: *"Can we re-use pre-trained deep convolutional networks for part discovery and detection? Does a deep model learned on ImageNet already include implicit detectors related to common parts found in fine-grained recognition tasks?"*

The answer to both questions is yes and to show this we present a novel part discovery and detection scheme using pre-trained deep convolution neural networks. Object representations for visual recognition are often part-based [8,9] and in several cases information about semantic parts is given. The parts of a bird, for example, include the belly, the wings, the beak and the tail. The benefit of part-based representations is especially notable in fine-grained classification tasks, in which the objects of different categories are similar in shape and general appearance, but differ greatly in some small parts. This is also the application scenario considered in our paper.

Our technique for providing such a part-based representation is based on computing gradient maps with respect to certain channel outputs and finding clusters of high activation within. This is followed by selecting channels which have their corresponding clusters closest to ground-truth positions of semantic parts or bounding boxes. An outline of our approach is given in Fig. 1. The most interesting aspect is that after finding these associations, parts can be reliably detected without much additional computational effort from the results of the deep CNN.

2 Related Work

CNN for Classification. The approach of Krizhevsky *et al.* [1] demonstrates the capabilities of multilayered architectures for image classification by achieving an outstanding error rate on the LSVRC2012 dataset. Donahue *et al.* [5] use a CNN with a similar architecture and analyze how well a network trained on ImageNet performs on other not related image classification datasets. They use the output of a hidden layer as feature representation followed by a SVM [10] learned on the new dataset. The authors have also published "DeCAF", an open source framework for CNNs [5], which we also use in our work. Similar studies have been done by [6,7]. In contrast to their work, we focus on part discovery with pre-trained CNNs rather than classification.

An important aspect of [4] is the qualitative analysis of the learned intermediate representations. In particular, they show that CNNs trained on ImageNet contain models for basic object shapes at lower layers and object part models at higher layers. This is exactly the property that we make use of in our approach. Although the CNN we use was not particularly trained on the fine-grained task we consider, it can be used for basic shape and part detection.

CNN for Object Detection. Motivated by the good results of CNNs in classification, several methods were proposed to apply this technique to object detection. Erhan *et al.* [11] use a deep neural network to directly predict the coordinates of a fixed number of bounding boxes and the corresponding confidence. They determine the category of the object in each bounding box using a second CNN. A main drawback of this approach is the fixed number of bounding box proposals once the network has been trained. In order to change the number of proposals, the whole networks needs to be trained again. An alternative to the direct prediction of the bounding box coordinates is presented in [12]. They train a deep neural network to predict an object mask at multiple scales. While the predicted mask is similar to our gradient maps, they need to train an additional CNN specifically for the object detection task. Simonyan *et al.* [13] perform object localization by analyzing the gradient of a deep CNN trained for classification. They compute the gradient of the winning class score with respect to the input image. By thresholding the absolute gradient values, seed background and seed foreground pixels are located and used as initialization for the GrabCut segmentation algorithm. We make use of their idea to use gradients. However, while [13] use the gradients for segmentation, we use them for part discovery. In addition to this, we introduce the idea of using intermediate layers and techniques like the aggregation of gradients of the same channel.

CNN for Part Localization. Many classification approaches in fine-grained recognition use part-based object models and hence also require part detection. At the moment, most part-based models use low-level features like histogram of oriented gradients [14] for detection and description. Examples are the deformable part model (DPM) [8], regionlets [15], and poselets [16]. Facing the success of features from deep CNN, a current line of research is the use of these features as a replacement for the low-level features of the part-based models. For example, [5] relies on deformable part descriptors [17], which is inspired by DPM. While the localization is still done with low-level features, the descriptor is calculated using the activations of a deep CNN for each predicted part. Zhang *et al.* [18] use poselets for part discovery as well as detection and calculate features for each region using a deep CNN. While DPM and regionlets work well on many datasets, they face problems on datasets with large intraclass variance and unconstrained settings especially due to the low-level features that are still used for localization. In contrast, our approach implicitly exploits all high-level features that a large CNN has learned already. It also allows us to solve part localization and the consequent classification within the same framework.

Entirely replacing the low-level features is difficult, because a CNN produces global features. Zou et al. [19] solves this by associating the output of a hidden layer with spatially related parts of the input. This allows them to apply the regionlets approach. However, their approach requires numerous evaluations of the CNN and the features are not arbitrarily dense. In contrast, our approach is working on the full resolution of the input.

The work of Jain et al. [20] uses the sliding window approach for part localization with CNNs. They evaluate a CNN at each position of the window in order to detect human body parts in images without using bounding box annotations. This requires hundreds or thousands of CNN evaluations. As sufficiently large CNNs take some time for prediction, this results in long run times. In contrast, only one forward- and one back-propagation pass per part is required for the localization with our approach. In [21,22], the part positions are estimated by a CNN specifically trained for this task. The outputs of their network are the coordinates of each part. In contrast to their work, our approach does not require any separately trained neural network but can exploit a CNN already trained for a different large-scale classification task.

3   Localization with Deep Convolutional Neural Networks

In the following, we briefly review the concept of deep CNNs in Sect. 3.1 and the use of gradient maps for object localization presented by Simonyan et al. [13] in Sect. 3.2 as these are the ideas our work is based on.

3.1   Deep Convolutional Architectures

A key idea of deep learning approaches is that the whole classification pipeline consists of one combined and jointly trained model. Many non-deep systems rely on hand-crafted features and separately trained machine learning algorithms. In contrast, no hand-crafted features are required in deep learning architectures as they are automatically learned from the training data and no separately trained machine learning algorithm is required as the deep architecture also covers this part. Most recent deep learning architectures for vision are based on a single CNN. CNNs are feed forward neural networks, which concatenate several layers of different types. These layers are often related to techniques that a lot of non-deep approaches for visual recognition used without joint parameter tuning:

1. Convolutional layers perform filtering with multiple filter masks, which is related to computing the distance of local features to a given codebook in the common bag-of-words (BoW) pipeline.

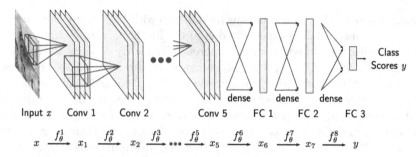

Fig. 2. Example of a convolutional neural network used for classification. Each convolutional layer convolves the output of the previous layer with multiple learned filter masks, applies an element-wise non-linear activation function, and optionally combines the outputs by a pooling operation. The last two layers are fully connected layers and multiply the input with a matrix of learned parameters followed by a non-linear activation function. The output of the network are scores for each of the learned categories.

2. Pooling layers spatially combine filter outputs, which is related to classical spatial pyramid matching [23].
3. Non-linear layers, such as the rectified linear unit used by [1], are related to non-linear encoding techniques for BoW [24].
4. Several fully connected layers at the end act as nested linear classifiers.

The final output of the CNN are scores for each object category. The architecture is visualized in a simplified manner in Fig. 2. For details about the network structure we refer to [1,5] since we use the same pre-trained CNN.

As visualized in the figure, we will denote the transformation performed by the CNN as a function $f_\theta(x)$, which maps the input image x to the classification scores for each category using the parameter vector θ. We omit θ in the following text since it is not relevant for our approach. The function f is a concatenation of functions $f(x) = f^{(n)} \circ f^{(n-1)} \circ \cdots \circ f^{(1)}(x)$, where the $f^{(1)}, f^{(2)}, \ldots, f^{(n)}$ correspond to the n layers of the network. Furthermore, let $g^{(k)}(x) := f^{(k)} \circ f^{(k-1)} \circ \cdots \circ f^{(1)}(x)$ be the output and $x^{(k)} := g^{(k-1)}(x)$ the input of the k-th layer. Please note that $f^{(j)}$ represents only the transformation of layer j, while $g^{(j)}$ includes all transformations from input image to layer j.

Furthermore and most importantly for our approach, the output of the first layers is organized in channels with each element in the channel being related to a certain area in the input image. The outputs of a channel are the result of several nested convolutions, non-linear activations and pooling operations applied to the input image. Therefore, we can view them as results of pooled detector scores, a connection that we make use of for our part discovery scheme in Sect. 4.

3.2 Localization Using Gradient Maps

Deep convolutional neural networks trained for classification can also be used for other visual recognition tasks like object localization. Simonyan *et al.* [13] present a method, which calculates the gradient of the winning class score with

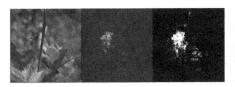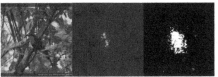

Fig. 3. Examples for the gradient maps (continuous and thresholded with the 95 %-quantile) that are calculated with respect to the winning class score.

respect to the input image. The intuition is that important foreground pixels have a large influence on the classification score and hence have a large absolute gradient value. Background pixels, however, do not influence the classification result and hence have a small gradient. The experiments in [13] support this intuition and it allows them to use this information for segmentation of foreground and background. The next paragraph briefly reviews the calculation of the gradients as we also use gradient maps in our system.

The calculation of the gradient $\frac{\partial f_i}{\partial x}$ of the model output $(f(x))_i$ with respect to the input image x is similar to the back-propagation of the classification error during training. Using the notation introduced in Sect. 3.1, the gradient can be computed using the chain rule as

$$\frac{\partial f_i}{\partial x} = \frac{\partial f_i}{\partial g^{(n-1)}} \frac{\partial g^{(n-1)}}{\partial g^{(n-2)}} \cdots \frac{\partial g^{(2)}}{\partial g^{(1)}} \frac{\partial g^{(1)}}{\partial x} = \frac{\partial g_i^{(n)}}{\partial x^{(n)}} \frac{\partial g^{(n-1)}}{\partial x^{(n-1)}} \cdots \frac{\partial g^{(1)}}{\partial x}. \qquad (1)$$

Each factor $\frac{\partial g^{(j)}}{\partial x^{(j)}}$ of this product is a Jacobian matrix of the output $g^{(j)}$ with respect to the input $x^{(j)}$ of layer j. This means that the gradient can be computed layer by layer. These factors are also calculated during back-propagation. The only difference is that the last derivative is with respect to x instead of θ.

The gradient $\frac{\partial f_i}{\partial x}$ can be reshaped such that it has the same shape as the input image. The result is called gradient map and Fig. 3 visualizes the gradient maps that are calculated with respect to the winning class score for two examples. At first glance, a gradient might seem very similar to a saliency map. However, while a saliency map captures objects that distinguish themselves from the background [25], the gradient values are only large for pixels, that influence the classification result. Hence, conspicuous background objects will be highlighted in a salient map but not in a gradient map as they do not influence the score of the winning class. The second image in Fig. 3 is a good example, whose strong background patterns are not highlighted in the gradient map.

4 Part Discovery in CNNs by Correspondence

Recent fine-grained categorization experiments have shown that the location of object parts is a valuable information and allows to boost the classification accuracy significantly [5,9,26]. However, the precise and fast localization of parts can be a challenging task due to the great variety of poses in some datasets.

In Sect. 4.1, we present a novel approach for automatically detecting parts of an object. Given a test image of an object from a previously known set of categories, the algorithm will detect visible parts and locate them in the image. This is followed by Sect. 4.2 presenting a part-based classification approach, which is used as an application of our part localization method in the experiments.

4.1   Part Localization

Gradient Maps for Part Discovery. Like the object localization system of the previous section, our algorithm requires a pre-trained CNN trained for image classification. The classification task it was trained for does not need to be directly related to the actual part localization task. For example, we used for our experiments the model of [5], which was trained on the ImageNet dataset. However, all our experiments are performed on the Caltech Birds dataset.

The part localization is done by calculating the gradient of the output elements of a hidden layer with respect to the input image. Suppose the selected layer has m output elements, then m gradients with respect to the input image and hence m gradient maps are computed. The calculation of the gradient maps for each element of a hidden layer is done in a similar way as the gradient of a class score. Let b denote the chosen hidden layer. Then, the gradient $\frac{\partial g_j^{(b)}}{\partial x}(x)$ of the j-th element of layer b with respect to the input image x is calculated as

$$\frac{\partial g_j^{(b)}}{\partial x} = \frac{\partial g_j^{(b)}}{\partial g^{(b-1)}} \frac{\partial g^{(b-1)}}{\partial g^{(b-2)}} \cdots \frac{\partial g^{(1)}}{\partial x} = \frac{\partial g_j^{(b)}}{\partial x^{(b)}} \cdot \frac{\partial g^{(b-1)}}{\partial x^{(b-1)}} \cdots \frac{\partial g^{(1)}}{\partial x}. \tag{2}$$

As before, we can also make use of the back-propagation scheme for gradients already implemented in most CNN toolboxes. The gradient maps of the same channel are added pixelwise in order to obtain one gradient map per channel. The intuition is that each element of a hidden layer is sensitive to a specific pattern in the input image. All elements of the same channel are sensitive to the same pattern but are focused on a different location of this pattern.

Part Discovery by Correspondence. We now want to identify channels, which are related to object parts. In the following, we assume that the ground-truth part locations z_i of the training images x_i are given. However, our method can be also provided with the location of the bounding box only as we will show later. We associate a binary latent variable h_k with each channel k, which indicates whether the channel is related to an object part. Our part discovery scheme can be motivated as a maximum likelihood estimation of these variables. First, let us consider the task of selecting the most related channel corresponding to a part which can be written as (assuming x_i are independent samples):

$$\hat{k} = \operatorname{argmax}_{1 \le k \le K} p(\boldsymbol{X} \mid h_k = 1) = \operatorname*{argmax}_{1 \le k \le K} \prod_{i=1}^{N} \frac{p(h_k = 1 | x_i) \, p(x_i)}{p(h_k = 1)}, \tag{3}$$

where $\boldsymbol{X}$ is the training data and K is the total number of channels. In the following, we assume a flat prior for $p(h_k = 1)$ and $p(x_i)$. The term $p(h_k = 1 | x_i)$

expresses the probability that channel k corresponds to the part currently under consideration given a single training example x_i. This is the case when the position p_i^k estimated using channel k equals the ground-truth part position z_i. However, the estimated position p_i^k is likely not perfect and we assume it to be a Gaussian random variable distributed as $p_i^k \sim \mathcal{N}(\mu_i^k, \sigma^2)$, where μ_i^k is a center of activation extracted from the gradient map of channel k. We therefore have:

$$p(h_k = 1|x_i) = p(p_i^k = z_i|x_i) = \mathcal{N}(z_i|\mu_i^k, \sigma^2) \tag{4}$$

Putting it all together, we obtain a very simple scheme for selecting a channel:

$$\hat{k} = \underset{1 \leq k \leq K}{\operatorname{argmax}} \sum_{i=1}^{N} \log p(h_k = 1|x_i) = \underset{1 \leq k \leq K}{\operatorname{argmin}} \sum_{i=1}^{N} \|\mu_i^k - z_i\|^2 \tag{5}$$

For all gradient maps of all training images, the center of activation μ_i^k is calculated as explained in the subsequent paragraph. These locations are compared to the ground-truth part locations z_i by computing the mean distance. Finally, for each ground-truth part, the channel with the smallest mean distance is selected. The result is a set of channels, which are sensitive to different parts of the object. There does not need to be a one-to-one relationship between parts and channels, because the neural network is not trained on semantic parts. We refer to this method as *part strategy*.

Part Discovery without Ground-Truth Parts. In many scenarios, ground-truth part annotations are not available. Our approach can also be applied in these cases by selecting relevant channels based on the bounding box of the training images only. We evaluate two different approaches related to different models for $p(h_k = 1|x_i)$. First, we count for every channel how often the activation center is within the bounding box $\mathrm{BB}(x_i)$ of the image x_i. We select the channels with the highest count, as these are most likely to correspond to the object of interest. It can be shown that this *counting strategy* is related to the following model for arbitrary $0 < \epsilon < 1$:

$$p(h_k = 1|x_i) = \begin{cases} 1 - \epsilon & \mu_i^k \in \mathrm{BB}(x_i) \\ \epsilon & \text{otherwise} \end{cases} \tag{6}$$

Second, we extend the first approach by taking the distance to the *bounding box* border into account. If the activation center of a channel is within the bounding box of a training image, the cost is 0. If it is outside, the cost equals to the Euclidean distance to the bounding box border.

Finding Activation Centers. The assumption for finding the center of activation μ_i is that high absolute gradient values are concentrated in local areas of the gradient maps and these areas correspond to certain patterns in the image. In order to robustly localize the center point of the largest area, we fit a Gaussian mixture model with K components to the pixel locations weighted by the normalized absolute gradient values. We then take the mean location of the most

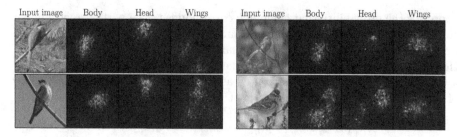

Fig. 4. Examples for gradient maps. Each group of images first shows the input image and then the gradient maps of the channels associated with the body, head and the wings. A light blue to red color means, that the gradient values of the corresponding pixel is high. A deep blue corresponds to a gradient value of zero (Color figure online).

prominent cluster in the mixture as the center of activation. In comparison to simply taking the maximum position in the gradient map, this approach is much more robust to noise as we show in the experiments.

Part Detection. In order to locate parts in a new image, the gradient maps for all selected channels are calculated. The activation center is estimated and returned as the location of the part. If the gradient map is equal to **0**, the part is likely not visible in the image and marked as occluded. Figure 4 visualizes the gradient maps for some test images used in our experiments. For each image, three channels are shown which are associated with semantic parts of a bird. In each group of images, the input is on the left followed by the normalized gradient maps of the channels associated with the body, head and the wings. A light blue to red color corresponds to a large absolute gradient value while a deep blue represents a zero gradient.

Why should this work? The results of [4] suggest that at least in the special case of deep CNNs, each element of a hidden layer is sensitive to specific patterns in the image. "Sensitive" means in this case that the occurrence of a pattern leads to a high change of the output. There is an implicit association between certain image patterns and output elements of a layer. In higher layers these patterns are increasingly abstract and hence might correspond to a specific part of an object. Our method automatically identifies channels with this property.

As an example, suppose the input of a deep architecture is a RGB color image and the first and only layer is a convolutional layer with two channels representing different local edge filters. If the first filter mask is a horizontal and the second one a vertical edge filter mask, then the first channel is sensitive to horizontal edge patterns and the second one to vertical edge patterns. This example also illustrates that at least in the case of convolutional layers any output element of the same channel reacts to the same pattern and that each element just focuses on a different area in the input image. Of course, the example only discusses low-level patterns without any direct connection to a specific part. However, experiments [4] indicate that in higher layers the patterns are more complex and correspond, for example, to wheels or an eye.

Implementation Details. At first, it might seem that simply adding the gradients of all elements of a channel causes a loss of information. Negative and positive gradients can cancel and might cause a close to zero gradient for a discriminative pixel. Possibly adding the absolute gradient values seems to be the better approach, but this is not the case. First, since each element of a channel focuses on a separate area in the input image, the cancellation of positive and negative gradients is negligible. A small set of experiments supports this. Second, calculating the sum of gradients requires only one back-propagation call per channel instead of one call for each element of the channel. In our experiments, each channel has 36 elements. Hence, there is a speedup of $36\times$ in our case.

The reason for this is the back-propagation algorithm which directly calculates the sum of gradients if initialized correctly. We have already showed how to calculate the gradient $\frac{\partial g_j^{(b)}}{\partial x}$ of a element with respect to the input image. It is possible to rewrite the calculation such that it shows more clearly how to apply the back-propagation algorithm. Let e_j be the j-th unit vector. Then

$$\frac{\partial g_j^{(b)}}{\partial x} = e_j \cdot \frac{\partial g^{(b)}}{\partial x} = e_j \cdot \frac{\partial g_\theta^{(b)}}{\partial g_\theta^{(b-1)}} \cdot \frac{\partial g_\theta^{(b-1)}}{\partial g_\theta^{(b-2)}} \cdot \ldots \cdot \frac{\partial g_\theta^{(2)}}{\partial g_\theta^{(1)}} \cdot \frac{\partial g_\theta^{(1)}}{\partial x}(x) \qquad (7)$$

where $\frac{\partial g^{(b)}}{\partial x}$ is the Jacobian matrix containing the derivatives of each output element (the rows) with respect to each input component of x (the columns). Here, e_j is the initialization for the back-propagation at layer b and all the other factors are applied during the backward pass. In other words, the initialization e_j selects the j-th row of the Jacobian matrix $\frac{\partial g^{(b)}}{\partial x}$. Suppose there would be more than one element of e_j equal to 1. Then the result is the sum of the corresponding gradient vectors. Let $s_c = (0, \ldots, 0, 1, 1, \ldots, 1, 0, 0, \ldots, 0)$ be such a "modified" e_j, where c is the channel index. s_c is 1 at each position that corresponds to an element of channel c and 0 for all remaining components. Replacing e_j in Eq. 7 by s_c consequently calculates the required sum of gradients which belong to the same channel. In contrast, the calculation of the sum of absolute gradients values requires multiple backward passes with a new e_j for each run.

4.2 Part-Based Image Classification

Part detection is only an intermediate step for most real world systems. We use the presented part discovery and detection method for part-based image classification. Our method adapts the approach of [26] replacing the SIFT and color name features by the activations of a deep neural network and the nonparametric part transfer by the presented part detection approach.

The feature vector consists of two types, the global and the part features. For the global feature extraction, we use the same CNN that is used for part detection. The whole image is warped in order to use it as input for the CNN. The activations of a hidden layer are then used to build a feature vector. For training as well as for testing, the part features are extracted from square shaped patches around the estimated part position. The width and height of the patches are calculated as $p = \sqrt{n \cdot m \cdot \lambda}$, where m and n is the width and height of the image, respectively, and λ is a parameter. We use $\lambda = 0.1$ in our experiments. Similar to the global feature extraction, the patches are resized in order to use them as input for the CNN. The activations of a hidden layer for all patches are then concatenated with the global feature. The resulting features are used to train a linear one-vs-all support vector machine for every category. We also tried various explicit kernel maps as demonstrated in [26], but none of these techniques lead to a performance gain.

5   Experiments

Experimental Setup. We evaluate our approach on Caltech Birds CUB200-2011 [27], a challenging dataset for fine-grained classification. The dataset consists of 11788 labeled photographs of 200 bird species in their natural environment. Further qualitative results are presented on the Columbia dogs dataset [28]. Besides class labels, both datasets come with semantic part annotations. The birds dataset also provides ground-truth bounding boxes.

We use the CNN framework DeCAF [5] and the network learned on the ILSVRC 2012 dataset provided by the authors of [5]. The CNN takes a 227×227 RGB color image as input and transforms it into a vector of 1000 class scores. Details about the architecture of the network are given in [5] as well as in [1] and we skip the details here, because our approach can be used with any CNN. For all experiments, we use the output of the last pooling layer to calculate the gradient maps with respect to the input image. It consists of 256 channels with 36 elements each and directly follows the last convolutional layer. For each gradient map, we use the GMM method as explained in Sect. 4 with $K = 2$ components, a maximum of 100 EM iterations, and three repetitions with random initialization to increase robustness.

In the classification experiments, the same CNN model as for the part detection is used. The activations of the last hidden layer are taken as a feature vector. For the part-based classification, the learned part detectors are used. From the estimated part positions of the training and test images, squared patches are extracted using $\lambda = 0.1$. Each patch is then warped to size 227×227 in order to be used as input for the CNN and the activations of the last hidden layer are used as a feature vector for this part.

Qualitative Evaluation. Figures 5 and 6 present some examples of our part localization applied to uncropped test images. For both datasets, relevant channels were identified using the ground-truth part annotations. In case of the dogs dataset, the three discovered detectors seem to correspond to the nose (red), head (green), and body (blue). Especially the nose is identified reliably. For the birds dataset, we present four challenging examples in which only a small portion of the image contains the actual bird. In addition to this, the bird is often partially occluded. Nevertheless, our approach is able to precisely locate the head (red) and the legs (white). While there is more variance in the body (blue), wing

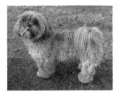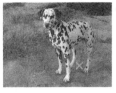

Fig. 5. Detections of the discovered part detectors on the dogs dataset. Green corresponds to the nose, red to the head and blue to the body of the dog. The last image is a failure case. Best viewed in color (Color figure online).

Table 1. Part localization error on the CUB-2011-200 dataset for our *part strategy* method w/ and w/o GMM for finding the activation centers, our method w/ and w/o restricting the localization to the bounding box (BB), and the method of [26]. In addition, we also show the performance of our approach for a CNN trained from scratch on CUB200-2011.

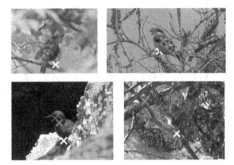

Method	Norm. error
Ours (GMM, BB)	**0.16**
Ours (GMM, Full)	0.17
Ours (MaxG, BB)	0.17
Part transfer [26] (BB)	0.18
Ours (CNN from scratch)	0.36

Fig. 6. Part localization examples from birds dataset. No bounding box and no geometric constraints for the part locations are used during the localization. The first three images are analyzed correctly, the belly and wing position are wrongly located in the fourth image. Best viewed in color (Color figure online).

(light blue), and tail (purple) location, they are still close to the real locations. The last example in Figs. 5 and 6 shows a failure case.

Evaluating the Part Localization Error. First, we are interested to what extent the learned part detectors relate to semantic parts. After identifying the spatially most related channel for each semantic part, we can apply our method to the test images to predict the location of semantic parts. The localization errors are given in Table 1. For calculating the localization error, we follow the work of [26] and use the mean pixel error normalized by the length of the diagonal of the ground-truth bounding box.

Our method achieves a significantly lower part localization error compared to [26] and a baseline using a CNN learned from scratch on the CUB200-2011 dataset only. A detailed analysis of the part localization error for each part is given in the supplementary material including several observations about the channel-part correspondences: there are groups of parts that are associated with the same channel and there are parts, such as the beak and the throat, where we are twice as accurate as [26]. This indicates that the system can distinguish

Table 2. Species categorization performance on the CUB200-2011 dataset. We distinguish between different experimental setups, depending on whether the ground-truth parts are used in training and whether the ground-truth bounding box is used during testing[a].

Training	Testing		Method	Recognition rate
Parts	BBox	Parts		
GT	GT		Baseline (BBox CNN features)	56.00 %
GT	GT	est	Berg et al. [9]	56.78 %
GT	GT	est	Goering et al. [26]	57.84 %
GT	GT	est	Chai et al. [29]	59.40 %
GT	GT	est	Ours (part strategy)	62.53 %
GT	GT	GT	Ours (part strategy)	62.67 %
GT	GT	est	Donahue et al. [5]	64.96 %
GT		est	Ours (part strategy)	60.17 %
GT		GT	Ours (part strategy)	60.55 %
			Baseline (global CNN features)	41.60 %
		est	Ours (counting)	51.93 %
		est	Ours (bounding box strategy)	53.75 %

[a] After submission, two additional publications [30,31] were published reporting 73.9 % and 75.7 % accuracy if part annotations are used only in training and no ground-truth bounding box is used during testing. Both of these works perform fine-tuning of the CNN models, which is not done in our case.

different bird body parts without direct training, which is a surprising fact given that we use a CNN trained for a completely different task.

Evaluation for Part-Based Fine-Grained Classification. We apply the presented part-based classification method to the CUB200-2011 dataset in order to evaluate to what extend the predicted part locations contribute to a higher accuracy. As can be seen in Table 2, our approach achieves a classification accuracy of 62.5 %, which is one of the best results on CUB-2011-200 without fine-tuned CNNs. Whereas the method of [26] heavily relies on the ground-truth bounding box for part estimation, our method can also perform fine-grained classification on unconstrained full images without a manual preselection of the area containing the bird. These results are also shown in Table 2.

As the main focus of this paper is the part localization, two more results are presented. First, the performance without using any part-based representation is a lower bound of our approach, since we also add global features to our feature representation. The recognition rate in this case is 56.0 % for the constrained and 41.6 % for the unconstrained setting. Second, the performance with ground-truth part locations is an upper bound, if we assume that human annotated semantic parts are also the best ones for automatic classification. In this case, the accuracy is 62.7 % and 60.6 %, respectively. The recognition rate of our approach with estimated part locations and the upper bound are nearly identical with a difference of only 0.2 % and 0.5 %, respectively. We also show the results in the case no ground-truth part annotations are provided for the training data. A baseline is provided by using CNN activations of the uncropped image for classification. The presented *counting strategy* as well as the *bounding box strategy* are able to significantly outperform this baseline by over 10 % accuracy. The *bounding box strategy* performs best with only 6 % less performance compared to the *part strategy*, which makes use of ground-truth part locations during training.

6   Conclusions

We have presented a novel approach for object part discovery and detection with pre-trained deep models. The motivation for our work was that deep convolutional neural network models learned on large-scale object databases such as ImageNet are already able to robustly detect basic shapes typically found in natural images. We exploit this ability to discover useful parts for a fine-grained recognition task by analyzing gradient maps of deep models and selecting activation centers related to annotated semantic parts or bounding boxes. After this simple learning step, part detection basically comes for free when applying the deep CNN to the image and detecting parts takes only a few seconds. Our experimental results show that in combination with a part-based classification approach this leads to an excellent performance of 62.5 % on the CUB-2011-200 dataset. In contrast to previous work [26], our approach is also suitable for situations when the ground-truth bounding box is not given during testing. In this scenario, we obtain an accuracy of 60.1 %, which is only slightly less than the result for the restricted setting with given bounding boxes. Furthermore, we also show how to learn without given ground-truth part locations, making fine-grained recognition feasible without huge annotation costs.

Future work will focus on dense features for the input image that can be obtained by stacking all gradient maps of a layer. This allows us to apply previous part-based models like DPM, which also include geometric constraints for the part locations. Furthermore, multiple channels can relate to the same part and our approach can be very easily modified to tackle these situations using an iterative approach.

References

1. Krizhevsky, A., Sutskever, I., Hinton, G.: Imagenet classification with deep convolutional neural networks. In: Advances in Neural Information Processing Systems (NIPS), pp. 1097–1105 (2012)
2. Bengio, Y., Courville, A.C., Vincent, P.: Representation learning: a review and new perspectives. IEEE Trans. Pattern Anal. Mach. Intell. (PAMI) **35**, 1798–1828 (2013)
3. Bengio, Y.: Learning deep architectures for AI. Found. Trends Mach. Learn. **2**, 1–127 (2009)

4. Zeiler, M.D., Fergus, R.: Visualizing and understanding convolutional networks. In: Fleet, D., Pajdla, T., Schiele, B., Tuytelaars, T. (eds.) ECCV 2014, Part I. LNCS, vol. 8689, pp. 818–833. Springer, Heidelberg (2014)

5. Donahue, J., Jia, Y., Vinyals, O., Hoffman, J., Zhang, N., Tzeng, E., Darrell, T.: Decaf: a deep convolutional activation feature for generic visual recognition (2013). arXiv preprint arXiv:1310.1531

6. Sermanet, P., Eigen, D., Zhang, X., Mathieu, M., Fergus, R., LeCun, Y.: Overfeat: integrated recognition, localization and detection using convolutional networks. In: International Conference on Learning Representations (ICLR). CBLS (2014). Preprint http://arxiv.org/abs/1312.6229

7. Razavian, A.S., Azizpour, H., Sullivan, J., Carlsson, S.: CNN features off-the-shelf: an astounding baseline for recognition (2014). arXiv preprint arXiv:1403.6382

8. Felzenszwalb, P.F., Girshick, R.B., McAllester, D., Ramanan, D.: Object detection with discriminatively trained part-based models. IEEE Trans. Pattern Anal. Mach. Intell. (PAMI) **32**, 1627–1645 (2010)

9. Berg, T., Belhumeur, P.: Poof: part-based one-vs.-one features for fine-grained categorization, face verification, and attribute estimation. In: IEEE Conference on Computer Vision and Pattern Recognition (CVPR), pp. 955–962 (2013)

10. Cortes, C., Vapnik, V.: Support-vector networks. Mach. Learn. **20**, 273–297 (1995)

11. Erhan, D., Szegedy, C., Toshev, A., Anguelov, D.: Scalable object detection using deep neural networks. In: IEEE Conference on Computer Vision and Pattern Recognition (CVPR) (2014). Preprint http://arxiv.org/abs/1312.2249

12. Szegedy, C., Toshev, A., Erhan, D.: Deep neural networks for object detection. In: Advances in Neural Information Processing Systems (NIPS), pp. 2553–2561. Curran Associates Inc (2013)

13. Simonyan, K., Vedaldi, A., Zisserman, A.: Deep inside convolutional networks: visualising image classification models and saliency maps (2013). arXiv preprint arXiv:1312.6034

14. Dalal, N., Triggs, B.: Histograms of oriented gradients for human detection. In: IEEE Conference on Computer Vision and Pattern Recognition (CVPR), pp. 886–893 (2005)

15. Wang, X., Yang, M., Zhu, S., Lin, Y.: Regionlets for generic object detection. In: IEEE International Conference on Computer Vision (ICCV), pp. 17–24 (2013)

16. Bourdev, L., Malik, J.: Poselets: Body part detectors trained using 3d human Pose annotations. In: IEEE International Conference on Computer Vision (ICCV), pp. 1365–1372 (2009)

17. Zhang, N., Farrell, R., Iandola, F., Darrell, T.: Deformable part descriptors for fine-grained recognition and attribute prediction. In: IEEE International Conference on Computer Vision (ICCV), pp. 729–736 (2013)

18. Zhang, N., Paluri, M., Ranzato, M., Darrell, T., Bourdev, L.: Panda: Pose aligned networks for deep attribute modeling. In: IEEE Conference on Computer Vision and Pattern Recognition (CVPR) (2014). Preprint http://arxiv.org/abs/1311.5591

19. Zou, W.Y., Wang, X., Sun, M., Lin, Y.: Generic Object Detection With Dense Neural Patterns and Regionlets. CoRR (2014). Preprint http://arxiv.org/abs/1404.4316

20. Jain, A., Tompson, J., Andriluka, M., Taylor, G.W., Bregler, C.: Learning human pose estimation features with convolutional networks. In: International Conference on Learning Representations (ICLR) (2014). Preprint http://arxiv.org/abs/1312.7302

21. Toshev, A., Szegedy, C.: Deeppose: human pose estimation via deep neural networks. In: IEEE Conference on Computer Vision and Pattern Recognition (CVPR) (2014). Preprint http://arxiv.org/abs/1312.4659
22. Sun, Y., Wang, X., Tang, X.: Deep convolutional network cascade for facial point detection. In: IEEE Conference on Computer Vision and Pattern Recognition (CVPR), pp. 3476–3483 (2013)
23. Lazebnik, S., Schmid, C., Ponce, J.: Beyond bags of features: spatial pyramid matching for recognizing natural scene categories. In: IEEE Conference on Computer Vision and Pattern Recognition (CVPR), pp. 2169–2178 (2006)
24. Coates, A., Ng, A.: The importance of encoding versus training with sparse coding and vector quantization. In: Proceedings of the 28th International Conference on Machine Learning (ICML), pp. 921–928. ACM (2011)
25. Borji, A., Itti, L.: State-of-the-art in visual attention modeling. IEEE Trans. Pattern Anal. Mach. Intell. (PAMI) **35**, 185–207 (2013)
26. Göring, C., Rodner, E., Freytag, A., Denzler, J.: Nonparametric part transfer for fine-grained recognition. In: IEEE Conference on Computer Vision and Pattern Recognition (CVPR) (2014)
27. Wah, C., Branson, S., Welinder, P., Perona, P., Belongie, S.: The Caltech-UCSD Birds-200-2011 dataset. Technical report CNS-TR-2011-001. California Institute of Technology (2011)
28. Liu, J., Kanazawa, A., Jacobs, D., Belhumeur, P.: Dog breed classification using part localization. In: Fitzgibbon, A., Lazebnik, S., Perona, P., Sato, Y., Schmid, C. (eds.) ECCV 2012, Part I. LNCS, vol. 7572, pp. 172–185. Springer, Heidelberg (2012)
29. Chai, Y., Lempitsky, V., Zisserman, A.: Symbiotic segmentation and part localization for fine-grained categorization. In: IEEE International Conference on Computer Vision (ICCV), pp. 321–328 (2013)
30. Zhang, N., Donahue, J., Girshick, R., Darrell, T.: Part-based R-CNNs for fine-grained category detection. In: Fleet, D., Pajdla, T., Schiele, B., Tuytelaars, T. (eds.) ECCV 2014, Part I. LNCS, vol. 8689, pp. 834–849. Springer, Heidelberg (2014)
31. Branson, S., Horn, G.V., Belongie, S., Perona, P.: Bird species categorization using Pose normalized deep convolutional nets. CoRR (2014). Preprint http://arxiv.org/abs/1406.2952

Performance Evaluation of 3D Local Feature Descriptors

Yulan Guo[1,2]($\boxtimes$), Mohammed Bennamoun[2], Ferdous Sohel[2], Min Lu[1],
Jianwei Wan[1], and Jun Zhang[1]

[1] College of Electronic Science and Engineering,
National University of Defense Technology, Changsha, China
yulan.guo@nudt.edu.cn
[2] School of Computer Science and Software Engineering,
The University of Western Australia, Crawley, Australia

Abstract. A number of 3D local feature descriptors have been proposed
in literature. It is however, unclear which descriptors are more appropriate for a particular application. This paper compares nine popular local
descriptors in the context of 3D shape retrieval, 3D object recognition,
and 3D modeling. We first evaluate these descriptors on six popular
datasets in terms of descriptiveness. We then test their robustness with
respect to support radius, Gaussian noise, shot noise, varying mesh resolution, image boundary, and keypoint localization errors. Our extensive
tests show that Tri-Spin-Images (TriSI) has the best overall performance
across all datasets. Unique Shape Context (USC), Rotational Projection
Statistics (RoPS), 3D Shape Context (3DSC), and Signature of Histograms of OrienTations (SHOT) also achieved overall acceptable results.

1 Introduction

Local features have proven to be very successful in many vision tasks such as
3D object recognition, 3D modeling, 3D shape retrieval, and 3D biometrics
[1–6]. Local features have been extensively investigated during the last few
decades with the aim to design descriptors which are distinctive, robust to occlusions and clutter [7]. A local feature based algorithm typically involves two major
phases: keypoint detection and feature description [8,9]. In the keypoint detection phase, keypoints with rich information contents are first identified and their
associated scales (spatial extents) are then determined [9]. In the feature description phase, local geometric information around a keypoint is extracted and stored
in a high-dimensional vector (i.e., feature descriptor) [10]. Finally, the feature
descriptors of one pointcloud (or range image and mesh) are matched against
the feature descriptors of other pointclouds of interest to yield point-to-point
feature correspondences [9].

A wide variety of 3D keypoint detectors and feature descriptors have been
proposed in the literature [8,9,11,12]. It is widely agreed that the evaluation
of feature detectors and descriptors is very important [13]. Several 3D keypoint
detector evaluations can be found in the literature, e.g., [9,11]. Descriptiveness

© Springer International Publishing Switzerland 2015
D. Cremers et al. (Eds.): ACCV 2014, Part II, LNCS 9004, pp. 178–194, 2015.
DOI: 10.1007/978-3-319-16808-1_13

and robustness have been considered as two important requirements for a qualified 3D feature descriptor (see more in Sect. 3.3) [14,15]. A feature descriptor is descriptive if it is capable of encapsulating the predominant information of the underlying surface. That is, it should provide sufficient descriptive richness to distinguish one local surface from another. A feature is robust if it is insensitive to a number of nuisances which can affect the data, e.g., noise and variations in the mesh resolution [9].

Although a large number of feature descriptors have been proposed, they were originally designed for various specific application scenarios and only tested on respective datasets. It is therefore very challenging for users to select the most appropriate and application independent descriptor. Beyond performance evaluations of 2D keypoint detectors [13,16–18], 2D local descriptors [7,17–19], and 3D keypoint detectors [9,11,20,21], several evaluations on 3D local feature descriptors can also be found in the literature. Bronstein et al. [11] and Boyer et al. [20] respectively proposed an experimental evaluation of three and four 3D local feature descriptors in the context of shape retrieval. Alexandre [22] evaluated both local and global feature descriptors on a clutter-free dataset for 3D object and category recognition. Kim and Hilton [23] presented an evaluation of 3D local feature descriptors for multi-modal data registration. Other related work include [14,24]. However, many of these evaluations tested only few 3D local feature descriptors and for a particular application domain. Besides, the robustness of the feature descriptors is ignored in most (if not all) of these papers.

In this paper, we present a comprehensive comparison of the state-of-the-art 3D local feature descriptors and extensively test their performance on six popular datasets. Our comparison is grounded on an established methodology which was previously adopted in the evaluation of 2D local feature descriptors in [7]. Our datasets contain a large variety of scene types acquired with different imaging techniques. The performance of these descriptors on these different datasets is analyzed and discussed. We also evaluate these descriptors in three different application contexts (namely, 3D shape retrieval, 3D modeling, and 3D object recognition). Moreover, we test the robustness of these descriptors with respect to a set of nuisances including support radius, Gaussian noise, shot noise, varying mesh resolutions, image boundary, and keypoint localization error (Sect. 3.3). The paper is different from the literature in several aspects. First, compared to [11,14,20,22,23], our paper includes more local feature descriptors and evaluates their performance for various applications. Second, compared to [24], our paper tested 6 additional feature descriptors and analyzed the robustness of local feature descriptors. Third, as opposed to [14,22–24], our paper compares the performance of each local feature descriptor based on criteria which only measure the performance of the feature matching of the descriptor, irrespective of any other parts of a pipeline in a specific context. Our evaluation therefore produces a performance measure for the descriptor itself rather than the whole pipeline (e.g., recognition accuracy), as commonly used in the evaluation for 2D feature descriptors (e.g., in [7,17–19]).

The rest of this paper is organized as follows. Section 2 presents the state-of-the-art of the 3D local feature descriptors. Section 3 describes the datasets, our evaluation criteria, and the implementation details of the tested descriptors. Section 4 presents our experimental results and analysis. Section 5 concludes this paper.

2   3D Local Feature Descriptors

A number of 3D local surface descriptors have been proposed in the literature [11,14,20,22,23]. Many algorithms use histograms to represent different characteristics of the local surface. Specifically, they describe the local surface by accumulating geometric or topological measurements (e.g., point numbers) into histograms according to a specific domain (e.g., point coordinates, geometric attributes). We therefore, categorize these algorithms into spatial distribution histogram based and geometric attribute histogram based descriptors. For a comprehensive review of the existing 3D local feature descriptors, the reader is referred to [8].

2.1   Spatial Distribution Histogram Based Descriptors

Spin Image (SI) [25]. The SI algorithm represents each neighboring point in the support region with two parameters α and β. The radial coordinate α is defined as the perpendicular distance to the line through the surface normal, the elevation coordinate β is defined as the signed perpendicular distance to the tangent plane of the keypoint. The $\alpha - \beta$ space is then discretized into a 2D array accumulator. Finally, the SI descriptor is generated by accumulating the neighboring points into each bin of the 2D array.

3D Shape Context (3DSC) [26]. The 3DSC algorithm places a 3D spherical grid at the keypoint, with the north pole of the grid being aligned with the surface normal of the keypoint. The support region is then divided into several bins along the radial, azimuth, and elevation dimensions. The 3DSC descriptor is generated by counting up the weighted number of points falling into each bin of the grid.

Unique Shape Context (USC) [27]. It is an extension of 3DSC with the goal to avoid the computation of multiple descriptors at a given keypoint. First, a Local Reference Frame (LRF) is constructed for each keypoint. Next, the local surface is aligned with the LRF in order to achieve invariance to rigid transformations. Finally, the USC descriptor is generated using the same approach as 3DSC.

Rotational Projection Statistics (RoPS) [10,28]. The algorithm first aligns the local surface with its LRF. The neighboring points on the local surface are then respectively rotated around the three coordinate axes. For each rotation, the neighboring points are projected onto the three coordinate planes to generate three distribution matrices. Each distribution matrix is further encoded with five statistics. Finally, the RoPS descriptor is generated by concatenating all these statistics from all rotations and projections.

Tri-Spin-Images (TriSI) [29]. It uses the same technique as in [10] to align the local surface with its LRF. Next, a spin image is generated using the x axis as its reference axis followed by the same procedure as the SI [25]. Then, another two spin images are also generated using the y and z axes as their reference axes. The three spin images are concatenated to form the TriSI descriptor.

2.2 Geometric Attribute Histogram Based Descriptors

THRIFT [30]. It is a 1D histogram over the deviation angles between the surface normal at the keypoint and the normals of the neighboring points. The contribution of each neighboring point to a particular bin of the histogram is determined by two factors: (1) the density of the point samples, and (2) the distance from the neighboring point to the keypoint.

Point Feature Histograms (PFH) [31]. It is a multi-dimensional histogram over several features of the neighboring point pairs. For each pair of neighboring points, four features are calculated using the Darboux frame and the surface normals. PFH is generated by accumulating the neighboring points in particular bins along the dimensions of the aforementioned four features. In their later work [32], one feature (i.e., distance) is excluded from the histogram of PFH to improve its robustness to the density variation of points.

Fast Point Feature Histograms (FPFH) [32]. A Simplified Point Feature Histogram (SPFH) is first formulated for each neighboring point by encoding the relationships between itself and its neighboring points. The FPFH descriptor is then generated as the weighted sum of the SPFH of the keypoint and the SPFHs of the neighboring points.

Signature of Histograms of OrienTations (SHOT) [33,34]. The SHOT algorithm first aligns the neighboring points of a keypoint with its LRF. Then, the support region is divided into several volumes along the radial, azimuth, and elevation axes. For each volume, a local histogram is generated by accumulating point counts into bins according to the angles between the normals at the neighboring points within the volume and the normal at the keypoint. Finally, the SHOT descriptor is generated by concatenating all local histograms.

2.3 Other Methods

Other descriptors include 3D Tensor [1], Variable-Dimensional Local Shape Descriptors (VD-LSD) [35], 2.5D SIFT descriptor [36], SI-SIFT descriptor [37], Exponential Map (EM) [38], and Integral Invariants [39,40]. However, 3D Tensor is defined at the center of two points rather than any point of the input mesh, it is difficult to generate 3D Tensor descriptors at a set of given keypoints. A complicated training stage is required for VD-LSD to select invariant properties. Furthermore, both 2.5D SIFT, SI-SIFT, and EM descriptors can only work on depth images with a lattice structure.

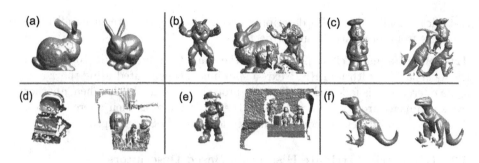

Fig. 1. Examples of models and scenes from the datasets. One model and one scene are shown for each dataset. (a) *Retrieval.* (b) *Random Views.* (c) *Laser Scanner.* (d) *Space Time.* (e) *Kinect.* (f) *2.5D Views.*

3   Experimental Setup

In this section, we describe the datasets and the evaluation criteria used in our tests to assess the performance of our selected descriptors in Sect. 2. We also present the implementation details of the evaluated descriptors.

3.1   Datasets

We evaluate the descriptors of Sect. 2 on six popular and publicly available datasets. Figure 1 shows some examples of models and scenes taken from these datasets. The first five datasets are the same as the ones used for the 3D keypoints evaluation in [9]. Therefore, our paper provides the possibility to select an appropriate combination of 3D keypoint detectors and feature descriptors for a particular application based on their respective performance on the same dataset. We also test the descriptors on an additional dataset, i.e., the *2.5D Views* dataset.

The details of these datasets are listed in Table 1. These datasets are selected based on three major considerations: diverse acquisition techniques (e.g., Minolta Vivid 910, SpaceTime Stereo, and Kinect), different application scenarios (e.g., 3D object recognition, 3D shape retrieval, and 3D modeling), and various image qualities.

Table 1. Datasets used in the evaluation. '-' means not relevant to that dataset.

No.	Dataset name	Acquisition	Quality	Occlusion	Clutter	Model	Scene	# Models	# Scenes	Scenario
1	*Retrieval* [9]	Synthetic	High	No	No	3D	3D	6	18	Retrieval
2	*Random Views* [9]	Synthetic	High	Yes	Yes	3D	2.5D	6	36	Recognition
3	*Laser Scanner*[1]	Vivid	High	Yes	Yes	3D	2.5D	5	10	Recognition
4	*Space Time* [9]	SpaceTime	Medium	Yes	Yes	2.5D	2.5D	6	12	Recognition
5	*Kinect* [9]	Kinect	Low	Yes	Yes	2.5D	2.5D	27	17	Recognition
6	*2.5D Views*[1]	Vivid	High	Yes	No	-	2.5D	-	75	Modeling

3.2 Ground-Truth

All datasets except *2.5D Views* consist of a number of models and scenes. The ground-truth rigid transformations (i.e., rotation and translation) between each model and its instance in the scene is known a priori. For more details on the generation of these ground-truth transformations, the reader is referred to [1,9, 33,34]. *2.5D Views* [1] contains only a set of 2.5D scenes from four objects for the reconstruction of 3D objects. The ground-truth transformation between any pair of pointclouds of the same object is first calculated by manual alignment and then refined using the iterative closest point algorithm [41].

3.3 Evaluation Criteria

We tested our selected descriptors (Sect. 2) in terms of both descriptiveness and robustness.

Descriptiveness. We use the *Recall* versus *1-Precision* Curve (RPC) to evaluate the descriptiveness of a feature descriptor. RPC is commonly used in the literature for the evaluation of local feature descriptors (in both 2D images and 3D pointclouds), for example in [7,10,30,33,34]. The process for generating a RPC is described in [7]. In this paper, the Euclidean distance is used to measure the similarity between feature descriptors (as in [10,33,34]). Then, the nearest neighbor distance ratio based matching strategy is adopted to generate the matching features (as in [7,10]).

In order to avoid the influence of keypoint detectors on the evaluation results, N_f keypoints are first randomly selected from each scene without keypoint detection ($N_f = 1000$ in this paper), their corresponding model keypoints are then determined and different surface descriptors are finally generated from these fixed keypoints (as in [10,33,34]). Since the same procedure is applied to all methods, we believe the comparison is fair and unbiased. For *2.5D Views*, we only consider the pointcloud pairs which have an overlap of more than 50 %.

Robustness. We test the robustness of each feature descriptor with respect to the following variations.

Support Radius ρ: We use different support radii to define the neighboring local surface of each keypoint. For a given radius ρ, points which are distant from the keypoint by less than ρ constitute the neighboring points of that keypoint. It should be noted that in the case of 3D data, "scale" corresponds to the "support radius" [9].

Gaussian Noise: We add Gaussian noise with standard deviations of 0.1 mr, 0.2 mr, 0.3 mr, 0.4 mr, and 0.5 mr to each scene, where 'mr' denotes the average mesh resolution of the models. For a given standard deviation, Gaussian noise is independently added to the x, y, and z axes of each scene point, as in [10].

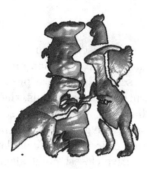

Fig. 2. A mesh with its boundary shown in red (Color figure online).

Shot Noise: We add shot noise with outlier ratios of 0.2 %, 0.5 %, 1.0 %, 2.0 %, and 5.0 % to each scene. Given an outlier ratio γ, a ratio γ of the total points in each scene are first selected and a displacement with an amplitude of 20 mr is then added to each selected point along its normal direction, as in [10,42]. Note that, shot noise usually exist in pointclouds acquired with low resolution scanners. It might be caused by miscalibration of the scanning device or image-based reconstruction of texture-less surfaces.

Varying Mesh Resolutions: We resample each scene to five levels such that only $1/2, 1/4, 1/8, 1/16$, and $1/32$ of their original points are left in the resampled scene, as in [10].

Distance to the Image Boundary: We classify the scene keypoints into six groups according to their distances to the image boundary (as shown in Fig. 2). Each group contains keypoints which are within a range of distances. For example, the 2nd group contains keypoints with distances larger than $1\rho/5$ and less than $2\rho/5$ (ρ is the support radius).

Keypoint Localization Error: For each pair of corresponding points $\left(\boldsymbol{p}_i^M, \boldsymbol{p}_i^S\right)$ in each scene-model pair, we randomly select another scene point $\boldsymbol{p}_{i'}^S$ such that the distance between $\boldsymbol{p}_i^S$ and $\boldsymbol{p}_{i'}^S$ is less than a threshold τ_d. We use these new corresponding points $\left(\boldsymbol{p}_i^M, \boldsymbol{p}_{i'}^S\right)$ to produce the RPC results. Six different distance thresholds τ_d (i.e., 1 mr, 3 mr, 5 mr, 7 mr, 9 mr, and 11 mr) are used in Sect. 4.2.

3.4   Implementation Details

We use 9 different descriptors for our performance evaluation. These descriptors are briefly described in Sect. 2 and include SI, 3DSC, THRIFT, PFH, FPFH, SHOT, USC, RoPS, and TriSI. Some other methods presented in Sect. 2 have specific requirements which make their inclusion in this comparison infeasible. 3DSC, PFH, FPFH, SHOT, and USC were implemented in C++ and they are available in the Point Cloud Library (PCL) [43], while the others were implemented in Matlab (as they are not available in PCL). Note that, although SI is available in PCL, its dimensionality is fixed to 153 and different from the original paper. We therefore implemented SI in Matlab using the same parameters (i.e., dimensionality of 225) as the original paper. In a similar manner to [9,16,24], the proposed default parameters in the original articles or PCL implementations were used for all selected descriptors. Unless stated otherwise in our experiments, the values of all the parameters of each descriptor were fixed when tested across all datasets. The support radius for all descriptors was set to 15 mr throughout this paper (except in Sect. 4.2 where the "Support Radius" was varied to assess the robustness of the selected descriptors). The surface normals of the points were calculated using the method described in [44], the directions of the normals in each scene are checked to ensure that they are the same as the normals of the models. Besides, the curvatures were estimated using the algorithm proposed in [45].

4 Performance Evaluation

4.1 Descriptiveness

We present the RPC results of these selected descriptors on the six datasets, as shown in Fig. 3.

Retrieval **Dataset.** The *Retrieval dataset* contains 18 scenes and 6 models. The scene meshes with three levels of noise are used in this experiment. USC achieves the best recall results, closely followed by TriSI, RoPS, and SHOT. 3DSC gives a moderate performance. Note that, the recall achieved by USC is much higher than 3DSC on the same dataset. This clearly demonstrates that the use of an LRF in USC not only reduces the memory requirements and the computational complexity of 3DSC, but also improves the matching accuracy of 3DSC [27]. Besides, FPFH, PFH, and SI have a similar performance, which is inferior to 3DSC.

Random Views **Dataset.** The *Random Views* dataset contains 36 scenes and 6 models. The scene meshes with three levels of noise are used in this experiment. 3DSC achieves the best performance, closely followed by TriSI. The next most performant descriptors are SHOT and USC. RoPS and SI achieve acceptable results, which are in fact much better compared to FPFH and PFH. As in the case of the *Retrieval* dataset, THRIFT gives the lowest scores. Note that, *Retrieval* and *Random Views* have the same models, with the major difference that *Random Views* contains occluded objects and clutter. Comparing the results in Fig. 3(a) and (b), three observations can be made. First, the recall on *Random Views* is significantly lower than the recall of *Retrieval* due to the more challenging conditions caused by occlusions and clutter. Second, when comparing the difference of the performance of each descriptor on these two datasets, USC, TriSI, RoPS, and SHOT have a larger drop compared to other descriptors. This is because these four descriptors are very sensitive to occlusions and clutter (see Sect. 4.2 under "Support Radius" and "Distance to the Image Boundary"). Third, the rankings of these descriptors on these two datasets are similar except

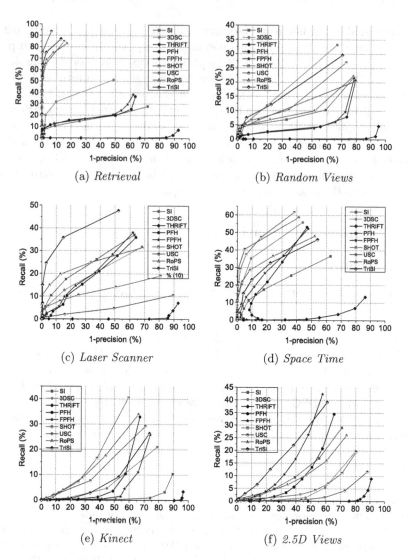

Fig. 3. Descriptiveness of the selected descriptors of Sect. 2 on the six datasets of Sect. 3.1 (Figure best seen in color) (Color figure online).

for SI, USC and 3DSC. USC is more suitable for the scenario of 3D shape retrieval, while 3DSC and SI are more suitable for 3D object recognition.

Laser Scanner Dataset. TriSI achieves the best results, showing a significant improvement compared to the other descriptors. RoPS and SI have a similar performance, followed by 3DSC, FPFH, and PFH. Note that, FPFH reduces the computational complexity of feature generation by an order of magnitude over PFH, while maintaining a similar performance in terms of feature matching accuracy. SHOT produces moderate results, which are better than those of USC. 3DSC performs much better than USC on this dataset at the cost of an increased computational complexity and storage requirement.

***Space Time* Dataset.** USC and SHOT outperform all the other descriptors, closely followed by 3DSC. It can be concluded that the shape context style descriptors (such as 3DSC and USC) are more suitable for applications with *Space Time*. The next performant descriptors are RoPS, TriSI, FPFH, and PFH. All these four descriptors produced a very close performance. SI achieves a moderate performance, with a lower recall compared to TriSI.

***Kinect* Dataset.** SHOT achieves the best performance, followed by RoPS and USC. PFH and TriSI produced a similar performance. Note that, the recall achieved by FPFH is lower than PFH. Similarly, the recall obtained by 3DSC is lower compared USC. We also observe that SI and THRIFT do not work well on this dataset, mainly due to its high sensitivity to noise (as shown in Sect. 4.2). SI and THRIFT are therefore more suitable for applications on images with low noise and high resolution (e.g., *Laser Scanner*).

***2.5D Views* Dataset.** TriSI gives the best results, followed by FPFH. PFH produced a much lower score compared to FPFH although the former requires more computational time. SI performs slightly better than PFH, which is followed by RoPS. 3DSC and SHOT have a very close performance, achieving a relatively low recall. Besides, the scores of USC and THRIFT are amongst the lowest. Note that, both *2.5D Views* and *Laser Scanner* were acquired with Minolta Vivid 910. The major difference between the two datasets is that *Laser Scanner* contains both occlusions and clutter while *2.5D Views* contains only occlusions. Compared to the results reported on *Laser Scanner* (Fig. 3(c)), several observations can be drawn. First, the rankings of these descriptors are similar on the two datasets. TriSI gives the best results, while SHOT, USC, and THRIFT achieve relatively low scores. Second, the superior performance of TriSI is more significant on *Laser Scanner* compared to *2.5D Views*. Third, FPFH performs better than PFH, and 3DSC achieved a better performance compared to USC on both of these two datasets. Fourth, RoPS is more suitable for object recognition compared to 3D modeling, FPFH and PFH are more suitable for 3D modeling compared to object recognition.

Descriptiveness Overall Performance. In order to directly compare the performance of these descriptors on each dataset, we calculate the recall at the precision of 50 % (denoted by $recall_{0.5p}$). $recall_{0.5p}$ is an established methodology previously adopted in [7] for the evaluation of a descriptor with a single number. The $recall_{0.5p}$ results of all these descriptors on the six datasets are presented in Table 2. We also present the average and median $recall_{0.5p}$ of the descriptors over all datasets. Several conclusions can be summarized as follows.

First, TriSI, SHOT, and RoPS are amongst the best descriptors. Specifically, SHOT achieves the best performance on the *Space Time* and *Kinect* datasets.

Table 2. The recall at 50 % precision of the descriptors of Sect. 2 on the six datasets of Sect. 3.1. The best performance is reported in bold face, and the highest results for each dataset are shown in blue (Table best seen in color).

Descriptor \ Dataset	SI	3DSC	THRIFT	PFH	FPFH	SHOT	USC	RoPS	TriSI
Retrieval	20.2	51.2	0.1	19.9	21.5	84.8	**93.5**	82.9	87.0
Random Views	9.1	**25.6**	0.2	4.2	3.8	17.1	14.3	9.9	22.2
Laser Scanner	31.6	25.2	0.1	27.0	29.5	14.0	4.8	28.0	**46.9**
Space Time	31.3	56.0	1.0	53.1	52.3	**61.7**	58.7	47.2	44.4
Kinect	0.3	7.1	0	4.3	1.1	**30.0**	17.3	22.0	8.2
2.5D Views	14.5	2.6	0	13.0	29.3	3.9	1.0	11.7	**31.0**
Average	17.8	27.9	0.2	20.2	23.0	35.3	31.6	33.6	**40.0**
Median	17.4	25.4	0.1	16.4	25.4	23.6	15.8	25.0	**37.7**

TriSI performs best on the *Laser Scanner* and *2.5D Views* datasets. Overall, TriSI has the highest average and median recall across all these datasets. It outperforms SHOT by a large margin, with average values of $recall_{0.5p}$ being 40.0 and 35.3, respectively. In contrast, THRIFT is the descriptor with the lowest performance on all these datasets.

Second, the performance of these descriptors depends on the dataset. It is clear that USC, 3DSC, TriSI, RoPS, and SHOT are the descriptors which produce the best performance on high resolution datasets (i.e., *Retrieval* and *Random Views*). Besides, SHOT, USC, and RoPS have a relatively better performance compared to all the others when tested on low resolution datasets (i.e., *Space Time* and *Kinect*). Moreover, TriSI, RoPS, SI, and FPFH are the top descriptors on the medium-level resolution datasets (i.e., *Laser Scanner* and *2.5D Views*).

Third, PFH, FPFH, TriSI, SI, and 3DSC generally show a more stable performance across datasets compared to all the others. In contrast, the performance of SHOT and USC varies significantly, as revealed by the large differences between their average and median values of $recall_{0.5p}$. This conclusion corroborates with the results in [14,23].

4.2 Robustness

In this section, we present the $recall_{0.5p}$ results of these descriptors with respect to different variations, as shown in Fig. 4. In this paper, we only present experimental results on the *Laser Scanner* dataset due to the limited number of pages. Note that, *Laser Scanner* is one of the most frequently used datasets in 3D computer vision [1,9,10,38,44].

Support Radius. The support radius affects both the feature's descriptiveness and its robustness to occlusions and clutter [10]. Two major observations can be made from the results in Fig. 4(a). First, the recall results of TriSI, FPFH,

PFH, RoPS, and SHOT improve rapidly when the support radius is increased. Their performance reaches the peak value with a support radius of about 15 mr. Their performance then decreases with an increase in the support radius. This is because these descriptors are highly sensitive to occlusions and clutter (as further demonstrated in Sect. 4.2 "Distance to the Image Boundary"). They produce the best performance when an optimal tradeoff is achieved between their descriptiveness and sensitivity. Second, for the descriptors which are less sensitive to occlusions and clutter (e.g., SI, 3DSC, and USC), their performance increases consistently with an increase in the support radius. This is because, the major factor which influences their performance is the encapsulated information of the underlying local surface rather than occlusions and clutter, as further explained in Sect. 4.2 "Distance to the Image Boundary".

Gaussian Noise. The performance of all descriptors decreases very rapidly when the standard deviation of the Gaussian noise increases. USC is the most robust descriptor with respect to Gaussian noise, its value is very stable under different levels of noise. RoPS, TriSI, and SHOT also have acceptable robustness with respect to Gaussian noise. On the other hand, SI, THRIFT, PFH, and FPFH are very sensitive to Gaussian noise, their recall drops significantly when the standard deviation of Gaussian noise increases to 0.1 mr. This is because they rely on first-order surface derivatives (i.e., surface normal), which are prone to noise.

Shot Noise. TriSI is highly robust to shot noise, achieving a high recall (close to 40 %) with an outlier ratio of shot noise of 5 %. USC and SHOT are also very robust to shot noise, their performances drop slowly when the shot noise increases. The other descriptors are more affected by shot noise. RoPS achieves similar results compared to PFH with low levels of shot noise. It then outperforms PFH when the level of shot noise is high. Both FPFH and PFH are highly sensitive to shot noise, their performance deteriorates dramatically even with a low level of shot noise. From Fig. 4(b) and (c), it is clear that TriSI, USC, and SHOT are robust while PFH and FPFH are sensitive to both Gaussian and shot noise.

Varying Mesh Resolutions. The recall of all these descriptors decreases as the level of mesh decimation increases. TriSI has the best performance under all levels of mesh decimation. PFH, FPFH, SI, TriSI are robust to varying mesh resolutions. Their drop in performance with respect to varying mesh resolutions is smaller compared to other descriptors. In contrast, THRIFT and USC are sensitive to varying mesh resolutions.

Distance to the Image Boundary. The performance of TriSI is significantly boosted by eliminating points which are close to the image boundary. Specifically, the $recall_{0.5p}$ is increased from about 10 % to about 60 % by removing points with

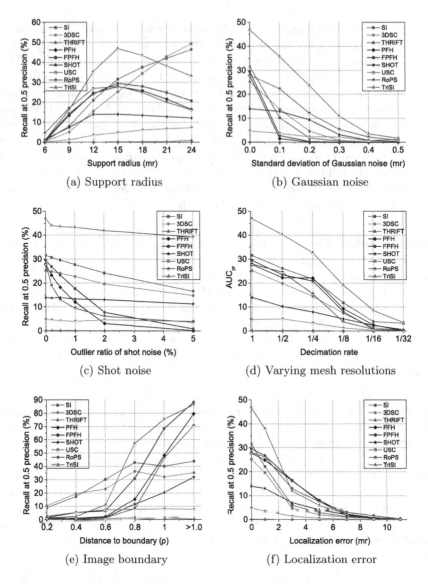

Fig. 4. Robustness of the selected descriptors of Sect. 2 on the *Laser Scanner* dataset (Figure best seen in color) (Color figure online).

distances less than 0.8ρ to the boundary. Similarly, the recall results of FPFH, PFH, RoPS, and SHOT are also significantly improved by removing boundary points. In contrast, SI, 3DSC, and USC are more robust to boundary points. SI and 3DSC achieve the best performance compared to all other descriptors when tested on keypoints with distances less than 0.7ρ to the boundary. Since the points close to the boundary include occlusions and clutter (as shown in Fig. 2) it can be concluded that TriSI, FPFH, PFH, RoPS, and SHOT are sensitive to occlusions and clutter. In contrast, SI, 3DSC, and USC are very robust to occlusions and clutter. This is consistent with the conclusions drawn in Sect. 4.2 "Support Radius".

Keypoint Localization Error. The recall decreases with increasing keypoint localization errors. The performance of TriSI, SI, and 3DSC drops faster than all the other descriptors, especially at keypoints with small localization errors. This indicates that these three descriptors are very sensitive to the accuracy of the keypoint localization. For keypoints with localization errors less than 3 mr, the superior performance of TriSI is highly significant compared to the other descriptors. For keypoints with localization errors of more than 5 mr, TriSI, RoPS, FPFH, PFH produce a very close performance. Their recall is the highest compared to the other descriptors. Besides, SI, SHOT, and 3DSC achieve the second best performance.

5 Conclusions

This paper presents a comprehensive evaluation of 3D local feature descriptors on a variety of datasets. It can serve as a "User Guide" for the selection of the most appropriate feature descriptor in the area of 3D computer vision. The descriptiveness of these descriptors was tested on six datasets in different application contexts. Generally, TriSI achieved the best overall results in terms of recall. USC, RoPS, and SHOT also produce good scores on some of these datasets. The robustness of these descriptors was also evaluated with respect to a number of nuisances. TriSI, SHOT, and USC are very robust to both Gaussian noise and shot noise, while PFH and FPFH are highly sensitive. SI and 3DSC are very robust to the distance to image boundary, while TriSI, RoPS, SHOT, PFH, and FPFH are all very sensitive. Moreover, the performance of TriSI, SI, and 3DSC dropped significantly when the localization error of the keypoints increased.

While these descriptors perform well on high resolution datasets (collected using costly scanners), their performance is rather weak with data from low-cost sensors (e.g., Kinect). Research should therefore be directed towards the design of suitable descriptors for low resolution and high-level noise data, or the design of higher resolution and low-cost RGBD cameras. In this paper, feature descriptors are extracted from the randomly selected ground-truth corresponding points between the scene and model. Therefore, the affect of keypoint detection algorithm on the feature matching performance of feature descriptors is not considered. In order to better resemble real applications, we will test these descriptors in combination with different 3D keypoint detectors in our future work.

Acknowledgement. This research was supported in part by the National Natural Science Foundation of China under Grant 61471371, and in part by the Australian Research Council under Grants DE120102960 and DP110102166.

References

1. Mian, A., Bennamoun, M., Owens, R.: Three-dimensional model-based object recognition and segmentation in cluttered scenes. IEEE Trans. Pattern Anal. Mach. Intell. **28**, 1584–1601 (2006)
2. Guo, Y., Wan, J., Lu, M., Niu, W.: A parts-based method for articulated target recognition in laser radar data. Opt. Int. J. Light Electron. Opt. **124**, 2727–2733 (2013)
3. Bronstein, A., Bronstein, M., Guibas, L., Ovsjanikov, M.: Shape google: geometric words and expressions for invariant shape retrieval. ACM Trans. Graph. **30**, 1–20 (2011)
4. Guo, Y., Sohel, F., Bennamoun, M., Wan, J., Lu, M.: An accurate and robust range image registration algorithm for 3D object modeling. IEEE Trans. Multimedia **16**, 1377–1390 (2014)
5. Lei, Y., Bennamoun, M., Hayat, M., Guo, Y.: An efficient 3D face recognition approach using local geometrical signatures. Pattern Recogn. **47**, 509–524 (2014)
6. Bennamoun, M., Guo, Y., Sohel, F.: 2D and 3D feature selection for face recognition. Encyclopedia of Electrical and Electronics Engineering (2015, in press)
7. Mikolajczyk, K., Schmid, C.: A performance evaluation of local descriptors. IEEE Trans. Pattern Anal. Mach. Intell. **27**, 1615–1630 (2005)
8. Guo, Y., Bennamoun, M., Sohel, F., Lu, M., Wan, J.: 3D object recognition in cluttered scenes with local surface features: a survey. IEEE Trans. Pattern Anal. Mach. Intell. **36**(11), 2270–2287 (2014)
9. Tombari, F., Salti, S., Di Stefano, L.: Performance evaluation of 3D keypoint detectors. Int. J. Comput. Vis. **102**, 198–220 (2013)
10. Guo, Y., Sohel, F., Bennamoun, M., Lu, M., Wan, J.: Rotational projection statistics for 3D local surface description and object recognition. Int. J. Comput. Vis. **105**, 63–86 (2013)
11. Bronstein, A., Bronstein, M., Bustos, B., et al.: SHREC 2010: robust feature detection and description benchmark. In: Eurographics Workshop on 3D Object Retrieval, vol. 2, p. 6 (2010)
12. Shah, S.A.A., Bennamoun, M., Boussaid, F., El-Sallam, A.: A novel local surface description for automatic 3D object recognition in low resolution cluttered scenes. In: IEEE International Conference on Computer Vision Workshops, pp. 638–643 (2013)
13. Schmid, C., Mohr, R., Bauckhage, C.: Evaluation of interest point detectors. Int. J. Comput. Vis. **37**, 151–172 (2000)
14. Restrepo, M.I., Mundy, J.L.: An evaluation of local shape descriptors in probabilistic volumetric scenes. In: British Machine Vision Conference, pp. 1–11 (2012)
15. Guo, Y., Bennamoun, M., Sohel, F., Lu, M., Wan, J.: An integrated framework for 3D modeling, object detection and pose estimation from point-clouds. IEEE Trans. Instrum. Measur. **64**(3), 683–693 (2015)
16. Mikolajczyk, K., Tuytelaars, T., Schmid, C., Zisserman, A., Matas, J., Schaffalitzky, F., Kadir, T., Gool, L.: A comparison of affine region detectors. Int. J. Comput. Vis. **65**, 43–72 (2005)
17. Moreels, P., Perona, P.: Evaluation of features detectors and descriptors based on 3D objects. In: 10th IEEE International Conference on Computer Vision, vol. 1, pp. 800–807 (2005)
18. Moreels, P., Perona, P.: Evaluation of features detectors and descriptors based on 3D objects. Int. J. Comput. Vis. **73**, 263–284 (2007)

19. Mikolajczyk, K., Schmid, C.: A performance evaluation of local descriptors. In: IEEE Conference on Computer Vision and Pattern Recognition, vol. 2, pp. II–257 (2003)

20. Boyer, E., Bronstein, A., Bronstein, M., et al.: SHREC 2011: robust feature detection and description benchmark. In: Eurographics Workshop on Shape Retrieval, pp. 79–86 (2011)

21. Salti, S., Tombari, F., Stefano, L.: A performance evaluation of 3D keypoint detectors. In: International Conference on 3D Imaging, Modeling, Processing, Visualization and Transmission, pp. 236–243 (2011)

22. Alexandre, L.A.: 3D descriptors for object and category recognition: a comparative evaluation. In: Workshop on Color-Depth Camera Fusion in Robotics at the IEEE/RSJ International Conference on Intelligent Robots and Systems (IROS) (2012)

23. Kim, H., Hilton, A.: Evaluation of 3D feature descriptors for multi-modal data registration. In: International Conference on 3D Vision, pp. 119–126 (2013)

24. Salti, S., Petrelli, A., Tombari, F., Di Stefano, L.: On the affinity between 3D detectors and descriptors. In: 2nd International Conference on 3D Imaging, Modeling, Processing, Visualization and Transmission (3DIMPVT), pp. 424–431 (2012)

25. Johnson, A.E., Hebert, M.: Using spin images for efficient object recognition in cluttered 3D scenes. IEEE Trans. Pattern Anal. Mach. Intell. 21, 433–449 (1999)

26. Frome, A., Huber, D., Kolluri, R., Bülow, T., Malik, J.: Recognizing objects in range data using regional point descriptors. In: Pajdla, T., Matas, J.G. (eds.) ECCV 2004. LNCS, vol. 3023, pp. 224–237. Springer, Heidelberg (2004)

27. Tombari, F., Salti, S., Di Stefano, L.: Unique shape context for 3D data description. In: ACM Workshop on 3D Object Retrieval, pp. 57–62 (2010)

28. Guo, Y., Bennamoun, M., Sohel, F., Wan, J., Lu, M.: 3D free form object recognition using rotational projection statistics. In: IEEE 14th Workshop on the Applications of Computer Vision, pp. 1–8 (2013)

29. Guo, Y., Sohel, F., Bennamoun, M., Wan, J., Lu, M.: A novel local surface feature for 3D object recognition under clutter and occlusion. Inf. Sci. 293(2), 196–213 (2015)

30. Flint, A., Dick, A., Van den Hengel, A.: Local 3D structure recognition in range images. IET Comput. Vis. 2, 208–217 (2008)

31. Rusu, R.B., Blodow, N., Marton, Z.C., Beetz, M.: Aligning point cloud views using persistent feature histograms. In: IEEE/RSJ International Conference on Intelligent Robots and Systems, pp. 3384–3391 (2008)

32. Rusu, R.B., Blodow, N., Beetz, M.: Fast point feature histograms (FPFH) for 3D registration. In: IEEE International Conference on Robotics and Automation, pp. 3212–3217 (2009)

33. Tombari, F., Salti, S., Di Stefano, L.: Unique signatures of histograms for local surface description. In: Daniilidis, K., Maragos, P., Paragios, N. (eds.) ECCV 2010, Part III. LNCS, vol. 6313, pp. 356–369. Springer, Heidelberg (2010)

34. Salti, S., Tombari, F., Stefano, L.D.: SHOT: unique signatures of histograms for surface and texture description. Comput. Vis. Image Underst. 125(8), 251–264 (2014)

35. Taati, B., Greenspan, M.: Local shape descriptor selection for object recognition in range data. Comput. Vis. Image Underst. 115, 681–694 (2011)

36. Lo, T., Siebert, J.: Local feature extraction and matching on range images: 2.5D SIFT. Comput. Vis. Image Underst. 113, 1235–1250 (2009)

37. Bayramoglu, N., Alatan, A.: Shape index SIFT: range image recognition using local features. In: 20th International Conference on Pattern Recognition, pp. 352–355 (2010)

38. Bariya, P., Novatnack, J., Schwartz, G., Nishino, K.: 3D geometric scale variability in range images: features and descriptors. Int. J. Comput. Vis. **99**, 232–255 (2012)

39. Pottmann, H., Wallner, J., Huang, Q.X., Yang, Y.L.: Integral invariants for robust geometry processing. Comput. Aided Geom. Des. **26**, 37–60 (2009)

40. Albarelli, A., Rodolà, E., Torsello, A.: Loosely distinctive features for robust surface alignment. In: Daniilidis, K., Maragos, P., Paragios, N. (eds.) ECCV 2010, Part V. LNCS, vol. 6315, pp. 519–532. Springer, Heidelberg (2010)

41. Besl, P.J., McKay, N.D.: A method for registration of 3-D shapes. IEEE Trans. Pattern Anal. Mach. Intell. **14**, 239–256 (1992)

42. Zaharescu, A., Boyer, E., Horaud, R.: Keypoints and local descriptors of scalar functions on 2D manifolds. Int. J. Comput. Vis. **100**, 78–98 (2012)

43. Rusu, R.B., Cousins, S.: 3D is here: point cloud library (PCL). In: IEEE International Conference on Robotics and Automation, pp. 1–4 (2011)

44. Mian, A., Bennamoun, M., Owens, R.: On the repeatability and quality of keypoints for local feature-based 3D object retrieval from cluttered scenes. Int. J. Comput. Vis. **89**, 348–361 (2010)

45. Chen, X., Schmitt, F.: Intrinsic surface properties from surface triangulation. In: Sandini, G. (ed.) ECCV 1992. LNCS, vol. 588. Springer, Heidelberg (1992)

Scene Text Detection Based on Robust Stroke Width Transform and Deep Belief Network

Hailiang Xu, Like Xue, and Feng Su$^{(\boxtimes)}$

State Key Laboratory for Novel Software Technology,
Nanjing University, Nanjing 210023, China
suf@nju.edu.cn

Abstract. Text detection in natural scene images is an open and challenging problem due to the significant variations of the appearance of the text itself and its interaction with the context. In this paper, we present a novel text detection method combining two main ingredients: the robust extension of Stroke Width Transform (SWT) and the Deep Belief Network (DBN) based discrimination of text objects from other scene components. In the former, smoothness-based edge information is combined with gradient for generating high quality edge images, and various edge cues are exploited in Connected Component (CC) analysis on basis of SWT to eliminate inter-character and intra-character errors. In the latter, DBN is exploited for learning efficient representations discriminating character and non-character CCs, resulting in the improved detection accuracy. The proposed method is evaluated on ICDAR and SVT public datasets and achieves the state-of-the-art results, which reveal the effectiveness of the method.

1 Introduction

Text detection in natural scene images is an open problem which has been attracting significant attention as a critical part in many computer vision applications like image retrieval, scene analysis, and robotic navigation in urban environments. Meanwhile, several contests have been held in the past years [1–4], and the winning method in the recent ICDAR 2013 contest [4] was reported capable of detecting 66 % words correctly from the testing images.

Numerous methods for text detection in natural scene images have been proposed [5–10] in recent years, which can be roughly divided into two groups: exhaustive search based methods and selective search based methods. The exhaustive search based methods [6,11,12] use a multiple-scale sliding window to extract features, such as the variance of intensity, HOG. However, the visual search space is huge, making an exhaustive search computationally expensive. Another group of text detection methods is based on the selective search [5,7,10,13–17]. These methods first extract candidate text regions based on certain text properties, such as stroke width or approximately constant color, then adopt heuristic filtering rules or trained classifiers to identify text regions. These methods are attractive since they can simultaneously detect texts at any scale and are not limited to

© Springer International Publishing Switzerland 2015
D. Cremers et al. (Eds.): ACCV 2014, Part II, LNCS 9004, pp. 195–209, 2015.
DOI: 10.1007/978-3-319-16808-1_14

horizontal texts. Meanwhile, they usually work fast due to the low number of candidate text regions. However, the recall rates of both categories of present methods are still far from satisfaction for complicated images.

Specifically, as one popular method for text detection in natural images lately, the method of B. Epstein et al. in [5] shows the great success with the innovative and effective Stroke Width Transform (SWT) algorithm, which achieves the high precision and recall rates with very short processing time. However, the SWT algorithm is sensitive to the defections of the edge images, and its ability of discriminating text components from ambiguous non-text components, which usually result from complicated object compositions like varying colors or unfavourable lighting conditions like shadows or low contrast, could be further improved.

In this paper, we present a novel text detection method combining two main ingredients: the robust extension of SWT and the Deep Belief Network (DBN) [18] based discrimination of text objects from other scene components. For the former, we propose a hybrid method combining both the gradient-based and smoothness-based edge information for generating high quality edge images. Meanwhile, we exploit various edge cues in Connected Component (CC) analysis to eliminate inter-character and intra-character errors. For the latter, we propose a DBN-based seed character extraction to discriminate between character and non-character CCs, followed by growing seed characters to the final text lines.

We evaluate the proposed method on the most cited public ICDARs and Street View Text (SVT) datasets. The method achieves state-of-the-art results in the experiments on all datasets, which show the effectiveness of the method for detecting texts in natural images. We describe the proposed text detection method in detail in Sect. 2 and present our experimental results in Sect. 3.

2   Proposed Method

In this section, we introduce the details of our method, which consists of five processing stages: (1) edge detection, (2) component extraction, (3) component filtering, (4) seed character extraction and (5) text line formation, as shown in Fig. 1 along with the sample results of each stage.

2.1   Edge Detection Combining Gradient and Smoothness Cues

The SWT algorithm tightly relies on the edge detection result, and the Canny method used by the original SWT-based implementation [5] usually failed to acquire robust edges from some complicated image regions like those with low contrast and shadows. Therefore, the first stage of our method is devoted to generating high quality edge images, for which we propose a hybrid edge detection algorithm with two ingredients - the gradient-based and smoothness-based edge detection. Correspondingly, our method will generate two edge images (as shown in Fig. 1(A)), the *gradient-based* edge image and the *smoothness-based*

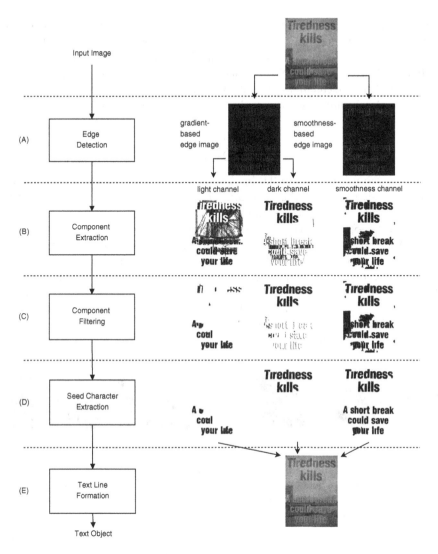

Fig. 1. The framework of the proposed approach (left) and illustration of the sample results of each processing stage (right).

edge image, in which the value of one no-edge pixel is 0 and that of an edge pixel is 255.

For gradient-based edge detection, to extract more complete edge information from the image, the most direct way is to use a lower threshold in edge detection algorithm like Canny, which may, however, also lead to more erroneous edges. To overcome this, we propose to generate the gradient-based edges with a locally adaptive thresholding mechanism. We first generate a gradient image using Sobel operator, then initialize all pixels of an edge image to 0 and set one pixel in the edge image to 255 if its corresponding gradient value (norm of the gradient) in the gradient image is larger than 50, which is a relatively low initial threshold to allow discovering more edge pixels, and the no-maximal suppression (NMS) is used to eliminate invalid edge pixels. Next, to acquire more accurate edges from the initial detection results, we calculate a locally adaptive threshold t for each edge pixel p as Eq. (1) using a sliding window of the size 16 * 16 with the step of 4.

$$t = \alpha * \frac{\sum_{i=1}^{n} \sum_{q \in S_i} G(q)}{\sum_{i=1}^{n} |S_i|} \tag{1}$$

where, α is empirically set to 0.9 in this paper, n is the number of the sliding windows passing through the edge pixel p, S_i is the set of edge pixels in the ith sliding window, $G(q)$ is the gradient value of an edge pixel q in S_i, $|S_i|$ is the size of set S_i. Furthermore, since the edges in a text region are typically sparse, for a pixel with more than 3 sliding windows passing it, in which the percentage of edge pixels exceeds 30 % (i.e. dense), we adjust its threshold t to $max(T_{den}, t)$, T_{den} is an empirical minimum threshold for dense edge regions, which is set to 120 in our method. Given the threshold t for each edge pixel, one edge is extracted starting from an edge pixel p with gradient value higher than t, then tracing from p with the deep traverse algorithm, until an edge pixel with gradient value lower than $t/2$ is met.

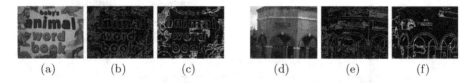

| (a) | (b) | (c) | (d) | (e) | (f) |

Fig. 2. Illustration of the gradient-based edge image (b, e) and the smoothness-based edge image (c, f) for the left sample image (a) with shadows and the right one (d) with low contrast. Note that the smoothness-based edge image better depicts the text contour than the gradient-based one.

Different from most edge extraction methods solely depending on the gradient information, we additionally introduce the smoothness-based edge image, based on the observation that the gradient-based edge image (as shown in Fig. 2(b) and (e)) cannot depict text objects well with shadows (Fig. 2(a)) or low contrast (Fig. 2(d)). To compute the smoothness-based edge image, we first select a set of seed pixels, which has less than 5 neighbouring pixels in the 5 * 5 window whose color distances (computed by CIE94[1] in Lab color space) with seed pixel exceed 4. Then, we identify *seed regions* by starting growing from the seed pixel to its 8-neighbouring pixels if their color distance does not exceed 4. Next, taking all pixels in the seed regions as seed points and increasing the color distance threshold to 7, we again run the region growing algorithm and repeat it

---

[1] http://en.wikipedia.org/wiki/Color_difference.

twice to acquire *color consistency regions (CCRs)*. CCRs of too big sizes will be eliminated for they are unlikely to be texts.

To further improve the completeness of CCRs, we apply two operations called smoothing and de-noising on CCRs. For the former, we traverse each pixel p in the CCR, if one of its neighbouring pixels q does not belong to any other CCRs and has a similar color (color distance less than 10) to p, then q is added to the CCR. On the other hand, the de-noising operation fills the small cavity (less than 30 pixels) in a CCR. Figure 3 illustrates the process of CCR extraction.

Based on the extracted CCRs, we compute the smoothness-based edge image by taking the contours of all CCRs as the edges, as shown in Fig. 2(c) and (f).

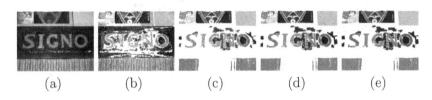

(a)   (b)   (c)   (d)   (e)

Fig. 3. Illustration of the color consistency region (CCR) extraction process: (a) original image, (b) seed regions, (c) CCRs. (d) CCRs after smoothing operation, (e) CCRs after de-noising operation.

2.2 Component Extraction by Robust SWT

We propose a robust SWT-based component extraction method, which is performed independently on the gradient-based edge image and the smoothness-based edge image. The method consists of two aspects: the modification of SWT for more complete retrieval of matching edges while reducing noises, and the CC analysis exploiting edge information to avoid inter-character and intra-character errors in CC extraction.

The Modified SWT. The SWT algorithm followed by CC analysis has been proved an effective and efficient way to detect texts in scene images [5,8]. However, the original SWT and CC algorithm are usually insufficient for complicated occasions like those distorted and interfered texts.

We propose two modifications to the SWT algorithm. First, since we observe in many situations that the gradient intersect angle of 30° used in the original SWT algorithm is not large enough to generate good character strokes, we increase the angle to 60° and in order to reduce the number of false rays between edge pixels in SWT, we introduce a heuristic rule for the admissible gradient value of edge pixels that, if the gradient intersect angle exceeds 30°, the ratio of gradient values of the pair of edge pixels must fall in $[\frac{1}{1.5}, 1.5]$.

Second, to reduce the noises of false rays yielded by the SWT (like those in Fig. 4(a)), we propose to locate and remove the isolated rays from the SWT output. One ray is considered isolated if more than 60 % of pixels on its path are isolated pixels, which in turn are defined as the pixels that have more than 3 neighboring pixels whose SWT value is ∞ (i.e. no passing ray). We remove all isolated rays in an iterative way since the operation may produce new isolated rays. The iteration stops if no more isolated rays are removed or the iteration number reaches 3. Similarly, since continuous isolated pixels are unlikely part of one character stroke, if there are 5 continuous isolated pixels in a ray, they are removed from the ray and this process is iterated until no more isolated pixels have been removed or the iteration number reaches 3. Figure 4(b) shows the result of eliminating such noises from Fig. 4(a).

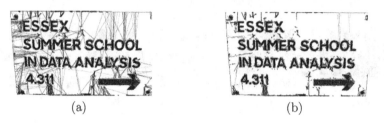

(a)   (b)

Fig. 4. Results of the original SWT (a) and our modified SWT algorithm (b) on the sample image.

Edge-Augmented Connected Component Analysis. The CC algorithm in [5] may produce two main types of errors - the intra-character and inter-character confusion, as illustrated in Fig. 5(a) and (b). To eliminate most of such errors, we propose to exploit the edge information to promote the accuracy of CC extraction. First, we sort each pixel into one of four categories - ES, E, S and $NONE$, as shown in Table 1, based on its corresponding value in the edge and SWT images.

Second, we propose a set of judgement conditions for the connectedness of two neighboring pixels in CC analysis and corresponding processing to avoid intra character and inter-character errors.

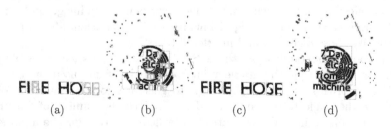

(a)   (b)   (c)   (d)

Fig. 5. Results of the original CC algorithm (left) on sample image with intra-character confusions (a) and sample image with inter-character confusions (b), and our edge-augmented CC algorithm (right) on the same sample images (c) and (d). Note that CCs colored in blue are false extraction results by the original algorithm (Color figure online).

Table 1. Categorization of pixels based on edge and SWT images.

Category	Edge image value	SWT image value
ES	255	Integer
E	255	∞
S	0	Integer
NONE	0	∞

1. Two *ES* pixels p and q are considered connected if the intersect angle of their gradient directions (noted as $AG(p, q)$ in rest of paper) is less than $\pi/6$, and the ratio between their stroke widths (noted as $RSW(p, q)$) is less than 5, and the color distance between the rays (noted as $RCD(p, q)$) passing the *ES* pixels does not exceed 10.
2. Two *S* pixels p and q are considered connected if $RSW(p, q) < 5$.
3. One *ES* pixel is considered connected with one *S* pixel if they belong to the same ray.
4. If there is an *E* pixel q around an *ES* pixel p (Fig. 6), we adopt 8-neighbouring deep traverse algorithm to search another *ES* pixel r whose $AG(p, r) < \pi/3$ and $RSW(p, r) < 5$ and $RCD(p, r) < 10$ and the length of the traverse path does not exceed two times of the largest stroke width of pixel p and r and the AG between each pair of two neighbouring *E* pixels in the path does not exceed $\pi/6$, and we add all *E* pixels to the component that pixel p belongs to. Otherwise, we abandon all *E* pixels in the path.

Figure 5(c) and (d) show the effectiveness of the edge-augmented CC algorithm, compared to the results by the original CC algorithm.

Note that, in order to detect both light text on dark background and vice-versa, we run the component extraction process twice on the gradient-based edge image, once using the normal gradient direction in SWT, producing the *light channel* of processing flow, and once using the inverse gradient direction

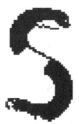 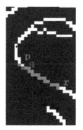

Fig. 6. Illustration of the proposed edge-augmented CC algorithm. Left is the SWT image with the intra-character error as the input of the algorithm. Right is the edge image, in which pixels in pink color correspond to the traversing path of the algorithm connecting the *ES* pixels p and r on the fragmented contour of the character (Color figure online).

in SWT, producing the *dark channel*. We also run the component extraction process on the smoothness-based edge image to produce the *smoothness channel*, as shown in Fig. 1(B).

2.3   Component Filtering

After component extraction processing, a large number of CCs will be extracted, from which we first exploit some characteristics of the CC to filter out non-character components:

- **Aspect ratio (AR)**.
- **Stroke width variation (SWV)**, defined by $\frac{s(c)}{u(c)}$, in which $u(c)$ and $s(c)$ are the mean and standard deviation, respectively, of the stroke widths in the component c.
- **Stroke count ratio (SCR)**, defined by the stroke count, which is the number of different rays within the component in the SWT process, divided by the component height.
- **Stroke width ratio (SWR)**, defined by the stroke width divided by the vertical height of the component.
- **SWT ratio (SWTR)**, defined by $\frac{|E_s|}{|E_{all}|}$, in which, E_s is the set of ES pixels of the component, and E_{all} is the merged set of ES and E pixels. Typically, a character component should have a high SWT ratio.
- **Surround edge ratio (SER)**, defined by $\frac{|n_e|}{|n_{all}|}$, in which, n_{all} is the set of pixels on the out-boundary contour of the component, and n_e is the set of edge pixels in n_{all}.

We learn the valid ranges of these characteristics from the training character components in experiment, by choosing proper thresholds in the histograms of these characteristics. Table 2 shows the valid ranges learned on the ICDAR 2003 training dataset. Figure 1(C) shows the sample results of the component filtering.

2.4   Seed Character Extraction Based on DBN

Deep Belief Network (DBN) [18] is a neural network consists of many layers of Restricted Boltzmann Machines (RBMs). One RBM has a single layer of hidden

Table 2. CC characteristics for component filtering and seed character extraction and their valid ranges.

Characteristics	Valid ranges for component filtering	Valid ranges for seed character extraction
AR	[0.1,4]	$[\frac{1}{3},2]$
SWV	[0, 1]	[0, 0.6]
SWR	[0.05, 0.75]	-
SCR	[0.8, ∞)	-
SWTR	[0.55, 1]	[0.75, 1]
SER	[0.65, 1]	[0.75, 1]

units that are not connected to each other and have undirected, symmetrical connections to a layer of visible units. The RBM is trained by a learning algorithm called Contrastive Divergence (CD) [18], which uses the Gibbs sampling and the reconstruction error to train the weights of RBM. The role of a RBM is to model the distribution of its input. The DBN is constructed by stacking many RBMs on top of each other and linking the hidden layer of one RBM to the visible layer of the next RBM. One way to use the DBN for classification is to simply use the hidden layer activation of the top level RBM as features for any standard classifier or to add a topmost label layer, and train the whole model as a feedforward-backpropagate neural network.

In this work, we exploit DBN to detect seed characters from CCs. Since the appearance of characters in complicated images could be very different from that of normal characters, which may be caused by merged characters or fragmentary edges, it's necessary to screen out candidate CCs corresponding to characters from similar non-character ones. However, the discrimination plane between character and non-character components is highly non-linear and complicated, simple classifiers with manually crafted features may be insufficient, resulting in a relatively low accuracy of detection. On the other hand, DBN provides the capability of generatively discovering and learning effective features from data as activations on intermediate hidden layers, and thus is exploited in this work.

Note that CCs corresponding to characters may have very variant appearances, some of them may preserve the relatively complete characteristic of the character, while the others may have degraded and ambiguous appearances that are hard to be discriminated, as shown in Fig. 7. Therefore, given the filtered components from the previous processing stage, we first pick out candidate seed characters by some pre-filtering rules, and next classify them by DBN to acquire the final seed characters, on basis of which we then detect characters with less representative appearances by growing from the seed characters.

To efficiently pick out potential seed characters from CCs, we first learn the valid ranges and proper thresholds of the four characteristics of CCs (SWV,

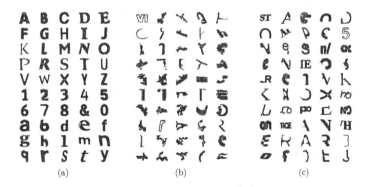

(a)   (b)   (c)

Fig. 7. Illustration of the training samples for seed character classification by DBN: (a) seed characters (positive samples), (b) non-character components (negative samples), (c) non-seed characters (also used as negative samples) for their vague appearance characteristics.

AR, SWTR and SER) from training samples of seed characters, then they are exploited to create a candidate seed character set SC by abandoning other CCs not satisfying the thresholds. Table 2 shows the set of valid ranges of characteristics for seed characters, which is learned from the ICDAR 2003 training dataset consisting of 8821 non-seed characters and 7449 seed characters.

Next, DBN is exploited to classify final seed characters from SC. Each candidate seed character in SC is first normalized to $48 * 48$ pixels, preserving the aspect of character, and is then used for the input layer of DBN. We add a top label layer of logistic regression to the DBN model for classification purpose and train the model with more than 100 configurations of parameter combinations. Table 3 shows the selected configuration yielding the best performance.

Table 3. Parameter settings of DBN in experiment.

Number of hidden layers	3
Units per layer	1400 600 100
Unsupervised learning rate	0.01
Number of unsupervised epochs	25
Supervised learning rate	2
Number of supervised epochs	50

Given the set of final seed characters SC_f found by DBN, we grow from SC_f to search for other degraded characters. Specifically, we search along the horizontal direction of each seed character for the non-seed characters, which have similar heights (difference ratio less than 2.0), stroke widths (difference ratio less than 2.0), gradient values (difference ratio less than 3.0), colors (color distance less than 8) and spatially close enough (distance less than 3 times of the width of the wider one) to the seed character. If found, the non-seed character is merged into SC_f. The process is repeated iteratively until no more such non-seed characters can be added to SC_f, then elements in SC_f are taken as the character components, as shown in Fig. 1(D).

2.5   Text Line Formation

The final stage of our method is to merge character components into text lines. Notice that we perform the previous processing stages independently in each of three channels: the dark channel, the light channel and the smoothness channel. Now, to combine characters detected in all three channels, we first merge the character components detected in the dark and the light channels into the so called *gradient-based* character component set C_g. Then, for each character component c_i in the smoothness channel, we add it to C_g if c_i does not intersects with any character components in C_g.

Finally, to combine character components into text lines, when two character components in C_g satisfy the same rules as used in the seed growing in Sect. 2.4, they are aggregated into a text line. Furthermore, two text lines can be merged together if they share one CC at one of their ends. Finally, we consider a character component not belonging to any text line as a special line containing only one character component, if it satisfies $SWV < 0.25$ and $SWTR > 0.9$ and $SER > 0.9$. Otherwise, the isolated character components are discarded.

Furthermore, to divide a text line into words, the word break algorithm is employed which estimates the typical word distance by computing the median value of character distances, and accordingly splits the text line at the inter-character gaps larger than the typical word distance. Figure 1(E) shows the example of text detection results.

3   Experiments

We evaluated our method on several public datasets, including ICDAR 2003 Text Locating Competition dataset [1], Robust Reading Competition datasets of ICDAR 2011 [3] and ICDAR 2013 (Challenge 2: Reading Text in Scene Images) dataset [4], and Street View Text (SVT) [19] dataset.

The ICDAR 2003 dataset contains 509 fully annotated text images including 258 images for training and 251 images for testing. The ICDAR 2011 dataset consists of 484 text images with 229 training images and 255 testing images. The ICDAR 2013 dataset contains 562 images including 229 images for training and 233 images for testing. All the images are full-color and vary in size from $307 * 93$ to $3888 * 2592$ pixels. For processing convenience, they are resized so that the maximum of height and width is equal to 1600 pixels, considering the trade-off of runtime and detection accuracy. The method proposed in this paper is implemented in C language with the DBN implementation based on the DeepLearnToolbox library [20]. The experiments are performed on a PC platform with one Intel Core i3 CPU at 3.30 GHz.

We first evaluate our algorithms for edge detection, modified SWT and CC extraction on the ICDAR 2003 dataset, and compare them to those used in

Table 4. Comparison of variant edge detection and component extraction methods. The 'Original SWT' and 'Original CC' algorithms are described in [5]. Filtered CCs are the CCs after the component filtering described in Sect. 2.3. Seed CCs are the seed characters extracted by the proposed method in Sect. 2.4. Indices p, r, f are the metrics for text word detection used in ICDAR 2003 dataset.

Edge Alg.	SWT and CC Alg.	# CCs	# Filtered CCs	# Seed CCs	p	r	f	Time
Canny	Original	68519	24966	4256	0.56	0.52	0.53	4 s
Canny	Modified	67925	26384	6109	0.68	0.63	0.64	4 s
Gradient-based	Original	190220	65436	6586	0.60	0.58	0.57	7 s
Gradient-based	Modified	169076	69133	11146	0.71	0.70	0.69	7 s
Hybrid	Original	212961	84146	12424	0.69	0.69	0.67	10 s
Hybrid	Modified	191817	88411	18614	0.70	0.74	0.70	10 s

Table 5. Comparison on ICDAR 2003 dataset

Methods	p	r	f
A. Mosleh [8]	**0.76**	0.66	**0.71**
Our method	0.70	**0.74**	0.70
X.B. Wang [9]	0.71	0.70	0.70
B. Epshtein [5]	0.73	0.60	0.66
H. Becker [2]	0.62	0.67	0.62

Table 6. Comparison on ICDAR 2011 dataset

Methods	p	r	f
X.C. Yin [21]	**0.86**	0.68	**0.76**
Our method	0.74	**0.74**	0.74
L. Neumann [10]	0.79	0.66	0.72
Kim's [3]	0.83	0.63	0.71
X.B. Wang [9]	0.73	0.67	0.70
L. Neumann [7]	0.73	0.65	0.69

Table 7. Comparison on ICDAR 2013 dataset

Methods	p	r	f
X.C. Yin [21]	**0.88**	0.66	**0.76**
Our method	0.75	**0.75**	0.75
Text Spotter [4]	0.88	0.65	0.75
CASIA NLPR [4]	0.79	0.68	0.73
Text Detector CASIA [4]	0.85	0.63	0.72

the original SWT work [5]. Table 4 shows the comparison results, along with the statistics of the outputs of the component filtering and the seed component selection processings. We can observe that the proposed method (with the hybrid edge detection and the modified SWT and CC algorithms) achieves the best results with f measure 0.70, although it is relatively slower than the original method. Comparatively, the original method [5] achieves the f measure 0.66.

Next, we evaluate and compare our text detection method with some other representative methods reported on the same ICDAR 2003, 2011 and 2013 datasets. We adopt the official evaluation protocol of ICDAR corresponding to the datasets. Notice that the evaluation protocol of ICDAR 2003 Text Locating Competition is different from that of Robust Reading Competition of ICDAR 2011 and ICDAR 2013. The f measure calculated by ICDAR 2003 evaluation protocol is lower than the harmonic mean value $\frac{2*p*r}{p+r}$ by definition, where p is the precision rate and r is the recall rate, while the f measures calculated by the ICDAR 2011 and ICDAR 2013 evaluation protocols are equal to the harmonic mean value.

Table 5 compares the performances of our method and some other methods evaluated on the ICDAR 2003 competition dataset. Among all methods, ours and that of Hinnerk Becker are evaluated with the official evaluation protocol of ICDAR 2003. The results show that our method performs overall much better than Hinnerk's. Since the other methods, however, used the different evaluation protocol from the official one, we focus on the precision and recall rates instead of the f measure obtained by these methods in comparison. Our method achieves the significantly higher recall rate than other methods, owing to the effectiveness of the proposed hybrid edge detection and seed character extraction algorithms.

In Tables 6 and 7, we compare the performances of our method with some other methods evaluated on the ICDAR 2011 and ICDAR 2013 competition datasets, respectively. Note that the evaluation protocol adopted is same for all methods being compared, in which the f measure is equal to the harmonic mean value. Our method achieves again the significantly highest recall rate (74 % and 75 % respectively), with its f measure slightly lower than the top one while better than all other methods.

Figure 8 shows the texts detected by the proposed method from some sample images of the ICDAR datasets, which were interfered by complicated illumination, shadow, low contrast or color variation. The proposed text detection method exhibits sufficient robustness to these interferences.

As another popular public dataset for text detection evaluation, SVT dataset contains 647 words and 3796 letters in 249 images harvested from Google Street View. Our method achieves a recall rate of 60 % and a precision rate of 34 % using the ICDAR 2003 evaluation protocol. Figure 9 shows the texts detected by the proposed method from some SVT sample images.

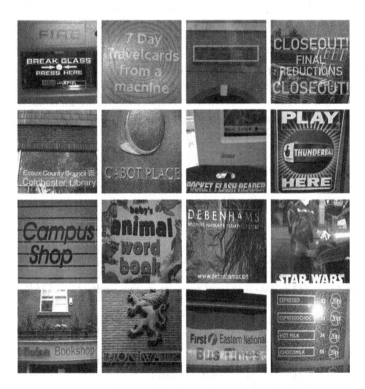

Fig. 8. Detected texts in some sample images from ICDAR 2003, 2011 and 2013 datasets. Only the cropped image regions containing the detected texts are shown.

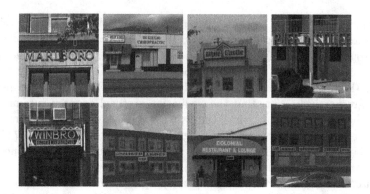

Fig. 9. Detected texts in some sample images from SVT dataset. Only the cropped image regions containing the detected texts are shown.

4   Conclusion

In this paper, we present a novel text detection method for natural scene images, which combines two main ingredients: the robust extension of the Stroke Width Transform algorithm and the Deep Belief Network based discrimination of text objects from other scene components. On the basis of SWT, we combine the gradient-based and smoothness-based edge information for generating high quality edge images, and further exploit various edge cues in connected component analysis to eliminate inter-character and intra-character errors. Given connected components extracted from the image, we exploit the DBN to discriminate character CCs from non-character ones and effectively aggregate multiple processing channels, yielding the overall improved detection performance in the experiments on ICDAR and SVT public datasets.

Acknowledgement. Research supported by the National Science Foundation of China under Grant Nos. 61003113, 61272218 and 61321491.

References

1. Lucas, S.M., Panaretos, A., Sosa, L., Tang, A., Wong, S., Young, R.: ICDAR 2003 robust reading competitions. In: ICDAR, pp. 682–687 (2003)
2. Lucas, S.M.: ICDAR 2005 text locating competition results. In: ICDAR, pp. 80–84 (2005)
3. Shahab, A., Shafait, F., Dengel, A.: ICDAR 2011 robust reading competition challenge 2: reading text in scene images. In: ICDAR, pp. 1491–1496 (2011)
4. Karatzas, D., Shafait, F., Uchida, S., Iwamura, M., Bigorda, L.G., Mestre, S.R., Mas, J., Mota, D.F., Almazan, J.A., Heras, L.P.: ICDAR 2013 robust reading competition. In: ICDAR, pp. 1484–1493 (2013)
5. Epsthtein, B., Ofek, E., Wexler, Y.: Detecting text in natural scenes with stroke width transform. In: CVPR, pp. 2963–2970 (2010)

6. Chen, X., Yuille, A.L.: Detecting and reading text in natural scenes. In: CVPR, pp. 366–373 (2004)
7. Neumann, L., Matas, J.: Real-time scene text localization and recognition. In: CVPR, pp. 3538–3545 (2012)
8. Mosleh, A., Bouguila, N.: Image text detection using a bandlet-based edge detector and stroke width transform. In: BMVC, pp. 1–12 (2012)
9. Wang, X.B., Song, Y.H., Zhang, Y.L.: Natural scene text detection with multi-channel connected component segmentation. In: ICDAR, pp. 1375–1379 (2013)
10. Neumann, L., Matas, J.: Scene text localization and recognition with oriented stroke detection. In: ICCV, pp. 97–104 (2013)
11. Mishra, A., Alahari, K., Jawahar, C.V.: Top-down and bottom-up cues for scene text recognition. In: CVPR, pp. 2687–2694 (2012)
12. Wang, K., Babenko, B., Belongie, S.: End-to-end scene text recognition. In: ICCV, pp. 1457–1464 (2011)
13. Neumann, L., Matas, J.: A method for text localization and recognition in real-world images. In: Kimmel, R., Klette, R., Sugimoto, A. (eds.) ACCV 2010, Part III. LNCS, vol. 6494, pp. 770–783. Springer, Heidelberg (2011)
14. Yi, C., Tian, Y.: Text detection in natural scene images by stroke gabor words. In: ICDAR, pp. 177–181 (2011)
15. Koo, H.I., Kim, D.H.: Scene text detection via connected component clustering and nontext filtering. IEEE TIP 22, 2296–2305 (2013)
16. Minetto, R., Thome, N., Cord, M., Stolfi, J., Precioso, F., Guyomard, J., Leite, N.: Text detection and recognition in Urban scenes. In: ICCVW, pp. 227–234 (2011)
17. Zhang, J., Kasturi, R.: A novel text detection system based on character and link energies. IEEE Trans. Image Process. 23, 4187–4198 (2014)
18. Hinton, G.E., Osindero, S., Teh, Y.: A fast learning algorithm for deep belief nets. Neural Comput. 18, 1527–1554 (2006)
19. Wang, K., Belongie, S.: Word spotting in the wild. In: Daniilidis, K., Maragos, P., Paragios, N. (eds.) ECCV 2010, Part I. LNCS, vol. 6311, pp. 591–604. Springer, Heidelberg (2010)
20. Palm, R.B.: Prediction as a candidate for learning deep hierarchical models of data. Master's thesis, Technical University of Denmark (2012)
21. Yin, X., Yin, X., Huang, K., Hao, H.: Robust text detection in natural scene images. IEEE Trans. PAMI 36, 970–983 (2014)

Cross-Modal Face Matching:
Beyond Viewed Sketches

Shuxin Ouyang[1]([✉]), Timothy Hospedales[2], Yi-Zhe Song[2], and Xueming Li[1]

[1] Beijing University of Posts and Telecommunications, Beijing, China
ouyangshuxin@gmail.com
[2] School of Electronic Engineering and Computer Science,
Queen Mary University of London, London E1 4NS, UK

Abstract. Matching face images across different modalities is a challenging open problem for various reasons, notably feature heterogeneity, and particularly in the case of sketch recognition – abstraction, exaggeration and distortion. Existing studies have attempted to address this task by engineering invariant features, or learning a common subspace between the modalities. In this paper, we take a different approach and explore learning a mid-level representation within each domain that allows faces in each modality to be compared in a domain invariant way. In particular, we investigate sketch-photo face matching and go beyond the well-studied viewed sketches to tackle forensic sketches and caricatures where representations are often symbolic. We approach this by learning a facial attribute model independently in each domain that represents faces in terms of semantic properties. This representation is thus more invariant to heterogeneity, distortions and robust to mis-alignment. Our intermediate level attribute representation is then integrated synergistically with the original low-level features using CCA. Our framework shows impressive results on cross-modal matching tasks using forensic sketches, and even more challenging caricature sketches. Furthermore, we create a new dataset with ≈59, 000 attribute annotations for evaluation and to facilitate future research.

1 Introduction

Cross-modal face recognition is an increasingly important research area that encompasses matching face images between different modalities: sketch, photo, infra-red, low/high resolution, 2D/3D and so on. Among all these, facial sketch based face recognition is perhaps the most important and the most well studied, due to its crucial role in assisting law enforcement. Facial sketches can be classified into three categories according to abstraction/deformation level compared to a corresponding photo: *viewed sketch*, *forensic sketch* and *caricature*, as shown in Fig. 1. Most existing studies have considered viewed sketches, which are drawn by artists while looking at a photo. This is the easiest (and most impractical) cross-modal task because the images are sufficiently similar and well aligned that extracting any grayscale descriptor from both is near sufficient

D. Cremers et al. (Eds.): ACCV 2014, Part II, LNCS 9004, pp. 210–225, 2015.
DOI: 10.1007/978-3-319-16808-1_15

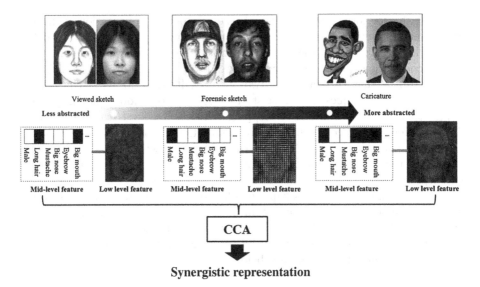

Fig. 1. Illustration of sketch abstraction level (top) and pipeline overview (below).

to bridge the cross-modal gap. As a result cross-modal matching rates for viewed sketch are saturated at near-perfect [1–7]. Therefore research focus has moved onto forensic sketches [1] and beyond (caricature) [8].

Contrast to viewed sketches, matching forensic sketches or caricatures to photos is significantly more challenging due to greater cross-modal gap. For forensic sketches, the witness may not exactly remember the appearance of a suspect – omitting, hallucinating or distorting individual details – or may not be able to communicate the visual memory clearly. As a result forensic sketches are often inaccurate and incomplete. In the case of caricatures, the sketch is a purposely exaggerated and distorted version of the original face. In both cases, the cross-modal gap is created by mismatch due to various factors: (i) feature heterogeneity, (ii) missing or additional facial details, (iii) distorted macro or micro proportions – which in turn affects alignment in a way that rigid registration cannot rectify. Despite these challenges, if the sketch subject is known to a human, they have no trouble identifying either forensic or caricature sketches. We are therefore motivated to study both caricature and forensic sketches, as contributions to matching caricature sketches will reflect robustness to the most challenging forensic sketch or other cross-modal recognition tasks.

In this paper, we aim to address the highlighted challenges in cross-modality matching of forensic sketches and caricatures to photos, by constructing a mid-level attribute representation of each facial modality. The idea is that this representation can be learned independently within each modality (thus completely avoiding any cross-modality challenge); but once learned, it is largely invariant to the cross-modal gap. That is, neither feature heterogeneity, nor non-linear cross-modal distortion affect this representation. Specifically, we train a bank of facial attribute detectors to produce low-dimensional semantic representation within each modality. Finally, although the attribute representation is invariant to the cross-modal gap, it does lose some detailed information encoded by the low-level features. We therefore develop a robust synergistic representation that encodes the best of both attributes and low-level features by learning a CCA subspace that correlates the two. The result outperforms feature-based face-matching techniques, as well as state of the art cross-modal matching techniques that focus on learning a mapping between low-level features without first building an invariant mid-level representation. Moreover, a new dataset combining common forensic [9] and caricature datasets [8] were annotated (≈59, 000 annotations in total) to learn and evaluate the proposed cross-modal face representation.

The remaining parts of this paper will be organised as follows: related works will be discussed in Sect. 2; the technical methodology to bridge large cross-modal gap, that is to say, the way to matching forensic sketches and caricatures is discussed in Sect. 3; all the experiments and analysis are shown in Sect. 4; and Sect. 5 details our attribute dataset before conclusions in Sect. 6.

2   Related Work

2.1   Sketch-Based Face Recognition

As we have discussed, sketch-based face recognition can be classified based on the type of sketch used as the probe: viewed, forensic and caricature-based. In each case, strategies to bridge the cross-modal gap broadly break down into four categories: (i) those that learn a cross-modal mapping to synthesise one modality from the other, and then perform within-modality matching [10,11], (ii) those that learn a common subspace where the two modalities are more comparable [12], (iii) those that learn discriminative models to maximise matching accuracy [1,13], and (iv) those that engineer features which are simultaneously invariant to the details of each modality, while being variant to person identity [4,14].

Viewed Sketches. Viewed sketches are the simplest type of sketch to match against facial photos because incorrect details and distortion are minimal. This is the most extensively studied type of heterogeneous face recognition. Studies taking synthesis strategies have used eigen-transform [10] and MRF [11] optimisation to map photos into sketches before within-modal matching. Alternative studies have used PLS [12] to synthesize a common subspace where the modalities are more comparable. Meanwhile, others have engineered new invariant descriptors, including histogram of averaged oriented gradients [14] and local radon binary patterns [4]. Recognition rates on viewed sketch benchmarks has saturated, reaching 100 % [14], thus research has moved on the more challenging and realistic setting of forensic sketches.

Forensic Sketches. One of the earliest studies to discuss automated matching forensic sketches with photos was [15]. Uhl and Lobo's study [15] proposed a theory, and the first simple method for matching a police artist sketch to a set of photographs. It highlighted the complexity and difficulties in forensic sketch based face recognition. One of the first major studies on forensic sketches was [1], which combined feature engineering (SIFT and LBP) with a discriminative (LFDA) method to learn a weighting that maximized identification accuracy. Later studies such as [13] improved these results, again combining feature engineering (Weber and Wavelet descriptors) plus discriminative learning (genetic algorithms) strategy to maximize matching accuracy; while [16] followed up also with feature engineering (LBP) and discriminative learning (RS-LDA).

All these strategies to bridge the cross-modal gap can largely address the feature heterogeneity problem, but the more fundamental problems of missing/additional details, and non-linear heteroskedastic distortion remain outstanding. Abstraction and distortion effects mean that any particular patch in a facial sketch image does not necessarily *correspond* to the associated patch in a facial sketch, an intrinsic problem that existing studies do not address. In this paper we avoid this issue by transforming both sketch and photo images into a mid-level semantic representation that does not depend on alignment or ability to find a patch correspondence, and is highly robust to missing/additional details.

Caricatures. An even more extreme cross-domain gap than in photo-forensic sketch is created by caricature-based matching. The extreme deformation and abstraction of caricatures seriously challenge all existing strategies: feature engineering methods as well as cross-domain mapping and synthesis methods are hamstrung by the impossibility of establishing patch correspondence, and mismatch of details. The main study so far addressing caricature-based matching is by Klare et al. [8]. This study proposed a semi-automated system to match caricatures to photographs based on *manually* specified facial properties for each image. However, how to *automatically* extract facial attributes is unaddressed. We address this question question here, as well as how best to synergistically integrate the extracted attributes with low-level features.

2.2 Cross-Modal Mapping

Learning cross-modal mappings is quite widely studied, as it is of broader relevance [17,18] than face recognition. Common approaches include using partial least squares (PLS) [12], Canonical correlation analysis (CCA) [17–19], or sparse coding [20] to map both modalities to common representation. These methods have all also been applied to cross-modal face recognition with some success. Nevertheless, in each case a fundamental assumption remains that a single linear mapping should relate the two domains. Clearly in the case of forensic sketches and caricatures with non-linear deformations, abstraction, and missing details, the assumptions of a single mapping between all sketches and all images, and that the mapping should be linear, are not met. In this paper we therefore focus on learning a semantic attribute representation, which maps low-level features to a mid-level semantic representation that is invariant to the domain gap [21] and alignment errors. Since the low-level feature to attribute transformation can be non-linear, overall this means that – unlike existing approaches – the learnable sketch-photo mapping can also be non-linear.

2.3   Semantic Attributes

Semantic attributes [22] have gained wide popularity as an effective represen-tation in the broader vision community with application to object recognition [22,23], person identification [21], and action recognition [24,25]. However appli-cation of attributes to faces [26] or face recognition [27] has been relatively limited, and their potential for bridging the cross-modal gap is not yet explored.

Psychologists have shown that the ability of humans to perform basic-level categorization (e.g. cats vs. dogs) develops well before their ability to perform subordinate-level or fine-grained visual categorization (e.g., species), or in our case, facial attribute detection [28]. Unlike basic-level recognition, even humans have difficulty with recognition of facial attributes. This is due to attributes, such as different types of noses and eyes being quite fine grained discrimination tasks. Models and algorithms designed for basic-level object or image categorization tasks are often unprepared to catch such subtle differences among different facial attributes. In this paper, we alleviate this problem by exploiting an ensemble of classifier regions with various shapes, sizes and locations [29].

2.4   Our Contributions

The contributions of the paper are summarized as follows: (1) we release a dataset with ≈59, 000 attribute annotations for the major caricature [8] and forensic photo-sketch datasets [1]; (2) we show how to automatically detect photo/sketch facial attributes as a modality-invariant semantic feature; (3) we show how to synergistically integrate attributes and low-level features for recog-nition; and (4) we demonstrate the efficacy of our approach on challenging foren-sic sketch and caricature sketch based recognition.

3   Matching Faces Across Modalities

Problem Setting. In the cross-modal face recognition problem, we are given a set of photo and sketch face images, $D^p = \{\mathbf{x}_i^p\}_{i=1}^N$ and $D^s = \{\mathbf{x}_i^s\}_{i=1}^N$ respec-tively. Each image is assumed to be represented by a fixed-length d-dimensional feature vector $\mathbf{x}$. The goal is to establish the correct correspondence between the photo set and the sketch set. Feature engineering approaches [4,14] focus on designing the representation $\mathbf{x}$ such that each 'probe' sketch $\mathbf{x}^s$ can be matched with its corresponding photo by simple nearest neighbour as in Eq. (1), where $|\cdot|$ indicates some distance metric such as L1, L2 [1] or $\mathcal{X}^2$ [13,14]. Going beyond feature engineering, studies have attempted to learn a mapping to make the modalities more comparable, such that mappings can be learned by synthesizing one modality from the other or discovering a new subspace. This typically results in NN matching in the form of Eq. (2), where the matrices W^s and/or W^p are learned, e.g., by CCA [19,30] or PLS [12]. Alternatively, matrices W may also be learned by discriminative models [1,8,13] to maximize matching rate.

$$i^*_{NN} = \underset{i}{\operatorname{argmin}} |\mathbf{x}^s - \mathbf{x}_i^p| \qquad (1)$$

$$i^*_{map} = \underset{i}{\operatorname{argmin}} |W^s\mathbf{x}^s - W^p\mathbf{x}_i^p| \qquad (2)$$

$$i^*_{attr} = \underset{i}{\operatorname{argmin}} |\mathbf{a}^s(\mathbf{x}^s) - \mathbf{a}^p(\mathbf{x}_i^p)| \qquad (3)$$

In this paper, we will go beyond existing approaches by learning a mid-level semantic attribute representation $\mathbf{a}$ for each modality. Since the attribute representation $\mathbf{a}$ is both (1) discriminative by design[1] [21,22,27] and (2) modality invariant, this means that NN matching as in Eq. (3) can be more powerful than previous while being robust to the modality gap approaches. In the next section we discuss how to compute a semantic attribute representation $\mathbf{a}(\cdot)$ for photos and sketches.

3.1   Attribute Detection

Training an Ensemble Classifier for Attribute Detection.   We assume an ontology of $j = 1 \ldots A$ attributes is provided (see Sect. 5 for details of the ontology). Each training image set D now also contains attribute annotation $\mathbf{a}$ as well as images, $D = \{\mathbf{x}_i, \mathbf{a}_i\}_{i=1}^N$. For each modality and for each attribute j we train an ensemble classifier $a_j(\cdot)$ as follows. Given the training data D, we randomly sample a set of M windows around the three annotated semantically relevant regions for each attribute. For all M regions, we then train a support vector machine (SVM) classifier to predict the presence of the current attribute j in the training set. The randomly sampled regions are evaluated for discriminativeness by their attribute-detection performance on a held out validation set. The top three most discriminative regions $r = 1, 2, 3$ are then selected for each attribute.

Detecting Attributes. The final evaluation of the classifier ensemble for attribute j on a test image $\mathbf{x}^*$ is $a_j(\mathbf{x}^*) = \sum_r f_{r,j}(\mathbf{x}^*) > 0$, where $f_{r,j}(\cdot)$ is the binary SVM classifier for attribute j trained on region r. That is, if any classifier in the ensemble predicts the attribute is present, then it is assumed to be present. This strategy has two key advantages: (i) by selecting relevant regions for each attribute it performs feature selection to focus on relevant sub windows thus increasing detection accuracy, (ii) by exploiting an ensemble of regions it is less sensitive to alignment or deformation, typical variations of these types will trigger at least one of the classifiers in the ensemble. Given the trained classifiers for each attribute, the A dimensional attribute representation for an sketch or photo $\mathbf{x}$ is represented by stacking them as $\mathbf{a}(\mathbf{x}) = [a_1(\mathbf{x}), \ldots, a_A(\mathbf{x})]$.

---

[1] Attributes are chosen to be properties that differentiate groups of the population, such as male/female, asian/white, young/old – thus an A-length attribute code can potentially differentiate 2^A people, providing a highly discriminative representation.

3.2   Learning a Synergistic Low+Mid Level Representation

The attribute representation derived in the previous section is robust and discriminative, but the original low-level features still retain some complementary information. A simple method to exploit both could be early fusion (concatenation $[\mathbf{x}, \mathbf{a}(\mathbf{x})]$), or score level fusion of the similarities obtained by each representation. As a significantly better alternative, we use canonical correlation analysis (CCA) to learn an embedding space that synergistically exploits both representations.

CCA For Representation Learning. Specifically, assuming that we have N images in total. Let X_x is be the $N \times d$ dimensional matrix stacking the low-level feature representations $\mathbf{x}$ for all images and X_a is a $N \times A$ dimensional matrix stacking the attribute representations $\mathbf{a}(\mathbf{x})$ for all images, then we find the projection matrices W_x and W_a such that:

$$\min_{W_x, W_a} \left\| X_a W_a - X_x W_x \right\|_F^2$$
$$subject\ to\ W_a^T \Sigma_{ax} W_x = I, w_{ak}^T \Sigma_{ax} w_{xl} = 0, \tag{4}$$
$$k, l = 1, \ldots, c$$

where Σ_{ax} is the covariance between X_a and X_x and w_{ak} is the kth column of W_a, and c is the dimensionality of the desired CCA subspace. To solve this optimization, we use the efficient generalized eigenvalue method of [18].

Note that this is a somewhat different use of CCA to some previous studies that used it to map across facial image domains [19, 20, 30]. Instead we use CCA to construct an embedding [18] to constructively fuse attribute and low-level feature representations.

Using the Representation.   In order to obtain the semantic embedding for a test image $\mathbf{x}^*$, we first obtain its estimated attributes $\mathbf{a}(\mathbf{x})$. Then we project both the original and semantic views of the image into the embedding space: $\mathbf{x}W_x$ and $\mathbf{a}(\mathbf{x})W_a$. Finally, we concatenate both views to give the final $2c$ dimensional representation: $R(\mathbf{x}) = [\mathbf{x}W_x, \mathbf{a}(\mathbf{x})W_a]$. Once our new robust and domain invariant representation is obtained for sketch and photo images, matching a sketch $\mathbf{x}^s$ against a photo dataset $D = \{\mathbf{x}_i^p\}_i^N = 1$ is then performed by nearest neighbor with L2 distance,

$$i^* = \operatorname*{argmin}_i |R^s(\mathbf{x}^s) - R^p(\mathbf{x}_i^p)| \tag{5}$$

Note that the representation R in Eq. (5) is indexed by (s)ketch or (p)hoto because the semantic attribute model $\mathbf{a}(\cdot)$ is independently trained for each modality, although the CCA mapping is shared.

4   Experimental Results

4.1   Datasets and Settings

Datasets: We evaluate our algorithm on two challenging datasets for photo-sketch face matching forensic [9] and caricature dataset [8]. For the forensic dataset we have 196 pairs of 200*160 pixel resolution face and photo images. For the caricature dataset, we have 207 pairs of caricatures and photographs of highly variable size. To obtain matching results, we perform 3-fold cross-validation, splitting the data into 2/3 s training, and test on the held out 1/3. Within the training set we use 4-fold cross-validation to both train the attribute representation (Sect. 3.1) and optimize dimensionality ($c = 250$ for both datasets) of the CCA subspace (Sect. 3.2).

Low-Level Features: For low-level feature representation, we densely extract histogram of gradients (HOG) and local binary patterns (LBP) on each image on a 16×16 grid, resulting in 4030 and 6960 dimensional descriptors respectively. We then use PCA to reduce the dimension of each to 350 and concatenate the result, producing a $d = 700$ dimensional descriptor for each image.

Training Attribute Detectors: Using the 73 attribute methodology defined in Sect. 5, and the training procedure in Sect. 3.1, we produce a 71 dimensional binary attribute vector for each image in the caricature dataset, and a 53 dimensional binary attribute vector for each image in the forensic dataset[2].

Baselines: We compare our method with the following four variants of our method: (i) use only HOG and LBP (**LLF**); (ii) use only the attribute representation in nearest neighbor matching (**Attribute**); (iii) use low-level features and attributes together with simple early (feature) level fusion (**Attribute+LLF**); (iv) our full method, using low-level features and attributes together through synergistic CCA space (Cross-modal Matching by Facial Attributes, **CMMFA**).

Additionally, we compare the following two previous state of the art approaches: (i) low-level features engineered for photo-caricature recognition followed by NN matching [8] (**Klare**); (ii) state of the art learned cross-modal mapping, learned based on our LLFs, followed by NN matching [19] (**CFS**).

Table 1. Attribute recognition results for caricature and forensic datasets, comparing our ensemble attribute classifier with flat-model ones (acc. is for average accuracy).

Dataset	Classifier	Acc. (sketch)	Acc. (photo)
Caricature	Flat-model	53.95 %	55.15 %
Forensic	Flat-model	56.23 %	54.43 %
Caricature	Ensemble	69.15 %	70.24 %
Forensic	Ensemble	65.19 %	65.28 %

---

[2] Both datasets (especially forensic) exhibits some degrees of lower diversity of attributes, so some attributes are always on or off rendering them meaningless for representation, so these are excluded for convenience.

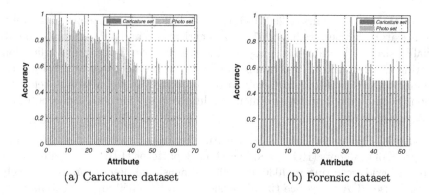

(a) Caricature dataset   (b) Forensic dataset

Fig. 2. Breakdown of per-attribute detection performance.

4.2   Attribute Detection

In this section, we first evaluate the performance of our automated attribute detection procedure (Sect. 3.1). In Table 1, we offer the average attribute detection accuracy for each of our datasets, and performance comparison between the proposed ensemble attribute detector and a flat-model variant where SVM classifiers are trained on whole images instead. Although many attributes are quite subtle (Sect. 5), the average accuracies in the range 65–70% clearly demonstrate that many of them can be reasonably reliably detected, especially when compared with flat-model performance (53–56%). Table 2 reports the top 5 most accurate attributes for each modality and dataset. The top 4 rows of Fig. 3 illustrate attribute detection results for the 1st ranked attributes (shown schematically) in each dataset/modality, the bottom 2 rows show failure examples of attribute detection (denoted by red cross), i.e., when automatic attribute detection disagrees with human annotated ground-truth.

To further investigate how these averages break down, we plot the per-attribute accuracy in Fig. 2 sorted by photo set accuracy. Clearly while there are some attributes which are too subtle to be reliably detected (some attributes at 50 % accuracy, e.g., slanted and sleepy eyes), others can be detected with near perfect accuracy (plots peak at around 100 % accuracy). Interestingly, while there is a general correlation of attribute reliability between datasets, it is relatively weak, so some of the best photo attributes don't work on sketch and vice-versa.

4.3   Matching Across Modalities

Given the attribute encoding as evaluated in the previous section, we next address the final goal of cross-modal face matching.

Caricature Dataset. The results for cross-modal face matching on the caricature dataset are shown in Fig. 4(a) and Table 3. For the caricature dataset our attribute encoding is significantly better than any of the LLF based approaches (Table 3, *Attribute versus HOG/LBP)*. This because the cross-modal gap for the

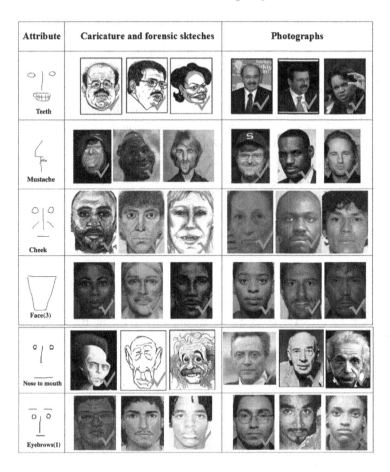

Fig. 3. Illustration of detections for the best performing attributes in Table 2 (top 4 rows) and 2 other average performing attributes (bottom 2 rows), Left: Schematic illustration of query attribute, middle and right: pairs of sketch/caricature (middle) and photograph (right) of the same identity (green tick for successful attribute detection, red cross otherwise) (Colour figure online).

caricature dataset is the most extreme, so low-level features cannot be effectively compared. CFS improves the results somewhat compared to LLFs, but due to the extreme gap between the domains, it offers limited improvement (Table 3, *CFS versus HOG/LBP*). For context, we also show the matching results obtained using the ground-truth attributes in the bottom row. Interestingly this is only a few percent above that obtained by using our inferred attributes, suggesting that we are already capturing most of the value in the current attribute methodology (Table 3, *Ground-truth attribute versus Attribute*).

With regards to strategies for combining attributes and LLFs, vanilla concatenation actually worsens the results somewhat compared to attributes alone (Table 3, *Attribute versus Attribute+LLF*). This is understandable, because the

Table 2. Top 5 attributes for caricature and forensic datasets

Caricature dataset			Forensic dataset		
Domain	Attribute	Accuracy	Domain	Attribute	Accuracy
Photo	Teeth	97.98 %	Photo	Cheeks(5)	100.00 %
	Cheeks(3)	96.96 %		No beard	98.68 %
	Glasses	96.43 %		Small forehead	92.86 %
	Small beard	94.87 %		Eyebrow(2)	92.50 %
	Big chin	93.12 %		No moustache	91.67 %
Caricature	Small mustache	100.00 %	Forensic	Face(3)	98.84 %
	Forehead(1)	100.00 %		No beard	96.97 %
	Square face	99.45 %		No moustache	96.67 %
	Big moustache	97.46 %		Thick eyebrow	94.57 %
	Big mouth	95.83 %		Small mouth	91.94 %

attributes are much stronger than the LLFs. In contrast, combining them in our CCA framework achieves the best result of all, 27.54 % at Rank 1. Finally, we compare with the results based on engineered image features reported in [8]. The features from [8] slightly outperform our LLFs alone. However our entire framework outperforms [8] by a noticeable margin.

We note that using everything together, [8]'s final result only slightly outperforms our CMMFA. However, this is using the critical but unrealistic cue of manually annotated ground-truth attributes at test time, which makes this approach not meaningful for a practical scenario that should be fully automated (Table 3, *Klare versus CMMFA*). In contrast, our CMMFA is computed based on image features alone without manual intervention.

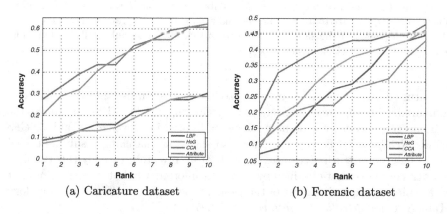

(a) Caricature dataset   (b) Forensic dataset

Fig. 4. CMC curves for cross-modality matching. Ranks = 1:10.

Table 3. Caricature dataset: comparison of all methods.

Methods	Rank1	Rank5
Dense HOG	7.25%	14.49%
Dense LBP	8.60%	15.94%
CFS [19] HOG+LBP	13.45%	
Attribute	20.29%	46.38%
Attribute+LLF	18.84%	46.38%
CMMFA (Attribute+LLF+CCA)	27.54%	43.48%
Klare et al. (image only) [8]	12.10%	52.10%
Klare et al. (method fusion and manual attributes) [8][a]	32.30%	–
Ground-truth attribute	23.19%	52.17%

[a] Not directly comparable due to use of manual intervention.

Forensic Dataset. The results for the forensic dataset are shown in Fig. 4(b) and Table 4. In this case our attribute encoding still outperforms LLF based approaches (Table 4, *Attribute versus HOG/LBP*), despite the fewer and weaker attributes in this case. CFS now improves the LLF results more significantly as expected since the cross-modal gap is more straightforward to model (Table 4, *CFS versus HOG/LBP*). However our full method still outperforms CFS (Table 4, *CMMFA versus CFS*).

Our CMMFA performance is slightly weaker on the forensic than the caricature dataset. This is somewhat surprising, because the caricature dataset might be considered 'harder' due to the bigger cross-modal gap. However, it is understandable because there are about 20 facial attributes which do not occur (or occur infrequently) in the forensic set, thus resulting in fewer working attribute detectors (Fig. 2); and because the process of caricature sketching often actually involves exaggerating facial attributes, thus making them easier to detect.

4.4 Attribute Description Search

As a final application of potential relevance to forensic search, we consider querying a mugshot database solely by attribute description. This is interesting and potentially useful for law enforcement, especially in situations where a trained forensic sketch expert is unavailable. In this application scenario, a witness would select all the attributes they recall from the full attribute list. A mugshot-database can then be queried directly by the attribute representation. We simulate this experiment by querying each person j's ground-truth attribute $\mathbf{a}_j^{gt}$ against the database of estimated attributes for the mugshots $\{\mathbf{a}(\mathbf{x}_i^p)\}_{i=1}^N$, $i^* = \arg\min_i \left| \mathbf{a}_j^{gt} - \mathbf{a}(\mathbf{x}_i^p) \right|$. With this setting, we achieve average of 10.3% rank 1 accuracy for the forensic dataset, and 20.7% rank 1 accuracy for the caricature dataset. Full CMC curves are shown in Fig. 5.

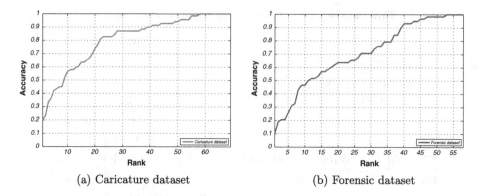

(a) Caricature dataset   (b) Forensic dataset

Fig. 5. CMC curves for attribute description search.

Table 4. Forensic dataset: comparison of all methods.

Methods	Rank1	Rank5
Dense HOG	8.60 %	34.48 %
Dense LBP	6.90 %	27.59 %
CFS [19] HOG+LBP	19.12 %	
Attribute	10.34 %	22.41 %
Attribute+LLF	18.97 %	36.21 %
CMMFA (Attribute+LLF+CCA)	20.69 %	41.38 %
Ground-truth attribute	15.52 %	44.83 %

5   Attribute Dataset

In this section we describe the dataset that was created in this study. Future studies comparing accuracies on this dataset should follow the protocol detailed in Sect. 4. We build our attribute dataset by annotating the caricature dataset[3] [8] and forensic dataset [9].

Caricature Dataset: The dataset consists of pairs of a caricature sketch and a corresponding facial photograph from 207 subjects. Two sources were used to collect these images. The first was through contacts with various artists who drew the caricatures. And the second source of caricature images was from Goolge Image searches. When selecting face photographs, care was taken to find images that had minimal variations in pose, illumination and expression, however, those images are hard to find. So, many of the factors still persist [8].

Forensic Dataset: The dataset consists of pairs of a forensic sketch and a corresponding mugshot from 196 subjects. Forensic sketches are drawn by a

---

[3] Reference [8] did not release their attributes. Our attributes and corresponding annotations are available at http://www.eecs.qmul.ac.uk/~yzs/heteroface/.

sketch artist from the description of an eyewitness based on his/her recollection of the crime scene. Two sources were used to collect these images. The first was through contact with various artists who drew the forensic sketches: Lois Gibson and Karen Taylor. The second was from Google Image searches [9].

Attribute Annotation. In our attribute dataset, each of the images (caricature, forensic sketch and photograph) is labeled with a set of facial attributes (categorical facial features). We start with the 63 facial attributes proposed by Klare et al [8], and add 10 additional attributes for a total of 73 attributes. Those 10 additional attributes include: wrinkles, glasses, ties, teeth, cheeks, black/while/asian, blonde hair and gender.

Each image (caricature, forensic sketch and photograph) was annotated for these 73 attributes. Each annotator labeled the entire set of image pairs with 3–4 facial attributes, being asked to label a single image with a single attribute at a time. Thus the annotator was shown an image of a caricature, a forensic sketch or a photograph, and the current attribute being labeled. If the attribute is present, then they label the image with '1', otherwise '0'. In total, we provided 58,838 labels on the 806 images. For each attribute (not each image), annotators are also asked to provide an estimate of three salient regions for that attribute, which were used to guide random sampling for attribute detection (Sect. 3.1).

6   Summary

In this work, going beyond viewed sketches, we address the challenging task of cross-modal face recognition for forensic and caricature sketches. To deal with the cross-modal gap due to heterogeneity, abstraction and distortion, we constructed an intermediate level attribute representation within each modality. To address the challenge of automated attribute detection within each image we introduce an ensemble of attribute detectors. Crucially, our semantic attribute representation is invariant to the details of the modality, and thus can be more directly compared across modalities than pixels or low-level features. Finally, we created a synergistic representation to integrate the semantic and low-level feature representations by learning an embedding subspace using CCA. As a result we are able to outperform several state of the art cross-domain mapping methods for both challenging datasets. We believe this is the first use of fully automated facial attribute analysis to improve cross-modal recognition.

Promising avenues for future research include integrating features at an abstraction level between pixels and attributes (e.g., facial interest points) along with our current framework of attributes and low-level image features. We also plan to investigate reasoning about attribute correlation; and extending our framework to apply to other modalities such as infra-red as well as sketch.

References

1. Klare, B., Li, Z., Jain, A.: Matching forensic sketches to mug shot photos. In: TPAMI, pp. 639–646 (2011)

2. Khan, Z., Hu, Y., Mian, A.: Facial self similarity for sketch to photo matching. In: Digital Image Computing Techniques and Applications (DICTA), pp. 1–7 (2012)
3. Kiani Galoogahi, H., Sim, T.: Face photo retrieval by sketch example. In: the 20th ACM International Conference on Multimedia, pp. 949–952 (2012)
4. Galoogahi, H., Sim, T.: Face sketch recognition by local radon binary pattern lrbp. In: ICIP, pp. 1837–1840 (2012)
5. Pramanik, S., Bhattacharjee, D.: Geometric feature based face-sketch recognition. In: Pattern Recognition, Informatics and Medical Engineering (PRIME), pp. 409–415 (2012)
6. Bhatt, H.S., Bharadwaj, S., Singh, R., Vatsa, M.: On matching sketches with digital face images. In: Biometrics: Theory Applications and Systems, pp. 1–7 (2010)
7. Choi, J., Sharma, A., Jacobs, D., Davis, L.: Data insufficiency in sketch versus photo face recognition. In: CVPR, pp. 1–8 (2012)
8. Klare, B., Bucak, S., Jain, A., Akgul, T.: Towards automated caricature recognition. In: The 5th IAPR International Conference on Biometrics Compendium, pp. 139–146 (2012)
9. Bhatt, H.S., Bharadwaj, S., Singh, R., Vatsa, M.: Memetic approach for matching sketches with digital face images. Indraprastha Institute of Information Technology Delhi, pp. 1–8 (2012)
10. Tang, X., Wang, X.: Face photo recognition using sketch. In: ICIP, pp. 257–260 (2002)
11. Wang, X., Tang, X.: Face photo-sketch synthesis and recognition. TPAMI **31**, 1955–1967 (2009)
12. Sharma, A., Jacobs, D.W.: Bypassing synthesis PLS for face recognition with pose, low-resolution and sketch. In: CVPR, pp. 593–600 (2011)
13. Bhatt, H., Bharadwaj, S., Singh, R., Vatsa, M.: Memetically optimized mcwld for matching sketches with digital face images. IEEE Trans. Inf. Forensics Secur. **7**, 1522–1535 (2012)
14. Galoogahi, H., Sim, T.: Inter-modality face sketch recognition. In: ICME (2012)
15. Uhl, R.G., Jr., da Vitoria Lobo, N.: A framework for recognizing a facial image from a police sketch. In: CVPR, pp. 586–593 (1996)
16. Bonnen, K., Klare, B., Jain, A.: Component-based representation in automated face recognition. IEEE Trans. Inf. Forensics Secur. **8**, 239–253 (2013)
17. Rasiwasia, N., Costa Pereira, J., Coviello, E., Doyle, G., Lanckriet, G.R., Levy, R., Vasconcelos, N.: A new approach to cross-modal multimedia retrieval. In: Proceedings of the international conference on Multimedia, pp. 251–260 (2010)
18. Gong, Y., Ke, Q., Isard, M., Lazebnik, S.: A multi-view embedding space for modeling internet images, tags, and their semantics. IJCV **106**, 210–233 (2014)
19. Wang, K., He, R., Wang, W., Wang, L., Tan, T.: Learning coupled feature spaces for cross-modal matching. In: ICCV, pp. 2088–2095 (2013)
20. Huang, D.A., Wang, Y.C.F.: Coupled dictionary and feature space learning with applications to cross-domain image synthesis and recognition. In: ICCV (2013)
21. Layne, R., Hospedales, T.M., Gong, S.: Person re-identification by attributes. In: BMVC, pp. 1–11 (2012)
22. Lampert, C.H., Nickisch, H., Harmeling, S.: Learning to detect unseen object classes by between-class attribute transfer. In: CVPR, pp. 951–958 (2009)
23. Fu, Y., Hospedales, T.M., Xiang, T., Fu, Z., Gong, S.: Transductive multi-view embedding for zero-shot recognition and annotation. In: Fleet, D., Pajdla, T., Schiele, B., Tuytelaars, T. (eds.) ECCV 2014, Part II. LNCS, vol. 8690, pp. 584–599. Springer, Heidelberg (2014)

24. Liu, J., Kuipers, B., Savarese, S.: Recognizing human actions by attributes. In: CVPR, pp. 3337–3344 (2011)
25. Fu, Y., Hospedales, T., Xiang, T., Gong, S.: Learning multimodal latent attributes. TPAMI **36**, 303–316 (2014)
26. Luo, P., Wang, X., Tang, X.: A deep sum-product architecture for robust facial attributes analysis. In: ICCV, pp. 2864–2871 (2013)
27. Kumar, N., Berg, A.C., Belhumeur, P.N., Nayar, S.K.: Attribute and simile classifiers for face verification. In: ICCV, pp. 365–372 (2009)
28. Johnson, K.E.: Effects of knowledge and development on subordinate level categorization. Cognitive Dev. **13**, 515–545 (1998)
29. Yao, B., Khosla, A., Fei-Fei, L.: Combining randomization and discrimination for fine-grained image categorization. In: CVPR, pp. 1577–1584 (2011)
30. Yi, D., Liu, R., Chu, R., Lei, Z., Li, S.Z.: Face matching between near infrared and visible light images. In: Lee, S.-W., Li, S.Z. (eds.) Advances in Biometrics. LNCS, vol. 4642. Springer, Heidelberg (2007)

3D Aware Correction and Completion of Depth Maps in Piecewise Planar Scenes

Ali K. Thabet[1], Jean Lahoud[1], Daniel Asmar[2],
and Bernard Ghanem[1(✉)]

[1] King Abdullah University of Science and Technology (KAUST),
Thuwal, Saudi Arabia
{ali.thabet,jean.lahoud,bernard.ghanem}@kaust.edu.sa
[2] American University of Beirut (AUB), Beirut, Lebanon
da02@aub.edu.lb

Abstract. RGB-D sensors are popular in the computer vision community, especially for problems of scene understanding, semantic scene labeling, and segmentation. However, most of these methods depend on *reliable* input depth measurements, while discarding unreliable ones. This paper studies how reliable depth values can be used to *correct* the unreliable ones, and how to *complete* (or extend) the available depth data beyond the raw measurements of the sensor (i.e. infer depth at pixels with unknown depth values), given a prior model on the 3D scene. We consider piecewise planar environments in this paper, since many indoor scenes with man-made objects can be modeled as such. We propose a framework that uses the RGB-D sensor's noise profile to adaptively and robustly fit plane segments (e.g. floor and ceiling) and iteratively complete the depth map, when possible. Depth completion is formulated as a discrete labeling problem (MRF) with hard constraints and solved efficiently using graph cuts. To regularize this problem, we exploit 3D and appearance cues that encourage pixels to take on depth values that will be compatible in 3D to the piecewise planar assumption. Extensive experiments, on a new large-scale and challenging dataset, show that our approach results in more accurate depth maps (with 20% more depth values) than those recorded by the RGB-D sensor. Additional experiments on the NYUv2 dataset show that our method generates more 3D aware depth. These generated depth maps can also be used to improve the performance of a state-of-the-art RGB-D SLAM method.

1 Introduction

Active RGB-D sensors are capable of directly capturing 3D structure from a scene, thus, avoiding the difficult task of inferring this information from the scene's appearance alone. Sensors like the MS Kinect are popular in computer

Electronic supplementary material The online version of this chapter (doi:10.1007/978-3-319-16808-1_16) contains supplementary material, which is available to authorized users.

D. Cremers et al. (Eds.): ACCV 2014, Part II, LNCS 9004, pp. 226–241, 2015.
DOI: 10.1007/978-3-319-16808-1_16

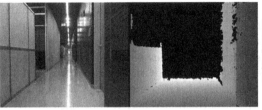 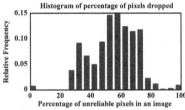

Fig. 1. Left: A sample RGB-D image pair. This is a single frame out of roughly 1000 that were recorded while walking through an indoor piecewise planar scene (*office corridor*). **Right:** The percentage of pixels per image of this walk-through that are unreliable because their depth values are above a certain threshold d_{rel} or are unknown.

vision applications, since they are relatively cheap, accessible, and well supported/maintained by manufacturers and third-party developers. There is a large amount of recent work that exploits RGB-D data to generalize and shed light on traditional vision problems, including semantic scene labeling [22], segmentation [13], scene understanding [1,11,19], object detection [20], visual SLAM (Simultaneous Localization And Mapping) [18,26], among others.

Most of the RGB-D methods above rely on the fact that the input depth image is largely comprised of pixels with *reliable* (accurate) depth measurements. This assumption might not always be valid, as most sensors only provide reliable measurements up to a maximum distance d_{rel} (usually of 3–4.5 m). Given this constraint, most RGB-D based methods either record images where the scene is within the d_{rel} range away from the sensor or disregard all pixels whose depth values exceed d_{rel}. This unreliability in depth measurement arises due to several reasons, including limitations in the depth sensor itself (e.g., the projected IR signal of a Kinect decays with squared distance and it is unable to image objects that are too close or too far) and the nature of the scene itself (e.g., IR absorbing or reflective surfaces). In Fig. 1 (*left*), we show a sample RGB-D image pair taken in an indoor office scene, with all the unreliable and unknown depth values set to zero (black pixels). Clearly, not all pixels are assigned depth values. Disregarding unreliable pixels limits the range and impedes the generality of methods using RGB-D data. This issue is even more pressing when general indoor scenes are considered, such as in open areas, office spaces, reasonably sized rooms, museums, etc. In these cases, much of the scene is at a distance larger than the maximum reliable depth value d_{rel}. We show empirical evidence of this in Fig. 1 (*right*). We histogram the average percentage of pixels discarded in an image because they were deemed unreliable ($d_{rel} = 4.5$ m) for a typical recording of a walk-through inside an office/lab environment. For this recording, roughly 60 % of pixels in each Kinect depth map are deemed unreliable. Discarding these pixels limits subsequent processing or learning modules, including RGB-D semantic labeling, scene understanding, and visual SLAM methods.

Interestingly, many of these unreliable pixels are projections of 3D scene points belonging to *objects* (e.g., floor, ceiling, walls, cabinets, etc.) that have extensions within the reliable range of depth pixels. So, it is important to study how reliable depth values can be used to judge and even *correct* unreliable ones, when a particular prior model is assumed on the 3D scene. In fact, this could also be used to *complete* (or extend) the depth values beyond the raw measurements of the sensor itself (i.e., infer depth at pixels with unknown depth). This paper studies this problem for 3D piecewise planar scenes and proposes a novel framework that makes use of both appearance and 3D cues from a *single* RGB-D image pair to correct and complete the depth image. This framework can enable subsequent scene processing and understanding even if the initial RGB-D data is deemed unreliable. Here, we define a piecewise planar scene to be one that comprises a set of intersecting planes (realistically plane segments). Piecewise planar scenes are valid descriptions of many indoor scenes containing man-made objects (e.g., building interiors, offices, homes, museums, etc.). This scene prior has been used in previous work for the purpose of stereo vision or 3D reconstruction [9,10], semantic labelling [22], and scene understanding from a single RGB-D image [8,19] or a single RGB image [14–16].

2   Related Work

This paper addresses the problem of correcting unreliable depth values and inferring unknown ones in RGB-D data of piecewise planar scenes. In data of this kind, large groups of contiguous pixels have either unreliable or unknown depth values. The most related work in the literature that address a similar problem (depth enhancement) is categorized as: **(1)** hole-filling (depth inpainting) methods or **(2)** depth upsampling methods.

Methods of category **(1)** attempt to infer depth at pixels that are not assigned depth values. These pixels tend to be projections of parts of surfaces that are IR absorbing, reflective, or too close to the RGB-D sensor. These pixels are small in number and tend not to cluster in the same portion of a depth image. Most hole-filling methods interpolate (or propagate) unknown depths from depths in pixel neighborhoods. To this end, joint bilateral filtering (JBF) has been extensively used to fill holes in depth images, especially due to its relatively attractive runtime [4,21]. Moreover, colorization techniques are also used to fill in unknown depth [23], as done in compiling the popular NYUv2 dataset [25]. In [6], the problem is formulated as a continuous Markov Random Field (MRF), where the latent variables are the depth values of all pixels, the unary (data) term is dependent on the known depth values, and the binary term encourages similar looking pixels in a local neighborhood to have similar depth values. In [5], a foreground depth model is assumed to be available and depth layers are inferred using a discrete MRF. Many other methods of this category exist (e.g., [27]); however, they all suffer from the same drawback that makes them infeasible and inappropriate for the problem of depth correction and completion tackled in this paper. Hole-filling (depth inpainting) methods assume that there is a strong correlation between depth discontinuities and image edges and that pixels with similar appearance have similar 3D geometry. In general, this assumption is a useful cue for interpolation but it does not always hold, especially in scenes where large portions of a depth image need to be filled.

Methods of category (2) attempt to generate a high resolution depth image from a low-resolution one and (usually) a registered high resolution RGB image. The low-resolution depth image is assumed to be complete and comprised of reliable depth values. Since a plethora of such methods abound in the literature, we mention a representative few here. In fact, JBF and MRF labeling are common techniques employed by methods of this category [6,21,24]. Similar to the problem of hole-filling, local assumptions of depth smoothness (except at color discontinuities) are made to propagate depth values from the low resolution image to a local neighborhood of unknown values in the higher resolution image. These assumptions break down in the case of large contiguous holes, which makes upsampling methods unsuitable for the problem addressed in this paper.

All previous methods apply local priors to depth values in RGB-D data, but they tend not to take into account the global 3D structure of the scene for unreliable depth correction and completion. These methods do *not* ensure that the processed depth maps lead to a 3D point cloud that has a compatible 3D structure (i.e. its structure does not lead to any 3D contradictions or impossibilities). Assuming a piecewise planar scene allows us to regularize the completion and correction process globally as well as locally. This regularization disallows certain depth assignments that lead to a 3D structure that is not compatible or does not respect the underlying planar assumption.

Contributions: They are three fold. (i) Unlike other depth enhancement methods, this paper addresses the problem of correction and completion of unreliable and unknown depth values in a single RGB-D image pair. To the best of our knowledge, this is the first work that makes use of local *and* global priors on the overall 3D scene to enable 3D aware depth prediction and correction. Here, the global prior on the scene is piecewise planarity. (ii) Instead of discarding unreliable depth information, we make use of its noisy (probabilistic) structure to perform adaptive depth smoothing and adaptive robust plane fitting. We model the depth correction/completion process as a discrete MRF (Markov Random Field), a labeling problem that can be efficiently solved using iterative interactive graph cuts. The unary and binary terms of the MRF go beyond traditional definitions to stress appearance and 3D cues that encourage a 3D structure compatible with the piecewise planar assumption. (iii) To evaluate our proposed approach and validate the importance of depth correction and completion, we compile a challenging, large-scale dataset with ground truth depth. Additionally, we qualitatively evaluate our method on the NYUv2 dataset. Also, we illustrate the merit of our solution in a real-world application, namely RGB-D SLAM. We show that replacing raw depth maps with our corrected and completed ones substantially improves the performance of a state-of-the-art visual SLAM approach.

3   Proposed Method

In this work, two images generated by an RGB-D sensor (the MS Kinect) are taken as input, where both RGB and depth sensors are assumed to be calibrated (i.e., their intrinsic and extrinsic parameters are estimated beforehand). Denote the RGB and depth images as $\mathbf{I}_c \in \mathbb{R}^{M \times N}$ and $\mathbf{I}_d \in \mathbb{R}^{M \times N}$ respectively. In the rest of the paper, we denote $\mathbf{I}_d$ as the *raw* depth image, since it contains the unprocessed depth values measured by the sensor directly.

3.1 Pre-processing

Before correcting and/or completing depth values in $\mathbf{I}_d$, we adaptively smooth them using a precomputed Kinect noise profile (see **Supplementary Material**) and we robustly extract planar segments from the smoothed 3D data. These segments constitute primitives for the piecewise planar scene, which will subsequently be filtered, grouped, and possibly extended.

Adaptive Depth Smoothing: To reduce the effect of sensor noise while preserving depth discontinuities, the projected 3D points are smoothed using the JBF defined in Eq. (1). This filter makes use of both the depth image $\mathbf{I}_d$ and RGB image $\mathbf{I}_c$, as in [5]. Since this filtering method is unaware of the underlying 3D scene, we only use it to smooth existing depth data but not fill unknown depth values in $\mathbf{I}_d$.

$$\hat{\mathbf{I}}_d(\mathbf{p}) = \frac{1}{k} \sum_{\mathbf{q} \in \Omega} \mathbf{I}_d(\mathbf{q}) F(\mathbf{p}, \mathbf{q}) G(\mathbf{I}_d(\mathbf{p}), \mathbf{I}_d(\mathbf{q})) H(\mathbf{I}_c(\mathbf{p}), \mathbf{I}_c(\mathbf{q})) \qquad (1)$$

In this filter, the smoothed depth at pixel $\mathbf{p}$ is a positive weighted sum of the raw depth values in the neighborhood Ω around $\mathbf{p}$. Each weight is a product of three similarity measures between $\mathbf{p}$ and its neighbor $\mathbf{q}$: within-image spatial closeness (defined by F), similarity in raw depth (defined by G), and similarity in appearance (defined by H). Similar to other methods, we take these three functions to be Gaussian. We model $G(\mathbf{I}_d(\mathbf{p}), \mathbf{I}_d(\mathbf{q}))$ as a Gaussian function $\mathcal{N}(\mathbf{I}_d(\mathbf{p}) - \mathbf{I}_d(\mathbf{q}), \sigma_d(\mathbf{I}_d(\mathbf{p})))$, where the standard deviation is depth dependent. By doing this, the JBF is made adaptive to varying depths, which specifically allows for more suitable smoothing at larger depths.

Adaptive and Robust Plane Fitting: After depth-adaptive smoothing, we aim to detect and fit 3D planes through the 3D projections of pixels in $\hat{\mathbf{I}}_d$ with known depth. Similar to previous methods, we use RANSAC for robust plane fitting. However, the criterion for a pixel to be an inlier (e.g. having the distance of its 3D projection to the plane be less than a threshold) should incorporate the noise in the sensor's depth measurements. Otherwise, fewer consistent planar segments can be detected at points that are farther away.

We start the RANSAC process at pixels with smoothed depth less than d_{rel}. We model the actual depth $d(\mathbf{p})$ at pixel $\mathbf{p}$ probabilistically as a Gaussian centered around the depth value $\hat{\mathbf{I}}_d(\mathbf{p})$ with a depth-varying standard deviation $\sigma_d(\hat{\mathbf{I}}_d(\mathbf{p}))$. Since the depth camera is calibrated, the 3D point corresponding to $\mathbf{p}$ is computed as $\mathbf{x}(\mathbf{p}) = d(\mathbf{p})\mathbf{K}^{-1}\tilde{\mathbf{p}} = d(\mathbf{p})\mathbf{t}(\mathbf{p})$, where $\tilde{\mathbf{p}}$ is $\mathbf{p}$ in homogenous coordinates and $\mathbf{K}$ is the camera matrix. It is easily shown that $\mathbf{x}(\mathbf{p})$ is a Gaussian random variable (centered around the observed 3D projection $\hat{\mathbf{I}}_d(\mathbf{p})\mathbf{t}(\mathbf{p})$). Similarly, the distance $D(\mathbf{x}(\mathbf{p})|(\mathbf{n}, n_0))$ between $\mathbf{x}(\mathbf{p})$ and a 3D plane parameterized by a unit normal $\mathbf{n}$ (pointing towards $\mathbf{x}(\mathbf{p})$) and offset n_0 also has a Gaussian distribution: $D(\mathbf{x}(\mathbf{p})|(\mathbf{n}, n_0)) \sim \mathcal{N}(\mu_D, \sigma_D^2)$, where

$$\mu_D = \hat{\mathbf{I}}_d(\mathbf{p})\mathbf{n}^T\mathbf{t}(\mathbf{p}) + n_0 \quad \text{and} \quad \sigma_D^2 = \sigma_d^2(\hat{\mathbf{I}}_d(\mathbf{p}))\|\mathbf{n} \circ \mathbf{t}(\mathbf{p})\|_2^2 \qquad (2)$$

Note that $\circ$ is the Hadamard product. As expected, the variance of $D(\mathbf{x}(\mathbf{p})|(\mathbf{n}, n_0))$ increases with depth and varies with the relative orientation of the plane with the camera plane. By representing this distance probabilistically, we replace the usual RANSAC inlier condition $D(\mathbf{x}(\mathbf{p})|(\mathbf{n}, n_0)) \leq a$ with $p(D(\mathbf{x}(\mathbf{p})|(\mathbf{n}, n_0)) \leq a) \geq \theta$. The latter probability can be computed straightforwardly using the CDF of a Gaussian. In this paper, we take $a = 2\,\text{cm}$ and $\theta = 0.8$. Also, normals of the observed 3D projections $\hat{\mathbf{I}}_d(\mathbf{p})\mathbf{t}(\mathbf{p})$ can be used to refine the inliers. Using this probabilistic rule allows a plane model $(\mathbf{n}, n_0)$ that is fit with 3D projections from pixels with reliable depth to extend into farther pixels with less reliable depth. This extension would not be possible and plane fragmentation would ensue, if the conventional RANSAC inlier condition is used.

Once the proposed plane-fitting method converges to a set of 3D plane equations and corresponding pixel inliers, we project the 3D projections of the inliers unto their respective planes and update $\hat{\mathbf{I}}_d$ to reflect this projection. This point-to-plane projection changes the depth values acquired by the sensor and, in the majority of cases, corrects their values when a piecewise planar scene is assumed. If a fitted plane exists such that the vast majority of projected points lie in the halfspace designated by its normal and the principal angle between its normal and the normal of the image plane is negative (clockwise), then this fitted plane is designated as the *floor*. A similar rule determines the ceiling plane, if it exists.

3.2   Depth Completion as an MRF

After pre-processing, the raw depth image $\mathbf{I}_d$ is transformed into $\hat{\mathbf{I}}_d$ and each pixel with a known depth value is assigned a label corresponding to the fitted plane it belongs to. We denote the resulting label image as $\mathbf{L}_0 \in \{0, 1, \ldots, l\}^{M \times N}$, where the 0 label designates pixels of unknown depth, 1 the floor (if it exists), and 2 the ceiling (if it exists). In this section, we describe how the initial label image $\mathbf{L}_0$ is relabelled through an iterative process that makes use of appearance and 3D cues from $\mathbf{I}_c$ and $\hat{\mathbf{I}}_d$. We denote the label image at iteration k as $\mathbf{L}_k$. As we will see, a consequence of this process is the iterative extension/completion of each plane label and the constriction of the 0 label. In other words, pixels with unknown depth values (labelled 0) can be assigned a plane label, if deemed likely from an appearance and 3D reasoning point of view. We formulate the relabeling process as an iterative *interactive graph cuts* problem, where regional (unary) and boundary (binary) terms are used to relabel all pixels in the image while enforcing the labels of pixels that already have plane labels.

Determining Background Pixels: Clearly, not all pixels in $\hat{\mathbf{I}}_d$ are projections of 3D points that belong to the l fitted planes. Due to sensor limitations and scene

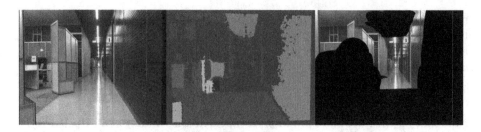

Fig. 2. Left: Original RGB image of a piecewise planar scene. **Middle:** Initial labeling of plane segments using our robust plane extraction in 3D (background *not* included). **Right:** The original RGB image showing only the pixels that are initially labelled in $\mathbf{L_0}$ as background.

structure, other planes might exist in the 3D scene but they are not imaged at all. To allow pixels not to belong to the l fitted planes, we construct a *background* label, denoted as $(l+1)$. Since no depth information exists for background pixels, we label them according to how their projection rays (3D rays connecting the pixels to the camera's optical center) relate to the fitted 3D planes, as follows. A pixel is given an $(l+1)$ label if **(i)** it cannot belong to any of the l fitted planes (i.e. its projection ray does not intersect any of the planes) or **(ii)** the intersection between its projection ray and each plane j is at least $d_{\max}$ far from the closest known 3D point of plane j. In our experiments, we take $d_{\max} = 1\,\text{m}$. Condition **(ii)** assumes that the farther away a point is from the observed points on the fitted planes, the more likely it belongs to the background label. Background pixels are labeled as $(l+1)$ and added to $\mathbf{L_0}$. Figure 2 shows an example of pixels labelled as background in a sample depth frame.

Discriminative Appearance Model: We discriminatively model the appearance of each label (i.e. pixels whose 3D points belong to the same fitted plane). All labelled pixels in the image are represented using a set of low-level image features that describe a pixel's color (local color histogram), neighborhood structure (HOG features), and texture information (LBP features). Using PCA, dimensionality reduction is performed to maintain 90 % variance in the labelled data. A discriminative appearance model is formed by training a multi-class RBF SVM classifier on all labelled pixels. This model is a vector scoring function $h(\mathbf{z}) \in \mathbb{R}^{l+1}$, where $h_i(\mathbf{z})$ is the SVM score of labelling feature vector $\mathbf{z}$ as i, for all $i \in \mathcal{L}$ such that $\mathcal{L} = \{1, \ldots, l+1\}$.

Vanishing Lines: Apart from appearance, other cues exist that shed light on the 3D structure of the scene. A widely used cue is the existence of vanishing line segments. This cue has been extensively used in scene recognition and understanding from single RGB images, especially in indoor piecewise planar scenes [14]. In an image, vanishing points are usually extracted through a process of clustering line segments that vanish to the same point. However, in our case, we can explicitly compute certain vanishing points without any need for clustering or line detection. In indoor scenes, many plane segments tend to be perpendicular to each other (e.g. the *floor* and *walls*), thus, many parallel 3D lines in the scene (belonging to the same or different planes) tend to be perpendicular to another plane in the scene. Therefore, we can easily estimate the vanishing point of 3D parallel lines that are perpendicular to fitted plane i by simply constructing at least two such lines (parallel to the normal of plane i) and projecting them unto the RGB image $\mathbf{I}_c$. We denote these vanishing points as $\mathcal{V}_1 = \{\mathbf{v}_i\}_{i=1}^l$, where $\mathbf{v}_i$ is the vanishing point of parallel 3D lines that are perpendicular to plane i. We also use a method similar to [2] to obtain another set of vanishing points $\mathcal{V}_2$ that is disjoint from $\mathcal{V}_1$. We maintain a record of the clustered line segments that vanish to points in $\mathcal{V}_1$ and $\mathcal{V}_2$. Obviously, the process of extracting line segments and clustering vanishing points in $\mathcal{V}_2$ is prone to error, but it provides an additional 3D cue that can be harnessed in the relabeling process.

MRF Formulation: Given the label image $\mathbf{L}_0$, we now aim to label all pixels in $\hat{\mathbf{I}}_d$, especially those with unknown depth values. We model this labelling problem with a discrete Markov Random Field (MRF), where $\mathcal{L} = \{1, \ldots, l + 1\}$ is the set of discrete labels, $\mathcal{P}$ is the set of all pixels, and $\mathcal{E}$ is the set of all connections defining local 8-connected neighborhoods around each pixel. We seek a labeling $\mathbf{f}^*$ that minimizes the energy in Eq. (3).

$$E(\mathbf{f}) = \sum_{\mathbf{p} \in \mathcal{P}} U(\mathbf{f}_p | \mathbf{p}) + \lambda \sum_{(\mathbf{p}, \mathbf{q}) \in \mathcal{E}} B(\mathbf{p}, \mathbf{q}) \tag{3}$$

Here, $U(\mathbf{f}_p | \mathbf{p})$ defines the unary (or data) term, which quantifies the cost incurred when pixel $\mathbf{p}$ is assigned to label $\mathbf{f}_p \in \mathcal{L}$. Alone, this term treats pixels in $\hat{\mathbf{I}}_d$ independently, so a binary (or smoothness) term $B(\mathbf{p}, \mathbf{q})$ is added for regularization, with tradeoff coefficient λ. This term quantifies the cost of assigning neighboring pixels $\mathbf{p}$ and $\mathbf{q}$ to different labels, i.e. $\mathbf{f}_p \neq \mathbf{f}_q$. This energy can be minimized efficiently using graph cuts [3]. Since some pixels in $\hat{\mathbf{I}}_d$ are already assigned to fitted planes with non-background labels, we use a version of graph cuts (popularly known as *interactive graph cuts*) to guarantee that the labels of these pixels, after optimization, remain the same. Other optimization methods could be used to solve the normalized version of this problem [12].

Unary (data) Term: Although interactive graph cuts is well-known and has been used for various labelling problems in the past, the quality of the final labeling is mainly determined by how appropriate and informative the unary and binary terms are. Here, the unary term is inversely proportional to the likelihood of a pixel belonging to a fitted plane. This term compares the appearance of a pixel to the discriminative appearance model of each plane and prevents label assignments that are incompatible in 3D under the piecewise planar assumption. In general, we set $U(i|\mathbf{p}) = -h_i(\mathbf{z}(\mathbf{p}))$ for each pixel $\mathbf{p} \in \mathcal{P}$ and each label $i \in \mathcal{L}$. This assumes that points belonging to the same plane look similar, which is usually a valid assumption. In what follows, we use 3D cues (from both $\hat{\mathbf{I}}_d$ and $\hat{\mathbf{I}}_c$) to regularize the labelling further.

To enforce the hard constraints, we follow a similar strategy as in [3], where $U(i|\mathbf{p}) = K \gg 0$ for each $i \in \mathcal{L} \backslash \{l + 1\}$ and $\mathbf{p}$ such that $\mathbf{L}_0(\mathbf{p}) = j \neq i$. This large cost K prevents a pixel that is already labelled in $\mathbf{L}_0$ to switch labels. This enforcement is done for all labels except background $(l + 1)$, which we allow to constrict or expand. Moreover, we set $U(i|\mathbf{p}) = K$ for any pixel $\mathbf{p}$ whose projection ray does not intersect plane i. Also, we enforce that all intersections between projection rays and planes occur *above* the floor plane (if it exists) and *below* the ceiling plane (if it exists). This prohibits label assignments that lead to 3D points, which tunnel into the floor or pierce the ceiling. For these pixels, we set $U(1|\mathbf{p}) = K$ and/or $U(2|\mathbf{p}) = K$. Lastly, the unary term should not lead to label assignments that are contradictory in 3D. As such, we set $U(i|\mathbf{p}) = K$ for any pixel $\mathbf{p}$, which belongs to a line segment that vanishes to $\mathbf{v}_i \in \mathcal{V}_1$. This discourages $\mathbf{p}$ from belonging to a fitted plane, if it lies on a line perpendicular to that plane. In this case, the points belonging to the intersection of two perpendicular planes will be assigned to only one of the two.

Binary (smoothness) Term: To allow for interactions between neighboring pixels, we define a binary term $B(\mathbf{p}, \mathbf{q})$, which encourages label smoothness among pixel neighbors that have similar appearance and/or that are likely to belong to the same plane in 3D. In general, we set $B(\mathbf{p}, \mathbf{q}) = \exp(-\Delta_c(\mathbf{p}, \mathbf{q})\Sigma_c^{-1}\Delta_c(\mathbf{p}, \mathbf{q}))$, where $\Delta_c(\mathbf{p}, \mathbf{q}) = \mathbf{I}_c(\mathbf{p}) - \mathbf{I}_c(\mathbf{p})$. The covariance matrix Σ_c is estimated from $\mathbf{I}_c$. Moreover, we make use of vanishing points to discourage pixels lying on the same vanishing line segment to belong to different planes. So, we set $B(\mathbf{p}, \mathbf{q}) = K$ when pixels $\mathbf{p}$ and $\mathbf{q}$ belong to the same line segment that vanishes to a point in $\mathcal{V}_1 \cup \mathcal{V}_2$. In our experiments and as suggested in [3], we set $K = 1 + \max_{\mathbf{p} \in \mathcal{P}} \sum_{\mathbf{q}:(\mathbf{p}, \mathbf{q}) \in \mathcal{E}} B(\mathbf{p}, \mathbf{q})$.

Iterative Solution: Once all unary and binary terms are computed for all pixels and labels, we solve the labeling problem using interactive graph cuts [3]. Upon convergence, we use the final labeling $\mathbf{f}^*$ to determine the depth value of each pixel with label $\mathbf{f}_p^* \in \{1, \ldots, l\}$. This is done by intersecting the projection ray of $\mathbf{p}$ with fitted plane $\mathbf{f}_p^*$. The depth of a pixel labeled as background (i.e. $\mathbf{f}_p^* = l+1$) remains unknown. Effectively, the original label image $\mathbf{L}_0$ has been relabelled to produce a modified version $\mathbf{L}_1$. Many pixels that had unknown depth values in $\mathbf{L}_0$ have been assigned depth values in $\mathbf{L}_1$. These depth values encourage conformity to appearance models of existing planes and non-contradictory 3D layouts in piecewise planar scenes. In fact, the relabeling process can be rerun with $\mathbf{L}_1$ replacing $\mathbf{L}_0$. Obviously, the plane equations can be refined, the appearance model for each label needs to be retrained, and the unary and binary terms should reflect the changes in hard constraints. The resulting iterative relabeling process converges at iteration k when the change in label image $\delta(\mathbf{L}_k, \mathbf{L}_{k-1})$ is negligible. As such, our proposed approach corrects (through robust plane fitting and projection) and completes (through appearance and 3D aware relabeling) raw depth values recorded by an RGB-D sensor in a piecewise planar scene. Figure 3 shows the end-to-end approach applied to a sample RGB-D image pair.

4   Experimental Results

In this section, we evaluate the effectiveness of our method in enhanceing/ correcting and completing depth measurements obtained by the Kinect. For

INPUT **PRE-PROCESSING** **OUTPUT**

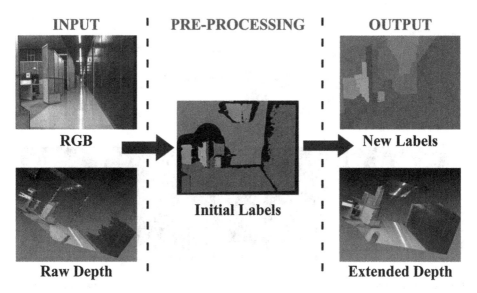

RGB **New Labels**

Initial Labels

Raw Depth **Extended Depth**

Fig. 3. End-to-end process. *Input:* The system takes as input an RGB-D image pair. *Pre-processing:* The input depth is smoothed using a JBF, after which, plane segments are extracted using the adaptive/robust RANSAC method described in this section. Using the extracted plane segments, an initial label image is created. In addition, background pixels are extracted and added as a new label. In the initial label image, each label is given a distinct color, and orange is used here to describe background pixels. These initial labels are fed to the Graph Cut solver. *Output:* The final output is a complete set of labels, which are converted to new depth values. We can observe how the depth range is extended from the original 3D point cloud to the final result of our correction/completion process.

a quantitative comparison between the depth maps generated by our method and the raw depth maps obtained from the sensor, we generate a large-scale 3D point cloud of a typical indoor scene, which we use to generate ground truth depth maps. Additionally, we show some quantitative results on the NYUv2 dataset. We also show how our method can be used in to enhance applications like RGB-D SLAM.

4.1 Dataset Compilation

To create the ground truth set, we scanned a large indoor area using 2 Kinect sensors mounted on a moving platform. The devices were pointed at different fields of view to avoid possible interference of their light patterns. We used 2 devices to be able to cover large areas in the scene, but each device reconstructs its view independently from the other. The relative movement of the platform was constrained to a fixed translation along a predefined direction perpendicular to the floor normal, and a rotation of 0 or $\pm 90°$ around the floor normal; such restrictions make the registration between frames trivial. A total of 700 frames were recorded,

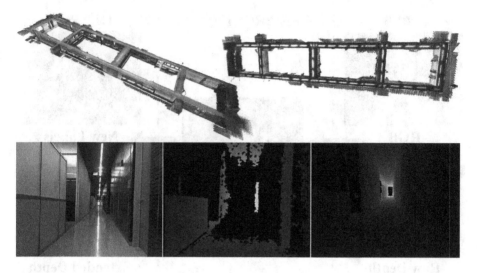

Fig. 4. Top: Different views of our large 3D reconstructed dataset. The point cloud covered a physical area of 220 m and comprised around 63 million points. It contains challenging images of reflective and transparent surfaces, where the Kinect fails to estimate depth values. The depth images obtained are comprised of large gaps with unknown depth as shown in Fig. 1. Bottom: RGB, raw depth, and ground truth depth. We notice the large amount of points missing in the raw depth image, due to the sensor's inability to process large dark areas and reflective surfaces. The ground truth depth frame shows a complete version of the view by back-projecting the large 3D point cloud aligned to this frame's view.

corresponding to 220 m of stretch inside a typical office space. In order to ensure data precision, we select from each frame depth values that only lie within a 0.8–4 m reliable range. Figure 4 shows 2 different views of the final point cloud, with a rough size of 63 million points, as well as a triplet of color, raw depth, and ground truth depth for the same image.

4.2   Quantitative Comparison

Using the ground truth set, we test the accuracy of our approach and compare it to the raw data provided by the Kinect. The result of our application is a new set of depth frames that improve the raw Kinect data in 2 ways, first by correcting depth values, particularly at large depths, and second by increasing the number of available depth pixels. In order to test for the first hypothesis, we compare the enhanced and raw depth with the ground truth 3D points. The comparison is done by converting the depth values of the enhanced and raw frames into 3D points, and calculating errors as Euclidean distances between closest points of these frames and the 3D point cloud of the scene. In order to do this computation in an efficient manner, we build a K-D tree for the ground truth point cloud once, and query the tree using the 3D points of each frame. Figure 5 *Left* plots these errors for both

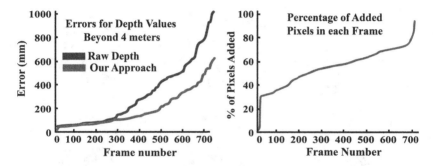

Fig. 5. Left: Comparison of raw depth values and depth values generated by our method w.r.t. ground truth for a large-scale piecewise planar scene. The plot shows the error per frame in increasing order of error. We notice the significantly lower errors obtained by applying our method. This improvement comes from a combination of correction and completion of the raw depth. **Right:** Percentage of depth values added to a single image. Our method is adding an average of 50 % of depth pixels, and sometimes as much as 80 % (Color figure online).

the raw depth data of the RGB-D sensor and our approach. Our method increases the accuracy of the depth values by an average of 0.5 m. We show a wide range of qualitative results on the **Supplementary Material**.

Since our method not only corrects but also extends the depth range of the sensor data; and thus increasing the number of depth pixels available, we also look at the average pixel increase as an additional measure of performance. Figure 5 *Right* shows a plot of percentage pixel increase per frame, calculated as the percentage of pixels added by the our correction/completion with respect to the original raw data available. The mean increase is around 40000 pixels, with standard deviation of around 20000 pixels. We note at this point that although an increase is present in more than 80 % of the cases, the amount of increase always scene-dependent, thus resulting in high standard deviations.

4.3   Result on NYUv2 Dataset

In addition to testing our proposed method on the set we compiled, we also make use of images from the popular NYUv2 dataset [25]. We choose images of piecewise planar environments (such as corridors or hallways) and apply our method on the raw depth images. We compare our corrected and completed depth map to that generated by the hole-filling (colorization) method in [23] used to colorize depth in NYUv2. We show some examples in Fig. 6, where we render 3D views of the raw depth data and the enhanced depth obtained by both techniques. Since the colorization technique is unaware of the 3D structure of the scene, depth points that were added by this method were not constrained to belong to any plane, leading to significant errors. As pointed out in Fig. 6, these errors come from bad depth predictions at large gaps as well as noise created ad depth discontinuities. Our method does not suffer from these drawbacks due

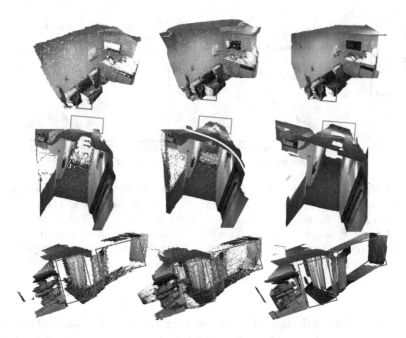

Fig. 6. Left to right: 3D renderings of the raw depth, depth after applying the colorization method in [23], depth from our proposed method. The depth colorization method creates unwanted artifacts at large depth gaps (red boxes), as well as a lot of noise at depth discontinuities (green boxes). these problems are not present in our method, since it provides a more 3D aware approach to estimating unknown depth (Color figure online).

to its 3D aware nature while estimating unknown depth. Further results are available in the **Supplementary Material**.

4.4 RGD-D SLAM

In order to substantiate the usage of the corrected depth data over regular raw sensor data, we test the performance of a well-known application, the RGBD SLAM, by using the enhanced depth. We tackle the problem of localization in feature-poor environments such as hallways. Such environments are challenging because of the low number of features (SIFTs or SURFs) within the range of the Kinect sensor that could be tracked to estimate the sensor motion. Moreover, using ICP algorithm to estimate the motion in those environments faces convergence to local minima solutions due to the lack of 3D cues. We use a method similar to the one used by [7] with SIFT features. This method can be complemented by other methods, such as RGBD ICP by [17], but the goal is to assess the advantages of providing the corrected depth as an input to any application that uses RGBD data. We compare our results to the ground truth data by measuring two errors: the drift in the sensor motion and that of the 3D point locations. The error in 3D point locations is computed as the distance between the predicated 3D point location and the true location where the predicted point location is calculated after movements of 2 m throughout the hallway. Results are shown in Fig. 7. The mean error in point locations is 682 mm when using the raw depth and 436 mm when using the corrected depth data. For translation, the average drift is 440 mm when using raw depth and 283 mm when using the our ones. Figure 7 also shows the difference in trajectory between the 2 methods, showing significant improvement when using the corrected/completed depth data.

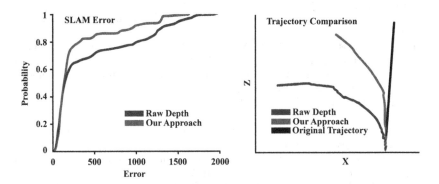

Fig. 7. RGB-D SLAM comparison. **Left:** A cumulative density distribution of the frame-to-frame SLAM error when using raw depth and our depth on 700 images. **Right:** We see in this plot the trajectory estimation of RGB-D SLAM using the raw depth (green), and using our depth (magenta), compared to the original trajectory (black). The improvement (after enhancement) in drift is substantial: 283 mm as opposed to 440 mm with the raw depth (Color figure online).

5   Conclusion

In this paper we presented a method to use the complete set of depth values provided by an RGB-D sensor to better represent Manhattan environment scenes. We showed that by properly analyzing the sensor error at large depth, we can correct the data given, and segment planar labels from the scene. By applying our method to a new large-scale ground truth data set, we show that our framework provides more accurate depth maps, having a larger number of pixels (20 % average increase) than those recorded by the RGB-D sensor. In addition, we qualitatively showed the power of our technique on the NYUv2 dataset. We also applied our methodology to improve the performance of RGB-D SLAM.

Acknowledgement. Research reported in this publication was supported by competitive research funding from King Abdullah University of Science and Technology (KAUST).

References

1. Barron, J.T., Malik, J., Berkeley, U.C.: Intrinsic scene properties from a single RGB-D image. In: CVPR (2013)
2. Bazin, J., Seo, Y.: Globally optimal line clustering and vanishing point estimation in manhattan world. In: CVPR (2012)
3. Boykov, Y., Funka-Lea, G.: Graph cuts and efficient N-D image segmentation. IJCV **70**(2), 109–131 (2006)
4. Camplani, M., Salgado, L.: Efficient spatio-temporal hole filling strategy for kinect depth maps. In: SPIE (2012)
5. Cheung, S.C.S.: Layer depth denoising and completion for structured-light RGB-D cameras. In: CVPR (2013)
6. Diebel, J., Thrun, S.: An application of markov random fields to range sensing. In: NIPS (2005)
7. Endres, F., Hess, J., Engelhard, N., Sturm, J., Cremers, D., Burgard, W.: An evaluation of the RGB-D SLAM system. In: ICRA (2012)
8. Flint, A., Murray, D., Reid, I.: Manhattan scene understanding using monocular, stereo, and 3D features. In: ICCV (2011)
9. Furukawa, Y., Curless, B., Seitz, S., Szeliski, R.: Manhattan-world stereo. In: CVPR (2009)
10. Furukawa, Y., Curless, B., Seitz, S.M., Szeliski, R.: Reconstructing building interiors from images. In: ICCV (2009)
11. Gallup, D., Frahm, J.M., Pollefeys, M.: Piecewise planar and non-planar stereo for urban scene reconstruction. In: CVPR (2012)
12. Ghanem, B., Ahuja, N.: Dinkelbach NCUT: An efficient framework for solving normalized cuts problems with priors and convex constraints. IJCV **89**(1), 40–55 (2010)
13. Gupta, S., Arbel, P., Malik, J., Berkeley, B.: Perceptual organization and recognition of indoor scenes from RGB-D images. In: CVPR (2013)
14. Hedau, V., Hoiem, D., Forsyth, D.: Recovering the spatial layout of cluttered rooms. In: CVPR (2009)
15. Hedau, V., Hoiem, D., Forsyth, D.: Thinking inside the box: using appearance models and context based on room geometry. In: Daniilidis, K., Maragos, P., Paragios, N. (eds.) ECCV 2010, Part VI. LNCS, vol. 6316, pp. 224–237. Springer, Heidelberg (2010)
16. Hedau, V., Hoiem, D., Forsyth, D.: Recovering free space of indoor scenes from a single image. In: CVPR (2012)
17. Henry, P., Krainin, M., Herbst, E., Ren, X., Fox, D.: RGB-D mapping: using kinect-style depth cameras for dense 3D modeling of indoor environments. IJRR **31**(5), 647–663 (2012)
18. Hu, G., Huang, S., Zhao, L.: A robust RGB-D SLAM algorithm. In: IROS (2012)
19. Jia, Z., Gallagher, A., Saxena, A., Chen, T.: 3D-based reasoning with blocks, support, and stability. In: CVPR (2013)
20. Kim, B.s., Arbor, A., Savarese, S.: Accurate localization of 3D objects from RGB-D data using segmentation hypotheses. In: CVPR (2013)
21. Kopf, J., Cohen, M.: Joint bilateral upsampling. In: SIGGRAPH (2007)
22. Koppula, H.S., Anand, A., Joachims, T., Saxena, A.: Semantic labeling of 3D point clouds for indoor scenes. In: NIPS (2011)
23. Levin, A., Lischinski, D., Weiss, Y.: Colorization using optimization. In: SIGGRAPH (2004)
24. Park, J., Kim, H., Brown, M.S., Kweon, I.: High quality depth map upsampling for 3D-TOF cameras. In: ICCV (2011)

25. Silberman, N., Hoiem, D., Kohli, P., Fergus, R.: Indoor segmentation and support inference from RGBD images. In: Fitzgibbon, A., Lazebnik, S., Perona, P., Sato, Y., Schmid, C. (eds.) ECCV 2012, Part V. LNCS, vol. 7576, pp. 746–760. Springer, Heidelberg (2012)
26. Sturm, J., Engelhard, N., Endres, F., Burgard, W., Cremers, D.: A benchmark for the evaluation of RGB-D SLAM systems. In: IROS (2012)
27. Wang, L., Jin, H., Yang, R., Gong, M.: Stereoscopic inpainting: joint color and depth completion from stereo images. In: CVPR (2008)

Regularity Guaranteed Human Pose Correction

Wei Shen$^{(\boxtimes)}$, Rui Lei, Dan Zeng, and Zhijiang Zhang

School of Communication and Information Engineering, Shanghai University,
149 Yanchang Road, Shanghai 200072, People's Republic of China
{wei.shen,cici_lr,dzeng,zjzhang}@shu.edu.cn

Abstract. Benefited from the advantages provided by depth sensors, 3D human pose estimation has become feasible. However, the current estimation systems usually yield poor results due to severe occlusion and sensor noise in depth data. In this paper, we focus on a post-process step, pose correction, which takes the initial estimated poses as the input and deliver more reliable results. Although the regression based correction approach [1] has shown its effectiveness in decreasing the estimated errors, it cannot guarantee the regularity of corrected poses. To address this issue, we formulate pose correction as an optimization problem, which combines the output of the regression model with a pose prior model learned on a pre-captured motion data set. By considering the complexity and the geometric property of the pose data, the pose prior is estimated by von Mises-Fisher distributions in subspaces following divide-and-conquer strategies. By introducing the pose prior into our optimization framework, the regularity of the corrected poses is guaranteed. The experimental results on a challenging data set demonstrate that the proposed pose correction approach not only improves the accuracy, but also outputs more regular poses, compared to the-state-of-the-art.

1 Introduction

With the invention of the low-cost high-speed depth sensor, such as Microsoft Xbox Kinect [2], marker-less human pose estimation from depth images becomes an increasingly active research topic in recent years [3]. By taking the advantages provided by depth data, including color and texture invariance and easy background subtraction, many reliable human pose estimation systems have been built, which output the locations of a certain number of joints to form the human skeleton. The estimated skeletons have been put into service in many real applications, especially the gaming industry. Although considerable progress and success have been achieved [4–9], pose estimation from a single depth image remains a challenging task. Various uncontrolled factors, such as occlusion, sensor noise and large articulation variation, may result in serious failures when estimating poses.

To achieve more robust pose estimation, several researchers perform an additional pose correction step which aims to recover poses from failure. The research devoted to this particular step usually makes use of the pose priors modeled from a motion capture data set and can be grouped into two broad categories:

© Springer International Publishing Switzerland 2015
D. Cremers et al. (Eds.): ACCV 2014, Part II, LNCS 9004, pp. 242–256, 2015.
DOI: 10.1007/978-3-319-16808-1_17

nearest neighbor (NN) search based approaches [6,10] and regression based approaches [1,11]. The former refines an initial estimated skeleton by directly merging it with the body configurations of its nearest neighbors in the motion capture data set. Such approaches can ensure that the corrected skeleton is regular. However, due to the significant differences between estimated skeletons and motion capture data, the merging procedure may decrease the accuracy of pose estimation. While the latter learns a regression function mapping a initial estimated skeleton to a corrected one by considering the systematic bias existing in the estimation step. Although regression based approaches are effective to improve the accuracy of pose estimation and efficient for both training and testing, they cannot guarantee the regularity of the corrected skeleton, as the errors across each joint are not homogeneous. For a better demonstration, we illustrate several pose examples belonging to a specific action domain, golf swing [1], in Fig. 1, in each of which we see the depth data, the ground truth skeleton, the initial estimated skeleton, the corrected skeleton obtained by a NN search based approach and the one obtained by a regression based approach [1]. Note that, the estimated skeletons obtained by the NN search based method are somewhat regular poses belonging to the action domain of golf swing. However, they can barely match their ground truths due to the serious errors existing in the initial estimated skeletons (as shown in the first row in Fig. 1) or the differences between the body configurations of different individuals (as shown in the second row in Fig. 1). On contrast, although the accuracy of the corrected skeletons obtained by the regression based approach (measured by the sum of joint errors) is obviously higher, they are quite weird w.r.t the action domain of golf swing. Consequently, neither of these two schemes are satisfactory in all aspects.

In this paper, we are concerned with the step of pose correction and try to address the problems discussed above. Toward this end, following hybrid strategies we formulate pose correction as an optimization problem by combining the output of the regression model proposed in [1] with a pose prior model learned on a pre-captured motion data set. Formulating problems by hybrid terms and inferring by optimization is a principal way for many vision tasks, such as object discovery [12] and manifold denoising [13]. In our case, the regression model provides the distribution of corrected skeletons on the searching space, while the pose prior model introduces a constraint to guarantee the regularity of the corrected poses. The data pose belonging to the action domain with high-speed motion, such as golf swing, is associated with complex data manifolds. Therefore, to learn a reliable pose prior model, data partition is first performed, and then the distribution of the pose data is modeled in each partitioned clusters. This is a divide-and-conquer strategy [14]. In order to eliminate the differences between the body configurations of different individuals, our pose prior is not modeled in the world coordinate space, but in a normalized skeleton feature space instead. By considering the intrinsic geometrical property of the skeleton feature, a new similarity measure is defined to cluster the skeleton data and a generative model based on the von Mises-Fisher distribution [15,16] is proposed to compute the pose prior. Consequently, by integrating a regression model, e.g., the random

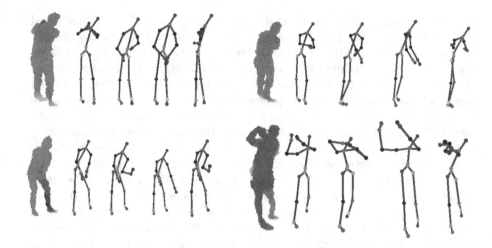

Fig. 1. Several pose examples selected from a golf swing data set [1]. In each example, we see the depth image, the ground truth skeleton, the initial estimated skeleton, the corrected skeleton obtained by a NN search based approach and the one obtained by a regression based approach. Note that, although the former corrected skeletons are regular, they are quite different from the ground truths. Conversely, the latter ones are more close to the ground truths, but they are not regular poses.

regression forest [1], with our prior model, the accuracy and regularity of the corrected poses can be guaranteed simultaneously.

Our contributions can be summarized into two aspects as follow. First, we propose an optimization framework for pose correction. Unlike the others who often take the temporal constraint into account, we consider the pose prior as a regularized term in our framework. This is attributed to the reason that the temporal constraint is usually not reliable in the actions with high-speed motion. Second, following the spirit of divide-and-conquer strategies, we propose a distribution estimation method by considering the intrinsic geometrical property of the skeleton data to properly model the pose prior.

The remainder of this paper is organized as follows. Section 2 reviews the related work to human pose estimation and correction from depth images. Section 3 introduces the skeleton data and ground truth used in our work as well as the procedure of data preprocessing. Section 4 describes the proposed approach to pose correction in detail, including the formulation and the inference. Experimental results on a challenge data set are given in Sect. 5. Finally, we draw the conclusion in Sect. 6.

2   Related Work

As one of the most active topics in computer vision, human pose estimated from depth images has attracted a lot of attention from the community [4–9]. A comprehensive survey on this topic can be found in [3]. Plagemann et al. [17] present a novel interesting point detector for depth data, which provides the candidate proposals for body parts, such as hand, foot and head, as they think the detected interesting points coincide with the salient points of the body. Then, the body parts can be identified and localized by applying a boosted classifier learned on the local shape descriptors extracted on the detected interesting points. Shotton et al. [4] present a remarkable work, which formulates pose estimation from a single depth image as a per-pixel body part classification problem. They apply randomized decision trees [18,19] to effectively inference the distribution of body parts, followed by estimating hypotheses of body joint positions by seeking the modes in the distribution. In order to handle the obstacle of occlusion, Girshick et al. [8] propose to predict the offset between each pixel and each joint by regression. The body joint positions are then estimated by aggregating of the weighted offset votes offered by relative pixels. Sun et al. [9] improve Girshick's method by learning the regression model conditioned on several global parameters, such as height and torso orientation. Hybrid strategies that combine generative and discriminative methods have proven to be a suitable methodology for pose estimation [5,7,20]. For example, Baak et al. [7] propose a data-driven hybrid strategy to optimize two hypotheses to yield the final pose, where the first one is retrieved from a 3D pose data set using sparse features extracted from depth data and the second one is generated based on the previous frame. Although we also follow hybrid strategies, our method differs from those in objective (pose estimation *vs* pose correction) and formulation (temporal constraint *vs* pose prior).

As the initial estimated pose usually yields poor results, the step of pose correction is vital [3]. Ye et al. [6] propose to perform pose correction through nonrigid registration between an estimated pose and its nearest neighbors searched from a motion capture data set. Shum et al. [10] also propose a NN search based pose correction method, in which a reliability confidence for each body part is defined to reweight the distances between poses. Shen et al. [1] propose to learn the systematic bias existing in the pose estimation stage by random forest regression to perform pose correction. Afterwards, they show that the performance can be further improved by learning the regression function conditioned on well-partitioned pose subspaces [11]. Although we also use the regression model, our pose prior is devoted for pose regularization and learned in an unsupervised manner. While in [11], the pose subspaces are obtained according to human annotated pose tags.

Pose prior models are quite general in 2D human pose estimation. Most of recent methods based on pictorial structure model [21] use a pairwise term that evaluates how each estimated pose fits with the pose prior model acquired by training data [22–27]. The proposed pose prior model is different from them. First, unlike those methods, e.g. Bayesian Network Prior model [28], which model a specific pose, such as wave, we model the distribution of the poses belonging to a domain-specific action which includes many types of poses, e.g., the action golf swing includes swing, hitting, standing etc. Therefore, we design a divide-and-conquer strategy for proper modeling. Second, we prefer using von Mises-Fisher distribution to model the prior on body part configuration rather than Gaussian distribution [24] by considering the geometric property of the skeleton feature.

3   Acquisition and Data Preparation

Skeleton Estimation. The Kinect camera is able to construct 640×480 depth images at 30 frames per second. In addition, the algorithm proposed in [4] has been ported into the XBOX Kinect SDK [2], which offers an advanced skeleton estimator for depth images in realtime. The human skeleton obtained by the XBOX Kinect SDK is the direct input for our approach and is called ES (Estimated Skeleton) for short in the rest of this paper. As shown in Fig. 2(a), a skeleton consists of rigid bones connecting a certain number of body joints. In our experiments, we are concerned with 20 body joints: hips, spine, shoulders, head, elbows, wrists, hands, knees, ankles, and feet.

Ground Truth. The recent works [4,8] suggest that the ground truth body joint positions can be recorded by marker-based motion capture (mocap) systems. By calibrating the mocap data to match the Kinect sensor, the **G**round truth **S**keleton (GS) for the ES from the Kinect depth data is obtained. Several examples of triplets of the depth image, the ES and the GS are shown in Fig. 1.

Skeleton Feature Computation. To remove the global translation and the variation caused by individual body differences from skeleton data, we adopt the normalized coordinates proposed in [1] as the skeleton feature. We briefly review this skeleton feature computation process here. Given a human skeleton $S = (\mathbf{x}_j^T; j = 1, \ldots, n)^T$, where $\mathbf{x}_i \in \mathbb{R}^3$ is the world coordinates of the j-th joints and n is the number of joints in the skeleton ($n = 20$ in this paper). Through forward kinematics [29], the skeleton joint C. Hip is selected as the root, and then the bones between the root and any other one joint form a kinematics chain. Such a chain determines an order for skeleton joints. For any two joints connected by a rigid bone, the one which is closer to the root in the kinematics chain is called the predecessor of the other, e.g., ankles and elbows are the predecessors of feet and wrists, respectively. The skeleton feature of S is defined according to kinematics, denoted by $h(S) = (\mathbf{r}_j^T; j = 1, \ldots, n)^T$, where

$$\mathbf{r}_j = \begin{cases} (0,0,0)^T, & j = 1 \\ \frac{\mathbf{x}_j - \mathbf{x}_{j_o}}{\|\mathbf{x}_j - \mathbf{x}_{j_o}\|_2}, & j = 2, \ldots, n \end{cases}, \tag{1}$$

In Eq. 1, $\mathbf{r}_1$ is the normalized coordinates of the root which is always on the origin (so that we drop it in our implementation) and j_o is the joint index of the predecessor of j-th joint. For notation simplicity, we define $h_j(S) = \mathbf{r}_j$.

The computation of the skeleton feature $h(S)$ is mapping the skeleton joints to a 3-dimensional unit sphere, as shown in Fig. 2(b), which actually represents the directions of the rigid bones in the skeleton.

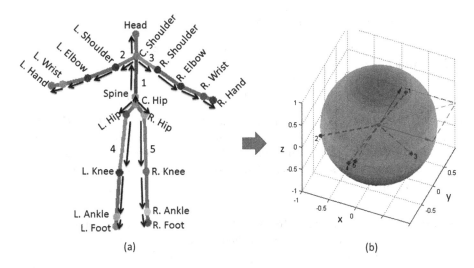

Fig. 2. (a) A skeleton and its joints. The C. Hip is the root of the kinematics chains formed by joints (marked by arrows). (b) An illustration for the skeleton feature computation. For better visualization, only 5 joints are shown in the unit sphere.

4 Problem Formulation

In this section, we give the formulation of our approach. Given a training data set $\{(\mathcal{E}_i, \mathcal{G}_i)\}_{i=1}^{N}$, where $\mathcal{G}_i$ is the ground truth of $\mathcal{E}_i$, our input is an ES $\mathcal{E} = (\hat{\mathbf{x}}_j^{\mathrm{T}}; j = 1,\ldots,n)^{\mathrm{T}}$ with n skeleton joints estimated from a single depth image by using XBOX Kinect SDK [2], and the goal is to predict the true position $\hat{\mathbf{x}}_i \to \mathbf{x}_i \in \mathbb{R}^3$ of each joint and obtain the GS $\mathcal{G} = (\mathbf{x}_j^{\mathrm{T}}; j = 1,\ldots,n)^{\mathrm{T}}$.

4.1 A Naive Bayesian Formulation

Given a input ES $\mathcal{E}$, to predict its true skeleton GS $\mathcal{G}$ is not easy, as the bias between the ES and the GS is non-linear. A solution to address this problem is to find the **C**orrected **S**keleton (CS) $\mathcal{C} = (\mathbf{z}_j^{\mathrm{T}}; j = 1,\ldots,n)^{\mathrm{T}}$ that maximize the probability of $\mathcal{C}$ given $\mathcal{E}$:

$$\hat{\mathcal{C}} = \arg\max_{\mathcal{C}} p(\mathcal{C}|\mathcal{E}) = \arg\max_{\mathcal{C}} p(\mathcal{E}|\mathcal{C})p(\mathcal{C}), \qquad (2)$$

where $p(\mathcal{E}|\mathcal{C})$ is the pose likelihood and $p(\mathcal{C})$ is the pose prior according to the Bayesian inference framework. Modeling the pose likelihood $p(\mathcal{E}|\mathcal{C})$ is quite intractable. Although a naive solution could model it by directly computing the similarity between $\mathcal{E}$ and $\mathcal{C}$, as $\mathcal{C}$ is refined from $\mathcal{E}$, not only should they be somewhat similar, but the the errors existing in $\mathcal{E}$ should be decreased in $\mathcal{C}$. Consequently, no existing generative models are able to guarantee this property. We therefore choose an alternative perspective which attempts to directly approximate the posterior probability $p(\mathcal{C}|\mathcal{E})$.

4.2   An Alternative Perspective

We can express the log posterior distribution $-\log p(\mathcal{C}|\mathcal{E})$ as an energy function $E(\mathcal{C}; \mathcal{E})$, which is defined by

$$E(\mathcal{C}; \mathcal{E}) = E_m(\mathcal{C}; \mathcal{E}, \{(\mathcal{E}_i, \mathcal{G}_i)\}_{i=1}^N) + \lambda E_r(\mathcal{C}; \{\mathcal{G}_i\}_{i=1}^N), \qquad (3)$$

where $E_m(\mathcal{C}; \mathcal{E}, \{(\mathcal{E}_i, \mathcal{G}_i)\}_{i=1}^N)$ is the mapping energy function between $\mathcal{C}$ and $\mathcal{E}$, $E_r(\mathcal{C}; \{\mathcal{G}_i\}_{i=1}^N)$ defines a pose prior to guarantee the regularity of $\mathcal{C}$, and λ is a weight factor between these two terms. Both of these two terms are leaned from the given training data set $\{(\mathcal{E}_i, \mathcal{G}_i)\}_{i=1}^N$. Next, we will explicitly describe how to learn them respectively.

Learning Mapping Energy. Instead of direct learning the mapping function from $\mathcal{E}$ to $\mathcal{C}$, we model the bias between them: $f : \mathcal{E} \to \Delta^1$, where $\Delta = \mathcal{C} - \mathcal{E}$. The reason lies in two folds: first, the biases between ESs and GSs are somewhat systematical, so that they are predicable; second, such systematical biases naturally map ESs into certain clusters on the data manifold, while directly approaching a GS requires exploring all possible ESs in the data space. Thus, we can rewrite $E_m(\mathcal{C}; \mathcal{E}, \{(\mathcal{E}_i, \mathcal{G}_i)\}_{i=1}^N) = E_m(\Delta; \mathcal{E}, \{(\mathcal{E}_i, \Delta_i)\}_{i=1}^N)$, where $\Delta_i = \mathcal{G}_i - \mathcal{E}_i$. The mapping function f can be obtained by minimizing the following objective function:

$$\min_f \sum_i \|\Delta_i - f(h(\mathcal{E}_i))\|_2^2. \qquad (4)$$

We use a randomized regression tree [1] to learn the mapping function f. The tree is learned recursively by splitting the training sample into left and right subsets under maximum information gain criterion. After training, each leaf node stores a bias vector that is the average of all the training samples falling into it. During testing, a sample $\mathcal{E}$ traverses the tree until it reaches a leaf node. Then the tree outputs the stored bias vector in the leaf node: $f(h(\mathcal{E}))$.

Independently training T randomized regression trees to form a regression forest could give us a pseudo distribution:

$$P(\Delta|h(\mathcal{E})) = \frac{1}{T} \sum_{t=1}^T \exp(-\|\frac{\Delta - f_t(h(\mathcal{E}))}{\sigma}\|_2^2), \qquad (5)$$

where σ is a learned bandwidth. Now, we can define the mapping energy by

$$E_m(\mathcal{C}; \mathcal{E}, \{(\mathcal{E}_i, \mathcal{G}_i)\}_{i=1}^N) = E_m(\Delta; \mathcal{E}, \{(\mathcal{E}_i, \Delta_i)\}_{i=1}^N) = -\log(P(\Delta|h(\mathcal{E}))). \qquad (6)$$

Learning Pose Prior. The pose prior measures how likely a CS $\mathcal{C}$ can be generated from the ground truth sets $\{\mathcal{G}_i\}_{i=1}^N$. Learning the pose prior is actually a distribution estimation (generative model learning) problem. As the variance

---

[1] The bias Δ should be normalized by the method proposed in [1] to eliminate the scale variances between individuals. While, for denotational simplicity, we do not involve the normalization factor in this paper.

in the skeleton data may be quite large, especially those captured from actions with high-speed motion, fitting a single model to them is not easy. To estimate the distribution of the skeleton data properly, a divide-and-conquer strategy is adopted here: cluster the training data first, followed by learning the distribution model in each cluster.

A key step leading to a reliable cluster result is to define a faithful distance/similarity measure in the data space. The most commonly used measure is Euclidean distance. However, as we have shown in Sect. 3, the skeleton feature consists of the directions of bones. Therefore, angle based measures are more suitable for our case. We define a cosine similarity based measure for two skeleton feature $h(\mathcal{S}_a)$ and $h(\mathcal{S}_b)$:

$$s(h(\mathcal{S}_a), h(\mathcal{S}_b)) = \frac{1}{n-1} \sum_{j=2}^{n} < h_j(\mathcal{S}_a), h_j(\mathcal{S}_b) >, \tag{7}$$

where $< \cdot, \cdot >$ denotes the dot product of two vectors. As both $h_j(\mathcal{S}_a)$ and $h_j(\mathcal{S}_b)$ are unit vectors, $< h_j(\mathcal{S}_a), h_j(\mathcal{S}_b) >$ is cosine of the included angle between them.

Based on the proposed similarity measure (Eq. 7), Normalized Cut [30] is applied to partition the ground truth sets $\{\mathcal{G}_i\}_{i=1}^{N}$ into K clusters. Let $\mathbb{1}(h(\mathcal{S}))$ denote the cluster index assigned to a skeleton $\mathcal{S}$. In each cluster $\{\mathcal{G}_i | \mathbb{1}(h(\mathcal{G}_i)) = k\}_{i=1}^{N}$, we consider each bone direction $h_j(\mathcal{G}_i)$ as a von Mises-Fisher distribution [15], which is a probability distribution on the $(p-1)$-dimensional sphere in $\mathbb{R}^p$:

$$p(h_j(\mathcal{G}_i), \mu_j^k, \kappa_j^k) \propto \exp(\kappa_j^k < h_j(\mathcal{G}_i), \mu_j^k >), \tag{8}$$

which μ_j^k and κ_j^k are the mean and a measure of concentration of all $h_j(\mathcal{G}_i)$s in the k-th cluster, respectively. κ_j^k characterizes how strongly the unit vector $h_j(\mathcal{G}_i)$ drawn according to $p(h_j(\mathcal{G}_i), \mu_j^k, \kappa_j^k)$ are concentrated around the mean μ_j^k. When $\kappa_j^k = 0$, $p(h_j(\mathcal{G}_i), \mu_j^k, \kappa_j^k)$ reduces to the uniform density, and if $k \to \infty$, $p(h_j(\mathcal{G}_i), \mu_j^k, \kappa_j^k)$ tends to a point density peaking at μ_j^k. By assuming each bone is independent, the parameter μ_j^k and κ_j^k can be estimated as follows. Let $\mathcal{I}_\nu$ denote the modified Bessel function of the first kind and order ν and define $A_p\left(\kappa_j^k\right) = \frac{\mathcal{I}_{p/2}\left(\kappa_j^k\right)}{\mathcal{I}_{p/2-1}\left(\kappa_j^k\right)}$, then the maximum likelihood estimation of μ_j^k and κ_j^k is given by [31]:

$$\mu_j^k = \frac{\sum_{i=1}^{N} h_j(\mathcal{G}_i)\delta(\mathbb{1}(h(\mathcal{G}_i)) = k)}{\| \sum_{i=1}^{N} h_j(\mathcal{G}_i)\delta(\mathbb{1}(h(\mathcal{G}_i)) = k)\|}$$
$$\kappa_j^k = A_p^{-1}\left(\bar{R}\right), \tag{9}$$

where $\delta(\cdot)$ is an indicator function and

$$\bar{R} = \frac{\| \sum_{i=1}^{N} h_j(\mathcal{G}_i)\delta(\mathbb{1}(h(\mathcal{G}_i)) = k)\|}{\sum_{i=1}^{N} \delta(\mathbb{1}(h(\mathcal{G}_i)) = k)}. \tag{10}$$

A simple approximation to κ_j^k is

$$\hat{\kappa}_j^k = \frac{\bar{R}\left(p - \bar{R}^2\right)}{1 - \bar{R}^2}. \tag{11}$$

In our case, $p = 3$, as our feature is obtained by mapping the skeleton joints to a 3-dimensional sphere.

After the estimation of μ_j^k and κ_j^k, the pose prior of a CS $\mathcal{C}$ is given by

$$P(\mathcal{C}) = \sum_{k=1}^{K} \prod_{j=2}^{n} p(h_j(\mathcal{C}), \mu_j^k, \kappa_j^k) \delta(\mathbb{1}(h(\mathcal{G}_i)) = k). \tag{12}$$

Thus, we obtain the regularization term by

$$E_r(\mathcal{C}; \{\mathcal{G}_i\}_{i=1}^{N}) = -\log(P(\mathcal{C})). \tag{13}$$

Energy Function Optimization. Given an input ES $\mathcal{E}$, we search the CS $\mathcal{C}$ which minimizes the energy function defined in Eq. 3, leading to an optimization problem:

$$\hat{\mathcal{C}} = \arg\min_{\mathcal{C}} E(\mathcal{C}; \mathcal{E}) \tag{14}$$

By combining Eqs. 3, 6 and 13, we have

$$\hat{\mathcal{C}} = \arg\min_{\mathcal{C}} -\log(P(\mathcal{C} - \mathcal{E}|h(\mathcal{E}))) - \lambda\log(P(\mathcal{C})). \tag{15}$$

As Eq. 15 does not have close-formed solutions, here we use coordinate descend [32] to infer an approximate solution for it.

We start the optimization process with an initial skeleton $\mathcal{C}^0 \in \mathbb{R}^{n \times 3}$, which can be obtained by $\mathcal{C}^0 = \mathcal{E} + \bar{\Delta} = \mathcal{E} + \sum_t^T f_t(h(\mathcal{E}))/T$. Then we generate a sequence of skeletons $\{\mathcal{C}^k\}_{k=0}^{\infty}$ by two-level iterations. We refer to the process from $\mathcal{C}^{k-1}$ to $\mathcal{C}^k$ as an outer iteration. In each outer iteration we have $n \times 3$ inner iterations, during which each dimension of $\mathcal{C}^{k-1}$ is sequentially updated: $c_{(i)}^k \leftarrow c_{(i)}^{k-1} (i = 1, \ldots, n \times 3)$. Thus, such an outer iteration generates skeleton $\mathcal{C}^k = \sum_i^{n \times 3} c_{(i)}^k \mathbf{e}_i$, where $\mathbf{e}_i = (0, \ldots, 0, 1, 0, \ldots, 0)^T$ is a basis vector, in which only the i-th element is one and others are zero. More specifically, to update $\mathcal{C}^{k-1}$ to $\mathcal{C}^k$, we solve the following one-variable sub-problem sequentially:

$$c_{(1)}^k = \arg\min_{c_{(1)}} E(c_{(1)}\mathbf{e}_1 + c_{(2)}^{k-1}\mathbf{e}_2 + \ldots + c_{(n \times 3)}^{k-1}\mathbf{e}_{n \times 3}; \mathcal{E})$$

$$c_{(2)}^k = \arg\min_{c_{(2)}} E(c_{(1)}^k\mathbf{e}_1 + c_{(2)}\mathbf{e}_2 + \ldots + c_{(n \times 3)}^{k-1}\mathbf{e}_{n \times 3}; \mathcal{E})$$

$$\vdots$$

$$c_{(i)}^k = \arg\min_{c_{(i)}} E(c_{(1)}^k\mathbf{e}_1 + c_{(2)}^k\mathbf{e}_2 + \ldots + c_{(i)}\mathbf{e}_i + \ldots + c_{(n \times 3)}^{k-1}\mathbf{e}_{n \times 3}; \mathcal{E}) \tag{16}$$

$$\vdots$$

$$c_{(n \times 3)}^k = \arg\min_{c_{(n \times 3)}} E(c_{(1)}^k\mathbf{e}_1 + c_{(2)}^k\mathbf{e}_2 + \ldots + c_{(n \times 3)}\mathbf{e}_{n \times 3}; \mathcal{E}).$$

As shown in Eq. 16, in each inner iteration, we optimize one dimension $c_{(i)}^{k-1}$ and update its value once for the next inner iteration. The outer iteration will be stopped when the bias between two sequentially obtained energies is no larger than a threshold: $\|E(\mathcal{C}^{k-1}; \mathcal{E}) - E(\mathcal{C}^k; \mathcal{E})\|_2 \leqslant \xi$. As the regression model usually provides a good initialization and the search space for each joint point is restricted within the range of the votes of the random forest, the optimization converges fast. It takes about 36 ms per frame.

5   Experimental Results

In this section, we show the experimental results and give the comparisons between alternative approaches. In the remainder of this section, unless otherwise specified, the parameters introduced in our method are set as follows: the weight factor $\lambda = 1.0$, the threshold for the stopping criterion $\xi = 0.001$, the number of clusters $K = 16$. We select optimal λ and K by grid search and the detail will be discussed in Sect. 5.3. For the parameters involved in the random forest regression model, we adopt the default setting given in [1]: The number of trees in random forest $T = 50$ and the bandwidth $\sigma = 0.01$ m.

In order to assess the performance of our algorithm, we evaluate our method on the data set constructed in [1]. This data set is quite challenge, which contains 15,815 poses belong to golf swing action. The estimated skeleton and ground truth skeleton of each pose are obtained by XBOX Kinect SDK [2] and a mopcap system, respectively. We use the same experimental setup as [1]: 3,720 poses are used for training and the rest 12,095 poses are used for testing. Several example poses of this data set are shown in Fig. 1.

5.1   Evaluation Measurement

Following the evaluation protocol proposed in [1], we use the mean of the sum of joint error as the quality assessment factor. Given a testing data set $\{(\mathcal{E}_i, \mathcal{G}_i)\}_{i=1}^M$, we obtain the corrected skeletons $\{\mathcal{C}_i\}_{i=1}^M$. We measure the accuracy of each CS $\mathcal{C} = (\mathbf{z}_j^T; j = 1, \ldots, n)^T$ by the sum of joint errors (sJE) to its GS $\mathcal{G} = (\mathbf{x}_j^T; j = 1, \ldots, n)^T$: $\varepsilon = \sum_j \|z_j - x_j\|_2$. To quantify the average accuracy on the whole testing data set, we report the mean sJE (msJE) across all testing skeletons: $\frac{\sum_i \varepsilon_i}{M}$ (unit:meter).

5.2   Comparisons

In this section, we compare the proposed method to other competing ones, including the NN search based and regression based. We also compare the proposed pose prior model with the one under Gaussian distribution assumption [24].

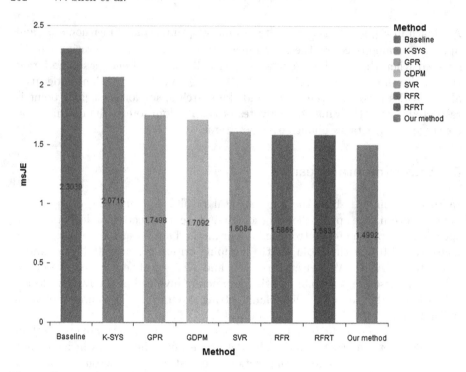

Fig. 3. Comparison with several methods on the golf swing data set [1] (Color figure online).

Current Kinect Approach. The current Kinect system for pose correction is complex, which employs several strategies such as temporal constraint and filtration. The main idea of this approach is actually nearest neighbor search. The approach finds the nearest neighbor of an input ES in the training set. The corrected skeleton is obtained by merging the corresponding GS of the nearest neighbor to the ES. We refer to the approach used in the current Kinect system as K-SYS. On the whole data set, K-SYS only achieves 2.0716 msJE, as the merging operation may damage the performance.

Regression Based Approaches. To show the significance of the introduced pose prior, we compared the random forest regression (RFR) based approaches [1]. As shown in Fig. 3, our method achieves better performance than RFR (1.499 *vs* 1.586). A interesting observation is that the introduction of the temporal constraint (RFRT) only leads to a tiny performance improvement (1.583 *vs* 1.586). This is because the temporal constraint makes use of the consistency between the current and previous predictions; While the errors in the ESs from the poses with severe occlusion or high-speed motion are usually quite large; In this case, the reliability of the previous prediction cannot be guaranteed. We also show that the proposed method outperforms other regression based methods, including Gaussian process regressor (GPR) [33], support vector regressor (SVR) [34].

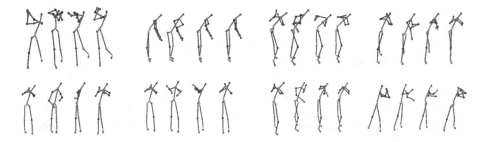

Fig. 4. Examples of corrected skeletons. In each example, we see the GS, the ES, the CS obtained by random forest regression [1], and the CS obtained by the proposed method. Note that, compared to the regression based method, the CSs obtained by our method are more similar to the GSs, and moreover, they are more regular.

In addition to the improvement in accuracy, more importantly, we emphasize that our method can generate more regular poses. As illustrated in Fig. 4, unlike the weird poses obtained by the regression based method, benefited from the constraint introduced by the well-learned pose prior, the poses obtained by our method are regularized and more similar to the ground truths.

Gaussian Distribution Based Prior Model (GDPM). Dantone et al. [24] proposed a prior model, which models pairwise part configuration by Gaussian distribution under the classical pictorial structure model [21]. To show the advantage of the proposed prior model, we instead use this Gaussian distribution based prior model in our pose correction framework for comparison. As shown in Fig. 3, our pose prior model achieves better performance than Dantone's (1.499 *vs* 1.709).

5.3   Parameter Discussion

We thoroughly investigate the effects of two involved parameters: the weight factor λ and the number of clusters K. As shown in Fig. 5(a), when λ become

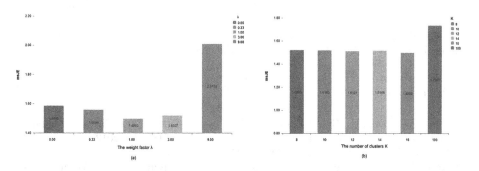

Fig. 5. Parameters versus performance. (a) The weight factor λ. (b) The number of clusters K (Color figure online).

quite large, our method tends to a NN search based method, which only achieves 2.010 msJE. While, when λ is small, our method reduces to a regression based method. We select a "good" λ to balance the output of the regression model and the pose prior. As shown in Fig. 5(b), the performance of our method would increase when the number of clusters become larger. The reason may be the poses in a compact cluster are more proper to fit the distribution model. But when the K is very large, the performance will decrease (e.g. $K = 100$, 1.7361 msJE). The reliability of the estimated distribution will be damaged due to the lack of samples in each cluster.

6   Conclusion and Future Work

We have presented an optimization framework for correcting the human poses estimated from Kinect depth images, which combines the output of a random forest regression model with a pose prior model learned on a motion capture data set. By considering the complexity and the geometric property of the pose data, the pose prior is modeled by von Mises-Fisher distributions learned on well-partitioned subspaces separately. The experimental results verify the superiority of the proposed pose correction framework and demonstrate that the introduction of the pose prior indeed generates more regular poses, compared to the current state-of-the-art approach.

In this paper, we only demonstrated the effectiveness of the proposed framework on the problem of correcting the human poses estimated from Kinect depth images. This idea is actually general and can be extended to other problems, such as correcting the human poses estimated from still images [24] and aligning the face images [35]. Besides, to port the proposed algorithm to mobile robots [36] equipped with kinect cameras is also our future work.

Acknowledgement. This work was supported in part by the National Natural Science Foundation of China under Grant 61303095, in part by Research Fund for the Doctoral Program of Higher Education of China under Grant 20133108120017, in part by Innovation Program of Shanghai Municipal Education Commission under Grant 14YZ018, in part by Innovation Program of Shanghai University under Grant SDCX2013012 and in part by Cultivation Fund for the Young Faculty of Higher Education of Shanghai under Grant ZZSD13005. We thank Microsoft Corporation for providing the skeleton data set used in our experiments.

References

1. Shen, W., Deng, K., Bai, X., Leyvand, T., Guo, B., Tu, Z.: Exemplar-based human action pose correction and tagging. In: Proceedings of CVPR (2012)
2. Microsoft Corp. Kinect for XBOX 360. Redmond WA
3. Han, J., Shao, L., Xu, D., Shotton, J.: Enhanced computer vision with microsoft kinect sensor: a review. IEEE Trans. Cybern. **43**, 1318–1334 (2013)

4. Shotton, J., Fitzgibbon, A., Cook, M., Sharp, T., Finocchio, M., Moore, R., Kipman, A., Blake, A.: Real-time human pose recognition in parts from a single depth image. In: Proceedings of CVPR (2011)
5. Ganapathi, V., Plagemann, C., Koller, D., Thrun, S.: Real time motion capture using a single time-of-flight camera. In: Proceedings of CVPR, pp. 755–762 (2010)
6. Ye, M., Wang, X., Yang, R., Ren, L., Pollefeys, M.: Accurate 3D pose estimation from a single depth image. In: Proceedings of ICCV (2011)
7. Baak, A., Müller, M., Bharaj, G., Seidel, H.P., Theobalt, C.: A data-driven approach for real-time full body pose reconstruction from a depth camera. In: Proceedings of ICCV (2011)
8. Girshick, R., Shotton, J., Kohli, P., Criminisi, A., Fitzgibbon, A.: Efficient regression of general-activity human poses from depth images. In: Proceedings of ICCV (2011)
9. Sun, M., Kohli, P., Shotton, J.: Conditional regression forests for human pose estimation. In: Proceedings of CVPR (2012)
10. Shum, H.P.H., Ho, E.S.L., Jiang, Y., Takagi, S.: Real-time posture reconstruction for microsoft kinect. IEEE Trans. Cybern. **43**, 1357–1369 (2013)
11. Shen, W., Deng, K., Bai, X., Leyvand, T., Guo, B., Tu, Z.: Exemplar-based human action pose correction. IEEE Trans. Cybern. **44**(7), 1053–1066 (2014)
12. Wang, X., Zhang, Z., Ma, Y., Bai, X., Liu, W., Tu, Z.: Robust subspace discovery via relaxed rank minimization. Neural Comput. **26**, 611–635 (2014)
13. Wang, B., Tu, Z.: Sparse subspace denoising for image manifolds. In: Proceedings of CVPR, pp. 468–475 (2013)
14. Bentley, J.L.: Multidimensional divide-and-conquer. Commun. ACM **23**, 214–229 (1980)
15. Fisher, N.I., Lewis, T., Embleton, B.J.J.: Statistical Analysis of Spherical Data. Cambridge University Press, Cambridge (1993)
16. Wang, X., Bai, X., Ma, T., Liu, W., Latecki, L.J.: Fan shape model for object detection. In: Proceedings of CVPR, pp. 151–158 (2012)
17. Plagemann, C., Ganapathi, V., Koller, D., Thrun, S.: Real-time identification and localization of body parts from depth images. In: Proceedings of ICRA, pp. 3108–3113 (2010)
18. Breiman, L.: Random forests. Mach. Learn. **45**, 5–32 (2001)
19. Quinlan, J.R.: Induction of decision trees. Mach. Learn. **1**, 81–106 (1986)
20. Ganapathi, V., Plagemann, C., Koller, D., Thrun, S.: Real-time human pose tracking from range data. In: Fitzgibbon, A., Lazebnik, S., Perona, P., Sato, Y., Schmid, C. (eds.) ECCV 2012, Part VI. LNCS, vol. 7577, pp. 738–751. Springer, Heidelberg (2012)
21. Felzenszwalb, P.F., Huttenlocher, D.P.: Pictorial structures for object recognition. Int. J. Comput. Vis. **61**, 55–79 (2005)
22. Ren, X., Berg, A.C., Malik, J.: Recovering human body configurations using pairwise constraints between parts. In: Proceedings of ICCV, pp. 824–831 (2005)
23. Ramanan, D.: Learning to parse images of articulated bodies. In: Proceedings of NIPS, pp. 1129–1136 (2006)
24. Dantone, M., Gall, J., Leistner, C., Gool, L.J.V.: Human pose estimation using body parts dependent joint regressors. In: Proceedings of CVPR, pp. 3041–3048 (2013)
25. Ladicky, L., Torr, P.H.S., Zisserman, A.: Human pose estimation using a joint pixel-wise and part-wise formulation. In: Proceedings of CVPR, pp. 3578–3585 (2013)

26. Yang, Y., Ramanan, D.: Articulated pose estimation with flexible mixtures-of-parts. In: Proceedings of CVPR, pp. 1385–1392 (2011)
27. Yao, C., Bai, X., Liu, W., Latecki, L.J.: Human detection using learned part alphabet and pose dictionary. In: Fleet, D., Pajdla, T., Schiele, B., Tuytelaars, T. (eds.) ECCV 2014, Part V. LNCS, vol. 8693, pp. 251–266. Springer, Heidelberg (2014)
28. Lehrmann, A.M., Gehler, P.V., Nowozin, S.: A non-parametric bayesian network prior of human pose. In: Proceedings of ICCV, pp. 1281–1288 (2013)
29. Murray, R.M., Li, Z., Sastry, S.S.: A Mathematical Introduction to Robotic Manipulation. CRC Press, Boca Raton (1994)
30. Shi, J., Malik, J.: Normalized cuts and image segmentation. IEEE Trans. Pattern Anal. Mach. Intell. **22**, 888–905 (2000)
31. Sra, S.: A short note on parameter approximation for von mises-fisher distributions: and a fast implementation of $i_s(x)$. Comput. Stat. **27**, 177–190 (2011)
32. Luo, Z.Q., Tseng, P.: On the convergence of the coordinate descent method for convex differentiable minimization. J. Optim. Theory Appl. **72**, 7–35 (1992)
33. Rasmussen, C.E., Williams, C.: Gaussian Processes for Machine Learning. MIT Press, Cambridge (2006)
34. Schölkopf, B., Smola, A., Williamson, R., Bartlett, P.L.: New support vector algorithms. Neural Comput. **12**, 1207–1245 (2000)
35. Cao, X., Wei, Y., Wen, F., Sun, J.: Face alignment by explicit shape regression. In: Proceedings of CVPR, pp. 2887–2894 (2012)
36. Zhou, Y., Yang, Y., Yi, M., Bai, X., Liu, W., Latecki, L.J.: Online multiple targets detection and tracking from mobile robot in cluttered indoor environments with depth camera. IJPRAI **28**(1) (2014)

Accelerated Kmeans Clustering Using Binary Random Projection

Yukyung Choi, Chaehoon Park, and In So Kweon[✉]

Robotics and Computer Vision Lab., KAIST, Daejeon, Korea
iskweon77@kaist.ac.kr

Abstract. Codebooks have been widely used for image retrieval and image indexing, which are the core elements of mobile visual searching. Building a vocabulary tree is carried out offline, because the clustering of a large amount of training data takes a long time. Recently proposed adaptive vocabulary trees do not require offline training, but suffer from the burden of online computation. The necessity for clustering high dimensional large data has arisen in offline and online training. In this paper, we present a novel clustering method to reduce the burden of computation without losing accuracy. Feature selection is used to reduce the computational complexity with high dimensional data, and an ensemble learning model is used to improve the efficiency with a large number of data. We demonstrate that the proposed method outperforms the-state of the art approaches in terms of computational complexity on various synthetic and real datasets.

1 Introduction

Image to image matching is one of the important tasks in mobile visual searching. A vocabulary tree based image search is commonly used due to its simplicity and high performance [1–6]. The original vocabulary tree method [1] cannot grow and adapt with new images and environments, and it takes a long time to build a vocabulary tree through clustering. An incremental vocabulary tree was introduced to overcome limitations such as adaptation in dynamic environments [4,5]. It does not require heavy clustering for the offline training process due to the use of a distributed online process. The clustering time of the incremental vocabulary tree is the chief burden in the case of realtime application. Thus, an efficient clustering method is required.

Lloyd kmeans [7] is the standard method. However, this algorithm is not suitable for high dimensional large data, because the computational complexity is proportional to the number and the dimension of data. Various approaches have been proposed to accelerate the clustering and reduce the complexity. One widely used approach is applying geometric knowledge to avoid unnecessary computations. Elkans algorithm [8] is the representative example, and this method does not calculate unnecessary distances between points and centers. Two additional strategies for accelerating kmeans are refining initial data and finding good initial clusters. The P.S Bradley approach [9] refines initial clusters as

© Springer International Publishing Switzerland 2015
D. Cremers et al. (Eds.): ACCV 2014, Part II, LNCS 9004, pp. 257–272, 2015.
DOI: 10.1007/978-3-319-16808-1_18

data close to the modes of the joint probability density. If initial clusters are selected by nearby modes, true clusters are found more often, and the algorithm iterates fewer times. Arthur kmeans [10] is a representative algorithm that chooses good initial clusters for fast convergence. This algorithm randomly selects the first center for each cluster, and then subsequent centers are determined with the probability proportional to the squared distance from the closest center.

The aforementioned approaches, however, are not relevant to high dimensional large data except for Elkans algorithm. This type of data contains a high degree of irrelevant and redundant information [11]. Also, owing to the sparsity of data, it is difficult to find the hidden structure in a high dimension space. Some researchers thus have recently solved the high dimensional problem by decreasing the dimensionality [12,13]. Others have proposed clustering the original data in a low dimensional subspace rather than directly in a high dimensional space [14–16]. Two basic types of approaches to reduce the dimensionality have been investigated: feature selection [14] and feature transformation [15,16]. One of the feature selection methods, random projection [17], has received attention due to the simplicity and efficiency of computation.

Ensemble learning is mainly used for classification and detection. Fred [18] first introduced ensemble learning to the clustering society in the form of an ensemble combination method. The ensemble approach for clustering is robust and efficient in dealing with high dimensional large data, because distributed processing is possible and diversity is preserved. In detail, the ensemble approach consists of the generation and combination steps. Robustness and efficiency of an algorithm can be obtained through various models in the generation step [19]. To produce a final model, multiple models are properly combined in the combination step [20,21].

In this paper, we show that kmeans clustering can be formulated by feature selection and an ensemble learning approach. We propose a two-stage algorithm, following the coarse to fine strategy. In the first stage, we obtain the sub-optimal clusters, and then we obtain the optimal clusters in the second stage. We employ a proposed binary random matrix, which is learned by each ensemble model. Also, using this simple matrix, the computational complexity is reduced. Due to the first ensemble stage, our method chooses the initial points nearby sub-optimal clusters in the second stage. Refined data taken from an ensemble method can be sufficiently representative because they are sub-optimal. Also, our method can avoid unnecessary distance calculation by a triangle inequality and distance bounds. As will be seen in Sect. 3, we show good performance with a binary random matrix, thus demonstrating that the proposed random matrix is suitable for finding independent bases.

This paper is organized as follows. In Sect. 2, the proposed algorithm to solve the accelerated clustering problem with high dimensional large data is described. Section 3 presents various experimental results on object classification, image retrieval, and loop detection.

2   Proposed Algorithm

The kmeans algorithm finds values for the binary membership indicator r_{ij} and the cluster center c_j so as to minimize errors in Eq. (1). If data point x_i is assigned to cluster c_j then $r_{ij} = 1$.

$$J = \sum_i^N \sum_j^K r_{ij} \|x_i - c_j\|_2 \tag{1}$$

We can do this through an iterative procedure in which each iteration involves two successive steps corresponding to successive optimizations with respect to r_{ij} and the c_j. The conventional kmeans algorithm is expensive for high dimensional large datasets, requiring $O(K*N*D)$ computation time, where K is the number of clusters, N is the number of input data and D is the maximum number of non-zero elements in any example vector. Large datasets of high dimensionality for kmeans clustering should be studied.

$$J \cong \sum_i^{\hat{N}} \sum_j^K r_{ij} \|\hat{x}_i - \hat{c}_j\|_2 \tag{2}$$

We proposed a novel framework for an accelerating algorithm in Eq. (2). The goal of our method is to find the refining data $\hat{x}$ that well represent the distribution of the original input x. Using the refining data obtained from Eq. (3), the final clustering process for K clusters is equal to the coarse to fine strategy for accelerated clustering. The number of $\hat{x}$, namely $\hat{N}$ is relatively small, but refined data $\hat{x}$ can sufficiently represent the original input data x. c and $\hat{c}$ represent the center of the clusters in each set of data.

$$J \cong \sum_i^N \sum_j^{\hat{N}} r_{ij} \|x_i - \hat{x}_j\|_2 \tag{3}$$

To obtain the refining data introduced in Eq. (2), this paper adopts a kmeans optimizer, as delineated in Eq. (3), because it affords simplicity and compatibility with variations of kmeans. The refining data $\hat{x}$ in Eq. (3) are used as the input data of Eq. (2) to calculate the K clusters. In the above, $\hat{x}$ denote refined data that have representativeness of the input x. $\hat{N}$ is the number of data $\hat{x}$. The $\hat{N}$ value is much smaller than N.

$$J \cong \sum_i^N \sum_j^{\hat{N}} r_{ij} \|A(x_i - \hat{x}_j)\|_2 \tag{4}$$

For estimating the refining data with the conventional kmeans optimizer, we propose a clustering framework that combines random selection for dimension reduction and the ensemble models. This paper proposes a way to minimize data loss using a feature selection method, binary random projection. Our approach can discover underlying hidden clusters in noisy data through dimension reduction. For these reasons, Eq. (3) is reformulated as Eq. (4). According to Eq. (4), the proposed method chooses $\hat{x}$ that best represents x. In the above, matrix A is the selection matrix of features. This matrix is called a random matrix.

$$J \cong \sum_{m}^{T} \sum_{i}^{\tilde{N}^m} \sum_{j}^{\tilde{K}^m} r_{ij}^m \| A^m (\tilde{x}_i^m - \hat{x}_j^m) \|_2 \tag{5}$$

Equation (4) is rewritten as Eq. (5) using ensemble learning models. Ensemble learning based our method reduces the risk of unfortunate feature selection and splits the data into small subset. Our work can select more stable and robust refining data $\hat{x}$ comparable with the results of Eq. (4) In the above, $\tilde{x}$ and $\tilde{N}$ denote sampling data of input x and the number of sampling data, and T and m denote the number and the order of ensemble models, respectively.

$$J \cong \sum_{m}^{T} \sum_{i}^{\tilde{N}^m} \sum_{j}^{\tilde{K}^m} r_{ij}^m \| (\tilde{x}_i^{'m} - \hat{x}_j^{'m}) \|_2 \tag{6}$$

Equation (6) can be derived from Eq. (5) by random selection instead of random projection. In the above, the prime symbol denotes that variables are projected by matrix A.

Finally, this paper approximates the kmeans clustering as both Eqs. (6) and (2). This approach presents an efficient kmeans clustering method that capitalizes on the randomness and the sparseness of the projection matrix for dimension reduction in high dimensional large data.

As mentioned above, our algorithm is composed of two phases combining Eqs. (3) and (2). In the first stage, our approach builds multiple models by small sub-samples of the dataset. Each separated dataset is applied to kmeans clustering, and it randomly selects arbitrary attribute-features in every iteration. As we compute the minimization error in every iteration, we only require sub-dimensional data. The approximated centroids can be obtained by smaller iterations than one phase clustering. These refined data from the first stage are used as the input of the next step. The second stage consists of a single kmeans optimizer to merge the distributed operations. Our algorithm adopts a coarse to fine strategy so that the product of the first stage is suitable to achieve fast convergence. The algorithm is delineated below in Algorithm 1.

2.1 Feature Selection in Single Model

$$\sum_{i}^{\tilde{N}^m} \sum_{j}^{\tilde{K}^m} r_{ij}^m \| A^m (\tilde{x}_i^m - \hat{x}_j^m) \|_2 \tag{7}$$

Equation (7) indicates the m_{th} single model in the ensemble generation stage. In each model, our algorithm finds values for r_{ij}^m, $\hat{x}_j^m$ and the A^m so as to minimize errors in Eq. (7). This problem is considered as a clustering problem in the high dimensional subspace. In this chapter, we describe basic concepts of the dimension reduction approaches, and we analyze the proposed algorithm with in comparison with others [14, 22].

Random Projection. Principal component analysis (PCA) is a widely used method for reducing the dimensionality of data. Unfortunately, it is quite expensive to compute in high dimensional data. It is thus desirable to derive a dimension reduction method that is computationally simple without yielding significant distortion.

As an alternative method, random projection (RP) has been found to be computationally efficient yet sufficiently accurate for the dimension reduction of high dimensional data. In random projection, the d-dimensional data in original spaces is projected to d'-dimensional sub-spaces. This random projection uses the matrix $A_{d' \times d}$, where the columns have unit lengths, and it is calculated through the origin. Using matrix notation, the equation is given as follows: $X^{RP}_{d' \times N} = A_{d' \times d} X_{d \times N}$. If a projection matrix A is not orthogonal, it causes significant distortion in the dataset. Thus, we should consider the orthogonality of matrix A, when we design the matrix A.

We introduce the random projection approach into the proposed method to improve the computational efficiency. The recent literature shows that a group among a set of high-dimensional clusters lies on a low-dimensional subspace in many real-world applications. In this case, the underlying hidden subspace can be retrieved by solving a sparse optimization problem, which encourages selecting nearby points that approximately span a low dimensional affine subspace. Most previous approaches focus on finding the best low-dimensional representation of the data for which a single feature representation is sufficient for the clustering task [23, 24]. Our approach takes into account clustering of high-dimensional complex data. It has more than a single subspace due to the extensive attribute variations over the feature space. We model the complex data with multiple feature representations by incorporating binary random projection.

Random Projection Matrix. Matrix A of Eq. (7) is generally called a random projection matrix. The choice of the random projection matrix is one of the key points of interest. According to [22], elements of A are Gaussian distributed (GRP). Achiloptas [14] has recently shown that the Gaussian distribution can be replaced by a simpler distribution such as a sparse matrix (SRP). In this paper, we propose the binary random projection (BRP) matrix, where the elements a_{ij} consist of zero or one value, as delineated in Eq. (8).

$$a_{ij} = \begin{cases} 1 & \text{with probability } \alpha \\ 0 & \text{with probability } 1 - \alpha \end{cases} \tag{8}$$

Given that a set of features from data is λ-sparse, we need at least λ-independent canonical bases to represent the features lying on the λ-dimensional subspace. Because BRP encourages the projection matrix to be λ-independent,

---

Algorithm 1. Proposed accelerated kmeans algorithm

1: X : input data, K : the number of clusters, $\hat{C}$: final centers of clusters
2: R : the binary membership indicator, C : the center of clusters
3: A : proposed random matrix
4: T : the number of ensemble models
5: $\widetilde{X}$: sampling data, $\widetilde{C}$: the center of clusters in single ensemble
6: $\widetilde{X}'$: sampling data in lower dimensional space
7: $\widetilde{C}'$: the center of clusters in lower dimensional space
8: N : the total number of sampling data
9: $\widetilde{N}$: the number of sampling data in single ensemble
10: $\hat{X}$: the refining sampling data from the first generation stage
11: ───

12: **procedure** ACCELERATEDKMEANS(X, K)
13:    **for** $m = 1 \rightarrow T$ **do**
14:        $\widetilde{X} = \textbf{Bootstrap}(X, \widetilde{N})$
15:        Initialize A, $\widetilde{X}'$, $\widetilde{C}'$ and R
16:        **while** the stop condition is satisfied **do**
17:            **if** the iteration is not first **then**
18:                $A_{new} = \textbf{GetBRP}()$
19:                **if** A_{new} reduce the error than A **then**
20:                    $A = A_{new}$, $\widetilde{X}' = A\widetilde{X}$, $\widetilde{C}' = A\widetilde{C}$
21:                **end if**
22:            **end if**
23:            $R = \textbf{MatchDataAndCluster}(\widetilde{X}', \widetilde{C}')$
24:            $\widetilde{C}' = \textbf{UpdateCluster}(\widetilde{X}', R)$
25:        **end while**
26:        **for** $j \rightarrow K$ **do**
27:            $\hat{x}_j^m = \frac{\sum r_{ij} \widetilde{x}_i}{\sum r_{ij}}$
28:            Add $\hat{x}_j^m$ to $\hat{X}$
29:        **end for**
30:    **end for**
31:    $\hat{C} = \textbf{kmeans}(\hat{X}, K)$
32: **end procedure**

---

the data are almost preserved to the extent of λ-dimensions even after the projection. If the projection vectors are randomly chosen regardless of the independence, it can be insufficient to accurately span the underlying subspace because of the rank deficiency of the projection matrix. This shows that SRP without imposing the independent constraint gives rise to representation errors when projecting onto a subspace.

Distance Bound and Triangle Inequality. Factors that can cause kmeans to be slow include processing large amounts of data, computing many point-center distances, and requiring many iterations to converge. A primary strategy of accelerating kmeans is applying geometric knowledge to avoid computing redundant distance. For example, Elkan kmeans [8] employs the triangle inequality to avoid many distance computations. This method efficiently updates the upper and lower bounds of point-center distances to avoid unnecessary distance calculations. The proposed method projects high dimensional data onto the lower dimensional subspace using the BRP matrix. It may be determined that each data of lower dimensional subspace cannot guarantee exact geometric information between data. However, our method is approximately preserved by the Johnson-Lindenstrauss lemma [25]: if points in a vector space are projected on to a randomly selected subspace of a suitably high dimension, then the distances between the points are approximately preserved. Our algorithm thus can impose a distance bound characteristic to reduce the computational complexity.

2.2 Bootstrap Sampling and Ensemble Learning

Our approach adopts an ensemble learning model because of statistical reasons and large volumes of data. The statistical reason is that combining the outputs of several models by averaging may reduce the risk of an unfortunate feature selection. Learning with such a vast amount of data is usually not practical. We therefore use a partitioning method that separates all dataset into several small subsets. Also, we learn each models with disjoint subdata. By adapting the ensemble approach to our work, we obtain diversity of models and decrease the correlation between ensemble models. The results of Eq. (5) thus are more stable and comparable to the results of Eq. (4).

To reduce the risk of an unfortunate feature selection, the diversity of each ensemble models should be guaranteed. The diversity of ensemble models can be generally achieved in two ways. The most popular way is to employ a different dataset in each model, and the other is to use different learning algorithms. We choose the first strategy, and the bootstrap is used for pre-processing of feature selection. We empirically show that our method produces sufficient diversity, even when the number of ensembles is limited.

As multiple candidate clusters are combined, our algorithm considers the compatibility with variants of kmeans methods and efficiency of the execution time. Our method simply combines multiple candidate clusters using the conventional kmeans algorithm to guarantee fast convergence. Finally, it affords K clusters by minimizing errors in Eq. (2) using the refined products of the generation stage, as mentioned above.

2.3 Time Complexity

The time complexity for three accelerated algorithms is described in Table 1. We use lower case letters n, d, and k instead of N, D, and K for the readability. The total time is the summation of elapsed time in each kmeans iteration without the initialization step. The proposed total time in Table 1, the first part of the or statement represents executed total time without geometric knowledge to avoid computing the redundant distance, while the second part indicates total time with geometric knowledge. Our algorithm shows the highest simplicity, since the $\alpha\beta * T$ term is much smaller than 1.

Table 1. The asymptotic total time for each examined algorithm.

	Total time
Kmeans	$O(ndk) * iter$
Elkan	$O(\underline{n}dk + dk^2) * iter$
Proposed	$\alpha\beta * T * O(ndk) * iter$ or $T * O(\widetilde{\underline{n}}d'k + d'k^2) * iter$

The underline notation comes from Elkans kmeans, and $\underline{n}$ denotes the number of data, which need to be updated in every distance calculation. $\widetilde{n}$ indicates the number of reduced data using bootstrap, and d' denotes the number of reduced features. Let α denote $\widetilde{n}/n$, β denote d'/d, and γ denote Tk/n, which is a ratio of the number of data used in the generation and combination stage. As will be seen in Sect. 3, these values are much smaller than 1.

3   Experiments

We extensively evaluate the performances on various datasets. Synthetic and real datasets are used for the explicit clustering evaluation in terms of accuracy and elapsed time. We also show offline and online training efficiency for building a vocabulary tree [1] and incremental vocabulary tree [5]. As mentioned earlier, the incremental vocabulary tree does not need heavy clustering in the offline training process due to the distributed online process. Thus, strict elapsed time is more important for online clustering.

Our algorithm has three parameters: α, β, and T. The default values of parameters are determined through several experiments. The values of α and β are set as [0.1, 0.3] and T is selected as [5, 7]. During the experiments, these values are preserved.

3.1   Data Sets

Synthetic data. We use synthetic datasets based on a standard cluster model using a multi-variated normal distribution. Synthetic data generation tool is available on the website[1]. This generator gives two datasets, Gaussian and ellipse cluster data. To evaluate the performance of the algorithm over various numbers of data (N), dimensions of data (D), and numbers of groups of data (K), we generated datasets having $N = 100\,K$, $K \in \{3, 5, 10, 100, 500\}$, and $D \in \{8, 32, 128\}$.

Tiny Images. We use the CIFAR-10 dataset, which is composed of labelled subsets of 80 million tiny images [26]. CIFAR-10 consists of 10 categories and it contains 6000 images for each category. Each image is represented as GIST feature of dimension 384.

RGBD Images. We collect about object images from the RGBD dataset [27]. RGBD images are randomly sampled with category information. We use a 384-dimensional GIST feature to represent each image.

---

[1] http://personalpages.manchester.ac.uk/mbs/Julia.Handl/generators.html.

Caltech101. It contains images of 101 categories of objects, gathered from the internet. This dataset is mainly used to benchmark classification methods. We extract dense multi-scale SIFT feature for each image, and randomly sample 1M features to form this dataset.

UKbench. This dataset is from the Recognition Benchmark introduced in [1]. It consists of 10200 images split into four-image groups, with each of the same scene/object taken at different viewpoints. The features of the dataset and ground truth are publicly available.

Indoor/Outdoor. One indoor and two outdoor datasets are used to demonstrate the efficiency of our approach. Indoor images are captured by a mobile robot that moves twice along a similar path in the building. This dataset has 5890 images. SURF features are used to represent each image. Outdoor datasets are captured by a moving vehicle. We refer to the datasets as small and large outdoor datasets for the sake of convenient reference. The vehicle moves twice along the same path in the small outdoor dataset. In the large outdoor dataset, the vehicle travels about 13 km while making many loops. This large dataset consists of 23812 images, and we use sub-sampled images for test.

3.2   Evaluation Metric

We use three metrics to evaluate the performance of various clustering algorithms, elapsed time, the within-cluster sum of squared distortions (WCSSD), and the normalized mutual information (NMI) [28]. NMI is widely used for clustering evaluation, and it is a measurement of how close clustering results are to the latent classes. NMI requires the ground truth of cluster assignments X for points in the dataset. Given clustering results Y, NMI is defined by $\text{NMI(X,Y)} = \frac{MI(X,Y)}{\sqrt{H(X)H(Y)}}$, where MI(X,Y) is the mutual information of X and Y and $H(\cdot)$ is the entropy.

To tackle a massive amount of data, distributed computing and efficient learning need to be integrated into vision algorithms for large scale image classification and image indexing. We apply our method to visual codebook generation for bag-of-models based applications. In our experiments, the precision/recall and similarity matrix are used for image indexing and the evaluation of classified images follows [29]. Our results show the quality and efficiency of the codebooks with all other parameters fixed, except the codebook.

3.3   Clustering Performance

We compare our proposed clustering algorithm with three variations: Lloyd kmeans algorithm, Athur kmeans algorithm, and Elkan kmeans algorithm. All algorithms are run on a 3.0 GHz, 8 GB desktop PC using a single thread, and are mainly implemented in C language with some routines implemented in Matlab. We use the public releases of Athur kmeans and Elkan kmeans. The time costs for initialization and clustering are included in the comparison.

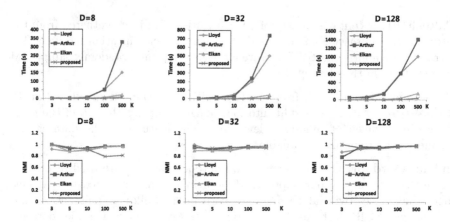

Fig. 1. Clustering performance in terms of elapsed time vs. the number of clusters and the clustering accuracy (N = 100,000)

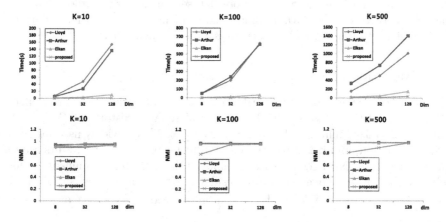

Fig. 2. Clustering performance in terms of elapsed time vs. the number of dimensions and the clustering accuracy (N = 100,000)

The results in Figs. 1 and 2 are shown for various dimensions of data and various numbers of clusters, respectively. The proposed algorithm is faster than Lloyds algorithm. Our algorithm consistently outperforms the other variations of kmeans in high dimensional large datasets. Also, our approach performs best regardless of K. However, from the results of this work, the accuracy of clustering in low dimensional datasets is not maintained. Hecht-Nielsens theory [30] is not valid in low dimensional space, because a vector having random directions might not be close to orthogonal.

Our algorithm is also efficient for real datasets. We use CIFAR10 and RGBD image sub-datasets without depth. Figures 3 and 4 show the clustering results in terms of WCSSD vs. time and NMI. As seen in these figures, the WCSSD of our algorithm is smaller than that of the earlier work and the NMI is similar.

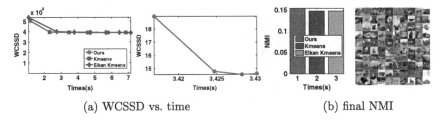

(a) WCSSD vs. time   (b) final NMI

Fig. 3. Clustering performance of CIFAR-10

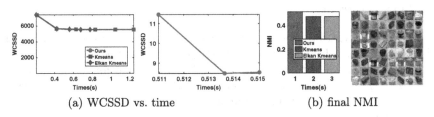

(a) WCSSD vs. time   (b) final NMI

Fig. 4. Clustering performance of RGBD objects

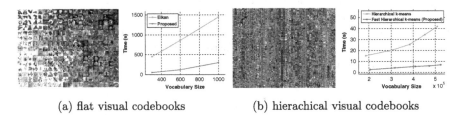

(a) flat visual codebooks   (b) hierachical visual codebooks

Fig. 5. The comparison of the clustering time with various vocabulary sizes. (a) Is the result on the Caltech101. (b) Is the result on the UKbench dataset.

From this, we can see that our approach provides faster convergence with a small number of iterations.

4   Applications

4.1   Evaluation Using Object Recognition

We compare the efficiency and quality of visual codebooks, which are respectively generated by flat and hierarchical clustering methods. A hierarchical clustering method such as HKM [1] is suitable for large data applications.

The classification and identification accuracy are similar and therefore we only present results in terms of elapsed time as increasing the size of visual words, namely vocabulary, in Fig. 5. We perform the experiments on the Caltech101 dataset, which contains 0.1M randomly sampled features. Following [29], we run the clustering algorithms used to build a visual codebook, and test only

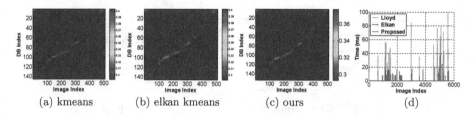

Fig. 6. The performance comparison on the indoor dataset. (a), (b), (c) Are the image similarity matrix of the conventional approach and the proposed algorithm. (d) Is the elapsed time of clustering.

the codebook generation process in the image classification. Results of the Caltech101 dataset are obtained by 0.3 K, 0.6 K, and 1 K codebooks, and a χ^2-SVM on top of 4×4 spatial histograms. From Fig. 5a, we see that for the same vocabulary size, our method is more efficient than the other approaches. However, the accuracy of each algorithm is similar. For example, when we use 1 K codebooks for clustering, the mAP of our approach is 0.641 and that of the other approach is 0.643.

In the experiment on the UKbench dataset, we use a subset of database images and 760 K local features. We evaluate the clustering time and the performance of image retrieval with various vocabulary sizes from 200 K to 500 K. Figure 5b shows that our method runs faster than the conventional approach with a similar mAP, about 0.75.

4.2   Evaluation Using Image Indexing

The vocabulary tree is widely used in vision based localization in mobile devices and the robot society [4–6]. The problem with the bag-of-words model lies in that a codebook built by each single dataset is insufficient to represent unseen images. Recently, the incremental vocabulary tree was presented for adapting to dynamic environments and removing offline training [4,5]. In this experiment, we use the incremental codebooks, as mentioned in AVT [5]. We demonstrate the accuracy of image indexing and the execution time for updating incremental vocabulary trees. Our visual search system follows [6], and we do qualitative evaluation by image to image matching. The clustering part of AVT is replaced by the state of the art kmeans and the proposed algorithms. We evaluate the online clustering process of modified AVT and show the performance of image matching for indoor and outdoor environments.

Three figures (from left to right) in Figs. 6 and 7 show the image similarity matrix that represents the similarity scores between training and test images. From this matrix, we can calculate the localization accuracy on each dataset, and diagonal elements show loop detection and the right-top part indicates loop closure. However, three similarity matrixes in each dataset have similar values and show similar patterns. These results mean that our clustering method runs well without losing accuracy. The last figure in Figs. 6 and 7 shows the execution time for the clustering process. This process runs when a test image is inserted.

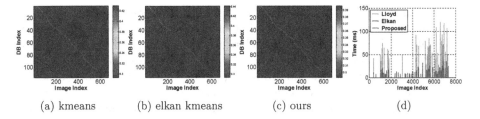

(a) kmeans   (b) elkan kmeans   (c) ours   (d)

Fig. 7. The performance comparison on the small outdoor dataset. (a), (b), (c) Are the image similarity matrix of the conventional approach and the proposed algorithm. (d) Is the elapsed time of clustering.

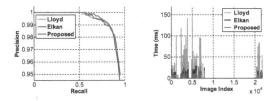

Fig. 8. The performance comparison on the large outdoor dataset. (a) Is the precision-recall of the loop detection. (b) Is the elapsed time of clustering.

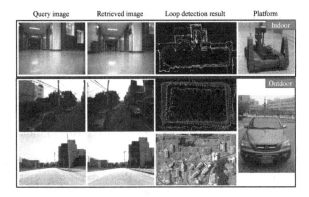

Fig. 9. Example images and the result of the loop detection in each dataset. Images of the first row belong to the indoor dataset, and images of the second and third rows belong to outdoor datasets (Color figure online).

If a test image is an unseen one, features of the image are inserted into the incremental vocabulary tree, and all histogram of images are updated. When adaptation of the incremental vocabulary tree occurs, the graph of the last figure has a value. As we can see in figure (d), the elapsed time of our method is smaller and the number of executions is greater.

In Fig. 8, we use the precision-recall curve instead of a similarity matrix. The tendency of both results is similar to that seen above.

Two images (from left) of each row in Fig. 9 are connected with each dataset: images of the first row belong to the indoor dataset, the second belong to the small outdoor dataset, and the third belong to the large outdoor dataset. Images of the third column show total localization results. There are three circles: green, the robot position; yellow, added image position; and red, a matched scene position. In order to prevent confusion, we should mention that the trajectories of the real position (green line) are slightly rotated to view the results clearly and easily.

5   Conclusions

In this paper, we have introduced an accelerated kmeans clustering algorithm that uses binary random projection. The clustering problem is formulated as a feature selection and solved by minimization of distance errors between original data and refined data. The proposed method enables efficient clustering of high dimensional large data. Our algorithm shows better performance on the simulated datasets and real datasets than conventional approaches. We demonstrate that our accelerated algorithm is applicable to an incremental vocabulary tree for object recognition and image indexing.

Acknowledgement. We would like to thank Greg Hamerly and Yudeog Han for their support. This work was supported by the National Research Foundation of Korea (NRF) grant funded by the Korea government (No. 2010-0028680).

References

1. Nister, D., Stewenius, H.: Scalable recognition with a vocabulary tree. In: International Conference on Computer Vision and Pattern Recognition, pp. 2161–2168 (2006)
2. Tsai, S.S., Chen, D., Takacs, G., Chandrasekhar, V., Singh, J.P., Girod, B.: Location coding for mobile image retrieval. In: Proceedings of the 5th International ICST Mobile Multimedia Communications Conference (2009)
3. Straub, J., Hilsenbeck, S., Schroth, G., Huitl, R., Möller, A., Steinbach, E.: Fast relocalization for visual odometry using binary features. In: IEEE International Conference on Image Processing (ICIP), Melbourne, Australia (2013)
4. Nicosevici, T., Garcia, R.: Automatic visual bag-of-words for online robot navigation and mapping. Trans. Robot. **99**, 1–13 (2012)
5. Yeh, T., Lee, J.J., Darrell, T.: Adaptive vocabulary forests br dynamic indexing and category learning. In: Proceedings of the International Conference on Computer Vision, pp. 1–8 (2007)
6. Kim, J., Park, C., Kweon, I.S.: Vision-based navigation with efficient scene recognition. J. Intell. Serv. Robot. **4**, 191–202 (2011)
7. Lloyd, S.P.: Least squares quantization in PCM. Trans. Inf. Theory **28**, 129–137 (1982)
8. Elkan, C.: Using the triangle inequality to accelerate k-means. In: International Conference on Machine Learning, pp. 147–153 (2003)

9. Bradley, P.S., Fayyad, U.M.: Refining initial points for k-means clustering. In: International Conference on Machine Learning (1998)
10. Arthur, D., Vassilvitskii, S.: K-means++: the advantages of careful seeding. In: ACM-SIAM Symposium on Discrete Algorithms (2007)
11. Parsons, L., Haque, E., Liu, H.: Subspace clustering for high dimensional data: a review. ACM SIGKDD Explorarions Newslett. **6**, 90–105 (2004)
12. Khalilian, M., Mustapha, N., Suliman, N., Mamat, A.: A novel k-means based clustering algorithm for high dimensional data sets. In: Internaional Multiconference of Engineers and Computer Scientists, pp. 17–19 (2010)
13. Moise, G., Sander: Finding non-redundant, statistically significant regions in high dimensional data: a novel approach to projected and subspace clustering. In: International Conference on Knowledge Discovery and Data Mining (2008)
14. Achlioptas, D.: Database-friendly random projections. In: ACM SIGMOD-SIGACT-SIGART Symposium on Principles of Database Systems, pp. 274–281 (2001)
15. Ding, C., He, X., Zha, H., Simon, H.D.: Adaptive dimension reduction for clustering high dimensional data. In: International Conference on Data Mining, pp. 147–154 (2002)
16. Hinneburg, A., Keim, D.A.: Optimal grid-clustering: towards breaking the curse of dimensionality in high-dimensional clustering. In: International Conference on Very Large Data Bases (1999)
17. Bingham, E., Mannila, H.: Random projection in dimensionality reduction: applications to image and text data. In: International Conference on Knowledge Discovery and Data Mining (2001)
18. Fred, A.L.N., Jain, A.K.: Combining multiple clusterings using evidence accumulation. Trans. Pattern Anal. Mach. Intell. **27**(6), 835–850 (2005)
19. Polikar, R.: Ensemble based systems in decision making. Circ. Syst. Mag. **6**(3), 21–45 (2006)
20. Fern, X.Z., Brodley, C.E.: Random projection for high dimensional data clustering: a cluster ensemble approach. In: International Conference on Machine Learning, pp. 186–193 (2003)
21. Kohavi, R., John, G.H.: Wrappers for feature subset selection. Artif. Intell. **97**, 273–324 (1997)
22. Indyk, P., Motwani, R.: Approximate nearest neighbors: towards removing the curse of dimensionality. In: ACM Symposium on Theory of Computing, pp. 604–613 (1998)
23. Elhamifar, E., Vidal., R.: Sparse subspace clustering. In: International Conference on Computer Vision and Pattern Recognition (2009)
24. Elhamifar, E., Vidal, R.: Sparse manifold clustering and embedding. Neural Inf. Process. Syst. **24**, 55–63 (2011)
25. Johnson, W.B., Lindenstrauss, J.: Extensions of lipschitz mapping into hilbert space. In: International Conference in Modern Analysis and Probability, vol. 26, pp. 90–105 (1984)
26. Krizhevsky, A.: Learning multiple layers of features from tiny images. Technical report (2009)
27. Lai, K., Bo, L., Ren, X., Fox, D.: A large-scale hierarchical multi-view RGB-D object dataset. In: International Conference on Robotics and Automation, pp. 1817–1824 (2012)
28. Strehl, A., Ghosh, J.: Cluster ensembles - a knowledge reuse framework for combining multiple partitions. J. Mach. Learn. Res. **3**, 583–617 (2003)

29. Lazebnik, S., Schmid, C., Ponce, J.: Beyond bags of features: spatial pyramid matching for recognizing natural scene categories. In: International Conference on Computer Vision and Pattern Recognition, pp. 2169–2178 (2006)
30. Hecht-Nielsen, R.: Context vectors: general purpose approximate meaning representations self-organized from raw data. In: Zurada, J.M., Marks II, R.J., Robinson, C.J. (eds.) Computational Intelligence: Imitating Life, pp. 43–56. IEEE Press, Cambridge (1994)

Divide and Conquer: Efficient Large-Scale Structure from Motion Using Graph Partitioning

Brojeshwar Bhowmick[1]($\boxtimes$), Suvam Patra[1], Avishek Chatterjee[2],
Venu Madhav Govindu[2], and Subhashis Banerjee[1]

[1] Indian Institute of Technology Delhi, New Delhi, India
{brojeshwar,suvam,suban}@cse.iitd.ac.in
[2] Indian Institute of Science, Bengaluru, India
{avishek,venu}@ee.iisc.ernet.in

Abstract. Despite significant advances in recent years, structure-from-motion (SfM) pipelines suffer from two important drawbacks. Apart from requiring significant computational power to solve the large-scale computations involved, such pipelines sometimes fail to correctly reconstruct when the accumulated error in incremental reconstruction is large or when the number of 3D to 2D correspondences are insufficient. In this paper we present a novel approach to mitigate the above-mentioned drawbacks. Using an image match graph based on matching features we partition the image data set into smaller sets or components which are reconstructed independently. Following such reconstructions we utilise the available epipolar relationships that connect images across components to correctly align the individual reconstructions in a global frame of reference. This results in both a significant speed up of at least one order of magnitude and also mitigates the problems of reconstruction failures with a marginal loss in accuracy. The effectiveness of our approach is demonstrated on some large-scale real world data sets.

1 Introduction

In structure from motion (SfM) we typically use many images of a scene to solve for both the 3D scene being viewed and the parameters of the cameras involved. Most contemporary large-scale SfM methods [1–5] use the bundle adjustment method [6] which simultaneously optimises for both structure and camera parameters using point correspondences in images by minimising a global cost function. However, being a joint optimisation over all cameras and 3D points, bundle adjustment often fails for large data sets. This is typically due to an accumulation of error in an incremental reconstruction or when cameras are weakly connected to 3D feature points. In addition, owing to the very large number of variables involved, bundle adjustment is also very computationally demanding and time consuming. In this paper we adopt a divide-and-conquer strategy that is designed to mitigate these problems. In essence, our approach partitions the full image data set into smaller sets that can each be independently reconstructed using a standard approach to bundle adjustment. Subsequently, by

© Springer International Publishing Switzerland 2015
D. Cremers et al. (Eds.): ACCV 2014, Part II, LNCS 9004, pp. 273–287, 2015.
DOI: 10.1007/978-3-319-16808-1_19

utilising available geometric relationships between cameras across the individual partitions, we solve a global registration problem that correctly and accurately places each individual 3D reconstructed component into a single global frame of reference.

In what follows we show that this approach is not only more robust with respect to failures in reconstruction but also gives significant improvements over the state-of-the-art techniques in terms of computational speed. The main contributions of our paper are:

1. A principled method based on normalised cuts [7] to partition the match graph of a large collection of images into disjoint connected components which can be independently and reliably reconstructed. This process also automatically identifies a set of connecting images between the components which can be used to register the independent reconstructions. Specifically, these are the image pairs specified by the cut edges in the graph.
2. A method for registering the point clouds corresponding to the independent connected components using pairwise epipolar geometry relationships. The epipolar based registration technique proposed in this paper is more robust than the standard techniques for registering point clouds using 3D-3D or 3D-2D correspondences. Registration methods based on 3D point correspondences do not use all available information (image correspondences) and may fail when the point clouds do not have sufficient number of 3D points in common. 3D-2D based methods, such as a sequential bundler [1,2,8], often result in broken reconstructions when the number of points available are inadequate for re-sectioning or when common 3D points are removed at the outlier rejection stage [1] (see Table 4). The proposed registration algorithm using pairwise epipolar geometry alleviates this problem as is shown in Fig. 1 and discussed in Sect. 4. Considered as an independent approach, the epipolar based algorithm can also be used to register independently reconstructed point clouds by introducing a few connecting images.

Matching all pairs of images in an iterative bundler is computationally expensive, especially when the number of images in the collection is large. There have been several attempts to reduce the number of images to be matched. Frahm et al. [9,10] try to find some representative "iconic images" from the image data set and then partition the iconic scene graph, reconstruct each cluster and register them using 3D similarity transformations. Snavely et al. [11,12] and Havlena et al. [13] compute skeletal sets from the match graph to reduce image matching. All these methods reduce the set of images on which they run SfM. Moreover, incremental bundle adjustment is also known to suffer from drift due to accumulation of errors which increase as the number of images increase [1,5,14]. Crandall et al. [5,14] propose an MRF based discrete formulation coupled with continuous Levenberg-Marquadt refinement for large-scale SfM to mitigate this problem. To reduce the matching time, Wu [1] (henceforth VSFM) proposed preemptive matching to reduce the number of pairs to be matched. Moreover, all cameras and 3D points are optimised only after a certain number of new

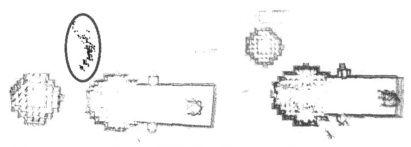

(a) Reconstruction failure by VSFM [1]. (b) Successful reconstruction by our method.

Fig. 1. Plan view of reconstruction of two temples at the Hampi site in India: (a) illustrates the failure of VSFM [1] due to inadequate points during re-sectioning (marked in red) whereas (b) our approach correctly solves the reconstruction problem. Please view this figure in color (Color figure online).

cameras are incorporated into the iterative bundler. Although VSFM demonstrates approximately linear running time, sometimes it fails for large data sets when the accumulated errors of iterative bundler become large [1]. Although there have been some recent global methods [15,16], to be able to solve large-scale SfM problems, global methods need to be exceedingly robust. Farenzena *et al.* [17] also propose to merge smaller reconstructions in a bottom up dendrogram. However, their largest datasets are of only 380 images and their use of reprojection errors of common 3D points for merging is unsuitable for very large datasets. In our approach, we propose to decompose the image set into smaller components so that the match graph of each component is densely connected. This is likely to yield correct 3D reconstructions, since fewer problems are encountered during the re-sectioning stage of a standard iterative bundler and the reconstruction is robust. Restricting pairwise image matching to within each component also yields a significant reduction in computation time. Moreover SfM based reconstruction of each component can be carried out in parallel. Our approach is conceptually depicted in Fig. 2.

The rest of the paper is organised as follows. Section 2 discusses our method of decomposing the image set into smaller groups and also determining the connecting images between individual groups. Section 3 provides the overview of our registration process. Section 4 reports the results of our experiments on different data sets, and Sect. 5 concludes the paper.

2   Data Set Decomposition Using Normalised Cuts

Images used for bundle adjustment can either be acquired from a site or aggregated from various sources on the internet. When the images are acquired from a site in an organised manner, the problem of decomposition into smaller sets becomes trivial. In what follows we provide an illustration. Figure 3 shows the Google Earth view of the Vitthala temple at Hampi in Karnataka, India, which

Normalised Cuts

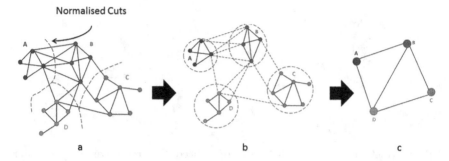

a   b   c

Fig. 2. (a) Original match graph where images (nodes) are connected by edges having similar image features. The edge weights represent similarity scores. (b) Normalised cut partitions the full image set into connected components which can be reconstructed independently. The "connecting images" across components are defined by the cut edges. (c) The individual cuts are now equivalent to individual nodes that represent independent rigid 3D reconstructions which are registered using pairwise epipolar relationship of the connecting images.

is a world heritage site maintained by the Archaeological Survey of India (Latitude: 15.342276, Longitude: 76.475287). Figure 4 shows a typical example where images of two buildings are captured separately and it also shows a typical *connecting* image which sees parts of both the buildings. We call such data sets *organised*.

In case such planned acquisition is not possible, the collection of images need to be automatically partitioned into smaller components. Unorganised data sets downloaded from the Internet are typical examples. In such cases a method for automatically grouping into visually similar sets and finding connecting images needs to be established. To this end, we train a vocabulary tree [18] using all image features (SIFTGPU [19]) and extract top p (typically p = 80) similar

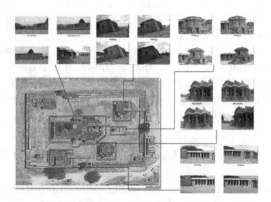

Fig. 3. Google Earth view of the Vitthala temple, Hampi, Karnataka, India. The red boxes denote different buildings of the temple. Images for each building were captured separately (Color figure online).

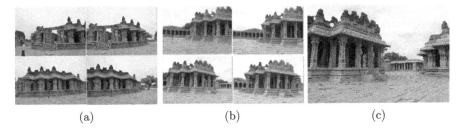

(a)   (b)   (c)

Fig. 4. (a) and (b) Two buildings of the Hampi temple complex, and (c) a typical connecting image.

images for each image in the set. We form a match graph where each node is an image and the edge weights between two nodes are the similarity values obtained from the vocabulary tree. We aim to partition the set of images such that each partition is densely connected. The partitions only capture dense connectivity of matched image features and need not represent a single physical structure. Here the dense connectivity ensures that SFM reconstruction is less likely to fail due to the paucity of reliable matches or accumulated error or drift.

We use the multi-way extension [7] of the normalised cut (NC) formulation to automatically partition the match graph $\mathbf{G} = (\mathbf{V}, \mathbf{E})$ into individual clusters. Since, in our case edge weights are based on visual similarity, the normalised cut would yield those connected components in which connected images are visibly similar. We use the images that belong to the cut as candidate connecting images. In Fig. 5 we show the result of our estimation upon applying the normalised cut to the set of images collected at the Hampi site illustrated in Fig. 3, i.e. when we treat the images as an unorganised dataset. Figure 5a shows the cameras partitioned into connected components in different colours. Figure 5b shows the plan view of the 3D reconstructions obtained for each component marked in corresponding colours. It should be noted that in this example, the graph weights are based only on pairwise image feature similarity scores. We can improve the quality of the graph by incorporating geometric information such as the robustness of computation of pairwise epipolar geometries of connected images. Such a scheme would not only ensure that the connected pairs of images can be reliably matched but would also ensure that the pairwise epipolar geometries can be robustly estimated. The corresponding result is provided in Fig. 8b and discussed in Sect. 4.

Extracting connecting images: The number of candidate connecting images are often very large. Reducing the number of connecting images will reduce the time for estimation of pairwise epipolar geometry. The connecting image extraction process is described below:

1. For each of the connecting images reject the outlier **out edges** (both within and across components) using a measure of the robustness of the epipolar computation (Eq. 6).
2. If the number of out edges retained is less than T (typically $T = 60\%$ of the original out degree) then remove the image from the set of connecting images.

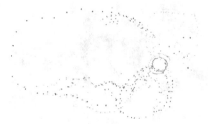
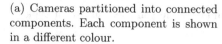

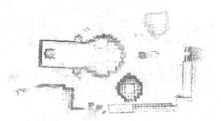

(a) Cameras partitioned into connected components. Each component is shown in a different colour.

(b) 3D reconstructions of each component marked in same colours.

Fig. 5. SfM results on the Hampi dataset (unorganised data) illustrating the effect of graph partitioning (Color figure online).

3. Compute the mean of the similarity scores of all the retained out edges for the current image.
4. If the similarity score for a cut edge exceeds the mean similarity values of the images they connect, then mark the images as connecting images.

3 Registration of Independent Component Reconstructions

In this Section, we describe how each of the individually reconstructed groups of cameras are aligned or registered to a single frame of reference. To register a pair of 3D reconstructions, we need to estimate the relative transformation between them. In what follows, we describe how we estimate relative rotation, translation and scale between a pair of reconstructions using epipolar relationships between the reconstructed cameras and the connecting cameras. While estimating epipolar geometry, we use focal lengths extracted from the EXIF information of the images.

Let us consider two independently reconstructed groups of cameras A and B[1]. Let $\mathbb{C}_{AB}$ be the set of connecting cameras between A and B. We first fix the relative scale between A and B using the approach described in Sect. 3.1. Once this relative scale is fixed, the two reconstructions A and B are now related by a rigid or Euclidean transformation which can be estimated using the method detailed in Sect. 3.2.

3.1 Relative Scale Estimation Between a Pair of Reconstructions

To estimate the relative scale between A and B, we first estimate the position of all the connecting cameras ($k \in \mathbb{C}_{AB}$) in the local frames of reference of both A and B separately. Then we compare the pairwise distances of common

---

[1] In this section, we use lower case letters to denote individual cameras and upper case letters to denote groups of reconstructed cameras.

cameras in the two reconstructions. If a connecting camera $k \in \mathbb{C}_{AB}$ shares common features with the cameras in A then, the rotation and translation of k can be found in the local reference frame of A. Let the unknown rotation and translation of k, with respect to the frame of reference of A be denoted by R_{Ak} and T_{Ak} respectively. Now, consider a camera i that belongs to the group A. Suppose, the rotation and translation of i with respect to the local frame of reference of A is R_{Ai} and T_{Ai} respectively (as estimated within A). If $i \in A$ and $k \in \mathbb{C}_{AB}$ share common features, then using epipolar relationships, we can find the relative rotation (R_{ik}) and the direction of relative translation (t_{ik}) between i and k. Clearly the following relations should hold:

$$R_{ik} = R_{Ak}R_{Ai}^{T} \Rightarrow R_{Ak} = R_{ik}R_{Ai} \tag{1}$$

$$t_{ik} \propto T_{Ak} - R_{ik}T_{Ai} \Rightarrow [t_{ik}]_{\times}(T_{Ak} - R_{ik}T_{Ai}) = 0 \tag{2}$$

where, $[.]_{\times}$ is the skew-symmetric matrix representation for vector cross product [20]. These relations hold for all $i \in A$ such that i and k share common features and the epipolar geometry between them can be estimated. Therefore, we take the geodesic mean [21] of all such estimates of the rotation R_{Ak} as,

$$\widehat{R}_{Ak} = \underset{i \in A}{\text{mean}}\,(R_{ik}R_{Ai}) \tag{3}$$

Similarly, the average estimate of the translation T_{Ak} is obtained as

$$\widehat{T}_{Ak} = \underset{T_{Ak}}{\text{argmin}} \sum_{i \in A} \frac{\left\| [t_{ik}]_{\times}(T_{Ak} - R_{ik}T_{Ai}) \right\|^{2}}{\left\| T_{Ak} - R_{ik}T_{Ai} \right\|^{2}} \tag{4}$$

which can be solved using the iterative method proposed in [22].

The center of projection of camera k, in the frame of reference of A, is given by $-\widehat{R}_{Ak}\widehat{T}_{Ak}$. Thus, we compute the camera centers $(-\widehat{R}_{Ak}\widehat{T}_{Ak})$ for all $k \in \mathbb{C}_{AB}$ in the frame of reference of A. Similarly, we compute the camera centers $(-\widehat{R}_{Bk}\widehat{T}_{Bk})$ for all $k \in \mathbb{C}_{AB}$ in the frame of reference of B. Then, the relative scale between A and B can be robustly estimated by comparing pairwise distances of common cameras in the two reconstructions as:

$$\widehat{s}_{AB} = \underset{k_{1},k_{2} \in \mathbb{C}_{AB}}{\text{median}} \frac{\left\| -\widehat{R}_{Bk_{1}}\widehat{T}_{Bk_{1}} + \widehat{R}_{Bk_{2}}\widehat{T}_{Bk_{2}} \right\|}{\left\| -\widehat{R}_{Ak_{1}}\widehat{T}_{Ak_{1}} + \widehat{R}_{Ak_{2}}\widehat{T}_{Ak_{2}} \right\|} \tag{5}$$

Once the relative scale between A and B is estimated, we scale the reconstruction of A to have the same scale as that of B. Therefore, the rotation of camera k in the frame of reference of A remains $\widehat{R}_{Ak}$ whereas, the translation of camera k becomes $\widehat{s}_{AB}\widehat{T}_{Ak}$ in the scaled local frame of reference of A. We do not change the scale of B. Hence the rotation ($\widehat{R}_{Ak}$) and the translation ($\widehat{T}_{Ak}$) of camera k in the frame of reference of B remains unaltered.

It should be noted here that the translation directions estimated using epipolar geometry may have outliers. To remove outliers, we check whether the two non-zero eigenvalues of the essential matrix have similar values [20]. We discard the estimated essential matrix as well as the corresponding translation direction if the ratio of the two largest eigenvalues (σ_2 and σ_1 in sorted order) is less than a threshold, i.e.

$$\frac{\sigma_2}{\sigma_1} < T \tag{6}$$

Typically we take T as 0.95 for our experiments.

3.2 Relative Rotation and Translation Estimation Between a Pair of Reconstructions

Once A is resized to have same scale as that of B, the two reconstructions are related by a rigid or Euclidean transformation. Earlier, we estimated the motion of k in the frame of reference of A to be a rotation and translation of $\widehat{R}_{Ak}$ and $\widehat{s}_{AB}\widehat{T}_{Ak}$ respectively. Similarly, the motion of k in the frame of reference of B is $\widehat{R}_{Bk}$ and $\widehat{T}_{Bk}$ respectively.

In the following we denote the 3D rotation and translation compactly as the Euclidean motion model

$$\mathbf{M} = \left[\begin{array}{c|c} R & T \\ \hline \mathbf{0} & 1 \end{array}\right] \tag{7}$$

where $\mathbf{0}$ denotes a 1×3 vector of zeros. Suppose the unknown motions that align A and B to the global frame of reference be $\mathbf{M}_A$ and $\mathbf{M}_B$ respectively. After applying these transformations to A and B, all common connecting cameras ($k \in \mathbb{C}_{AB}$) between A and B should have the same motion parameters. Therefore, after A and B are registered with the global frame of reference, we have

$$\widehat{\mathbf{M}}_{Ak}\mathbf{M}_A = \widehat{\mathbf{M}}_{Bk}\mathbf{M}_B \tag{8}$$

where we reiterate that the translation component of $\widehat{\mathbf{M}}_{Ak}$ is the scaled version, i.e. $\widehat{s}_{AB}\widehat{T}_{Ak}$. Therefore, the relative motion between A and B is

$$\mathbf{M}_{AB} = \mathbf{M}_B\mathbf{M}_A^{-1} = \widehat{\mathbf{M}}_{Bk}^{-1}\widehat{\mathbf{M}}_{Ak} \tag{9}$$

From Eq. 9 we can see that we have

$$R_{AB} = R_B R_A^T = \widehat{R}_{Bk}^T \widehat{R}_{Ak} \tag{10}$$

If there are many connecting cameras between A and B, then we have many estimates of R_{AB}, which we average to provide the estimate:

$$\widehat{R}_{AB} = \underset{k \in \mathbb{C}_{AB}}{\text{mean}} \left(\widehat{R}_{Bk}^T \widehat{R}_{Ak} \right) \tag{11}$$

Similarly, from Eq. 9, the relative translation between A and B can be seen to be given by:

$$T_{AB} = T_B - R_B R_A^T T_A = \widehat{s}_{AB}\widehat{R}_{Bk}^T \widehat{T}_{Ak} - \widehat{R}_{Bk}^T \widehat{T}_{Bk} \tag{12}$$

Therefore, we estimate relative translation between A and B by robustly averaging all pairwise estimates from different connecting cameras as:

$$\widehat{T}_{AB} = \underset{T}{\operatorname{argmin}} \sum_{k \in \mathbb{C}_{AB}} \left\| T - \left(\widehat{s}_{AB} \widehat{R}_{Bk}^T \widehat{T}_{Ak} - \widehat{R}_{Bk}^T \widehat{T}_{Bk} \right) \right\|_1 \tag{13}$$

In our implementation, we start the process of global registration using the largest reconstruction (with maximum number of images) as the seed and register all other reconstructions which are connected to this seed and merge them into a single model. We also remark that the motion models required for registering individual reconstructions connected to the current model can be estimated in parallel.

4 Experimental Results

We present our results on both *organised* and *unorganised* image data sets. For our experiments, we used an Intel i7 quad core machine with 16 GB RAM and GTX 580 graphics card. We first present our result on an *organised* image set acquired from Hampi (see Fig. 3). The data set consists of 2337 images covering 4 temple buildings. The physical footprint of these 4 buildings covers an area of approximately 160×94 m.[2] For reconstructing the images in each individual set we use VSFM [1] as the iterative bundler. We merge each of these reconstructions using the method described in Sect. 3 into a common frame of reference. Figure 6a shows our reconstruction after registration superimposed on a view from Google Earth. As we do not have ground truth for such real-world data, to analyse the quality of our reconstruction we use the output of VSFM applied on the entire data set using all pairs matching as our baseline reconstruction. We note that all pairs matching is necessitated here as the scheme of preemptive matching suggested in [1] fails on this data set. Figure 6b shows the comparison where the red point cloud is obtained from VSFM and the green points are obtained using our method. VSFM took 5760 min to reconstruct the data set using all pairs matching. In contrast our method takes 2578 min (using all pairs matching) to reconstruct the same data set. The computation time of our method is calculated by considering the time required for reconstruction of the largest component and the total time for registration, since the reconstruction of each component is done in parallel. We also compare the 3D camera rotations and positions (i.e. translations) obtained by our method against the 'ground truth' provided by VSFM. As the two camera estimates are in different frames of reference and may also differ in scale, we align them in a common Euclidean reference frame by computing the best similarity (Euclidean transformation

---

[2] We point out here that these buildings are far more complex compared to urban buildings and even heritage sites such as the Notre Dame cathedral reconstructed in [4]. Specifically, these temples have fluted pillars, are repleted with ornate carvings and sculptures, repeated patterns as well as layered cupola. The complexity of these structures can also be judged from the building footprint as seen in the plan view presented in Fig. 6a.

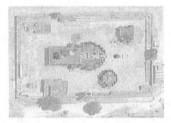 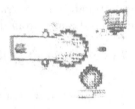

(a) Reconstruction overlaid on Google map.   (b) Comparison between VSFM (red) and our method (green).

Fig. 6. Validation of reconstruction of Hampi data set (organised data) (Color figure online).

Table 1. Comparison of total reconstruction by VSFM against individual reconstructions being registered by our method

Error entity	Error unit	Mean error	Median error	RMS error
Camera rotation	Degrees	1.93	1.57	2.66
Camera translation	Ratio of graph diameter	0.012	0.0091	0.041

and a global scale) transformation between them. The results of our comparison are presented in Table 1. Here, while the rotation error is in absolute degrees, since the overall scale of the reconstruction is arbitrary, we present the errors in translation (position) estimates as a fraction of the graph diameter of the full reconstruction. As can be seen, apart from being much faster than VSFM, our result is qualitatively similar to that obtained by VSFM.

For experimenting with unorganised image datasets we consider a total of 3017 images from the Hampi data set. We train a vocabulary tree [18] using SIFT [19,23] features and take 80 most similar images from vocabulary tree for each image in the set to construct a match graph. Normalised cut is applied on this match graph and connected components are obtained. In our experiments, the expected number of connected components is decided intuitively and is used as an input parameter for the number of components needed using normalised cut. We use the process described in Sect. 2 to find the connecting images. We then run VSFM on individual connected components and merge them into a single coordinate frame. Figure 7 shows a frontal view of the reconstruction by our method. Figure 5b shows the 3D reconstructions corresponding to each of the connected components registered and in different colors. To validate our result, we overlay our reconstruction on the corresponding site map from Google Earth and Fig. 8c shows that the registration is accurate. We also run VSFM with all 3017 images and compare the results. Figure 8a shows the comparison results where the VSFM output is marked in red and the output obtained using our method is marked in green. Figure 8b shows the corresponding results using a measure of robustness of epipolar estimation as edge weights in normalised cut. It can be noted that the results are marginally superior to that of Fig. 8a especially near the top left corner of the plan view. This is because the images

Table 2. Data sets used in our experiments

Data set	No. of images	No. of components	No. of images reconstructed
Rome	13783	24	10534
Hampi	3017	7	2584
St Peter's Basilica	1275	5	1236
Colosseum	1164	3	1032

Table 3. Time statistics of our method on different data sets compared with VSFM

Data set	Match graph creation using vocabulary tree (mins)	Pairwise matching (mins)	Reconstruction and registration (mins)	Total time by us (mins)	Pairwise matching by VSFM (mins)	Reconstruction by VSFM (mins)	Total time by VSFM (mins)
Rome	768	502	27	1297	N/A	N/A	N/A
Hampi	481	424	8	913	9522	59	9581
St Peter's Basilica	98	22	4	124	1385	10	1395
Colosseum	83	24	3	110	1394	9	1403

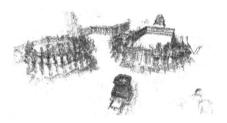

Fig. 7. Frontal view of the Hampi reconstruction (considered as unorganised data).

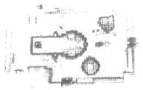 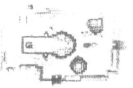 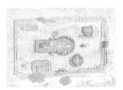

(a) Comparison with VSFM (red) and our method (green).

(b) Comparison with VSFM (red) and our method with epipolar robustness (green).

(c) Overlaid on Google map.

Fig. 8. Reconstruction of the Hampi data set (considered as unorganised data) validated against VSFM reconstruction and Google Earth (Color figure online).

corresponding to this region are no longer distributed across different segments by normalised cut.

We also tested our algorithm on some standard *unorganised* data sets downloaded from the Internet. We downloaded approximately 13 K images of Central Rome from Flickr and tested our algorithm on this data set. Figure 9 shows the reconstruction using our method. This data set could not be reconstructed using

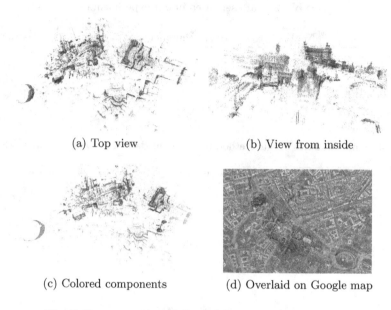

(a) Top view

(b) View from inside

(c) Colored components

(d) Overlaid on Google map

Fig. 9. Reconstruction of Central Rome using our method.

VSFM with our hardware resources. Figure 9d shows the reconstruction over-laid on Google map. We also ran our algorithm on the St Peter's Basilica and Colosseum data sets obtained from [1], the results of which are shown in Figs. 10 and 11 respectively. Table 2 shows the total number of connected components and the total number of images reconstructed for each of the data sets. The time statistics of our algorithm for different data sets are presented in Table 3. For most of the cases we had to use all pairs matching in VSFM as preemp-tive matching was causing the reconstruction to break in the middle, which is also reported in [1]. In our case we used the initial match graph obtained from vocabulary tree. It is evident that most of the time is consumed for matching. The reconstruction and the total registration time taken by our approach is significantly less than the reconstruction time of VSFM. The overall speed up achieved is at least one order of magnitude superior. We also note that iterative bundle adjustment schemes often results in broken reconstruction even within a component. In Table 4 we present statistics of such breaks. In all such cases we have been able to register the broken components using pairwise epipolar geometry on the connecting images in the broken components identified auto-matically from the match graph. Finally, we also remark in passing that we also experimented with the method presented in [17] using the author's code. On the Hampi dataset, [17] failed to reconstruct in more than 24 h. While [17] is faster than original BA, its runtime complexity is far inferior to the $O(n)$ complexity of VSFM. In an additional test, for a 300 image subset of the Hampi dataset, [17] was 10 times slower than VSFM and produced a significantly poorer result.

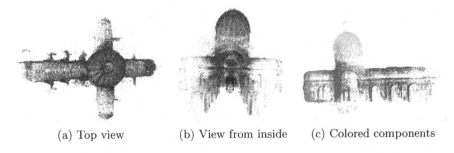

(a) Top view   (b) View from inside   (c) Colored components

Fig. 10. Reconstruction of St Peter's Basilica using our method (1275 images used).

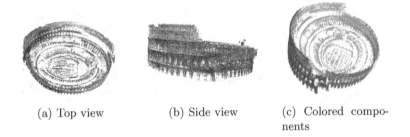

(a) Top view   (b) Side view   (c) Colored components

Fig. 11. Reconstruction of Colosseum using our method.

Table 4. Statistics of breaks in reconstruction of the data sets

Data set	No. of components	No. of components broken by VSFM	Total no. of components including broken sub-components
Rome	24	5	33
Hampi	7	2	9
St Peter's Basilca	5	1	6
Colosseum	3	2	6

5 Conclusion

We have presented a new pipeline for automatic 3D reconstruction from a large collection of images. We have demonstrated the utility of partitioning the images into clusters that can be independently and reliably reconstructed and then aligned in a global frame of reference. Results on a number of large data sets demonstrates that our method results in large speed improvements compared to the state-of-the-art without any significant loss of accuracy.

Acknowledgement. The authors affiliated with the Indian Institute of Technology Delhi (BB, SP and SB) acknowledge the support of the Department of Science and Technology, Government of India under the Indian Digital Heritage programme.

References

1. Wu, C.: Towards linear-time incremental structure from motion. In: Proceedings of the International Conference on 3D Vision, 3DV 2013, pp. 127–134 (2013)
2. Agarwal, S., Snavely, N., Seitz, S.M., Szeliski, R.: Bundle adjustment in the large. In: Daniilidis, K., Maragos, P., Paragios, N. (eds.) ECCV 2010, Part II. LNCS, vol. 6312, pp. 29–42. Springer, Heidelberg (2010)
3. Snavely, N., Seitz, S., Szeliski, R.: Modeling the world from internet photo collections. Int. J. Comput. Vis. **80**, 189–210 (2008)
4. Snavely, N., Seitz, S., Szeliski, R.: Photo tourism: exploring photo collections in 3D. In: Proceedings of ACM SIGGRAPH, pp. 835–846 (2006)
5. Crandall, D.J., Owens, A., Snavely, N., Huttenlocher, D.P.: Discrete-continuous optimization for large-scale structure from motion. In: Proceedings of IEEE Conference on Computer Vision and Pattern Recognition, pp. 3001–3008 (2011)
6. Triggs, B., McLauchlan, P.F., Hartley, R.I., Fitzgibbon, A.W.: Bundle adjustment – a modern synthesis. In: Triggs, B., Zisserman, A., Szeliski, R. (eds.) ICCV-WS 1999. LNCS, vol. 1883, pp. 298–372. Springer, Heidelberg (2000)
7. Shi, J., Malik, J.: Normalized cuts and image segmentation. IEEE Trans. Pattern Anal. Mach. Intell. **22**, 888–905 (2000)
8. Wu, C., Agarwal, S., Curless, B., Seitz, S.: Multicore bundle adjustment. In: Proceedings of IEEE Conference on Computer Vision and Pattern Recognition, pp. 3057–3064 (2011)
9. Frahm, J.-M., Fite-Georgel, P., Gallup, D., Johnson, T., Raguram, R., Wu, C., Jen, Y.-H., Dunn, E., Clipp, B., Lazebnik, S., Pollefeys, M.: Building rome on a cloudless day. In: Daniilidis, K., Maragos, P., Paragios, N. (eds.) ECCV 2010, Part IV. LNCS, vol. 6314, pp. 368–381. Springer, Heidelberg (2010)
10. Raghuram, R., Wu, C., Frahm, J., Lazebnik, S.: Modeling and recognition of landmark image collections using iconic scene graphs. Int. J. Comput. Vis. **95**, 213–239 (2011)
11. Agarwal, S., Snavely, N., Simon, I., Seitz, S., Szeliski, R.: Building rome in a day. In: Proceedings of the International Conference on Computer Vision, pp. 72–79 (2009)
12. Snavely, N., Seitz, S., Szeliski, R.: Skeletal graphs for efficient structure from motion. In: Proceedings of IEEE Conference on Computer Vision and Pattern Recognition, pp. 1–8 (2008)
13. Havlena, M., Torii, A., Pajdla, T.: Efficient structure from motion by graph optimization. In: Daniilidis, K., Maragos, P., Paragios, N. (eds.) ECCV 2010, Part II. LNCS, vol. 6312, pp. 100–113. Springer, Heidelberg (2010)
14. Crandall, D.J., Owens, A., Snavely, N., Huttenlocher, D.P.: SfM with MRFs: discrete-continuous optimization for large-scale reconstruction. IEEE Trans. Pattern Anal. Mach. Intell. **35**, 2841–2853 (2013)
15. Moulon, P., Monasse, P., Marlet, R.: Global fusion of relative motions for robust, accurate and scalable structure from motion. In: Proceedings of IEEE International Conference on Computer Vision, pp. 3248–3255 (2013)

16. Jiang, N., Cui, Z., Tan, P.: A global linear method for camera pose registration. In: Proceedings of IEEE International Conference on Computer Vision, pp. 481–488 (2013)
17. Farenzena, M., Fusiello, A., Gherardi, R.: Structure-and-motion pipeline on a hierarchical cluster tree. In: Proceedings of IEEE International Conference on Computer Vision Workshop on 3-D Digital Imaging and Modeling, pp. 1489–1496 (2009)
18. Nister, D., Stewenius, H.: Scalable recognition with a vocabulary tree. In: Proceedings of IEEE Conference on Computer Vision and Pattern Recognition, vol. 2, pp. 2161–2168 (2006)
19. Wu, C.: SiftGPU: a GPU implementation of scale invariant feature transform (SIFT) (2007). http://cs.unc.edu/ccwu/siftgpu
20. Hartley, R., Zisserman, A.: Multiple View Geometry in Computer Vision, 2nd edn. Cambridge University Press, New York (2004)
21. Govindu, V.M.: Lie-algebraic averaging for globally consistent motion estimation. In: Proceedings of IEEE Conference on Computer Vision and Pattern Recognition (2004)
22. Govindu, V.: Combining two-view constraints for motion estimation. In: Proceedings of IEEE Conference on Computer Vision and Pattern Recognition, pp. 218–225 (2001)
23. Lowe, D.: Distinctive image features from scale-invariant keypoints. Int. J. Comput. Vis. **60**, 91–110 (2004)

A Homography Formulation to the 3pt Plus a Common Direction Relative Pose Problem

Olivier Saurer[1], Pascal Vasseur[2], Cedric Demonceaux[3],
and Friedrich Fraundorfer[4]([✉])

[1] ETH, Zürich, Switzerland
[2] LITIS - Université de Rouen, Rouen, France
[3] Le2i, UMR CNRS 6306, Université de Bourgogne, Bourgogne, France
[4] Remote Sensing Technology, Technische Universität München, Munich, Germany
friedrich.fraundorfer@tum.de

Abstract. In this paper we present an alternative formulation for the minimal solution to the 3pt plus a common direction relative pose problem. Instead of the commonly used epipolar constraint we use the homography constraint to derive a novel formulation for the 3pt problem. This formulation allows the computation of the normal vector of the plane defined by the three input points without any additional computation in addition to the standard motion parameters of the camera. We show the working of the method on synthetic and real data sets and compare it to the standard 3pt method and the 5pt method for relative pose estimation. In addition we analyze the degenerate conditions for the proposed method.

1 Introduction

Reducing the number of required points to be matched or to be tracked in order to estimate the egomotion of a visual system can be very interesting in terms of computation time efficiency and of robustness improvement. In the case of an uncallbrated camera, eight points are at least necessary for estimating the fundamental matrix [1] while only five are sufficient in the calibrated case for the essential matrix [2]. It appears clearly that this point number reduction is only possible if some hypotheses or supplementary data are available. For example, some recent works proposed to use only one point to perform a structure from motion method [3] by supposing a non-holonomic motion or to estimate the metric velocity of a single camera [4] in combining with accelerometer and attitude measurements.

In our method, we propose to use a known common direction between two images. Thus, this knowledge of a common direction reduces the number of rotations from three to one. Obtaining a common direction can be performed either by the use of an IMU (Inertial Measurement Unit) or by some information extracted from the images such as vanishing points or horizon. IMUs are nowadays used in many devices such as smart phones or robotic platforms. The coupling with a camera is then very easy and can then be used for different

© Springer International Publishing Switzerland 2015
D. Cremers et al. (Eds.): ACCV 2014, Part II, LNCS 9004, pp. 288–301, 2015.
DOI: 10.1007/978-3-319-16808-1_20

computer vision tasks [5–9]. However, even if a complete rotation is available from an IMU, it appears nevertheless that the heading is generally less accurate than the two other angles [10]. Let us note, in the case of a pure vision approach (without external sensor), this common direction can be obtained by one vanishing point in man made environment [11] or by the detection of the horizon line [12] in the case of natural scene.

Recently, it has been shown that only three points are needed to compute the pose between two cameras if we know a common direction [10,13,14]. This method derives the epipolar constraint to compute the essential matrix with only 3 degrees of freedom. In this paper we propose to use the homography constraint between two views. We show, contrary to the general case where 4 points are needed, that we can compute the pose with only 3 matching points. Let us note, as we need only 3 points in the scene, our method works even if these 3D points do not belong physically to the same plane. Thus the derived formulation using the homography constraint can be used in the same settings as the standard 3pt method using the epipolar constraint.

Moreover, if we assume the existence of a dominant plane in the scene, our method can be included in a RANSAC process in order to estimate the normal of the plane and the pose of the cameras in presence of noise. Compared to the classical algorithm of homography estimation which needs 4 points, we use only 3 points and thus allows to decrease the number of iterations in the RANSAC. Indeed, as presented in Fig. 1, for a probability of success of 0.99 and a rate of outliers equal to 0.5, the number of trials is divided by two for a robust implementation with RANSAC compared to the 4 points algorithm. Using the co-planarity constraint in order to simplify the SFM problem is not new [15,16]. Moreover, if we know roll and pitch of the camera, Saurer et al. [17] prove that we need only 2 points to estimate the full pose of the camera if we also know the normal of the plane. In this paper, we show that only 3 points are needed if roll and pitch angles are known and if the normal is unknown.

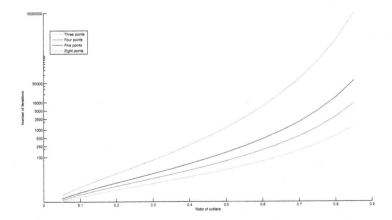

Fig. 1. Comparison of the RANSAC iteration numbers for a 99 % probability of success

2   Related Works

When the camera is not calibrated, at least 8 points are needed to recover the motion [1]. It's now well known that, if this camera is calibrated, only 5 feature points in the scene can be sufficient. Reducing this number of points can be very interesting in order to reduce the computation time and to increase the robustness. To do this, we have to add some hypotheses about the motion of the camera, on the extracted feature points or use supplementary sensors.

For example, if all the 3D points belong on a plane, we need a minimum of 4 points to estimate the motion of the camera between two-views [1]. On the other hand, if the camera is embedded on a mobile robot which moves on a planar surface we need 2 points to recover the motion [18] and if moreover the mobile robot has non-holonomic constraints only one point is necessary [3]. In the same way, if the camera moves in a plane perpendicular to the gravity, Troiani et al. [19] have also shown that one point is enough.

The number of points needed to estimate the ego motion can also be reduced if we have some information about the relative rotation between two poses. This information can be given by vanishing points extraction in the images [20] or in taking into account extra information given by an other sensor. Thus, Li et al. [21] show if we use an IMU mounted to the sensor only 4 points are sufficient to estimate the relative motion even if we don't know the extrinsic calibration between the IMU and the camera.

Similarly, some different algorithms have been recently proposed in order to estimate the relative pose between two cameras by knowing a common direction. We can show that if we know the roll and pitch angles of the camera at each time, we need only three points to recover the yaw angle and the translation of the camera motion [10,13,14]. In these approaches, only the formulation of the problem is different and consequently the way to solve it. All these works start with a simplified essential matrix in order to derive a polynomial equation system. For example, in [10], their parametrization leads to 12 solutions by using the Macaulay matrix method. The good solution has then to be found among this set of solutions. The approach presented in [13] permits to obtain a 4th-order polynomial equation and consequently leads to a more efficient solution. In contrast to the method of [13] the proposed algorithm directly solves for rotation and translation parameters. In [13] the essential matrix is estimated first and to solve for rotation and translation parameters the essential matrix has to be decomposed by an additional step typically involving SVD. In [14], the authors propose a closed-form solution to the 4th-order polynomial equation that allows a faster computation.

If we want to reduce again the number of points, stronger hypotheses have to be added. When the full rotation between the two views are known, we have only 2 degrees of freedom to estimate corresponding to the translation up-to-scale. In this strong hypothesis, 2 points can be use to solve the problem [22]. In this case, the authors compute the translation vector by epipolar geometry with a rotation equal to identity. Thus, these approaches allow to reduce the number of points but the knowledge of the complete rotation between two views makes these

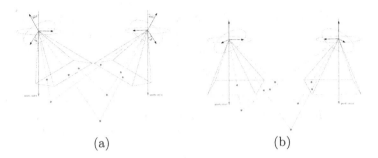

(a)   (b)

Fig. 2. (a) 3D scene with two camera frames in general position. (b) Cameras after de-rotation such that both camera frames are aligned with the vertical direction (gravity direction).

methods really sensitive to IMU accuracy. More recently, Martinelli [23] proposes a closed-form solution for structure from motion knowing the gravity axis of the camera in a multiple views scheme. He shows that we need at least 3 features points belong on a same plane and 3 consecutive views to estimate the motion of the camera. In the same way, the plane constraint has been used for reducing the complexity of the bundle adjustment (BA) in a visual simultaneous localization and mapping (SLAM) embedded on a micro-aerial vehicle (MAV) [24].

In [17] a strong assumption about the environment is made to reduce the number of necessary points for motion estimation. Within the Manhattan world assumption any scene plane is either parallel or vertical to a gravity aligned camera plane. Thus only 2 points are necessary to estimate relative camera pose using a homography formulation. This paper also describes the possibility of propagating relative scale by utilizing the recovered distance to the scene plane used for motion estimation as an alternative to the standard way of propagating scale through 3D reconstruction of feature points. As our proposed method also recovers the distance to scene planes this method for scale propagation can also be used when using our proposed method for motion estimation, in particular when a dominant scene plane is present (e.g. ground plane).

3 Relative Pose with the Knowledge of a Common Direction

Knowing a common direction in images will simplify the estimation of camera pose and camera motion, which are fundamental methods in 3D computer vision. It is then possible to align every camera coordinate system using the known common direction, e.g. aligning them to the vertical direction such that the z-axis of the camera is parallel to the vertical direction and the x-y-plane of the camera is orthogonal to the vertical direction (illustrated in Fig. 2) or any other arbitrary alignment. This alignment can just be done as a coordinate transform for motion estimation algorithms, but also be implemented as image warping such that feature extraction method benefit from it. Relative motion between two such aligned cameras reduces to a 3-DOF motion, which consists of 1 remaining rotation and a 2-DOF translation vector. A general relative pose between two images is represented using the following epipolar constraint

$$p_j^T E p_i = 0, \tag{1}$$

where E is the essential matrix representing a 5-DOF relative pose. Aligning transformations R_i, R_j for the point measurements p_i, p_j can be computed from the known common direction and lead to the aligned measurements q_i, q_j.

$$q_i = R_i p_i \tag{2}$$
$$q_j = R_j p_j \tag{3}$$

This leads to the simplified epipolar constraint

$$q_j^T \hat{E} q_i = 0, \tag{4}$$

where the essential matrix $\hat{E}$ represents the simplified 3-DOF relative pose between the aligned cameras. The general relative pose R, t can then be computed by reversing the alignment with $R = R_j^T \hat{R} R_i$ and $t = R_j^T \hat{t}$.

For the case of points on a plane the relative pose can also be written by using the homography constraint:

$$q_j = H_{ij} q_i \tag{5}$$

The homography is composed of

$$\mathbf{H} = \mathbf{R} - \frac{1}{d} \mathbf{t} \mathbf{n}^T, \tag{6}$$

where $\mathbf{R} = \mathbf{R_z R_y R_x}$ is a rotation matrix representing the relative camera rotations around the x, y, and z-axis, $\mathbf{t} = [t_x, t_y, t_z]^T$ represents the relative motion, $\mathbf{n} = [n_x, n_y, n_z]^T$ is the plane normal and d is the distance from the first camera center to the plane.

For the 3-DOF relative pose between two aligned cameras the homograpy simplifies as well and writes as

$$H_{ij} = R_z - \frac{1}{d} \mathbf{t} \mathbf{n}^T, \tag{7}$$

where R_z is the remaining rotation around a single axis between the aligned cameras.

3.1   Previous Approaches - 3pt Relative Pose Using the Epipolar Constraint

All the previous approaches that solve the 3pt + 1 problem [10, 13, 14] have in common that they utilize the epipolar constraint to set up the equations for relative pose estimation.

$$q_j^T E_{ij} q_i = 0 \tag{8}$$

where E_{ij} is the essential matrix composed of $E_{ij} = [t_{ij}]_\times R_{ij}$.

However, for this case, when only 3 point correspondences are necessary, one can consider to use the homography constraint alternatively. 3 points by definition are always co-planar and form a plane. For any such 3 points the homography constraint will hold. It is therefore possible to use the homography constraint instead of the epipolar constraint to solve the 3pt + 1 problem. In the next section we show the derivation of the solution to this novel idea.

3.2   3pt Relative Pose Using the Homography Constraint

The general homography relation for points belonging to a 3D plane and projected in two different views is defined as follows :

$$q_j = H_{ij}q_i \tag{9}$$

with $q_i = \begin{bmatrix} x_i\ y_i\ w_i \end{bmatrix}^T$ and $q_j = \begin{bmatrix} x_j\ y_j\ w_j \end{bmatrix}^T$ the projective coordinates of the points between the views i and j. H_{ij} is given by :

$$H_{ij} = R_{ij} - \frac{1}{d}\mathbf{t}\mathbf{n}^T \tag{10}$$

where R_{ij} and $\mathbf{t}$ are respectively the rotation and the translation between views i and j and where d is the distance between the camera i and the 3D plane described by the normal $\mathbf{n}$.

In our case, we assume that the camera intrinsic parameters are known and that the points q_i and q_j are normalized. We also consider that the attitude of the cameras for both views are known and that these attitude measurements have been used to align the camera coordinate system with the vertical (gravity) direction. In this way, only the yaw angle θ between the views remains unknown.

$$\mathbf{H} = \mathbf{R_z} - \frac{1}{d}[t_x, t_y, t_z]^T[n_x, n_y, n_z] \tag{11}$$

Without loss of generality Eq. 11 can be written as

$$\mathbf{H} = \mathbf{R_z} - \hat{d}[\hat{t_x}, \hat{t_y}, 1]^T[n_x, n_y, n_z]. \tag{12}$$

In Eq. 12 the scale of the parameter t_z has been included in $\hat{d}$ and thus the z-component of the translation can be set to 1. This reformulation of the parameters proves useful for the used Groebner basis technique for solving the equation system. For the case of very small z-motions this choice could lead to numerical instability but in such cases any other motion direction could be set to 1 instead. However, in practice we did not notice such an instability.

The homography matrix then consists of the following entries:

$$\mathbf{H} = \begin{bmatrix} \cos(\theta) - \hat{d}n_x\hat{t_x} & -\sin(\theta) - \hat{d}n_y\hat{t_x} & -\hat{d}n_z\hat{t_x} \\ \sin(\theta) - \hat{d}n_x\hat{t_y} & \cos(\theta) - \hat{d}n_y\hat{t_y} & -\hat{d}n_z\hat{t_y} \\ -\hat{d}n_x & -\hat{d}n_y & 1 - \hat{d}n_z \end{bmatrix} \tag{13}$$

The unknowns that we are seeking for are the motion parameters $\cos(\theta)$, $\sin(\theta)$, $\hat{d}$, $\hat{t}_x$, $\hat{t}_y$ as well as the plane normals n_x, n_y, n_z of the plane defined by the 3 point correspondences. This is a significant difference to the standard 3pt which does not solve for the plane normals. The proposed 3pt also solves for the plane normals for free.

By utilizing the homography constraints of point correspondences, an equation system to solve for these unknowns can be set up.

$$q_j \times H_{ij} q_i = 0 \qquad (14)$$

In this $\times$ denotes the cross product and by expanding the relation we obtain

$$\begin{bmatrix} w_i y_j - \cos(\theta) w_j y_i - \sin(\theta) w_j x_i - \hat{d} n_z w_i y_j - \hat{d} n_x x_i y_j - \hat{d} n_y y_i y_j + \hat{d} n_z \hat{t}_y w_i w_j + \hat{d} n_x \hat{t}_y w_j x_i + \hat{d} n_y \hat{t}_y w_j y_i \\ \cos(\theta) w_j x_i - w_i x_j - \sin(\theta) w_j y_i + \hat{d} n_z w_i x_j + \hat{d} n_x x_i x_j + \hat{d} n_y x_j y_i - \hat{d} n_z \hat{t}_x w_i w_j - \hat{d} n_x \hat{t}_x w_j x_i - \hat{d} n_y \hat{t}_x w_j y_i \end{bmatrix} = 0$$

$$(15)$$

The third equation being a linear combination of the two others is being omitted.

Each point correspondence gives 2 linearly independent equations and there are two additional quadratic constraints in the unknowns that can be utilized.

$$\cos^2 \theta + \sin^2 \theta - 1 = 0 \qquad (16)$$
$$n_x^2 + n_y^2 + n_z^2 - 1 = 0 \qquad (17)$$

The total number of unknowns is 8 and the two quadratic constraints together with the equations from 3 point correspondences will give a total of 8 polynomial equations in the unknowns. Finding a solution to such a polynomial equation system can be difficult. Most monomials are mixed terms of the unknowns. One way of solving such an equation system in closed form is by using the Groebner basis technique [25]. By computing the Groebner basis a univariate polynomial in a single variable can be found which allows to find the value of this variable by root solving. The remaining variables can then be computed by back-substitution. To solve our problem we utilize the automatic Groebner basis solver by Kukelova et al. [26]. This solver automatically computes Matlab-code to solve for the unknowns of the given polynomial equation system.

The analysis of the Groeber basis solutions shows, that the final univariate polynomial has degree 8, which means that there are up to 8 real solutions to our problem.

3.3   Degenerate Conditions

In this section we discuss the degenerate conditions for the proposed 3pt homography method. The degenerate conditions for the standard 3pt method have been discussed in detail in [10,13,14]. In these papers it is pointed out that a collinear configuration of 3D points is in general not a degenerate condition for the 3pt method, while it is one for the 5pt method. Degenerate conditions for the standard 3pt algorithm however are collinear points that are parallel to the translation direction and points that are coplanar to the translation vector.

We investigated if these scenarios also pose degenerate conditions for the proposed 3pt homography method by conducting experiments with synthetic data. Degenerate cases could be identified by a rank loss of the action matrix within the Groebner basis solver. These tests showed that the proposed method shares the degenerate conditions of the standard 3pt method but in addition also has a degenerate condition for the case of collinear points. This is understandable as the 3pt homography method also solves for the plane normal which then has an undefined degree of freedom around the axis of the collinear points. The results of the comparison are summarized in Table 1.

Table 1. Comparison of the degenerate conditions for the standard 3pt method and the proposed 3pt homography method.

	3pt	3pt-homography
Collinear points	no	yes
Collinear points parallel to translation direction	yes	yes
Points coplanar to translation vector	yes	yes

4 Experiments

The proposed method is evaluated on both synthetic and real datasets.

4.1 Synthetic Evaluation

The synthetic evaluation is conducted under the following setup. Focal length of the camera is 1000 pixel with a field of view of 45 degrees. The first camera is set to the origin of the coordinate frame and kept fixed. The base-line between the first and second camera is set to 0.2 i.e., 20 % of the average scene depth. The scene consists of 200 randomly sampled points. The algorithm is evaluated under varying image noise and increasing IMU noise (roll and pitch) on two configurations, sideways and forward motion of the camera. Each configuration is evaluated on 100 randomly sampled cameras. For the evaluation of the synthetic data we use the following error measure:

- Angle difference in $\mathbf{R}$: $\xi_R = cos^{-1}((Tr(\mathbf{R}\dot{\mathbf{R}}^\top) - 1)/2)$
- Direction difference in $\mathbf{t}$: $\xi_t = cos^{-1}((\mathbf{t}^\top \dot{\mathbf{t}})/(\|\mathbf{t}\|\|\dot{\mathbf{t}}\|))$

Where $\mathbf{R}, \mathbf{t}$ denote the ground-truth transformation and $\dot{\mathbf{R}}, \dot{\mathbf{t}}$ are the corresponding estimated transformations.

Figures 3, 4 compare the 3-point homography based algorithm to the general 5-point [2] and the 3-point algorithms [13]. The evaluation shows that the proposed method outperforms the 5pt algorithm, in terms of accuracy. Under perfect IMU measurements the algorithm is robust to image noise and performs significantly better than the 5pt algorithm and equally good as the 3pt algorithm. With increasing IMU noise the performance of the 3pt and 3pt-homography (proposed) algorithm are still comparable to the 5pt algorithm.

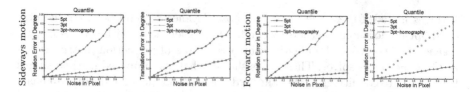

Fig. 3. Evaluation of the 3 point algorithm under varying image noise for two different motion settings (sideways and forward motion)

4.2   Experiments on Real Data with Vicon Ground-Truth

In order to have a practical evaluation of our algorithm, several real datasets have been collected with reliable ground-truth data. The ground-truth data has been obtained by conducting experiments in a room equipped with a Vicon motion capture system made of 22 cameras. Synchronization between visual and ground-truth data has been obtained by a pre-processing step. We used the VICON data as inertial measures and scale factor in the different experiments. The sequences have been acquired with a perspective camera mounted on a mobile robot and on an handheld system in order to have planar and general trajectories. The lengths of these trajectories are between 20 and 50 meters and the number of images are between 200 and 350 per sequence. We propose a comparison with the five-point algorithm and the general three-point algorithm (implemented after [13] in order to prove the efficiency of the proposed method. Both methods use the same matched feature point sets as input and apply RANSAC algorithm in order to select the inliers. For the case of the 5pt algorithm and the standard 3pt algorithm a least squares estimation is performed on the inlier sets for the estimation of the motion parameters, while for the proposed 3pt method this was not possible.

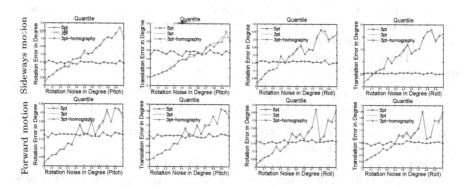

Fig. 4. Evaluation of the 3-point algorithm under different IMU noise and constant image noise of 0.5 pixel standard deviation. First row: sideways motion of the camera with varying pitch angle (left) and varying roll angle (right). Second row: forward motion of the camera with varying pitch angle (left) and varying roll angle (right).

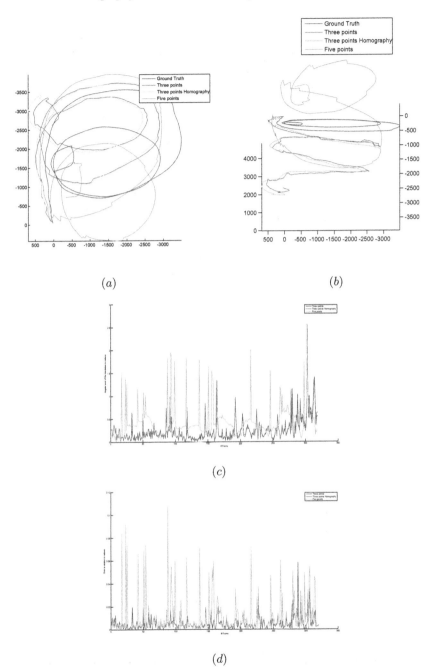

Fig. 5. Results for sequence GT1 - (a) Top view of the trajectories estimated with general three-point (red curve), homography three-point (yellow curve), five-point (green curve) algorithms compared to the Vicon ground-truth (blue curve) (axis in mm) - (b) Side view - (c) Angular error in translation between consecutive frames during the sequence - (d) Rotation error between consecutive frames during the sequence

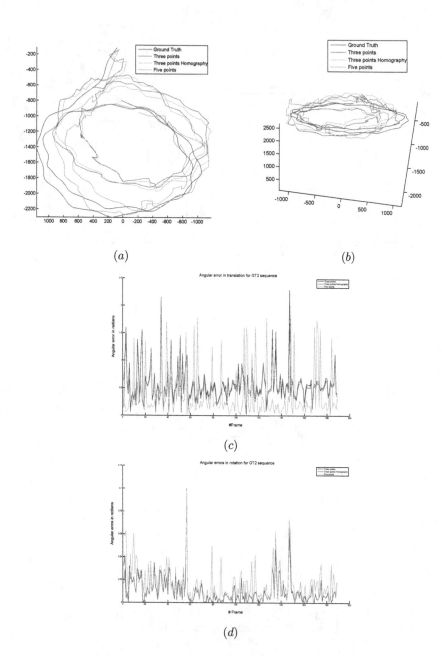

Fig. 6. Results for sequence GT2 - (a) Top view of trajectories estimated with general three-point (red curve), homography three-point (yellow curve), five-point (green curve) algorithms compared with the Vicon ground-truth (blue curve) (axis in mm) - (b) Side view - (c) Angular error in translation between consecutive frames during the sequence - (d) Rotation error between consecutive frames during the sequence

Figure 5 shows the results for the GT1 sequence. For this sequence the camera has been mounted on a mobile robot in forward direction the z-axis of the camera parallel to the ground plane. The robot was mainly moving forward which poses a difficult situation for a visual odometry system. We can note that all the algorithms show trajectories with a strong drift in z direction (height) even if the global shapes of the trajectories are quite similar. The mean angular error of the translation and the mean error of the rotation of consecutive frames during the sequence are respectively equal to 0.2399 and 0.0052 for the general three-point, 0.2455 and 0.0048 for the three-point homography and 0.4302 and 0.0112 for the five-point methods. The details of these errors during the complete sequence are given in Figs. 5 (c) and (d). The three-point homography method presents the best results and also the minimum drift at the end of the motion. Such drift as visible in the plots is typical for visual odometry systems without structure triangulation and local optimization. It is however noticeable that the purely vision based 5pt algorithm has much more difficulties with this sequence than the 3pt methods that use an additional common direction.

Figure 6 shows the results for the GT2 sequence. In this sequence the camera has been handheld, pointing toward the ground in a 45 degree angle and was moved sideways in a circular trajectory. This comprised a less difficult setting than for GT1. In this case, the five-point algorithm presents globally better results but the three-point homography algorithm is better than the general three-point approach. As previously, the details of the rotation and translation errors between consecutive images are given in Figs. 6 (c) and (d). We can note that the rotation error of the three-point homography is smaller than the two other approaches.

5   Conclusion

In this paper we presented a new formulation for the 3pt plus common direction relative pose problem using a homography formulation. We show that it is possible to utilize the homography constraint for an alternative formulation for the 3pt problem. With the same number of input point correspondences the homography formulation also solves for the plane normal in addition to the motion parameters. In experiments with synthetic data and real image sequences we show that the alternative formulation produces similar results to the standard 3pt and also demonstrate that additional information in kind of a common direction allows to get better visual odometry results in certain configurations.

Acknowledgment. This work has been partially supported by Projet ANR Blanc International DrAACaR-ANR-11-IS03-0003 and a Google Award.

References

1. Hartley, R., Zisserman, A.: Multiple View Geometry in Computer Vision, 2nd edn. Cambridge University Press, Cambridge (2004). ISBN: 0521540518

2. Nistér, D.: An efficient solution to the five-point relative pose problem. IEEE Trans. Pattern Anal. Mach. Intell. **26**, 756–777 (2004)

3. Scaramuzza, D.: 1-point-ransac structure from motion for vehicle-mounted cameras by exploiting non-holonomic constraints. Int. J. Comput. Vis. **95**, 74–85 (2011)

4. Kneip, L., Martinelli, A., Weiss, S., Scaramuzza, D., Siegwart, R.: Closed-form solution for absolute scale velocity determination combining inertial measurements and a single feature correspondence. In: IEEE International Conference on Robotics and Automation, ICRA 2011, pp. 4546–4553. Shanghai, China, 9–13 May 2011

5. Viéville, T., Clergue, E., Facao, P.D.S.: Computation of ego-motion and structure from visual and inertial sensors using the vertical cue. In: Proceedings, Fourth International Conference on Computer Vision, pp. 591–598. IEEE (1993)

6. Corke, P.: An inertial and visual sensing system for a small autonomous helicopter. J. Rob. Syst. **21**, 43–51 (2004)

7. Lobo, J., Dias, J.: Vision and inertial sensor cooperation using gravity as a vertical reference. IEEE Trans. Pattern Anal. Mach. Intell. **25**, 1597–1608 (2003)

8. Weiss, S., Siegwart, R.: Real-time metric state estimation for modular vision-inertial systems. In: 2011 IEEE International Conference on Robotics and Automation (ICRA), pp. 4531–4537. IEEE (2011)

9. Domke, J., Aloimonos, Y.: Integration of visual and inertial information for egomotion: a stochastic approach. In: Proceedings 2006 IEEE International Conference on Robotics and Automation. ICRA 2006, pp. 2053–2059. IEEE (2006)

10. Kalantari, M., Hashemi, A., Jung, F., Guédon, J.P.: A new solution to the relative orientation problem using only 3 points and the vertical direction. J. Math. Imaging Vis. **39**, 259–268 (2011)

11. Antone, M.E., Teller, S.J.: Automatic recovery of relative camera rotations for urban scenes. In: CVPR, pp. 2282–2289. IEEE Computer Society (2000)

12. Oreifej, O., da Vitoria Lobo, N., Shah, M.: Horizon constraint for unambiguous uav navigation in planar scenes. In: IEEE International Conference on Robotics and Automation, ICRA 2011, pp. 1159–1165. Shanghai, China, 9–13 May 2011

13. Fraundorfer, F., Tanskanen, P., Pollefeys, M.: A minimal case solution to the calibrated relative pose problem for the case of two known orientation angles. In: Daniilidis, K., Maragos, P., Paragios, N. (eds.) ECCV 2010, Part IV. LNCS, vol. 6314, pp. 269–282. Springer, Heidelberg (2010)

14. Naroditsky, O., Zhou, X.S., Gallier, J.H., Roumeliotis, S.I., Daniilidis, K.: Two efficient solutions for visual odometry using directional correspondence. IEEE Trans. Pattern Anal. Mach. Intell. **34**, 818–824 (2012)

15. Chum, O., Werner, T., Matas, J.: Two-view geometry estimation unaffected by a dominant plane. In: CVPR (1), pp. 772–779. IEEE Computer Society (2005)

16. Szeliski, R., Torr, P.: Geometrically constrained structure from motion: points on planes. In: Koch, R., Van Gool, L. (eds.) SMILE 1998. LNCS, vol. 1506, pp. 171–186. Springer, Heidelberg (1998)

17. Olivier Saurer, F.F., Pollefeys, M.: Homography based visual odometry with known vertical direction and weak manhattan world assumption. In: IEEE/IROS Workshop on Visual Control of Mobile Robots (ViCoMoR 2012) (2012)

18. Ortin, D., Montiel, J.: Indoor robot motion based on monocular images. Robotica **19**, 331–342 (2001)

19. Troiani, C., Martinelli, A., Laugier, C., Scaramuzza, D.: 1-point-based monocular motion estimation for computationally-limited micro aerial vehicles. In: 2013 European Conference on Mobile Robots (ECMR), pp. 13–18. IEEE (2013)

20. Bazin, J.C., Demonceaux, C., Vasseur, P., Kweon, I.: Rotation estimation and vanishing point extraction by omnidirectional vision in urban environment. Int. J. Robot. Res. **31**, 63–81 (2012)
21. Li, B., Heng, L., Lee, G.H., Pollefeys, M.: A 4-point algorithm for relative pose estimation of a calibrated camera with a known relative rotation angle. In: Proceedings of IEEE/RSJ International Conference on Intelligent Robots and Systems, IROS 2013, Tokyo, Japan (2013)
22. Troiani, C., Martinelli, A., Laugier, C., Scaramuzza, D.: 2-point-based outlier rejection for camera-imu systems with applications to micro aerial vehicles. In: IEEE InternationalConference on Robotics and Automation (ICRA), Hong Kong (2014)
23. Martinelli, A.: Closed-form solution of visual-inertial structure from motion. Int. J. Comput. Vis. **106**, 138–152 (2014)
24. Lee, G.H., Fraundorfer, F., Pollefeys, M.: Mav visual slam with plane constraint. In: ICRA, pp. 3139–3144. IEEE (2011)
25. Cox, D.A., Little, J., O'Shea, D.: Ideals, Varieties, and Algorithms: An Introduction to Computational Algebraic Geometry and Commutative Algebra, 3/e (Undergraduate Texts in Mathematics). Springer-Verlag, Secaucus (2007)
26. Kukelova, Z., Bujnak, M., Pajdla, T.: Automatic generator of minimal problem solvers. In: Forsyth, D., Torr, P., Zisserman, A. (eds.) ECCV 2008, Part III. LNCS, vol. 5304, pp. 302–315. Springer, Heidelberg (2008)

MoDeep: A Deep Learning Framework Using Motion Features for Human Pose Estimation

Arjun Jain[⊠], Jonathan Tompson, Yann LeCun, and Christoph Bregler

New York University, New York, USA
{ajain,tompson,yann,bregler}@cs.nyu.edu

Abstract. In this work, we propose a novel and efficient method for articulated human pose estimation in videos using a convolutional network architecture, which incorporates both color and motion features. We propose a new human body pose dataset, *FLIC-motion* (This dataset can be downloaded from http://cs.nyu.edu/~ajain/accv2014/.), that extends the FLIC dataset [1] with additional motion features. We apply our architecture to this dataset and report significantly better performance than current state-of-the-art pose detection systems.

1 Introduction

Human body pose recognition in video is a long-standing problem in computer vision with a wide range of applications. However, body pose recognition remains a challenging problem due to the high dimensionality of the input data and the high variability of possible body poses. Traditionally, computer vision-based approaches tend to rely on appearance cues such as texture patches, edges, color histograms, foreground silhouettes or hand-crafted local features (such as histogram of gradients (HoG) [2]) rather than motion-based features. Alternatively, psychophysical experiments [3] have shown that motion is a powerful visual cue that alone can be used to extract high-level information, including articulated pose.

Previous work [4,5] has reported that using motion features to aid pose inference has had little or no impact on performance. Simply adding high-order temporal connectivity to traditional models would most often lead to intractable inference. In this work we show that deep learning is able to successfully incorporate motion features and is able to out-perform existing state-of-the-art techniques. Further, we show that by using motion features alone our method outperforms [6–8] (see Fig. 9(a) and (b)), which further strengthens our claim that information coded in motion features is valuable and should be used when available.

This paper makes the following contributions:

- A system that successfully incorporates motion-features to enhance the performance of pose-detection 'in-the-wild' compared to existing techniques.
- An efficient and tractable algorithm that achieves close to real-time frame rates, making our method suitable for wide variety of applications.

© Springer International Publishing Switzerland 2015
D. Cremers et al. (Eds.): ACCV 2014, Part II, LNCS 9004, pp. 302–315, 2015.
DOI: 10.1007/978-3-319-16808-1_21

– A new dataset called **FLIC-motion**, which is the FLIC dataset [1] augmented with 'motion-features' for each of the 5003 images collected from Hollywood movies.

2   Prior Work

Geometric Model Based Tracking: One of the earliest works on articulated tracking in video was Hogg [9] in 1983 using edge features and a simple cylinder based body model. Several other model based articulated tracking systems have been reported over the past two decades, most notably [10–16]. The models used in these systems were explicit 2D or 3D jointed geometric models. Most systems had to be hand-initialized (except [12]), and focused on incrementally updating pose parameters from one frame to the next. More complex examples come from the HumanEva dataset competitions [17] that use video or higher-resolution shape models such as SCAPE [18] and extensions. We refer the reader to [19] for a complete survey of this era. Most recently such techniques have been shown to create very high-resolution animations of detailed body and cloth deformations [20–22]. Our approach differs, since we are dealing with single view videos in unconstrained environments.

Statistical Based Recognition: One of the earliest systems that used no explicit geometric model was reported by Freeman et al. in 1995 [23] using oriented angle histograms to recognize hand configurations. This was the precursor for the bag-of-features, SIFT [24], STIP [25], HoG, and Histogram of Flow (HoF) [26] approaches that boomed a decade later, most notably including the work by Dalal and Triggs in 2005 [2]. Different architectures have since been proposed, including "shape-context" edge-based histograms from the human body [27,28] or just silhouette features [29]. Shakhnarovich et al. [30] learn a parameter sensitive hash function to perform example-based pose estimation. Many techniques have been proposed that extract, learn, or reason over entire body features, using a combination of local detectors and structural reasoning (see [31] for coarse tracking and [32] for person-dependent tracking).

Though the idea of using "Pictorial Structures" by Fischler and Elschlager [33] has been around since the 1970s, matching them efficiently to images has only been possible since the famous work on 'Deformable Part Models' (DPM) by Felzenszwalb et al. [34] in 2008. Many algorithms that use DPM for creating the body part unary distribution [6,7,35,36] with spatial-models incorporating body-part relationship priors have since then been developed. Johnson and Everingham [37], who also proposed the 'Leeds Sports Database', employ a cascade of body part detectors to obtain more discriminative templates. Almost all best performing algorithms since have solely built on HoG and DPM for local evidence, and yet more sophisticated spatial models. Pishchulin [38] proposes a model that augments the DPM unaries with *Poselet* conditioned [39] priors. Sapp and Taskar [1] propose a model where they cluster images in the pose-space and then find the mode which best describes the input image. The pose of this mode then acts as a strong spatial prior, whereas the local evidence is again based on HoG and gradient features. Following the *Poselets* approach [39], the *Armlets* approach by Gkioxari et al. [40] incorporates edges, contours, and color histograms in addition to the HoG features. They employ a semi-global classifier for part configuration and show good performance on real-world data. However, they only show their results on arms. The major drawback of all these approaches is that both the local evidence and the global structure is hand crafted, whereas we jointly learn both the local features and the global structure using a multi-resolution convolutional network.

Shotton et al. [41] use an ensemble of random trees to perform per-pixel labeling of body parts in depth images. As a means of reducing overall system latency and avoiding repeated false detections, their work focuses on pose inference using only a single depth image. By contrast, we extend the single frame requirement to at least 2 frames (which we show considerably improves pose inference), and our input domain is unconstrained RGB images rather than depth.

Pose Detection Using Image Sequences:

Deep Learning Based Techniques: Recently, state-of-the-art performance has been reported on many vision tasks using deep learning algorithms [42–47]. References [48–50] also apply neural networks for pose recognition, specifically Toshev et al. [48] show better than state-of-the-art performance on the 'FLIC' and 'LSP' [51] datasets. In contrast to Toshev et al., in our work we propose a translation invariant model which improves upon their method, especially in the high-precision region.

3   Body-Part Detection Model

We propose a Convolutional Network (ConvNet) architecture for the task of estimating the 2D location of human joints in video (Sect. 3.2). The input to the network is an RGB image and a set of *motion features*. We investigate a wide variety of motion feature formulations (Sect. 3.1). Finally, we will also introduce a simple Spatial-Model to solve a specific sub-problem associated with evaluation of our model on the FLIC-motion dataset (Sect. 3.3).

3.1   Motion Features

The aim of this section is to incorporate features that are representative of the true *motion-field* (the perspective projection of the 3D velocity-field of moving surfaces) as input to our detection network so that it can exploit motion as a cue for body part localization. To this end, we evaluate and analyze four motion features which fall under two broad categories: those using simple derivatives of the RGB video frames and those using optical flow features. For each RGB image pair f_i and $f_{i+\delta}$, we propose the following features:

- RGB image pair - $\{f_i, f_{i+\delta}\}$
- RGB image and an RGB difference image - $\{f_i, f_{i+\delta} - f_i\}$

- Optical-flow[1] vectors - $\{f_i, \text{FLOW}(f_i, f_{i+\delta})\}$
- Optical-flow magnitude - $\{f_i, \|\text{FLOW}(f_i, f_{i+\delta})\|_2\}$

The RGB image pair is by far the simplest way of incorporating the relative motion information between the two frames. However, this representation clearly suffers from a lot of redundancy (i.e. if there is no camera movement) and is extremely high dimensional. Furthermore, it is not obvious to the deep network what changes in this high dimensional input space are relevant temporal information and what changes are due to noise or camera motion. A simple modification to this representation is to use a difference image, which reformulates the RGB input so that the algorithm sees directly the pixel locations where high energy corresponds to motion (alternatively the network would have to do this implicitly on the image pair). A more sophisticated representation is optical-flow, which is considered to be a high-quality approximation of the true *motion-field*. Implicitly learning to infer optical-flow from the raw RGB input would be non-trivial for the network to estimate, so we perform optical-flow calculation as a pre-processing step (at the cost of greater computational complexity).

FLIC-motion Dataset: We propose a new dataset which we call **FLIC-motion**[2]. It is comprised of the original FLIC dataset of 5003 labeled RGB images collected from 30 Hollywood movies, of which 1016 images are held out as a test set, augmented with the aforementioned motion features.

We experimented with different values for δ and investigated the above features with and without camera motion compensation; we use a simple 2D projective motion model between f_i and $f_{i+\delta}$, and warp $f_{i+\delta}$ onto f_i using the inverse of this best fitting projection to approximately remove camera motion. A comparison between image pairs with and without warping can be seen in Fig 1.

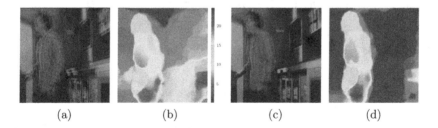

(a)   (b)   (c)   (d)

Fig. 1. Results of optical-flow computation: (a) average of frame pair, (b) optical flow on (a), (c) average of frame pair after camera compensation, and (d) optical-flow on (c)

To obtain $f_{i+\delta}$, we must know where the frames f_i occur in each movie. Unfortunately, this was non-trivial as the authors Sapp et al. [1] could not provide

---

[1] We use the algorithm proposed by Weinzaepfel et al. [47] to compute optical-flow.
[2] This dataset can be downloaded from http://cs.nyu.edu/~ajain/accv2014/.

us with the exact version of the movie that was used for creating the original dataset. Corresponding frames can be very different in multiple versions of the same movie (4:3 vs wide-screen, director's cut, special editions, etc.). We estimate the best similarity transform S between f_i and each frame f_j^m from the movie m, and if the distance $|f_i - Sf_j^m|$ is below a certain threshold (10 pixels), we conclude that we found the correct frame. We visually confirm the resulting matches and manually pick frames for which the automatic matching was unsuccessful (e.g. when enough feature points were not found).

3.2   Convolutional Network

Recent work [48,49] has shown ConvNet architectures are well suited for the task of human body pose detection, and due to the availability of modern Graphics Processing Units (GPUs), we can perform Forward Propagation (FPROP) of deep ConvNet architectures at interactive frame-rates. Similarly, we realize our detection model as a deep ConvNet architecture. The input is a 3D tensor containing an RGB image and its corresponding motion features, and the output is a 3D tensor containing *response-maps*, with one response-map for each joint. Each response-map describes the per-pixel energy for the presence of the corresponding joint at that pixel location.

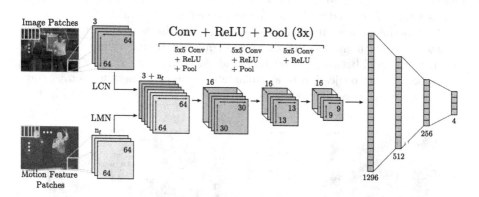

Fig. 2. Sliding-window with image and flow patches

Our ConvNet is based on a *sliding-window* architecture. A simplified version of this architecture is shown in Fig. 2. The input patches are first normalized using Local Contrast Normalization (LCN [52]) for the RGB channels and a new normalization method for the motion features we call *Local Motion Normalization* (LMN). We formulate LMN as the local subtraction with the response from a Gaussian kernel with large standard deviation followed by a divisive normalization. The result is that it removes some unwanted background camera motion as well as normalizing the local intensity of motion (which helps improve network generalization for motions of varying velocity but with similar pose). Prior to processing through the convolution stages, the normalized motion channels are concatenated along the feature dimension with the normalized RGB channels, and the resulting tensor is processed though 3 stages of convolution.

The first two convolution stages use rectified linear units (ReLU) and Max-pooling, and the last stage incorporates a single ReLU layer. The output of the last convolution stage is then passed to a three stage fully-connected neural-network. The network is then applied to all 64 × 64 sub-windows of the image, stepped every 4 pixels horizontally and vertically. This produces a dense response-map output, one for each joint. The major advantage of this model is that the learned detector is translation invariant by construction.

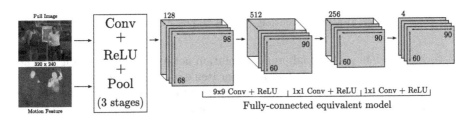

Fig. 3. Efficient sliding window model

Because the layers are convolutional, applying two instances of the network in Fig. 2 to two overlapping input windows leads to a considerable amount of redundant computation. Recent work [53,54] eliminates this redundancy and thus yields a dramatic speed up. This is achieved by applying each layer of the convolutional network to the entire input image. The fully connected layers for each window are also replicated for all sub-windows of the input. This formulation allows us to back-propagate though this network for all windows simultaneously. Due to the two 2 × 2 subsampling layers, we obtain one output vector every 4 × 4 input pixels. An equivalent efficient version of the sliding window model is shown in Fig. 3.

Note that an alternative model (such as in Tompson et al. [50]) would replace the last 3 convolutional layers with a fully-connected neural network whose input context is the feature activations for the entire input image. Such a model would be appropriate if we knew a priori that there existed a strong correlation between skeletal pose and the position of the person in the input frame since this alternative model is not invariant with respect to the translation of the person within the image. However, the FLIC dataset has no such strong pose-location bias (i.e. a subject's torso is not always in the same location in the image), and therefore a sliding-window based architecture is more appropriate for our task.

We extend the single resolution ConvNet architecture of Fig. 3 by incorporating a *multi-resolution* input. We do so by down-sampling the input (using appropriate anti-aliasing), and then each resolution image is processed through either a LCN or LMN layer using the same normalization kernels for each bank producing an approximate Laplacian pyramid. The role of the Laplacian Pyramid is to provide each bank with non-overlapping spectral content which minimizes

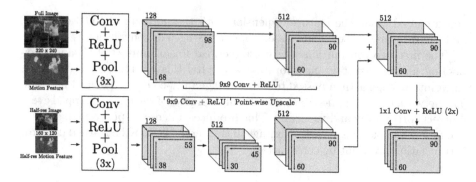

Fig. 4. Multi-resolution efficient sliding window model

network redundancy. Our final, multi-resolution network is shown in Fig. 4. The outputs of the convolution banks are concatenated (along the feature dimension) by point-wise up-scaling of the lower resolution bank to bring the feature maps into canonical resolution. Note that in our final implementation we use 3 resolution banks.

We train the Part-Detector network using supervised learning via Back Propagation and Stochastic Gradient Descent. We minimize a mean squared error criterion for the distance between the inferred response-map activation and a ground truth response-map, which is a 2D Gaussian distribution centered at the target joint location and with small standard deviation (1px). We use Nesterov momentum to reduce training time [55] and we randomly perturb the input images each epoch by randomly flipping and scaling the images to prevent network overtraining and improve generalization performance.

3.3 Simple Spatial Model

Our model is evaluated on our new FLIC-motion dataset (Sect. 3.1). As per the original FLIC dataset, the test images in FLIC-motion may contain multiple people, however, only a single actor per frame is labeled in the test set. As such, a rough torso location of the labeled person is provided at test time to help locate the "correct" person. We incorporate this information by means of a simple and efficient Spatial-Model.

The inclusion of this stage has two major advantages. Firstly, the correct feature activation from the Part-Detector output is selected for the person for whom a ground-truth label was annotated. An example of this is shown in Fig. 5. Secondly, since the joint locations of each part are constrained in proximity to the single ground-truth torso location, then (indirectly) the connectivity between joints is also constrained, enforcing that inferred poses are anatomically viable (i.e. the elbow joint and the shoulder joint cannot be to far away from the torso, which in turn enforces spatial locality between the elbow and shoulder joints).

The core of our Spatial-Model is an empirically calculated *joint-mask*, shown in Fig. 5(b). The joint-mask layer describes the possible joint locations, given

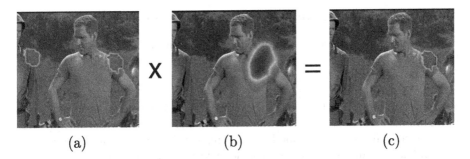

Fig. 5. Simple spatial model used to mask-out the incorrect shoulder activations given a 2D torso position

that the supplied torso position is in the center of the mask. To create a mask layer for body part A, we first calculate the empirical histogram of the part A location, x_A, relative to the torso position x_T for the training set examples; i.e. $x_{\text{hist}} = x_A - x_T$. We then turn this histogram into a Boolean mask by setting the mask amplitude to 1 for pixels for which $p(x_{\text{hist}}) > 0$. Finally, we blur the mask using a wide Gaussian low-pass filter which accounts for body part locations not represented in the training set (but which might be present in the test set).

During test time, this joint-mask is shifted to the ground-truth torso location and the per-pixel energy from the Part-Model (Sect. 3.2) is then multiplied with the mask to produce a filtered output. This process is carried out for each body part independently.

It should be noted that while this Spatial-Model does enforce some anatomic consistency, it does have limitations. Notably, we expect it to fail for datasets where the range of poses is not as constrained as the FLIC dataset (which is primarily front facing and standing up poses).

4   Results

Training time for our model on the FLIC-motion dataset (3957 training set images, 1016 test set images) is approximately 12 hours, and FPROP of a single image takes approximately 50 ms[3]. For our models that use optical flow as a motion feature input, the most expensive part of our pipeline is the optical flow calculation, which takes approximately 1.89 s per image pair. (We plan to investigate real-time flow estimations in the future).

Section 4.1 compares the performance of the motion features from Sect. 3.1. Section 4.2 compares our architecture with other techniques and shows that our system significantly outperforms existing state-of-the-art techniques. Note that for all experiments in Sect. 4.1 we use a smaller model with 16 convolutional features in the first 3 layers. A model with 128 instead of 16 features for the first 3 convolutional layers is used for results in Sect. 4.2.

---

[3] Analysis of our system was on a 12 core workstation with an NVIDIA Titan GPU.

4.1   Comparison and Analysis of Proposed Motion Features

Figure 6 shows a selection of example images from the FLIC test set which highlights the importance of using motion features for body pose detection. In Fig. 6(a), the elbow position is occluded by the actor's sling, and no such examples exist in the training set; however, the presence of body motion provides a strong cue for elbow location. Figure 6(b) and (d) have extremely cluttered backgrounds and the correct joint location is locally similar to the surrounding region (especially for the camouflaged clothing in Fig. 6(d)). For these images, motion features are essential in correct joint localization. Finally, Fig. 6(c) is an example where motion blur (due to fast joint motion) reduces the fidelity of RGB edge features, which results in incorrect localization when motion features are not used.

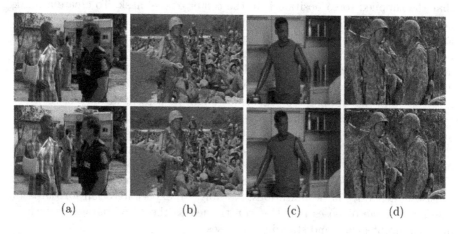

(a)   (b)   (c)   (d)

Fig. 6. Predicted joint positions on the FLIC test-set. Top row: detection with motion features (L2 motion flow). Bottom row: without motion features (baseline).

Figure 7(a) and (b) show the performance of the motion features of Sect. 3.1 on the FLIC-motion dataset for the Elbow and Wrist joints respectively. For evaluating our test-set performance, we use the criterion proposed by Sapp et al. [1]. We count the percentage of the test-set images where joint predictions are within a given radius that is normalized to a 100 pixel torso size. Surprisingly, even the simple frame-difference temporal feature improves upon the baseline result (which we define as a single RGB frame input) and even outperforms the 2D optical flow input (see Fig. 6(b) inset).

Note that stable and accurate calculation of optical-flow from arbitrary RGB videos is a very challenging problem. Therefore, incorporating motion flow features as input to the network adds non-trivial localization cues that would be very difficult for the network to learn internally with limited learning capacity. Therefore, it is expected that the best performing networks in Fig. 7 are those that incorporate motion flow features. However, it is surprising that using the magnitude of the flow vectors performs as well as - and in some cases outperforms - the full 2D motion flow. Even though the input data is richer, we hypothesize that when using 2D flow vectors the network must learn invariance to the direction of joint movement; for instance, the network should predict the same head position whether a person is turning his/her head to the left or right on the next frame. On the other hand, when the L2 magnitude of the flow vector is used, the network sees the high velocity motion cue but cannot over-train to the direction of the movement.

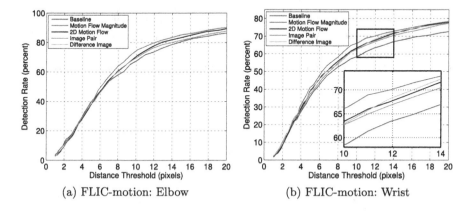

(a) FLIC-motion: Elbow   (b) FLIC-motion: Wrist

Fig. 7. Model performance for various motion features

Figure 8(a) shows that the performance of our network is relatively agnostic to the frame separation (δ) between the samples for which we calculate motion flow; the average precision between 0 and 20 pixel radii degrades 3.9 % from -10 pixels offset to -1 pixel offset. A frame difference of 10 corresponds to approximately 0.42 s (at 24fps), and so we expect that large motions over this time period would result in complex non-linear trajectories in input space for which a single finite difference approximation of the pixel velocity would be inaccurate. Accordingly, our results show that performance indeed degrades as a larger frame step is used.

Similarly, we were surprised that our camera motion compensation technique (described in Sect. 3.1) does not help to the extent that we expected, as shown in Fig. 8(b). Likely this is because either LMN removes a lot of constant background motion or the network is able to learn to ignore the remaining foreground-background parallax motion due to camera movement.

4.2   Comparison with Other Techniques

Figure 9(a) and (b) compares the performance of our system with other state-of-the-art models on the FLIC dataset for the elbow and wrist joints respectively.

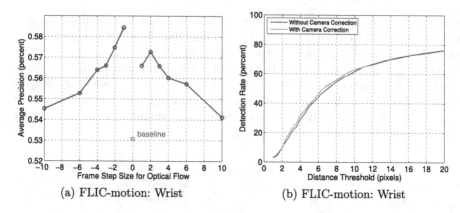

(a) FLIC-motion: Wrist   (b) FLIC-motion: Wrist

Fig. 8. Model performance for (a) varying motion feature frame offsets (b) with and without camera motion compensation

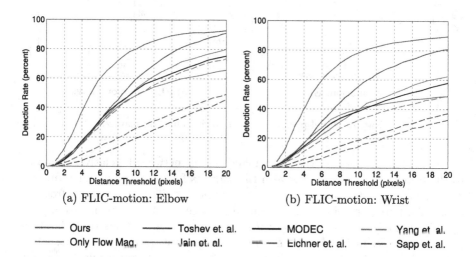

(a) FLIC-motion: Elbow   (b) FLIC-motion: Wrist

Fig. 9. Our model performance compared with our model using only flow magnitude features (no RGB image), Toshev et al. [48], Jain et al. [49], MODEC [1], Eichner et al. [6], Yang et al. [7] and Sapp et al. [8].

Our detector is able to significantly outperform all prior techniques on this challenging dataset. Note that using only motion features already outperforms [6–8]. Also note that using only motion features is less accurate than using a combination of motion features and RGB images, especially in the high accuracy region. This is because fine details such as eyes and noses are missing in motion features. Toshev et al. [48] suffers from inaccuracy in the high-precision region, which we attribute to inefficient direct regression of pose vectors from images. MODEC [1], Eichner et al. [6] and Sapp et al. [8] build on hand crafted HoG features. They all suffer from the limitations of HoG (i.e. they all discard color information, etc.). Jain et al. [49] do not use multi-scale information and evaluate their model in a sliding window fashion, whereas we use the 'one-shot' approach. Finally, we believe that increasing the complexity of our simple spatial model will improve performance of our model, specifically for large radii.

5 Conclusion

We have shown that when incorporating both RGB and motion features in our deep ConvNet architecture, our network is able to outperform existing state-of-the-art techniques for the task of human body pose detection in video. We have also shown that using motion features alone can outperform some traditional algorithms [6–8]. Our findings suggest that even very simple temporal cues can greatly improve performance with a very minor increase in model complexity. As such, we suggest that future work should place more emphasis on the correct use of motion features. We would also like to further explore higher level temporal features, potentially via learned spatiotemporal convolution stages and we hope that using a more expressive temporal-spatial model (using motion constraints) will help improve performance significantly.

Acknowledgments. The authors would like to thank Tyler Zhu for his help with the data-set creation. This research was funded in part by the Office of Naval Research ONR Award N000141210327.

References

1. Sapp, B., Taskar, B.: Modec: multimodal decomposable models for human pose estimation. In: CVPR (2013)
2. Dalal, N., Triggs, B.: Histograms of oriented gradients for human detection. In: CVPR (2005)
3. Johansson, G.: Visual perception of biological motion and a model for its analysis. Percept. Psychophys. **14**, 201–211 (1973)
4. Ferrari, V., Marin-Jimenez, M., Zisserman, A.: Progressive search space reduction for human pose estimation. In: CVPR (2008)
5. Weiss, D., Sapp, B., Taskar, B.: Sidestepping intractable inference with structured ensemble cascades. In: NIPS (2010)
6. Eichner, M., Ferrari, V.: Better appearance models for pictorial structures. In: BMVC (2009)
7. Yang, Y., Ramanan, D.: Articulated pose estimation with flexible mixtures-of-parts. In: CVPR (2011)
8. Sapp, B., Toshev, A., Taskar, B.: Cascaded models for articulated pose estimation. In: Daniilidis, K., Maragos, P., Paragios, N. (eds.) ECCV 2010, Part II. LNCS, vol. 6312, pp. 406–420. Springer, Heidelberg (2010)
9. Hogg, D.: Model-based vision: a program to see a walking person. Image Vis. Comput. **1**, 5–20 (1983)
10. Rehg, J.M., Kanade, T.: Model-based tracking of self-occluding articulated objects. In: Computer Vision (1995)

11. Kakadiaris, I.A., Metaxas, D.: Model-based estimation of 3d human motion with occlusion based on active multi-viewpoint selection. In: CVPR (1996)
12. Wren, C.R., Azarbayejani, A., Darrell, T., Pentland, A.P.: Pfinder: Real-time tracking of the human body. IEEE Trans. Pattern Anal. Mach. Intell. **19**, 780–785 (1997)
13. Bregler, C., Malik, J.: Tracking people with twists and exponential maps. In: CVPR (1998)
14. Deutscher, J., Blake, A., Reid, I.: Articulated body motion capture by annealed particle filtering. In: CVPR (2000)
15. Sidenbladh, H., Black, M.J., Fleet, D.J.: Stochastic tracking of 3D human figures using 2D image motion. In: Vernon, D. (ed.) ECCV 2000. LNCS, vol. 1843, pp. 702–718. Springer, Heidelberg (2000)
16. Sminchisescu, C., Triggs, B.: Covariance scaled sampling for monocular 3d body tracking. In: CVPR (2001)
17. Sigal, L., Balan, A., Black, M.J.: HumanEva: synchronized video and motion capture dataset and baseline algorithm for evaluation of articulated human motion. Int. J. Comput. Vis. **87**, 4–27 (2010)
18. Anguelov, D., Srinivasan, P., Koller, D., Thrun, S., Rodgers, J., Davis, J.: Scape: shape completion and animation of people. In: TOG (2005)
19. Poppe, R.: Vision-based human motion analysis: an overview. Compu. Vis. Image Underst. **108**, 4–18 (2007)
20. De Aguiar, E., Stoll, C., Theobalt, C., Ahmed, N., Seidel, H.P., Thrun, S.: Performance capture from sparse multi-view video. ACM Trans. Graph. **27**, 1–9 (2008)
21. Jain, A., Thormählen, T., Seidel, H.P., Theobalt, C.: Moviereshape: tracking and reshaping of humans in videos. In: TOG (2010)
22. Stoll, C., Hasler, N., Gall, J., Seidel, H., Theobalt, C.: Fast articulated motion tracking using a sums of gaussians body model. In: ICCV (2011)
23. Freeman, W.T., Roth, M.: Orientation histograms for hand gesture recognition. In: International Workshop on Automatic Face and Gesture Recognition (1995)
24. Lowe, D.G.: Distinctive image features from scale-invariant keypoints. Int. J. Comput. Vis. **60**, 91–110 (2004)
25. Laptev, I.: On space-time interest points. Int. J. Comput. Vis. **64**, 107–123 (2005)
26. Dalal, N., Triggs, B., Schmid, C.: Human detection using oriented histograms of flow and appearance. In: Leonardis, A., Bischof, H., Pinz, A. (eds.) ECCV 2006. LNCS, vol. 3952, pp. 428 441. Springer, Heidelberg (2006)
27. Mori, G., Malik, J.: Estimating human body configurations using shape context matching. In: Heyden, A., Sparr, G., Nielsen, M., Johansen, P. (eds.) ECCV 2002. LNCS, vol. 2352, pp. 666–680. Springer, Heidelberg (2002)
28. Agarwal, A., Triggs, B., Rhone-Alpes, I., Montbonnot, F.: Recovering 3D human pose from monocular images. IEEE Trans. Pattern Anal. Mach. Intell. **28**, 44–58 (2006)
29. Grauman, K., Shakhnarovich, G., Darrell, T.: Inferring 3d structure with a statistical image-based shape model. In: ICCV (2003)
30. Shakhnarovich, G., Viola, P., Darrell, T.: Fast pose estimation with parameter-sensitive hashing. In: ICCV (2003)
31. Ramanan, D., Forsyth, D., Zisserman, A.: Strike a pose: Tracking people by finding stylized poses. In: CVPR (2005)
32. Buehler, P., Zisserman, A., Everingham, M.: Learning sign language by watching TV (using weakly aligned subtitles) (2009)
33. Fischler, M.A., Elschlager, R.: The representation and matching of pictorial structures. IEEE Trans. Comput. **22**, 67–92 (1973)

34. Felzenszwalb, P., McAllester, D., Ramanan, D.: A discriminatively trained, multi-scale, deformable part model. In: CVPR (2008)
35. Andriluka, M., Roth, S., Schiele, B.: Pictorial structures revisited: people detection and articulated pose estimation. In: CVPR (2009)
36. Dantone, M., Gall, J., Leistner, C., Gool., L.V.: Human pose estimation using body parts dependent joint regressors. In: CVPR (2013)
37. Johnson, S., Everingham, M.: Learning effective human pose estimation from inaccurate annotation. In: CVPR (2011)
38. Pishchulin, L., Andriluka, M., Gehler, P., Schiele, B.: Poselet conditioned pictorial structures. In: CVPR (2013)
39. Bourdev, L., Malik, J.: Poselets: body part detectors trained using 3d human pose annotations. In: ICCV (2009)
40. Gkioxari, G., Arbelaez, P., Bourdev, L., Malik, J.: Articulated pose estimation using discriminative armlet classifiers. In: CVPR (2013)
41. Shotton, J., Sharp, T., Kipman, A., Fitzgibbon, A., Finocchio, M., Blake, A., Cook, M., Moore, R.: Real-time human pose recognition in parts from single depth images. ACM (2013)
42. Zeiler, M., R., F.: Visualizing and understanding convolutional neural networks. In: arXiv preprint arXiv:1311.2901. (2013)
43. Razavian, A.S., Azizpour, H., Sullivan, J., Carlsson, S.: Cnn features off-the-shelf: an astounding baseline for recognition (2014)
44. Yaniv Taigman, Ming Yang, M.R., Wolf, L.: Deepface: closing the gap to human-level performance in face verification. In: CVPR (2014)
45. Deng, L., Abdel-Hamid, O., Yu, D.: A deep convolutional neural network using heterogeneous pooling for trading acoustic invariance with phonetic confusion. In: ICASSP (2013)
46. Sermanet, P., Kavukcuoglu, K., Chintala, S., LeCun, Y.: Pedestrian detection with unsupervised multi-stage feature learning. In: CVPR (2013)
47. Weinzaepfel, P., Revaud, J., Harchaoui, Z., Schmid, C.: Deepflow: large displacement optical flow with deep matching. In: ICCV (2013)
48. Toshev, A., Szegedy, C.: Deeppose: Human pose estimation via deep neural networks. In: CVPR (2014)
49. Jain, A., Tompson, J., Andriluka, M., Taylor, G., Bregler, C.: Learning human pose estimation features with convolutional networks. In: ICLR (2014)
50. Tompson, J., Stein, M., LeCun, Y., Perlin, K.: Real-time continuous pose recovery of human hands using convolutional networks. In: TOG (2014)
51. Johnson, S., Everingham, M.: Clustered pose and nonlinear appearance models for human pose estimation. In: BMVC (2010)
52. Collobert, R., Kavukcuoglu, K., Farabet, C.: Torch7: a matlab-like environment for machine learning. In: BigLearn, NIPS Workshop (2011)
53. Giusti, A., Ciresan, D.C., Masci, J., Gambardella, L.M., Schmidhuber, J.: Fast image scanning with deep max-pooling convolutional neural networks. In: CoRR (2013)
54. Sermanet, P., Eigen, D., Zhang, X., Mathieu, M., Fergus, R., LeCun, Y.: Overfeat: Integrated recognition, localization and detection using convolutional networks. In: ICLR (2014)
55. Sutskever, I., Martens, J., Dahl, G., Hinton, G.: On the importance of initialization and momentum in deep learning. In: ICML (2013)

Accelerating Cost Volume Filtering Using Salient Subvolumes and Robust Occlusion Handling

Mohamed A. Helala$^{(\boxtimes)}$ and Faisal Z. Qureshi

Faculty of Science, University of Ontario Institute of Technology,
Oshawa, ON, Canada
{Mohamed.Helala,Faisal.Qureshi}@uoit.ca

Abstract. Several fundamental computer vision problems, such as depth estimation from stereo, optical flow computation, etc., can be formulated as a discrete pixel labeling problem. Traditional Markov Random Fields (MRF) based solutions to these problems are computationally expensive. Cost Volume Filtering (CF) presents a compelling alternative. Still these methods must filter the entire cost volume to arrive at a solution. In this paper, we propose a new CF method for depth estimation by stereo. First, we propose the Accelerated Cost Volume Filtering (ACF) method which identifies salient subvolumes in the cost volume. Filtering is restricted to these subvolumes, resulting in significant performance gains. The proposed method does not consider the entire cost volume and results in a marginal increase in unlabeled (occluded) pixels. We address this by developing an Occlusion Handling (OH) technique, which uses superpixels and performs label propagation via a simulated annealing inspired method. We evaluate the proposed method (ACF+OH) on the Middlebury stereo benchmark and on high resolution images from Middlebury 2005/2006 stereo datasets, and our method achieves state-of-the-art results. Our occlusion handling method, when used as a post-processing step, also significantly improves the accuracy of two recent cost volume filtering methods.

1 Introduction

Computing dense depth maps from a pair of stereo images is one of the fundamental problems in computer vision. In the last few years, several pixel-labeling techniques have been proposed to estimate depth maps from a pair of stereo images [3]. The goal here is to assign a depth value (or label) to each pixel, given a pair of stereo images. Pixel labeling problems are typically cast within an optimization framework, where the cost is defined for assigning a label $l \in L$ to a pixel $p \in P$. The solution to the labeling assignment problem $f : L \to P$ is then found by minimizing the overall assignment cost. Often times the desired solution is (i) spatially smooth, (ii) obeys label costs and (iii) preserves the discontinuities at image edges. Markov Random Fields (MRFs) provide a robust framework for modeling such labeling problems [5]. Overall assignment cost is modeled as an energy function that accounts for both assigning a label to a particular pixel

© Springer International Publishing Switzerland 2015
D. Cremers et al. (Eds.): ACCV 2014, Part II, LNCS 9004, pp. 316–331, 2015.
DOI: 10.1007/978-3-319-16808-1_22

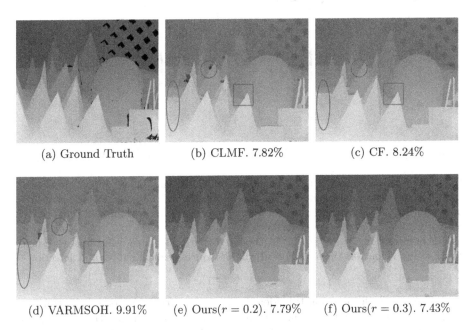

(a) Ground Truth   (b) CLMF. 7.82%   (c) CF. 8.24%

(d) VARMSOH. 9.91%   (e) Ours($r = 0.2$). 7.79%   (f) Ours($r = 0.3$). 7.43%

Fig. 1. Comparison on Middlebury Cones dataset [1]: (a) Ground truth, (b) CLMF [2], (c) CF [3], (d) VARMSOH [4], and (e,f) our method ACF+OH. r determines the size of local windows during salient subvolume detection. For $r = 2$, ACF+OH achieves 2.2 speedup over CF, and for $r = 3$, ACF+OH achieves 1.7 times speedup over CF. Percentage errors shown next to each figure are calculated using the default error threshold of 1.0. Ellipses and squares in CLMF, CF and VARMSOH indicate regions that exhibit large errors.

and assigning a label pair to a pair of neighboring pixels. The pairwise term enforces spatially smooth, edge-aligned solutions. Standard energy minimization inference algorithms, such as graph cut [6] and belief propagation [7–9] yield acceptable results; however, these schemes are computationally expensive and do not fare well when dealing with large label sets or high-resolution images.

Recently local filtering methods [2,3,10] have been developed as an alternative to energy-based approaches. These filtering methods are designed to achieve (spatially) locally smooth label assignments, as opposed to globally smooth label assignments in the case of MRFs. Despite this simplifying assumption, recent work shows that filtering methods are able to achieve high-quality results. A benefit of these filtering methods is that their complexity is linear in the number of labels for each pixel. An early application of filtering methods for stereo appeared in [11,12]. Method presented in [11] was slow and did not offer any real advantage over energy-minimization methods. [12], on the other hand, employed an approximate (and fast) implementation of the filter, which resulted in a considerable speed gain at the cost of accuracy. Hosni *et al.* [3] used edge-aware *guided filters* to achieve high-quality results for multi-label problems, including stereo. Here the complexity is independent of the size of the filter, resulting in good runtime

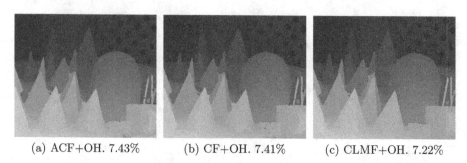

(a) ACF+OH. 7.43%   (b) CF+OH. 7.41%   (c) CLMF+OH. 7.22%

Fig. 2. The proposed OH, when used in place of the RF gap-filling [3] post-processing step, improves the performance of ACF, CF, and CLMF methods. When using OH, instead of RF, ACF($r = 0.3$) all pixel percentage error reduces from 8.49 % to 7.43 %. Similarly, all pixel percentage error for CF reduces from 8.24 % to 7.41 %, and that of CLMF reduces from 7.82 % to 7.22 %. These errors are calculated using error threshold equal to 1.0. r controls the size of local windows during salient subvolume detection.

performance. Building upon this idea, Lu *et al.* [2] further improved the runtime performance by formalizing the filtering process as a local multi-point regression problem. A latter work by the same authors combined *PatchMatch* with edge-aware filtering in order to further speed up the inference process [10]. The complexity of this method is sublinear in the number of labels.

Filtering methods mentioned above rely upon a post-processing step to deal with gaps present in the initial solution.[1] These gaps exist in mismatched or non-overlapping areas. Energy minimization schemes explicitly model these gaps; whereas, filtering methods refine the initial label assignments and fill these gaps using a row-filling strategy described in [3]. These gaps seem to play a larger role in filtering methods, perhaps because these methods ignore global smoothing. This suggests that one way to increase the accuracy of filtering methods is to implement a better algorithm for gap filling. In the case of stereo, gap filling is typically referred to as occlusion handling.

Within this backdrop, this paper develops a new method for dense stereo estimation. First, we present an extension of the Cost Filter (CF) [3] method, called Accelerated Cost Filtering (ACF) (see Fig. 1). ACF uses feature matching to identify *salient subvolumes* within the cost volume and restrict filtering to these subvolumes. For stereo pairs with large disparity, this results in a significant speed up. ACF runtime performance, for example, provides a speedup of up to 4 times over CF on five high resolution images from the Middlebury 2005/2006 stereo datasets [13]. Since ACF restricts filtering to the selected subvolumes, initial label assignments show a marginal increase in the gaps as compared to those returned from CF. We develop an Occlusion Handling (OH) (or gap filling) method that uses superpixels [14] and a label propagation algorithm inspired by simulated annealing [15] to propagate the labels to pixels within the occluded

---

[1] Gap here refers to pixels with no label assignments.

regions (see Fig. 2). Our occlusion handling method gives better results than the Row Filling (RF) method described in [3].

The following hypotheses underpin our work on ACF: (1) each slice in the cost volume can be partitioned into visible and non-visible regions, where the visible regions indicate areas where input images agree (*visibility hypothesis*) and (2) matched keypoints in the stereo image pair can be used to define the visible regions within a slice of the cost volume (*selection hypothesis*). Edge aware filtering methods implicitly assume that the visibility hypothesis stands. Good feature point matches between the two images is needed for the second hypothesis to hold. For this work, we use Lowe's Scale Invariant Feature Transform (SIFT) keypoints [16,17] to find matches between the two images. Given a matched keypoint between the left and right images, it is possible to compute the disparity for its location and use it to define a salient subvolume within the cost volume.

Our algorithm for occlusion handling uses superpixels. Superpixels are robust to noise, respect object boundaries and encode within them a higher-level of image representation. We use the SLIC algorithm that was proposed in [18] to generate superpixels. Label propagation to pixels in the occluded regions is modeled as *simulated annealing*, where appearance similarity between neighboring superpixels determine the temperature. Initially temperature is high and labels are propagated to most similar neighboring superpixels. However, by decreasing the temperature, it is possible to propagate labels to superpixels with lower similarity values. We show that this has the advantage of assigning consistent labels that preserve edge discontinuities in the resulting disparity maps.

We have compared our ACF+OH method with the Cost Filter (CF) [3], Cross-based Local Multipoint Filtering (CLMF) [2], and a recent global energy minimization method (VARMSOH) that appeared in [4] on the Middlebury stereo benchmark dataset [1]. We also compare ACF+OH with CF [3] on five high resolution images (Rocks1, Rocks2, Dolls, Moebius, and Books) from Middlebury 2005/2006 stereo datasets [13], and our method achieves state-of-the-art results. The results also demonstrate that our occlusion handling method improves the accuracy of CF on all error measures and that of CLMF on the error percentage of all and non-occluded image regions. We have not compared our method with [10], which uses slanted surfaces.

1.1 Contributions and Outline

Our contributions are threefold. First, we develop an algorithm for computing salient subvolumes within the cost volume for label assignment problems via filtering. Second, we present a gap filling (occlusion handling) algorithm that gives better results than existing gap filling strategy proposed in [3]. We show that our gap filling algorithm can be used as a post-processing step to refine the initial label assignments in other filtering methods. We used our gap filling technique to refine the label assignments returned by CF [3] and CLMF [2] and show that our method is superior to the row-filling method for occlusion handling. Third, we extend the CF method incorporating ideas developed in this work and show

that our algorithm achieves state-of-the-art results on the Middlebury benchmark dataset [1], beating [2–4]. We also beat [3] on high resolution images from
the Middlebury 2005/2006 stereo datasets [13].

The rest of the paper is organized as follows. We discuss related work in
the next section. The following section describes the methodology. We present
experimental results in Sec. 4 and concludes the paper with a summary and
discussion in the following section.

2   Literature Review

MRF global energy minimization techniques [4,5,19] are popular approaches for
solving pixel labeling problems. These approaches, however, do not scale well
with large cost volumes. Edge-aware filtering methods [20,21] have contributed
to the development of fast alternative techniques for solving pixel labeling problems [2,3]. These technique are broadly referred to as cost volume filtering methods. Hosni et al. [3], for example, provide a framework that uses a guided filter
[20] for cost volume filtering. The complexity of their approach is independent
of the size of the filter. Lu et al. [2] further speed up the filtering process by
aggregating cost estimates for a set of points. Cost volume filtering methods—
although more efficient than MRF global energy minimization schemes—scale
linearly with the size of the cost volume, which is undesirable when dealing with
large cost volumes.

There have been several attempts to reduce the complexity of cost volume
filtering. For example, Min et al. [22] proposed the histogram-based disparity
pre-filtering scheme that reduces the cost aggregation by estimating the set of
most likely candidate disparities for each pixel. This method, however, requires
a pre-scanning of the entire cost volume. Lu et al. [10] proposed a method that
combines EAF with the randomized search of PatchMatch to speed up the filtering process. This method has sublinear complexity in the label space size.
Boufama et al. [23] developed a fast method for dense matching, which can
perhaps be used for disparity map calculation.

A number of occlusion handling techniques have been proposed for gap filling.
For example, Sun et al. [24] formulated stereo matching as a global energy minimization problem and added an extra term to enforce smoothness of occlusions.
Min et al. [19] proposed an energy minimization method that filled occluded
regions through label propagation. Yang et al. [25] formulated an energy minimization problem that used an iterative refinement step to fit planes to color
segmented regions. It then filled occluded regions by minimizing the difference
to the fitted planes. The work of Ben-Ari et al. [4] also provided an energy
minimization formulation that explicitly model occlusions using an energy term,
which was optimized by an iterative scheme. Hosni et al. [3] proposed a post-
processing method for occlusion handling. This method performs row scanning
and assigns each occluded pixel the lowest disparity value among its neighbouring
non-occluded pixels. Weighted median filtering is employed to remove undesirable artifacts in the resulting disparity map.

3   Methodology

We begin by discussing the cost volume filtering method for estimating disparity $D(x, y)$ from stereo image pair (I_1, I_2). It is straightforward to estimate the depth of a pixel given a disparity map. Without the loss of generality we treat I_1 as the reference image I_{ref} and disparity map $D(x, y)$ assigns a disparity value to every pixel (x, y) in the reference image. We will also denote I_2 as I_k to keep open the possibility of using more than two images for estimating the disparity maps.

3.1   Cost Volume Filtering

Depth estimation given a stereo image pair can be reformulated as a discrete label assignment problem, where each pixel p with coordinates (x, y) is assigned a label l_p. Here $l_p \in L$ and L is the set of pixel disparities. Disparity space image, often referred to as cost volume, $C(x, y, l)$ is defined over pixels and the set of possible labels [1,3]. Cost volume stores the costs of assigning a label l to a pixel at (x, y). Each slice of the cost volume is filtered, i.e., the cost of assigning a label l to a pixel at (x, y) is the weighted average of the costs of assigning label l to the neighboring pixels. Mathematically,

$$C'(x, y, l) = \sum_{(u,v) \in [-\frac{w}{2}, \frac{w}{2}]} W_{I_{\text{ref}}(x,y)}(u, v) C(x + u, y + v, l), \tag{1}$$

where w is the size of the kernel, $W_{I_{\text{ref}}(x,y)}(u, v)$ are weights determined using the guidance image for each pixel location (x, y), and $C'(x, y, l)$ represent the filtered costs of assigning label l to the pixel at location (x, y). In the case of stereo, the guidance image is the reference image. Various filtering techniques exist to select $W_{I_{\text{ref}}(x,y)}(u, v)$ while preserving the intensity changes of the guidance image during the filtering process [20,21]. Finally, a *winner-takes-all* scheme is applied to assign a label l_p to a pixel p at (x, y). Specifically,

$$l_p = \arg \min_l C'(x, y, l). \tag{2}$$

Aside: Although edge aware filtering techniques can provide accurate results in a fast and efficient manner, they need to process the entire cost volume. Therefore, the complexity of edge aware filtering is linear in the number of cost volume slices (or labels). [10] attempted to remedy this situation and combined edge aware filtering with randomized search; however, their runtime performance is similar to that of [2] on the Middlebury dataset. An obvious strategy to improve runtime performance is to restrict filtering to small sections of the cost volume.

3.2   Salient Regions in the Cost Volume

We now describe our algorithm for selecting salient subvolumes within a cost volume. Filtering is restricted to these subvolumes, resulting in reduced processing

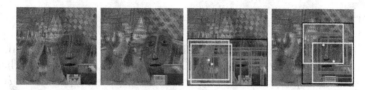

Fig. 3. Using feature matching to identify salient regions in the cost volume. The first two images from left show projections at disparities 10.8 and 14.4, respectively. For each image, we show how plane keypoints (shown as blue) indicate best matching locations for each depth. The next two images show local windows (red squares) around each plane keypoint and the final salient region (black rectangle) for these planes. We also show the expanded windows from neighboring planes as white rectangles centered on white keypoints from these planes. The width of local windows around each keypoint is equal to $r \times I_{\text{width}}$. For this figure r is set to .2 (Color figure online).

times and better runtime performance. Our method constructs the cost volume $C(x, y, l)$ using the fronto-parallel plane sweep algorithm from [26]. The family of depth planes is defined within the coordinate system of the reference image I_{ref}. The depths l of the planes fall within the expected disparity range. For the *Teddy* dataset, 187 equally spaced fronto-parallel planes were constructed with depths ranging between 1 and 57. In order to compute $C(x, y, l)$, the pixel (x, y) in the reference image I_{ref} is projected to the other image(s) I_k using homography that relates I_{ref} to I_k via the fronto-parallel plane at depth l (for details, please see [26]). Similar to [3], if pixel (x, y) is mapped to location (x_k, y_k) in image I_k then

$$C(x, y, l) = (1 - \beta) \min(\|I_{\text{ref}}(x, y) - I_k(x_k, y_k)\|, \gamma_1)$$
$$+ \beta \min(\|\nabla_x I_{\text{ref}}(x, y) - \nabla_x(I_k(x_k, y_k))\|, \gamma_2). \quad (3)$$

$\beta \in [0, 1]$, γ_1 and γ_2 are user-defined thresholds. The intuition behind this formulation is that when the surface projected to pixel (x, y) intersects the plane at l, $I_{\text{ref}}(x, y)$ and $I_k(x_k, y_k)$ should have similar appearances under the Lambertian surface assumption.

Salient regions are defined within the cost volume by inspecting each plane in the cost volume and identifying sections where $I_{\text{ref}}(x, y)$ agrees well with $I_k(x, y)$. One scheme to find such sections in a plane at l is to use already computed $C(x, y, l)$. A better method, however, is to employ feature matching. Our method extracts SIFT keypoints from the input images (I_{ref} and I_k) and compares these using the ratio test to find matches between the two images [16,17]. It is easy to calculate the disparity values between matched points' pairs, identifying locations (x, y, l') within the cost volume that correspond to each matched points' pair. The salient region for the plane at depth l' is constructed as follows: (1) define local windows $b_{l'}(x, y)$ centered around each (x, y, l') and (2) construct the smallest window $b_{l'}$ that encloses all $b_{l'}(x, y)$ defined in the previous step. The dimensions of local windows $b_{l'}(x, y)$ is typically a small fraction r of the dimensions of the reference image. For the experiments presented

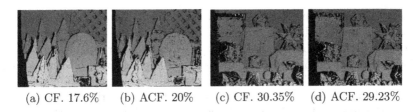

(a) CF. 17.6%   (b) ACF. 20%   (c) CF. 30.35%   (d) ACF. 29.23%

Fig. 4. Initial disparity maps computed by our ACF method shows a slight increase in the percentage of occluded pixels; black regions are occluded pixels. (Cones): (a) and (b) show the disparity maps computed by CF and ACF($r = .3$), respectively, without any gap filling. (Moebius): (c) and (d) show high resolution disparity maps computed by CF and ACF($r = .3$), respectively, without any gap filling. It is interesting to note that for Moebius dataset, ACF creates disparity maps with less occluded pixels. One explanation might be that filtering reduced cost volume may be better for some scenes. More work is needed to investigate this behavior. The width of local windows used for constructing salient regions is equal to $r \times I_{\text{width}}$.

here, the widths of the local windows are roughly 0.2 to 0.3 times the image width I_{width}.

Often times the depths l' of (x, y, l') locations corresponding to the matched points' pairs do not match exactly with a depth plane available for the cost volume (remembering that depth planes are simply a discrete representation of the cost volume). Such situations are dealt with by considering (x, y, l') for more than one neighboring depth planes. Specifically, each location (x, y, l') is used during computing the salient regions b_l for planes with depths l, such that $\|l - l'\| \leq u$. u is a user-defined parameter that controls the expansion within the disparity range. Note that, the definition of salient regions does not depend on the cost volume $C(x, y, l)$. So, a better strategy is to pre-compute the salient regions and only build the cost volume for these regions.

Figure 3 illustrates our method for identifying salient regions in the cost volume. The two images on the left show the results of projecting stereo image pair from the Cones dataset on the planes at different depths (assuming different disparities) in the cost volume. Notice that different regions of the projection appear to be in focus at different depths as expected. We also show the locations of the (matched) keypoints (as blue dots). Notice that disparity calculated for a matched keypoint agrees with the depth at which the neighboring area is in focus. The two images on right show the final salient region (black rectangle) for the two depth levels. The final salient region is determined by computing the minimum bounding box for the local windows around the keypoints whose disparity agrees with the depth level, and the expanded local windows from the neighboring depth planes.

Together the salient regions for neighboring depth levels define a cuboid within the cost volume. This process results in (ideally) a sparse set of cuboids within the cost volume, and the subsequent filtering is restricted to these subvolumes, which results in an increased runtime performance. A side effect of restricting filtering to these subvolumes is that resulting disparity maps show a fractional increase in the number of unlabeled pixels. Parallax effects manifest themselves as unlabeled pixels. Similarly boundary regions that are missing from one or the other image of the stereo pair also lead to gaps or unlabeled pixels. We employ the method proposed in [3] to identify the pixels with missing or incorrect disparity values. Given a stereo pair, two disparity maps are constructed. The first disparity map D_1 is constructed treating I_1 as the reference image; whereas, the second disparity map D_2 is constructed using I_2 as the reference image. A pixel (x, y) is considered unlabeled if its disparity values in D_1 and D_2 do not agree. For the remaining of this discussion, we will refer to the unlabeled pixels as occluded pixels. By extension, pixels that are correctly labeled will be henceforth referred to as non-occluded pixels. Figure 4 shows the disparity maps constructed using our method compared to the ones constructed by [3]. For our disparity maps, filtering is only performed for the selected subvolumes within the cost volume. The black regions indicate occluded pixels.

3.3   Gap Filling

We now describe our gap filling method for computing disparity values for occluded pixels. Our gap filling algorithm relies upon superpixels. The intuition behind our framework stems from the following three observations: (1) the solutions of pixel-labeling problems are spatially smooth and preserve discontinuities at image edges; (2) spatially compact superpixels preserve boundaries and increase the chance that neighboring pixels within a superpixel share similar labels (or disparity values); and (3) using superpixels as primitive units boosts the runtime performance. In this work, we use the SLIC superpixel segmentation algorithm that appeared in [18] to segment an input image I into a set $S = \{S_1, S_2, S_3, \cdots, S_K\}$ of K non-overlapping superpixels. The SLIC method scales linearly with the size of the image and creates compact superpixels that respect image edges. Each superpixel is defined over a set of contiguous coordinates (x, y) and $(x, y) \in S$ denotes that pixel at (x, y) belongs to superpixel S. $(x, y) \in [1, I_{\text{width}}] \times [1, I_{\text{height}}]$, and I_{width} and I_{height} represent the width and the height of image I.

The proposed method begins by assigning occlusion probabilities $p_{\text{occ}}(S)$ to each superpixel $S \in S$. These probabilities are determined using the disparity map $D(x, y)$ computed in the previous step. A superpixel is said to be non-occluded if none of its pixels are occluded. Say $Occ(x, y) = 1$ for pixels that are occluded and zero otherwise. We can then define the occlusion probability of a superpixel as follows:

$$p_{\text{occ}}(S) = \frac{\sum_{(x,y)\in S} Occ(x, y)}{|S|}, \tag{4}$$

$|S|$ denotes the number of pixels in the superpixel $S \in S$. $p_{\text{occ}}(S)$ is 0 if the superpixel is not occluded. Function $h(S)$ returns the most likely label for a superpixel S when $p_{\text{occ}}(S) < 1$. $h(S)$ is simply the most frequent label $D(x, y)$ where $(x, y) \in S$. Unlabeled pixels $(x, y) \in S$ when $p_{\text{occ}}(S) < \tau_{\text{fill}}$ are set equal to

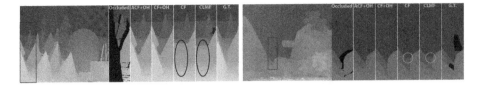

Fig. 5. Depth estimation using cost filtering with and without our OH method on the Cones (left) and Teddy (right) Middlebury benchmark datasets. For each dataset, the left-most figure shows the depth map computed by our method (ACF+OH). The other columns show a close-up of the section highlighted as the red rectangle. Occluded column shows the depth map computed by ACF without any post-processing. ACF+OH post-processes depth computed by ACF using OH. Similarly, CF+OH indicates the result of CF after post-processing using OH. CF and CLMF show depth maps computed by these algorithms, respectively. The last column shows the Ground Truth (G.T.). Ellipses in CF and CLMF indicate regions that exhibit large errors.

$h(S)$. After this step $\forall S \in \mathcal{S}_{\text{occ}}$, $p_{\text{occ}}(S) \geq \tau_{\text{fill}}$. τ_{fill} is a user-defined threshold. In our examples, it is set to either 0.5 or 0.6. The set of superpixels can be partitioned into occluded $\mathcal{S}_{\text{occ}}$ and non-occluded $\mathcal{S}_{\text{nocc}}$ superpixel sets, such that $\mathcal{S} = \mathcal{S}_{\text{occ}} \cup \mathcal{S}_{\text{nocc}}$.

Label Propagation via Simulated Annealing. Superpixels provide a good starting point for label propagation. Pixels within the same superpixels tend to have similar labels (under the local smoothness assumption) and the superpixels align with scene intensity edges. The label propagation method defines an adjacency graph $G = (\mathcal{S}, \mathcal{S} \times \mathcal{S})$ over the set of superpixels. The graph has as its nodes, the superpixels, with edges between any two superpixels if they share a part of their boundaries. Given a superpixel S, $N_{\text{nocc}}(S)$ is the possibly empty set of its neighboring non-occluded superpixels. It is straightforward to construct $N_{\text{nocc}}(S)$ given G. Let $sim(S, S') = 1 - \|col(S) - col(S')\|_2 \in [0, 1]$ defines a similarity value between two neighboring superpixels, where $col(S)$ and $col(S')$ return the normalized average colors for superpixels S and S', respectively. The label propagation algorithm is inspired by *simulated annealing* [15]. The similarity threshold T at which labels are propagated to neighboring superpixels is slowly reduced over time by ΔT. The labels for non-occluded superpixels are never updated. The following algorithm describes our label propagation algorithm:

Require: $\mathcal{S}_{occ}, \mathcal{S}_{nocc}, T, \Delta T$
Ensure: $\mathcal{S}_{occ} = \Phi$ and $\mathcal{S} = \mathcal{S}_{nocc}$
 1: $T = 1.0$;
 2: **while** $\mathcal{S}_{occ} \neq \Phi$ **do**
 3:    **for all** $S \in \mathcal{S}_{occ}$ **do**
 4:      **if** $N_{\text{nocc}}(S) = \Phi$ **then**
 5:        continue
 6:      **end if**
 7:      $S^* = \arg\max\limits_{S'} sim(S, S')$, where $S' \in N_{\text{nocc}}(S)$

8:      **if** $sim(S, S^*) > T$ **then**
9:          $\forall(x, y) \in S$, **if** $Occ(x, y)$ **then** $D(x, y) = h(S^*)$
10:         $S_{nocc} = S_{nocc} \cup \{S\}$
11:         $S_{occ} = S_{occ} - \{S\}$
12:     **end if**
13:    **end for**
14:    $T = \max(T - \Delta T, 0.0)$
15: **end while**

As a final enhancement step, we apply the weighted median filtering used in [3]. Figure 5 shows results for our occlusion handling method. Note that the results from ACF+OH method are closer to the ground truth than those of CF and CLMF. Furthermore, the proposed OH, when used as a post-processing step for CF, improves its results.

4   Results

We have compared our ACF+OH method against CF [3], CLMF [2], VARM-SOH [4] methods on the Middlebury stereo benchmark dataset [1]. We also compared our method against CF [3] on the Rocks1, Rocks2, Moebius, Dolls, and Books high resolution Middlebury 2005/2006 datasets [13]. Note that, VARM-SOH applies global energy minimization for occlusion handling; whereas, CF and CLMF use Row Filling (RF) [3]. In our results, we will indicate CF and CLMF, as CF+RF and CLMF+RF.

Table 1 lists quantitative stereo evaluation results on Middlebury benchmark. It shows rank and average percentage error corresponding to two error thresholds: 1 and 0.5 (default error threshold is 1.0). Notice that our method ACF+OH outranks CF+RF, CLMF+RF, and VARMSOH methods on the default threshold. For error threshold equal to 0.5, our method performs slightly worse than CF+RF and VARMSOH. This is because currently our method does not support slanted planes. We plan to address this limitation in the future. The table also shows the importance of occlusion handling for our method. Notice that ACF+RF's rank drops to 60 and 64 for $r = .2$ and $r = .3$, respectively, for the default error threshold. The table also shows that the proposed OH method improves the performance of CF algorithm—CF+OH's rank is 25 as compared to that of CF+RF, which is 42 for the default threshold. CLMF+OH and CLMF+RF achieve similar performance. Furthermore, on high-resolution Middlebury datasets, ACF+OH and CF+RF achieve average percentage of all pixel errors of 10.57 % and 11.13 %, respectively. These results support the central premise of this paper: it is possible to filter sub-volumes in the cost volume and achieve accuracy comparable to schemes that filter the entire cost volume.

Table 2 compares ACF and CF without any post-processing steps on the Middlebury standard and high resolution datasets. Notice that while average percentage of occluded pixels for ACF and CF are comparable, ACF's runtime performance is significantly better than that of CF's, especially on high resolution datasets. This table also lists runtimes for RF and OH post-processing steps. Our post-processing method outperforms RF on high resolution datasets.

Table 1. Quantitative evaluation on Middlebury benchmark datasets [1]. These results are aggregated over Cones, Teddy, Venus, and Tsukuba datasets.

Algorithm	Error threshold = 1		Error threshold = 0.5	
	Rank	% error	Rank	% error
CF+OH	**25**	5.22	30	12.9
CLMF+OH	38	5.14	66	16.9
ACF+OH ($r = .3$)	30	5.26	33	13
ACF+OH ($r = .2$)	39	5.45	37	13.3
CF+RF [3]	42	5.55	27	12.8
CLMF+RF [2]	37	**5.13**	64	16.7
ACF+RF($r = .3$)	64	5.99	45	13.4
ACF+RF($r = .2$)	60	5.92	42	13.6
VARMSOH [4]	116	8.17	**21**	**11.8**

Table 2. A comparison of ACF and CF without any post-processing steps on Middlebury standard and high-resolution datasets. Runtimes for RF and OH post-processing steps are also provided.

Algorithm	Average % occluded pixels		Run-time (seconds)	
	Standard	High resolution	Standard	High resolution
ACF($r = 0.2$)	14.2	-	16.117	-
ACF($r = 0.3$)	14.39	26.1	18.717	159.82
CF	13.6	26.9	28.2	505
RF	-	-	0.11	1.4
OH	-	-	0.131	0.2

Table 3 shows the stereo evaluation results on the Middlebury benchmark datasets for the default error threshold 1.0. For each dataset, we list the values for the three popular error measures: (1) nocc, which measures the error percentage of non-occluded regions, (2) all, which calculates the error percentage of all regions, (3) disc, which provides the error percentage of regions near depth discontinuities. Notice that our method ACF+OH outperforms CF+RF and CLMF+RF on nearly every error measure when $r = .3$, and on the error percentage of all regions when $r = .2$. It also outperforms VARMSOH on all measures. The results also show that the proposed OH method improves ACF over the RF scheme—E.g. for the Cones dataset, ACF+OH has an all error of 7.79 % and 7.43 % for $r = .2$ and $r = .3$, respectively; however, for ACF+RF, these errors are 9.06 % and 8.49 %. Additionally OH significantly improves the accuracy of CF on every error measure, and that of CLMF on the nocc and all error measures.

Table 3. Stereo evaluation results on Middlebury benchmark with error threshold equal to 1.0.

Algorithm	Tsukuba			Venus			Teddy			Cones		
	nocc	all	disk	nocc	all	disk	nocc	all	disc	nocc	all	disk
CF+OH	**1.45**	**1.75**	7.37	**0.19**	**0.37**	2.24	5.85	10	16.1	2.6	7.41	7.31
CLMF+OH	2.39	2.69	6.53	0.26	**0.37**	2.23	**5.49**	10.7	**14.2**	2.46	**7.22**	7.10
ACF+OH ($r = .3$)	1.45	1.75	7.37	0.19	0.37	2.24	5.94	10.1	16.4	2.61	7.43	7.23
ACF+OH ($r = .2$)	1.45	1.75	7.37	0.19	0.37	2.24	6.64	10.7	16.3	2.82	7.79	7.74
CF+RF [3]	1.51	1.85	7.61	0.2	0.39	2.42	6.16	11.8	16	2.71	8.24	7.66
CLMF+RF [2]	2.46	2.78	**6.26**	0.27	0.38	**2.15**	5.50	10.6	**14.2**	**2.34**	7.82	**6.80**
ACF+RF ($r = .3$)	1.51	1.85	7.61	0.2	0.39	2.42	6.94	11.3	18.5	3.38	8.49	9.3
ACF+RF ($r = .2$)	1.51	1.85	7.61	0.2	0.39	2.42	6.96	11.1	17.1	3.66	9.06	9.8
VarMSOH [4]	3.97	5.23	14.9	0.28	0.76	3.78	9.34	14.3	20	4.14	9.91	11.4

Table 4. Parameters for OH procedure. $\Delta T = 0.0001$.

Dataset	#superpixels	τ_{fill}	Dataset	#superpixels	τ_{fill}	Dataset	#superpixels	τ_{fill}
Cones	1600	0.6	Teddy	2000	0.6	Tsukuba	500	0.5
Venus	1000	0.5	Rocks1	700	0.5	Rocks2	700	0.5
Moebius	1600	0.5	Dolls	1600	0.5	Books	1600	0.5

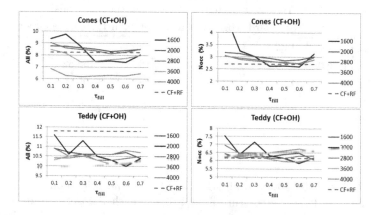

Fig. 6. The accuracy of CF+RF and CF+OH against τ_{fill} threshold for OH method. The dashed (red) line indicate the accuracy of CF+RF. It is independent of the choice of τ_{fill}. Solid lines indicate the all (left column) and nocc (right column) percentage errors for different values of the number of superpixels K. The top row shows plots for Cones dataset and the bottom row shows plots for Teddy dataset. *This figure is best viewed in color* (Color figure online).

Table 4 list the OH parameters used for results presented here. ΔT is set to 0.0001 in all cases. While the performance of our occlusion handling depends upon these parameters, plots in Fig. 6 suggest that the proposed OH method is able to achieve good accuracy over a range of these parameters. Expansion

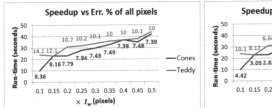
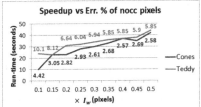

Fig. 7. Run-time vs. accuracy comparison for our ACF+OH method using different values for the r parameter that controls the size of local window used for defining salient regions. The numbers printed next to the plots represent average percentage errors. *This figure is best viewed in color* (Color figure online).

factor u is chosen to be 6 and 2, respectively, for the standard and high-resolution datasets. Figure 6 plots the accuracy of CF+RF and CF+OH methods against the τ_{fill} user-selected threshold (for OH method) for the Cones (top-row) and Teddy (bottom-row) datasets. Accuracies are plotted for different values of the number of superpixels K. These plots suggest that the proposed OH method improves both all and nocc errors, over a range of values for τ_{fill} and K.

Figure 7 shows a run-time vs. accuracy comparison for our ACF+OH method while varying the size of local windows used for defining salient regions. The local window size is expressed as a fraction $r \times I_{width}$ (along x-axis). The y-axis represents run-times in seconds. As expected the accuracy increases when using large window sizes for computing salient regions. The good news is that the accuracy does not change much when using window sizes that are more than $0.3 \times I_{width}$.

5   Conclusions

This paper develops accelerated cost volume filtering for disparity estimation from a stereo image pair. Feature matching is used to identify salient subvolumes within the cost volume and filtering is restricted to these subvolumes, resulting in increased runtime performance. We have also developed an occlusion handling method, which acts as a post-processing step and refines the disparity maps computed via filtering. The occlusion handling technique relies upon superpixels and uses a simulated annealing inspired method for label propagation between superpixels, preserving edge discontinuities in the process. The proposed method is evaluated on the Middlebury stereo datasets and it outperforms state-of-the-art techniques: CF [3], CLMF [2] and VARMSOH [4]. Our occlusion handling method also improves the accuracy of CF on all error measures and that of CLMF on the error percentage of all and non-occluded image regions. In the future we intend to explore the use of slanted surfaces during detecting salient subvolumes. We also hope to apply our method to other discrete labeling problems, such as optical flow computation, etc.

References

1. Scharstein, D., Szeliski, R.: A taxonomy and evaluation of dense two-frame stereo correspondence algorithms. Int. J. Comput. Vis. **47**, 7–42 (2002)
2. Lu, J., Shi, K., Min, D., Lin, L., Do, M.: Cross-based local multipoint filtering. In: Proceedings of the IEEE CVPR, pp. 430–437 (2012)
3. Hosni, A., Rhemann, C., Bleyer, M., Rother, C., Gelautz, M.: Fast cost-volume filtering for visual correspondence and beyond. IEEE Trans. Pattern Anal. Mach. Intell. **25**, 504–511 (2013)
4. Ben-Ari, R., Sochen, N.: Stereo matching with mumford-shah regularization and occlusion handling. IEEE Trans. Pattern Anal. Mach. Intell. **32**, 2071–2084 (2010)
5. Delong, A., Osokin, A., Isack, H., Boykov, Y.: Fast approximate energy minimization with label costs. Int. J. Comput. Vis. **96**, 1–27 (2012)
6. Boykov, Y., Veksler, O., Zabih, R.: Fast approximate energy minimization via graph cuts. IEEE Trans. Pattern Anal. Mach. Intell. **23**, 1222–1239 (2001)
7. Weiss, Y., Freeman, W.: On the optimality of solutions of the max-product belief propagation algorithm in arbitrary graphs. IEEE Trans. Inf. Theory **47**, 723–735 (2001)
8. Sun, J., Zheng, N., Shum, H.: Stereo matching using belief propagation. IEEE Trans. Pattern Anal. Mach. Intell. **25**, 787–800 (2003)
9. Felzenszwalb, P., Huttenlocher, D.: Efficient belief propagation for early vision. Int. J. Comput. Vis. **70**, 41–54 (2006)
10. Lu, J., Yang, H., Min, D., Do, M.: Patch match filter: efficient edge-aware filtering meets randomized search for fast correspondence field estimation. In: Proceedings of the IEEE CVPR, pp. 1854–1861 (2013)
11. Yoon, K.J., Kweon, I.S.: Adaptive support-weight approach for correspondence search. IEEE Trans. Pattern Anal. Mach. Intell. **28**, 650–656 (2006)
12. Richardt, C., Orr, D., Davies, I., Criminisi, A., Dodgson, N.A.: Real-time spatiotemporal stereo matchingusing the dual-cross-bilateral grid. In: Daniilidis, K., Maragos, P., Paragios, N. (eds.) ECCV 2010, Part III. LNCS, vol. 6313, pp. 510–523. Springer, Heidelberg (2010)
13. Hirschmuller, H., Scharstein, D.: Evaluation of cost functions for stereo matching. In: Proceedings of the IEEE CVPR, pp. 1–8 (2007)
14. Schick, A., Bauml, M., Stiefelhagen, R.: Improving foreground segmentations with probabilistic superpixel markov random fields. In: Proceedings of the IEEE CVPRW, pp. 27–31 (2012)
15. Granville, V., Krivanek, M., Rasson, J.: Simulated annealing: a proof of convergence. IEEE Trans. Pattern Anal. Mach. Intell. **16**, 652–656 (1994)
16. Lowe, D.: Distinctive image features from scale-invariant keypoints. Int. J. Comput. Vis. **60**, 91–110 (2004)
17. Brown, M., Hua, G., Winder, S.: Discriminative learning of local image descriptors. IEEE Trans. Pattern Anal. Mach. Intell. **33**, 43–57 (2011)
18. Achanta, R., Shaji, A., Smith, K., Lucchi, A., Fua, P., Susstrunk, S.: SLIC superpixels compared to state-of-the-art superpixel methods. IEEE Trans. Pattern Anal. Mach. Intell. **34**, 2274–2282 (2012)
19. Min, D., Sohn, K.: Cost aggregation and occlusion handling with WLS in stereo matching. IEEE Trans. Image Process. **17**, 1431–1442 (2008)
20. He, K., Sun, J., Tang, X.: Guided image filtering. IEEE Trans. Pattern Anal. Mach. Intell. **35**, 1397–1409 (2013)

21. Paris, S., Kornprobst, P., Tumblin, J., Durand, F.: Bilateral filtering: theory and applications. Found. Trends Comput. Graph. Vis. **4**, 1–73 (2009)
22. Min, D., Lu, J., Do, M.: A revisit to cost aggregation in stereo matching: how far can we reduce its computational redundancy? In: Proceedings of the IEEE ICCV, pp. 1567–1574 (2011)
23. Boufama, B., Jin, K.: Towards a fast and reliable dense matching algorithm. Soc. Manuf. Eng. J. (2003)
24. Sun, J., Li, Y., Kang, S., Shum, H.Y.: Symmetric stereo matching for occlusion handling. In: Proceedings of the IEEE CVPR, vol. 2, pp. 399–406 (2005)
25. Yang, Q., Wang, L., Yang, R., Stewenius, H., Nister, D.: Stereo matching with color-weighted correlation, hierarchical belief propagation, and occlusion handling. IEEE Trans. Pattern Anal. Mach. Intell. **31**, 492–504 (2009)
26. Gallup, D., Frahm, J.M., Mordohai, P., Qingxiong, Y., Pollefeys, M.: Real-time plane-sweeping stereo with multiple sweeping directions. In: Proceedings of the IEEE CVPR, pp. 1–8 (2007)

3D Human Pose Estimation from Monocular Images with Deep Convolutional Neural Network

Sijin Li[✉] and Antoni B. Chan

Department of Computer Science, City University of Hong Kong,
Kowloon Tong, Hong Kong
sijin.li@my.cityu.edu.hk

Abstract. In this paper, we propose a deep convolutional neural network for 3D human pose estimation from monocular images. We train the network using two strategies: (1) a multi-task framework that jointly trains pose regression and body part detectors; (2) a pre-training strategy where the pose regressor is initialized using a network trained for body part detection. We compare our network on a large data set and achieve significant improvement over baseline methods. Human pose estimation is a structured prediction problem, i.e., the locations of each body part are highly correlated. Although we do not add constraints about the correlations between body parts to the network, we empirically show that the network has disentangled the dependencies among different body parts, and learned their correlations.

1 Introduction

Human pose estimation is an active area in computer vision due to its wide potential applications. In this paper, we focus on estimating 3D human pose from monocular RGB images [1–3]. In general, recovering 3D pose from 2D RGB images is considered more difficult than 2D pose estimation, due to the larger 3D pose space, more ambiguities, and the ill-posed problem due to the irreversible perspective projection. Although using depth maps has been shown to be effective for 3D human pose estimation [4], the majority of the media on the Internet is still in 2D RGB format. In addition, monocular pose estimation can be used to aid multi-view pose estimation.

Human pose estimation approaches can be classified into two types—model-based generative methods and discriminative methods. The pictorial structure model (PSM) is one of the most popular generative models for 2D human pose estimation [5,6]. The conventional PSM treats the human body as an articulated structure. The model usually consists of two terms, which model the appearance of each body part and the spatial relationship between adjacent parts. Since the

---

Electronic supplementary material The online version of this chapter (doi:10.1007/978-3-319-16808-1_23) contains supplementary material, which is available to authorized users. Videos can also be accessed at http://www.springerimages.com/videos/978-3-319-16807-4.

D. Cremers et al. (Eds.): ACCV 2014, Part II, LNCS 9004, pp. 332–347, 2015.
DOI: 10.1007/978-3-319-16808-1_23

length of a limb in 2D can vary, a mixture of models was proposed for modeling each body part [7]. The spatial relationships between articulated parts are simpler for 3D pose, since the limb length in 3D is a constant for one specific subject. Reference [8] proposes to apply PSM to 3D pose estimation by discretizing the space. However, the pose space grows cubicly with the resolution of the discretization, i.e., doubling the resolution in each dimension will octuple the pose space.

Discriminative methods view pose estimation as a regression problem [4,9–11]. After extracting features from the image, a mapping is learned from the feature space to the pose space. Because of the articulated structure of the human skeleton, the joint locations are highly correlated. To consider the dependencies between output variables, [11] proposes to use structured SVM to learn the mapping from segmentation features to joint locations. Reference [9] models both the input and output with Gaussian processes, and predicts target poses by minimizing the KL divergence between the input and output Gaussian distributions.

Instead of dealing with the structural dependencies manually, a more direct way is to "embed" the structure into the mapping function and learn a representation that disentangles the dependencies between output variables. In this case models need to discover the patterns of human pose from data, which usually requires a large dataset for learning. Reference [4] uses approximately 500,000 images to train regression forests for predicting body part labels from depth images, but the dataset is not publicly available. The recently released Human3.6M dataset [12] contains about 3.6 million video frames with labeled poses of several human subjects performing various tasks. Such a large dataset makes it possible to train data-driven pose estimation models.

Recently, deep neural networks have achieved success in many computer vision applications [13,14], and deep models have been shown to be good at disentangling factors [15,16]. Convolutional neural networks are one of the most popular architectures for vision problems because it reduces the number of parameters (compared to fully-connected deep architectures), which makes training easier and reduces overfitting. In addition, the convolutional and max-pooling structure enables the network to extract translation invariant features.

In this paper, we consider two approaches to train deep convolutional neural networks for monocular 3D pose estimation. In particular, one approach is to jointly train the pose regression task with a set of detection tasks in a heterogeneous multi-task learning framework. The other approach is to pre-train the network using the detection tasks, and then refine the network using the pose regression task alone. To the best of our knowledge, we are the first to show that deep neural networks can be applied to 3D human pose estimation from single images. By analyzing the weights learned in the regression network, we also show that the network has discovered correlation patterns of human pose.

2   Related Work

There is a large amount of literature on pose estimation, and we refer the reader to [17] for a review. In the following, we will briefly review recent regression networks and pose estimation techniques.

In [18] trains convolutional neural networks to classify whether a given window contains one specific body-part, and then detection maps for each body-part are calculated by sliding the detection window over the whole image. A spatial model is applied to enforce consistencies among all detection results. Reference [19] applies random forests for joint point regression on depth maps. The tree structures are learned by minimizing a classification cost function. For each leaf node, a distribution of 3d offsets to the joints is estimated for pixels reaching that node. Given a test image, all the pixels are classified into leaf nodes, and offset distributions are used for generating the votes for joint locations.

In [20], a cascade neural network is proposed for stage-by-stage prediction of facial points. Networks in the later stages will take inputs centered at the predictions of the previous stage, and it was shown that cascading the networks helps to improve the accuracy. Similarly, [21] cascades 3 stages of neural networks for estimating 2D human pose from RGB images. In each stage, the network architecture is similar to the classification network in [13], but is applied to joint point prediction in 2D images. The networks in the later stages take higher resolution input windows around the previous predictions. In this way, more details can be utilized to refine the previous predictions. The cascading process assumes that the prediction can be made accurately by only looking at a relatively small local window around the target joints. However, this is not the case for 3D pose estimation. To estimate the joint locations in 3D, the context around the target joints must be considered. For example, by looking at the local window containing an elbow joint, it is very difficult to estimate its position in 3D. In addition, when body parts are occluded, local information is insufficient for accurate estimation. Therefore, our networks only contain one stage. To take into account contextual features, we design the network so that each node in the output layer receives contributions from all the pixels in the input image.

Previous works on using neural networks for 3D pose estimation from images mainly focuses on rigid objects or head pose. Reference [22] uses fully connected networks for estimating the pose parameters of 3D objects in single images. However, [22] is only applicable to 3D rigid objects, such as cups and plates, which are very different from 3D articulated objects such as humans. Reference [23] uses convolutional neural networks to detect faces, and estimates the head pose using a manually-designed low-dimensional manifold of head pose. In contrast to these previous works, we train our network to estimate the 3D pose of the whole human, which is a complex 3D articulated object. Finally, [24] uses an implicit mixture of conditional restricted Boltzmann machines to model the motion of 3D human poses (i.e., predicting the next joint points from the previous joint points), and applies it as the transition model in a Bayesian filtering framework for 3D human pose tracking. In contrast, here we focus on estimating the 3D pose directly from the image, and do not consider temporal information.

Previous works have demonstrated that learning body part labels could help to find better features for pose estimation [4, 25]. In [4], random forests are used for estimating the body part labels from depth images. Given the predictions of labels, mean shift is applied to obtain the part locations. Reference [25] trains a multi-task deep convolutional neural network for 2D human pose estimation, consisting of the pose regression task and body part detection tasks. All tasks share the same convolutional feature layers, and it was shown that the regression network benefits from sharing features with the detection network. In this work, we also introduce an intermediate representation, body joint labels, for learning intermediate features within a multi-task framework. In contrast to [25], here we focus on 3D pose estimation.

Pre-training has also been shown to be effective in training deep neural networks [26,27]. Reference [26] empirically shows that the early stages of training with stochastic gradient descent have a large impact on the network's final performance. Pre-training "regularizes" the network by leaving it in a basin of attraction with better generalization. In this work, we propose a strategy to pre-train the regression network using the detection network.

In the literature, deep convolutional neural networks have mainly been used for classification tasks [13,14,28], and have achieved state-of-art performances on many vision problems. Importantly, given sufficient data, deep convolutional neural networks can learn good features from randomly initialized weights. In addition, features learned by classification networks can also be used for other tasks – [29] feeds the output of the last convolutional layer of a trained classification neural network into a regression network for predicting bounding boxes for object detection.

3   Deep Network for 3D Pose Estimation

In this paper, we use two strategies to train a deep convolutional neural network for 3D pose estimation. Our framework consists of two types of tasks: (1) a joint point regression task; and (2) joint point detection tasks. The input for both tasks are the bounding box images containing human subjects. The goal of the regression task is to estimate the positions of joint points relative to the root joint position. We define a set of detection tasks, each of which is associated with one joint point and one local window. The aim of each detection task is to classify whether one local window contains the specific joint or not.

3.1   Notation

Let $J_i = (J_{i,x}, J_{i,y}, J_{i,z})$ be the location of the i-th joint in the camera coordinate system. Let P be the articulated skeleton model for the human body, which specifies the parent-child relationship between joints. For example, $P(i)$ specifies the parent joint of the i-th joint. To simplify notation, we let the parent of the root joint to be itself.

3.2   Joint Point Regression Task

The goal of joint point regression is to predict the positions of the joints relative to the root location, $\tilde{J}_i = J_i - J_{root}$. Similar to [9,12], we assume that the bounding box of the human is provided, and hence it is not necessary to estimate the root location of the person. However, rather than predict the relative joint positions with respect to root joint, which is a common formulation as in [9,11,12], we instead aim to predict the joint positions relative to their *parents* joints,

$$R_i = J_i - J_{P(i)}. \tag{1}$$

This representation can be interpreted as the unnormalized orientation of limbs. There are several reasons why this representation may be advantageous: (1) the variance of R_i is much smaller than $\tilde{J}_i$, which makes it easier to learn – for example, the distance between the wrist and elbow (i.e., $\|R_{wrist}\|$) is constant (for the same person), whereas the distance between the wrist and root position (i.e., $\|\tilde{J}_i\|$) has a wide range of possible values; (2) Since the human body is symmetric, information can be shared between different joints, e.g., the left arm and right arm have the same length. In addition, this representation makes it easier to infer the locations of occluded joints given its opposite part.

The joint point regressor is trained by minimizing the squared difference between the prediction and the ground-truth position,

$$E_r(R_i, \hat{R}_i) = \|R_i - \hat{R}_i\|_2^2 \tag{2}$$

where R_i and $\hat{R}_i$ are the ground-truth and estimated relative position for the i-th joint.

3.3   Joint Point Detection Task

Inspired by [25], we define a set of detection tasks for each joint i and each window l, where the goal is to predict the indicator variable,

$$h_{i,l} = \begin{cases} 1, & \text{if } B_i \text{ is inside window } l, \\ 0, & \text{otherwise,} \end{cases} \tag{3}$$

where B_i is the 2D image location of the i-th joint in the input bounding box. B_i is calculated by projecting J_i into the image and calculating its relative positions with respect to the bounding box. In this work, we do not consider whether the joints are visible or not, i.e., the indicator variables are calculated regardless if the joint is occluded. The reason for doing this is to train the network to learn features for pose estimation even in the presence of occlusions, which might enable the network to predict valid poses when occlusion occur.

As in [25], the detection tasks are trained by minimizing the cross-entropy between the ground-truth label $h_{i,l}$ and the estimated label $\hat{h}_{i,l}$,

$$E_d(\hat{h}_{i,l}, h_{i,l}) = -h_{i,l} \log(\hat{h}_{i,l}) - (1 - h_{i,l}) \log(1 - \hat{h}_{i,l}). \tag{4}$$

The relationship between the regression tasks and detection tasks is illustrated in Fig. 1.

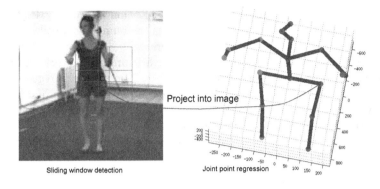

Fig. 1. Illustration of detection tasks and regression task.

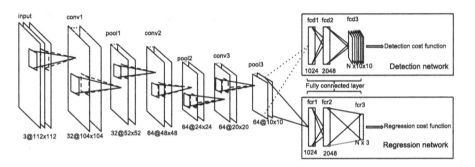

Fig. 2. Network architecture. For network training using multi-task learning, the `pool3` layer is connected to both the `fcd1` and `fcr1` layers. For pre-training with detection tasks, `pool3` is only connected to `fcd1` layer. After pre-training, this connection is removed and `pool3` is connected to `fcr1`. N is the number of joints ($N = 17$ for Human3.6M).

3.4 Network Architecture and Multi-task Training

Our network architecture for 3D pose estimation is displayed in Fig. 2. The whole network consists of 9 trainable layers – 3 convolutional layers that are shared by both regression and detection networks, 3 fully connected layers for the regression network, and 3 fully connected layers for the detection network. Rectified linear units (ReLu) [30] are used for `conv1`, `conv2`, and the first two fully connected layers for both regression and detection networks. We use tanh as the activation function for the last regression layer. To make the network robust to pixel intensity, we add a local response normalization layer after `conv2`, which applies the following function to calculate the output values,

$$f(u_{x,y}) = \frac{u_{x,y}}{(1 + \frac{\alpha}{|W_x| \cdot |W_y|} \sum_{x' \in W_x} \sum_{y' \in W_y} u^2_{x',y'})^\beta} \qquad (5)$$

where $u_{x,y}$ is the value of the previous layer at location (x,y), (W_x, W_y) are the neighborhood of locations (x,y), $|W|$ represents the number of pixels within the neighborhood, and $\{\alpha, \beta\}$ are hyper-parameters.

We train the network within a multi-task learning framework. As in [25], we allow features in the lower layers to be shared between the regression and detection tasks during joint training. During the training, the gradients from both networks will be back-propagated to the same shared feature network, i.e., the network with layers from conv1 to pool3. In this case, the shared network tends to learn features that will benefit both tasks. The global cost function for multi-task training is

$$\Phi_M = \frac{1}{2} \sum_{t=1}^{T} \sum_{i=1}^{N} E_r(R_i^{(t)}, \hat{R}_i^{(t)}) + \frac{1}{2} \sum_{t=1}^{T} \sum_{i=1}^{N} \sum_{l=1}^{L} E_d(h_{i,l}^{(t)}, \hat{h}_{i,l}^{(t)}), \qquad (6)$$

where the superscript t is the index of the training sample, N is the number of joints, and T is the number of training samples.

3.5   Pre-training with the Detection Task

As an alternative to the multi-task training discussed earlier, another approach is to train the pose regression network using pre-trained weights from the detection network. Firstly we train the detection network alone, i.e., the connections between the pool3 layer and the fcr1 layer are blocked. In this stage, we only minimize the second term in (6).

After training the detection tasks, we block the connection between pool3 and fcd1 (thus removing the detection task), and reconnect pool3 to fcr1 layer. Using this strategy, the training for pose regression is initialized using the feature layer weights (conv1-conv3) learned from the detection tasks. Finally, the pose regression is trained using the first term in (6) as the cost function. Note that we do not use the weights of the fully-connected layers of the detectors (fcd1 and fcd2) to initialize fully-connected layers of the regression task (fcr1 and fcr2). The reason is that the target for the detection and regression tasks are quite different, so that the higher-level features used by the detection tasks might not be useful for regression.

3.6   Training Details

For both the multi-task and pre-training approaches, we use back-propagation [31] to update the weights during training. In multi-task training, the pool3 layer forwards its values to both fcd1 and fcr1, and receives the average of the gradients from fcd1 and fcr1 when updating the weights. To reduce overfitting, we use "dropout" [32] in fcr1 and fcd1, and set the dropout rate to 0.25. The hyper-parameters for the local response normalization layer are set to $\alpha = 0.0025$ and $\beta = 0.75$. More training details can be found in [13].

4 Experiment

In this section we present experiments using our deep convolutional neural network for monocular 3d pose estimation (DconvMP).

4.1 Human3.6M Dataset

The Human3.6M dataset [12] contains around 3.6 million frames of video with 11 human subjects performing 15 actions. The subjects are recorded from 4 different views with RGB cameras, and the joint positions of the subjects were measured by a MoCap system. The calibration parameters are available for the RGB cameras and MoCap system. In our experiments, we use 5 subjects (S1, S5, S6, S7, S8) for training and validation, and 2 subjects (S9, S11) for testing.

Since our method is based on monocular images, we treat the 4 camera views of each pose as separate examples. The ground-truth poses for each camera view are obtained by transforming the joint locations into that camera's coordinate system. Therefore, the input for our method is a single image from one view, and the targets are the joint locations under that view. Test samples from the same frame but different views are evaluated separately, which follows the same setup as [12].

4.2 Data Augmentation

We use data augmentation to improve the robustness of the network. After obtaining the bounding box of the human subject (provided by the Human3.6M dataset), we resize the bounding box to 128×128, such that the aspect ratio of the image is maintained. In order to make the network robust to the selection of the bounding box, in each iteration, a sub-window of size 112×112 is randomly selected as the training image (the 2D joint point projections are also adjusted accordingly).

Random pixel noise is also added to each input image during training to make the network robust to small perturbations of pixel values. As in [13] we apply PCA on the RGB channels over the whole training samples. In the training stage, we add random noise to all the pixels in each image,

$$\hat{\mathbf{p}} = \mathbf{p} + [\mathbf{e_1}, \mathbf{e_2}, \mathbf{e_3}] \cdot [g_1\sqrt{\alpha_1}, g_2\sqrt{\alpha_2}, g_3\sqrt{\alpha_3}]^T, \tag{7}$$

where $[\mathbf{e_1}, \mathbf{e_2}, \mathbf{e_3}]$ and $[\alpha_1, \alpha_2, \alpha_3]$ are the eigenvectors and eigenvalues of the 3×3 RGB covariance matrix of the training set, and $\{g_c\}_{c=1}^3$ are each Gaussian distributions with zero mean and variance 0.1. In each iteration, all the pixels within one training sample will share the same random values $\{g_c\}_{c=1}^3$.

4.3 Experiment Setup

To generate the sliding window for joint point detection, we set the window size to 10×10 and the step size to 10 pixels. Experiments are run on a machine with

two 6-core Intel(R) Xeon(R) CPUs and an Nvidia Tesla K20. It takes 1–2 days
to train one action in the Human3.6M dataset (around 100,000 samples after
augmentation).

4.4   Evaluation on Human3.6M

Since there is sufficient data in Human3.6M, we train the network for each
action separately, which follows the same action-specific protocol as [12]. We
selected six representative actions that ranged from easy to difficult (according
to previous results in [12]), which include "Walking", "Discussion", "Eating",
"Walking Dog", "Greeting" and "Taking Photos". There were 132,744 training
samples for "Walking", 158,788 for "Discussion", 109,424 for "Eating", 79,412
for "Walking Dog", 72,436 for "Greeting" and 76,048 for "Taking Photos".

We test networks trained with the heterogeneous multi-task learning framework (denoted as DconvMP-HML), and using pre-training (denoted as DconvMP).
Since training detection and regression separately takes more time, we only run
DconvMP for 3 actions, namely "Walking", "Eating" and "Taking Photo". We
compare against the best performing method, LinKDE, from [12], using the
code provided in Human3.6M. We use the code provided by Human 3.6M to generate the bounding box for each image sample. Pose predictions are evaluated using
the mean per joint position error (MPJPE) [12],

$$\text{MPJPE} = \frac{1}{T}\frac{1}{N}\sum_{t=1}^{T}\sum_{i=1}^{N}\|(J_i^{(t)} - J_{root}^{(t)}) - (\hat{J}_i^{(t)} - \hat{J}_{root}^{(t)})\|_2. \tag{8}$$

The pose prediction results are reported in Table 1. We also show the MPJPE
accuracy versus error threshold for all methods in Fig. 3. Compared with the
baseline method LinKDE [12], our network obtains significant improvement for
all the actions evaluated. In our experiments, the DconvMP network achieves
roughly the same performance as DconvMP-HML, but takes longer to train.

Figure 4 shows several examples of pose estimation (also see supplemental).
We observe that our methods perform better when there are occlusions (e.g.,
row 3 in Fig. 4). In addition, our model performs well at distinguishing between
the left and right body parts (e.g., row 2 in Fig. 4). In the case where the error
is large, our model still outputs a "valid" rough pose.

Table 1. The MPJPE results on Human3.6 dataset. The unit is millimeters. The
numbers in parenthesis is the standard deviation of the MPJPE for samples in the
testing set.

Action	Walking	Discussion	Eating	Taking Photo	Walking Dog	Greeting
DconvMP	80.09 (23.45)	-	103.31 (37.33)	190.37 (90.64)	-	-
DconvMP-HML	77.60 (23.54)	148.79 (100.49)	104.01 (39.20)	189.08 (93.99)	146.59 (75.38)	127.17 (51.10)
LinKDE (BS) [12]	97.07 (37.14)	183.09 (116.74)	132.50 (72.53)	206.45 (112.61)	177.84 (122.65)	162.27 (88.43)

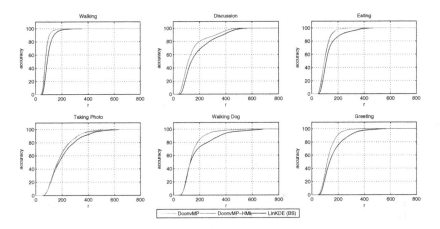

Fig. 3. MPJPE accuracy for error threshold r.

5 Visualization of Learned Structures

In this section, we explore whether the network has learned the structure of the human skeleton by analyzing the weights in the last layers of the joint regression network. Let F be a $m \times 3 \times N$ matrix of weights between the penultimate and last layers, where m is the dimension of the penultimate layer. We use F_i to denote the $m \times 3$ matrix for predicting the i-th joint, and $F_{i,x}$ to denote the weights for predicting the x-coordinate of the i-th joint (see Fig. 5). In the following section, we examine the weights learned on the "Walking" action in the Human3.6M dataset. The weights learned for other actions show similar patterns.

5.1 Pearson Correlation Between Joints

We first examine the correlation between the weights of pairs of joints, i.e., whether two joints use the same high-level features. To this end, we calculate the Pearson correlation between the weights for each pair of joints (i, j),

$$\rho_{i,j}^x = \frac{\text{cov}(F_{i,x}, F_{j,x})}{\sigma(F_{i,x})\sigma(F_{j,x})}, \qquad (9)$$

where $\text{cov}(X, Y)$ is the covariance of X and Y, $\sigma(X)$ is the standard derivation of X. The Pearson correlation is calculated for each dimension (x, y, and z).

Figure 6 (top) shows the correlation matrices between the regression weights. Firstly, the correlation matrices show that the learned weights for the left and right hips (also left and right shoulders) are negative correlated. This explains why the network can correctly predict the left hip when only the right side of the body is visible (see row 1 of Fig. 4). Also note that the left hip and left shoulder (also right hip and right shoulder) are positively correlated in the x- and z-dimensions, but not the y-dimension; i.e., the left hip and left shoulder

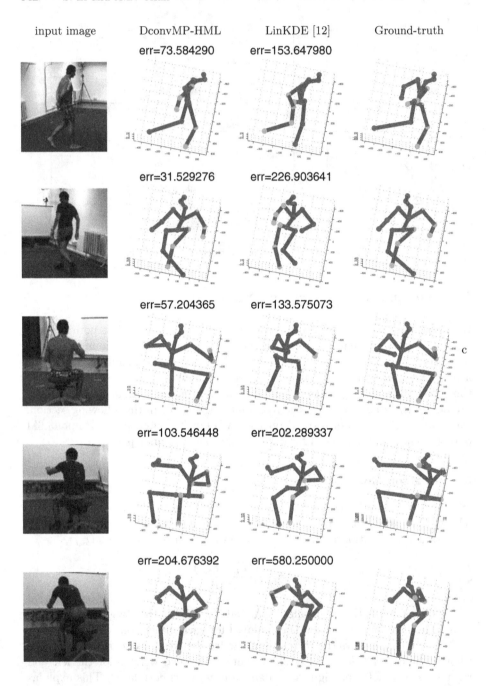

Fig. 4. Examples of pose estimation on Human3.6M. The first two rows are taken from the "Walking" action. The last three rows are taken from "Eating" action. The joints on the right-side are represented by blue balls, while the remaining joints are represented by red balls (Color figure online).

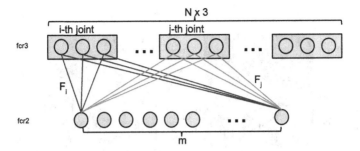

Fig. 5. Illustration of weights F_i and F_j in the final fully-connected layer for regression. For clarity, all the connections are not shown.

share the same internal feature for predicting their x- and z-coordinates. This suggests that the network has an internal representation for the positions of the left (or right) side of the person, as delineated by the hip and shoulders.

For comparison, Fig. 6 (bottom) shows the correlation matrices between the ground-truth relative joint positions. Interestingly, these correlation matrices share similar patterns to those calculated using the regression weights.

5.2 Sparsity Measure with LP Norm

We next examine the degree to which the internal features are shared in the regression network. To do this, we measure the sparsity (number of zero entries) of weight pairs. Reference [33] showed that the negative l^p norm can be used for measuring the sparsity of a vector. We calculate the "co-sparsity" between the regression weights of two joints (i, j) using

$$S_p(F_{i,x}, F_{j,x}) = -\sum_k \left(\left| \frac{F_{i,x,k}}{\sigma(F_{i,x})} \right|^p + \left| \frac{F_{j,x,k}}{\sigma(F_{j,x})} \right|^p \right)^{\frac{1}{p}}, \tag{10}$$

where $(F_{i,x,k}, F_{j,x,k})$ are the weights for joints i and j corresponding to the same feature k. The S_p measure will be high if entries in the weight pair $(F_{i,x,k}, F_{j,x,k})$ are zero.

The sparsity measures for each pair of joints are shown in Fig. 7. We observe that pairing wrists (or ankles) with other parts yields sparser weight pairs, i.e., the prediction for wrists (or ankles) do not share high-level features with other parts. One possible reason is that these extremal joints have the most variance, and thus are the most difficult to predict. As a result, the network has learned specific features for ankles and wrists, which are not shared with other body parts.

6   Conclusion

In this work, we used a deep convolutional neural network for estimating 3D human pose from monocular images. We considered two strategies for training

correlation between weights in the last regression layer

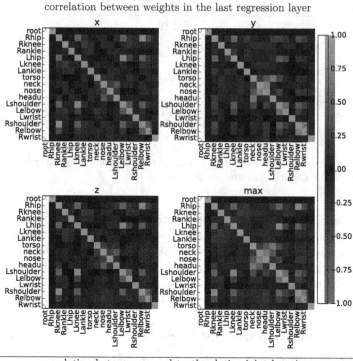

correlation between ground-truth relative joint locations

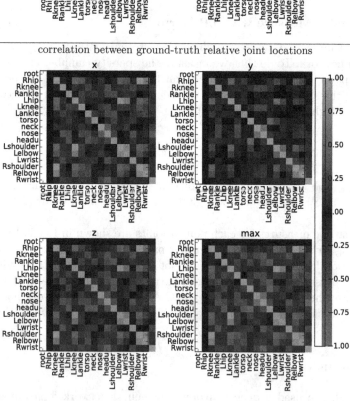

Fig. 6. Pairwise Pearson correlation. Each group of four matrices shows the correlation for the x-, y-, and z-dimensions, as well as the maximum magnitude over all dimensions.

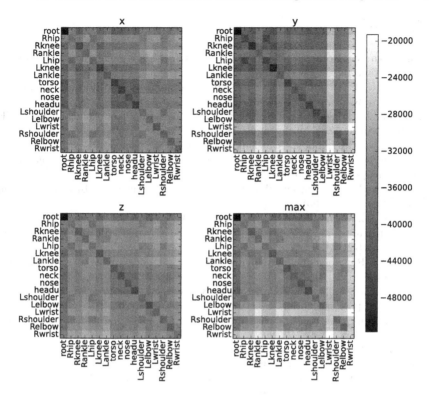

Fig. 7. The LP norm ($p = 0.2$) of the weights for joint pairs.

the network: (1) multi-task framework that simultaneously trains the regression and detection tasks; (2) and pre-training the regression task with detection tasks. These two strategies yield networks that achieve approximately the same performance, although pre-training has longer running time. When either using pre-training or sharing features, the detection tasks helps to regularize the training of the regression network and guides it to better local minimums. We evaluated our methods on the Human3.6M dataset, and the network achieves significant improvement over baseline methods in [12]. We empirically showed that the deep convolutional network has disentangled dependencies between body parts and learned the correlation between output variables. In this work we have examined how the network encodes structural dependencies in its weights. Future work will explore how such structural dependencies can be induced in the network a priori.

Acknowledgement. This work was supported by the Research Grants Council of the Hong Kong Special Administrative Region, China (CityU 123212 and CityU 110513).

References

1. Andriluka, M., Roth, S., Schiele, B.: Monocular 3d pose estimation and tracking by detection. In: CVPR (2010)
2. Wei, X.K., Chai, J.: Modeling 3d human poses from uncalibrated monocular images. In: ICCV, pp. 1873–1880 (2009)
3. Agarwal, A., Triggs, B.: Recovering 3d human pose from monocular images. IEEE Trans. Pattern Anal. Mach. Intell. **28**, 44–58 (2006)
4. Shotton, J., Fitzgibbon, A., Cook, M., Sharp, T., Finocchio, M., Moore, R., Kipman, A., Blake, A.: Real-time human pose recognition in parts from single depth images. In: CVPR (2011)
5. Felzenszwalb, P.F., Huttenlocher, D.P.: Pictorial structures for object recognition. IJCV **61**, 55–79 (2005)
6. Eichner, M., Marin-Jimenez, M., Zisserman, A., Ferrari, V.: 2d articulated human pose estimation and retrieval in (almost) unconstrained still images. IJCV **99**, 190–214 (2012)
7. Yang, Y., Ramanan, D.: Articulated pose estimation with flexible mixtures-of-parts. In: CVPR (2011)
8. Burenius, M., Sullivan, J., Carlsson, S.: 3d pictorial structures for multiple view articulated pose estimation. In: CVPR, pp. 3618–3625 (2013)
9. Bo, L., Sminchisescu, C.: Twin gaussian processes for structured prediction. Int. J. Comput. Vis. **87**, 28–52 (2010)
10. Dantone, M., Gall, J., Leistner, C., van Gool, L.: Human pose estimation from still images using body parts dependent joint regressors. In: CVPR (2013)
11. Ionescu, C., Li, F., Sminchisescu, C.: Latent structured models for human pose estimation. In: ICCV, pp. 2220–2227 (2011)
12. Ionescu, C., Papava, D., Olaru, V., Sminchisescu, C.: Human3.6m: Large scale datasets and predictive methods for 3d human sensing in natural environments. IEEE Trans. Pattern Anal. Mach. Intell. **36**, 1325–1339 (2014)
13. Krizhevsky, A., Sutskever, I., Hinton, G.E.: Imagenet classification with deep convolutional neural networks. In: NIPS 25 (2012)
14. Farabet, C., Couprie, C., Najman, L., LeCun, Y.: Learning hierarchical features for scene labeling. IEEE TPAMI **32**, 1744–1757 (2013)
15. Bengio, Y.: Deep learning of representations: Looking forward. CoRR abs/1305.0445 (2013)
16. Glorot, X., Bordes, A., Bengio, Y.: Domain adaptation for large-scale sentiment classification: A deep learning approach. In: ICML (2011)
17. Moeslund, T.B., Hilton, A., Krüger, V.: A survey of advances in vision-based human motion capture and analysis. CVIU **104**, 90–126 (2006)
18. Jain, A., Tompson, J., Andriluka, M., Taylor, G.W., Bregler, C.: Learning human pose estimation features with convolutional networks. In: International Conference on Learning Representations (ICLR) (2014)
19. Girshick, R., Shotton, J., Kohli, P., Criminisi, A., Fitzgibbon, A.: Efficient regression of general-activity human poses from depth images. In: ICCV, pp. 415–422 (2011)
20. Sun, Y., Wang, X., Tang, X.: Deep convolutional network cascade for facial point detection. In: CVPR (2013)
21. Toshev, A., Szegedy, C.: Deeppose: Human pose estimation via deep neural networks. In: IEEE Conference on Computer Vision and Pattern Recognition (2014)

22. Yuan, C., Niemann, H.: Neural networks for the recognition and pose estimation of 3d objects from a single 2d perspective view. Image Vis. Comput. **19**, 585–592 (2001)
23. Osadchy, M., Cun, Y.L., Miller, M.L.: Synergistic face detection and pose estimation with energy-based models. JMLR **8**, 1197–1215 (2007)
24. Taylor, G.W., Sigal, L., Fleet, D.J., Hinton, G.E.: Dynamical binary latent variable models for 3d human pose tracking. In: CVPR, pp. 631–638 (2010)
25. Li, S., Liu, Z.Q., Chan, A.B.: Heterogeneous multi-task learning for human pose estimation with deep convolutional neural network. In: CVPR: DeepVision Workshop (2014)
26. Erhan, D., Bengio, Y., Courville, A., Manzagol, P.A., Vincent, P., Bengio, S.: Why does unsupervised pre-training help deep learning? J. Mach. Learn. Res. **11**, 625–660 (2010)
27. Hinton, G.E., Osindero, S., Teh, Y.W.: A fast learning algorithm for deep belief nets. Neural Comput. **18**, 1527–1554 (2006)
28. Le, Q., Ranzato, M., Monga, R., Devin, M., Chen, K., Corrado, G., Dean, J., Ng, A.: Building high-level features using large scale unsupervised learning. In: ICML (2012)
29. Sermanet, P., Eigen, D., Zhang, X., Mathieu, M., Fergus, R., LeCun, Y.: Overfeat: Integrated recognition, localization and detection using convolutional networks. CoRR abs/1312.6229 (2013)
30. Nair, V., Hinton, G.E.: Rectified linear units improve restricted boltzmann machines. In: ICML (2010)
31. Lecun, Y., Bottou, L., Bengio, Y., Haffner, P.: Gradient-based learning applied to document recognition. Proc. IEEE **86**, 2278–2324 (1998)
32. Hinton, G.E., Srivastava, N., Krizhevsky, A., Sutskever, I., Salakhutdinov, R.: Improving neural networks by preventing co-adaptation of feature detectors. CoRR (2012)
33. Hurley, N., Rickard, S.: Comparing measures of sparsity. IEEE Trans. Inf. Theor. **55**, 4723–4741 (2009)

Plant Leaf Identification via a Growing Convolution Neural Network with Progressive Sample Learning

Zhong-Qiu Zhao[1,2](✉), Bao-Jian Xie[1], Yiu-ming Cheung[2,4],
and Xindong Wu[1,3]

[1] College of Computer Science and Information Engineering,
Hefei University of Technology, Hefei, China
z.zhao@hfut.edu.cn
[2] Department of Computer Science, Hong Kong Baptist University,
Hong Kong SAR, China
[3] Department of Computer Science, University of Vermont, Burlington, USA
[4] United International College, Beijing Normal University–Hong Kong
Baptist University, Zhuhai, China

Abstract. Plant identification is an important problem for ecologists, amateur botanists, educators, and so on. Leaf, which can be easily obtained, is usually one of the important factors of plants. In this paper, we propose a growing convolution neural network (GCNN) for plant leaf identification and report the promising results on the ImageCLEF2012 Plant Identification database. The GCNN owns a growing structure which starts training from a simple structure of a single convolution kernel and is gradually added new convolution neurons to. Simultaneously, the growing connection weights are modified until the squared-error achieves the desired result. Moreover, we propose a progressive learning method to determine the number of learning samples, which can further improve the recognition rate. Experiments and analyses show that our proposed GCNN outperforms other state-of-the-art algorithms such as the traditional CNN and the hand-crafted features with SVM classifiers.

1 Introduction

Plant identification is a basic work of plant research and development, and is very important for plant protection and exploration of distinction and genetic relationship between plant species. Usually, the leaves can be easily gotten from plant and have sufficient visible characteristics for differentiating between many species. Currently, plant identification mainly relies on plant scientists with specialized knowledge. However, there exist a large number of plant species, which are hard to be fully identified by a plant scientist. Thus, an automatic plant species identification system by computers and related machine learning algorithms is desired.

The existing state-of-the-art methods of plant leaf identification usually use hand-crafted features such as shape [1], local binary patterns (LBP) [2], pyramid

D. Cremers et al. (Eds.): ACCV 2014, Part II, LNCS 9004, pp. 348–361, 2015.
DOI: 10.1007/978-3-319-16808-1_24

histograms of oriented gradients (PHOG) [3] and their combinations [4], followed by a trainable classifier such as support vector machine (SVM) [5,6], neural networks [7–9], and so on. However, the performances of these methods largely depend on an appropriate set of features, which are varying and need a special design for specific tasks. Moreover, low-level features can be successfully achieved directly, but mid-level and high-level features are difficult to be achieved without any learning procedures [10]. The convolution neural network (CNN) [11] is such a system that can learn generic features for different tasks, directly acting on the two-dimensional image pixels without changing the topology of the input image.

The CNN has received much attention and has been used in lots of applications such as face detection [12], handwriting recognition [13], speech recognition [14], and pedestrian detection [15]. Garcia and Delakis adopted a three-layer CNN structure to detect human face [16], and later they further improved the collecting samples algorithm in the training process [17]. Hinton et al. [18] have proved that increasing the number of feature detectors can significantly improve the performance of the CNNs on various tasks. This particular kind of neural network has no requirement for image preprocessing or feature extraction, and it implements future extraction and pattern classification simultaneously [19].

The CNNs have much fewer parameters to be trained, compared to traditional neural networks. Further, because of the weight sharing technology, the CNNs are easier to be trained. However, there are still some problems in the traditional CNNs. First, the traditional CNNs have fixed structures, which are usually not applicable to all practical problems or the learning of subsequent samples, because the learning of subsequent sample learning often needs to overthrow early learning to establish new weights. Second, it is difficult to determine the number of training samples in the traditional CNNs because too few samples can cause the under-fitting of network learning, while too many may result in over-learning [20].

Addressing the problems mentioned above, this paper proposes a novel approach to construct a growing convolution neural network (GCNN) with a varying architecture for plant leaf identification. The construction and training start with the simplest architecture with a single neuron for each layer, and add new neural cells into each layer, accompanied by modifying the corresponding weights, until the training target is reached. This approach can automatically adjust the CNN structure to fit any specific task. In addition, this paper also proposes a progressive learning method to determine the appropriate number of learning samples for the GCNN. Compared to the traditional CNN, the proposed GCNN model is more effective.

The reminder of the paper is organized as follows. Section 2 reviews the traditional convolution neural network. Section 3 describes the proposed growing convolution neural network. Section 4 presents the details of the progressive sample learning method. Then, Sect. 5 shows the experimental results and makes some discussions. Finally, a conclusion is drawn in Sect. 6.

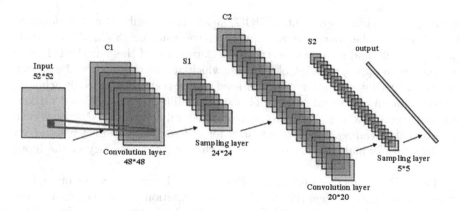

Fig. 1. The structure of a traditional CNN

2   A Review of Convolution Neural Network

The CNN [5] is a feed-forward neural network which can extract the eigen feature from a two-dimensional image. It can directly process grayscale images, and allows image shift and distortion.

2.1   The CNN Structure

Figure 1 shows a traditional CNN structure, consisting of an input layer, several convolution layers, several sampling layers, and an output layer. There are unknown weight parameters needed to be trained between two adjacent layers, the feature maps in S2 layer are fully connected to the output layer, otherwise, the feature maps are not fully connected between two layers. Convolution layers are interspersed with sampling layers to reduce computation time and to gradually improve spatial and configural invariance. A sampling layer produces downsampled version of the input maps. At a convolution layer, the features from the previous layer are convolved with learnable kernels and then fed to an activation function to form the output feature maps. In general, the output of convolution layers is computed as follows:

$$x_j^l = f \left(\sum_{i \in M_j} x_j^{l-1} * k_{ij}^l + b_j^l \right) \tag{1}$$

where M_j represents the set of input maps, x_j^l is an output map, which is given an additive bias b_j^l, l denotes the layer index, k_{ij}^l denotes convolution kernels, and $'*'$ denotes the convolution operator.

As shown in Fig. 1, an input image with simple preprocessing including size normalization (52*52) and graying. Then a convolution operation with a window (5*5) from all directions extracts the features of the input image, and there by features are obtained at the C1 layer. The sampling layer S1 produces downsampled version of the input to eliminate the deviation and image distortion. The size of feature map (48*48) in C1 becomes (24*24) by sampling operation of S1, and the size of sampling window of S1 is 2*2. The output of the sampling layers is computed as follows.

$$x_j^l = f\left(\frac{1}{n}\sum_{i \in M_j} x_i^{l-1} + b^l\right) \qquad (2)$$

where n is the size of window from the convolution layer to the sampling layer so that the output image is n-times smaller along both spatial dimensions.

2.2   The Connections and Weights of the Network

In traditional neural networks, there is an unknown parameter with respect to each connection. However, the CNN uses a weight-sharing technology. Units at a layer are organized in planes, sharing the same set of weights. This technology can greatly reduce the number of free parameters and can be used to detect the representation of the same characteristics in different angles. For the example in Fig. 1, each unit in one feature map has 25 inputs connected to a 5*5 area in one feature map of the convolution layer. This unit is called the receptive field [21]. Therefore, there are 25 tunable weights and a trainable bias for each unit. Layer C1 is a convolutional layer with six feature maps, and the size of the feature maps of C1 is 48*48. So there are $6 * 26 = 156$ tunable parameters and $26*6*48*48 = 359{,}424$ connections between the input and C1 layers. Layer S1 is a sampling layer with the sampling window of (2*2), which produces six feature maps of (24*24). Four pixels in C1 are sampled into one pixel in S1, and there is one tunable weight and a tunable bias for each feature map between C1 and S1. So there are $2*6 = 12$ tunable parameters and $6 * [(2*2) * (24*24) + (24*24)] = 17280$ connections between C1 and S1. Similarly, there are $16*26 = 416$ tunable parameters and $26 * 16 * 24 * 24 = 166400$ connections between S1 and C2, $2 * 16 = 32$ tunable parameters and $16 * [(4*4) * (5*5) + (5*5)] = 6800$ connections between C2 and S2, and $16*5*5+5 = 2005$ tunable parameters and $16*5*5+5 = 2005$ connections between S2 and the output layer. So the network in Fig. 1 totally contains 551,909 connections, but only 2,621 free parameters need learning. The tunable parameters are updated by iteration based on the back-propagation (BP) algorithm [22].

3   The Proposed Growing Convolution Neural Network (GCNN)

The performance of CNN depends greatly on the number of neurons. The recognition rate of the network increases with the growth of the number of neurons, but the computation cost also increases accordingly. Current researches mainly rely on prior knowledge to design the network structure. In this paper, we propose a growth algorithm to construct the CNN, in which the network grows up itself until it solves the target problem. Thereby, the best tradeoff can be achieved between classification accuracy and computation cost.

3.1 Initialization of the Network

The initial network structure is set very simple, as shown in Fig. 2. The initial network consists of two layers of convolution (C1,C2) and two layers of sampling (S1,S2), each of which contains two feature maps. The initial network consists of two branches (branch 1 and branch 2). There are 367 parameters in the convolution network 'Net0' needed to be trained. The weights are updated by the output and the corresponding errors at previous iteration, and the weight updating route is marked by a dotted line in Fig. 2. When the errors converge to be lower than a threshold value, the network learning is stopped. If the error convergence speed becomes smaller than a threshold value, then the training process enters the first round of growth.

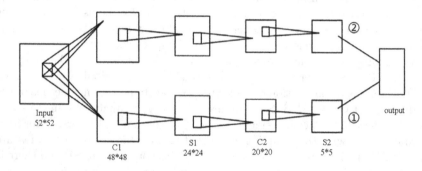

Fig. 2. The initial convolution neural network 'Net0'

3.2 The First Round of Growth

Branch 3 sprouts at the first round of grows on the basis of network 'Net0', which results in the network 'Net1' shown in Fig. 3. The growth rule is as follows. The two feature maps contained in the sampling layer S1 are combined to constitute the third feature map in the convolution layer C2, and the number of feature maps in the convolution layer C2 and sampling layer S2 feature map is increased by one to three. The feature map combination can increase the diversity of features. We initialize the new neurons while the weights in Branches 1 and 2 remain unchanged. The learning route only goes through the output layer and Branch 3 at the new growth round. The connection weights of Branch 3 are modified iteratively until the overall error of the network converges to a small value. If the error convergence speed becomes smaller than a threshold value, then the training process enters the second round of growth.

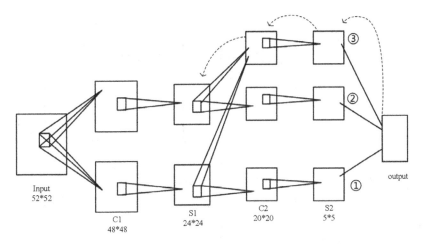

Fig. 3. The first round of growth: the network 'Net1'

3.3 The Second Round of Growth

The second growth of the network adds a feature map to each layer, producing Branch 4 as shown in Fig. 4. Thereby, there are three feature maps in the C1 or S1 layer, while four in the C2 or S2 layer. All learning outcomes of network Net1 are kept unchanged, and the weight modification by back-propagation algorithm only involves Branch 4. The weights of Branch 4 are updated until the overall error of the network converges to a small value. If the error convergence speed becomes smaller than a threshold value, then the training process continues to grow according to the following algorithm.

3.4 The Whole Growth Algorithm and Back-Propagation Algorithm

The whole growing algorithm of the GCNN is shown in Algorithm 1. And Fig. 5 shows an example of a maturing GCNN network with six branches.

Back-Propagation Algorithm

Feedforward Pass. Let l denote the layer index, and then the output of the lth layer is defined as [23]:

$$x^l = f\left(W^l x^{l-1} + b^l\right) \tag{3}$$

where $f(\cdot)$ is an activation function, which is usually set to be sigmoid function or hyperbolic tangent function. The outcomes of layer $l-1$, namely x^{l-1}, pass forward the activation function to produce the final output. Given N training samples $\{x_n\}_{n=1,...,N}$ and the corresponding target vectors $\{t_n\}_{n=1,...,N}$, for a

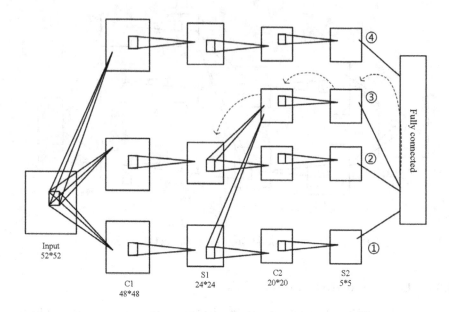

Fig. 4. The second round of growth: the network 'Net2'

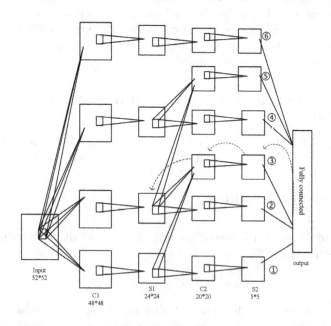

Fig. 5. An example of the CNN network structure of six branches

Algorithm 1. The Whole Growing Algorithm

SET:
E denotes the squared error for training samples;
$E0$ denotes the squared error threshold;
s denotes the convergence speed of BP;
$s0$ denotes the convergence speed threshold;
Nb denotes the number of current network branches;
Initialize: $E0$, $s0$, η(the learning rate of BP), $Net0$;

```
 1: if E > E0 then
 2:    (continue to grow the network:)
 3:    if s > s0 then
 4:       train the network with the BP algorithm;
 5:    else
 6:       (add a new branch to the current network:)
 7:       if Nb is an even number then
 8:          add a new branch starting from the S1 layer, and the feature maps in S1
             layer are merged as a new starting point of the new branch;
 9:          Nb = Nb + 1;
10:       else
11:          add a new branch starting from the input layer;
12:          Nb = Nb + 1;
13:       end if;
14:    end if;
15: else
16:    stop growing;
17: end if
```

Output: A matured CNN.

multiclass classification problem with c classes, we have the following squared-error loss function:

$$E^N = \frac{1}{2} \sum_{n=1}^{N} \sum_{k=1}^{c} (t_k^n - y_k^n)^2 \tag{4}$$

where y^n is the output with respect to the input vector x_n. In training process, the targets of multiclass problems are organized as "one-of-c" codes where the kth element of t_n is positive if the pattern x_n belongs to class k.

Backpropagation Pass. The errors propagate backward through the network, which can be considered as 'sensitivities' of each unit with respect to perturbations of the bias b. The derivative of the error can be defined

$$\delta = \frac{\partial E}{\partial b} \tag{5}$$

It is this derivative that is backpropagated from higher layers to lower layers using the following propagation rule:

$$\delta^l = \left(W^{l+1}\right)^T \delta^{l+1} \cdot f'\left(W^l x^{l-1} + b^l\right) \tag{6}$$

Finally, the delta rule is used to update the weight of a given neuron. For the layer of l, the delta of the error with respect to each weight of this layer is computed by the vector of inputs and the vector of sensitivities:

$$\frac{\partial E}{\partial W^l} = x^{l-1} \left(\delta^l \right)^T \tag{7}$$

$$\Delta W^l = -\eta \frac{\partial E}{\partial W^l} \tag{8}$$

where η is the learning rate.

4   The Progressive Sample Learning Method

It is difficult to determine the proper number of training samples for traditional CNNs. Too few can lead to under-fitting of network learning, while too many may result in over-learning. Therefore, we propose a progressive sample learning method (PSLM) which is self-organizing. The method starts with learning a small amount of samples from each class and then adds to the training set the samples from the classes whose errors are larger until the whole squared-error is satisfactory. This method not only reduces the number of training samples and simplifies learning, but also allows adding new categories. The details of the PSLM is shown in Algorithm 2. The misclassification rate threshold in this algorithm is set as $\varepsilon = 0.3$.

Algorithm 2. The Progressive Sample Learning Method

SET:
E denotes the squared error for training samples;
$E0$ denotes the squared error threshold;
A_i denotes the current training set for class i;
A_i' denotes an additional small sample set from class i excluding A_i;
e_i denotes the misclassification rate for class i;
ε denotes a misclassification rate threshold.

1: **while** $E > E0$ **do**
2:     Train the CNN using the training set $\bigcup_i A_i$;
3:     Compute e_i of the CNN for all i;
4:     **for** each i **do**
5:        **if** $e_i > \varepsilon$ **then**
6:           $A_i = A_i \bigcup A_i'$;
7:        **else**
8:           $A_i = A_i$;
9:        **end if**
10:    **end for**
11: **end while**

Output: A learned CNN.

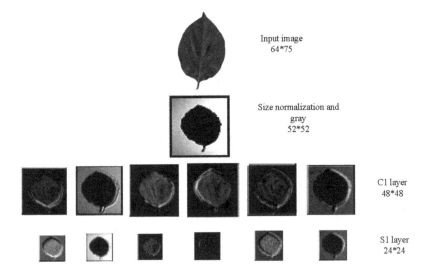

Fig. 6. An example of 2D feature maps of a plant leaf image in the CNN

5   Experiments and Analyses

The experiments includes four parts: (1) The traditional CNNs to classify plant leaf images; (2) The CNN with growing structure to classify plant leaf images; (3) The CNN with growing structure and progressive sample learning method to classify leaf images; (4) Other state-of-the-art methods such as HSV+SVM, Phog+SVM, HSV+Phog+SVM. We evaluate various algorithms on the dataset of the ImageCLEF2012 [24] Plant Identification task. The database comes from the ImageCLEF2012 competition, and it contains 126 tree species in the French Mediterranean area, and the images for each species are contributed by various people, but taken from the same individual plant. The database consists of three kinds of images: scans, scan-like photos (called pseudo-scans) and natural photos. We select 40 classes from ImageCLEF2012 database, each of which contains 60 leaf images of scans and scan-like for evaluations. And 40 images of each class are selected for training and the remaining for test. The evaluation indexes include MCR (misclassification rate), recognition time, RSME (root mean square error), and recognition rate. We set the sample average error threshold $E0 = 0.2$, the predetermined threshold of error convergence speed $s0 = 0.05$ and the learning rate $\eta = 0.0002$. All experiments are implemented by the MATLAB7.1.0.183 (R14) Service Pack 3 running on a computer with the CPU of 8 Quad-Core AMD, memory of 4 194 304 kB, and the WIN7 OS.

Figure 6 shows an example of 2D feature maps of a plant leaf image in the CNN. Figure 7 shows the RMSE and MCR variations of the growing CNN by iteration, respectively, from which we can see that the RMSE and MCR both decrease by iteration. Table 1 shows the comparison of recognition rate

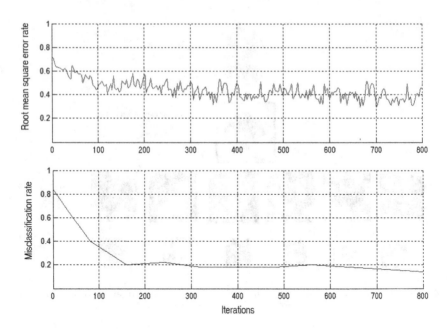

Fig. 7. The MCR and RMSE variations of the CNN of 7 branches in training process

Table 1. The comparison of recognition rate and recognition time between different algorithms

Algorithms	Recognition rate (%)	Recognition time per image (s)	Number of parameters in network
CNN	80.34	0.53	2621
CNN+PLSM	82.05	0.51	2621
HSV+SVM	65.11	0.29	–
Phog+SVM	78.10	0.31	–
HSV+Phog+SVM	83.04	0.41	–
GCNN (5 branches)	66.53	0.43	906
GCNN (5 branches)+PLSM	71.85	0.41	906
GCNN (6 branches)	79.71	0.49	1087
GCNN (6 branches)+PLSM	81.06	0.48	1087
GCNN (7 branches)	86.42	0.61	1266
GCNN (7 branches)+PLSM	87.22	0.60	1266
GCNN (8 branches)	87.68	0.78	1447
GCNN (8 branches)+PLSM	87.89	0.78	1447
GCNN (9 branches)	87.94	0.95	1626
GCNN (9 branches)+PLSM	88.14	0.95	1626

and recognition time between different algorithms. And the number of unknown parameters needed learning for each CNN network is also listed in Table 1.

From Table 1, we can see that traditional CNN performs better than any single feature with an SVM classifier, but has no advantages over fusion of several features such as HSV and Phog. The recognition rate of the GCNN increases with the expansion of the network scale, but the recognition time increases at the same time. When the CNN grows to 9 branches, the recognition rate reaches 87.94 %, and the PLSM helps to further improve the recognition rate, which reaches 88.14 %. However, for the CNN of 7 branches, the recognition rate already reaches 86.42 %, and 87.22 % with the PLSM method, which is significantly higher than that of traditional CNN. And the recognition time of the CNN of 7 branches is much less than that of 9 branches. So the CNN of 7 branches may be a good choice, considering the tradeoff between the recognition rate and recognition time in real applications. In addition, the results in Table 1 also show that our proposed GCNN involves much fewer unknown parameters needed learning than the traditional CNN, which indicates that the GCNN owns simpler structure and is easier to train.

6   Conclusion

In this paper, we have proposed GCNN with a variable topology structure, and evaluated it on plant leaf recognition. The GCNN automatically grows to a proper size according to the complexity of specific classification task. Also, we have presented a progressive sample learning algorithm for the GCNN, which can automatically determine the proper number of training samples, avoiding under-learning or over-fitting. The experiments and analyses on the ImageCLEF2012 plant Identification Dataset show that our proposed GCNN outperforms the other state-of-the-art algorithms such as traditional CNN and hand-crafted features with SVM classifiers.

Acknowledgments. This research was supported by the National Natural Science Foundation of China (Nos. 61375047 and 61272366), the 973 Program of China (No. 2013CB329604), the 863 Program of China (No. 2012AA011005), the Program for Changjiang Scholars and Innovative Research Team in University of the Ministry of Education of China (No. IRT13059), the US National Science Foundation (NSF CCF-0905337), the Faculty Research Grant of Hong Kong Baptist University (No. FRG2/12-13/082), the Hong Kong Scholars Program (No. XJ2012012), China Postdoctoral Science Foundation (No. 2013M540510), and the Fundamental Research Funds for the Central Universities of China.

References

1. Arora, A., Gupta, A., Bagmar, N., Mishra, S., Bhattacharya, A.: A plant identification system using shape and morphological features on segmented leaflets: Team iitk, clef 2012. In: CLEF (Online Working Notes/Labs/Workshop) (2012)

2. Ren, X.-M., Wang, X.-F., Zhao, Y.: An efficient multi-scale overlapped block LBP approach for leaf image recognition. In: Huang, D.-S., Ma, J., Jo, K.-H., Gromiha, M.M. (eds.) ICIC 2012. LNCS, vol. 7390, pp. 237–243. Springer, Heidelberg (2012)

3. Chen, J., Bai, Y.: Classification of smile expression using hybrid phog and gabor features. In: Computer Application and System Modeling (ICCASM), vol. 12, pp. V12–417. IEEE (2010)

4. Ma, L.-H., Zhao, Z.-Q., Wang, J.: ApLeafis: an android-based plant leaf identification system. In: Huang, D.-S., Bevilacqua, V., Figueroa, J.C., Premaratne, P. (eds.) ICIC 2013. LNCS, vol. 7995, pp. 106–111. Springer, Heidelberg (2013)

5. Cortes, C., Vapnik, V.: Support-vector networks. Mach. Learn. **20**, 273–297 (1995)

6. Sun, B.-Y., Huang, D.-S., Guo, L., Zhao, Z.-Q.: Support vector machine committee for classification. In: Yin, F.-L., Wang, J., Guo, C. (eds.) ISNN 2004. LNCS, vol. 3173, pp. 648–653. Springer, Heidelberg (2004)

7. Zhao, Z.Q., Huang, D.S.: A mended hybrid learning algorithm for radial basis function neural networks to improve generalization capability. Appl. Math. Modell. **31**, 1271–1281 (2007)

8. Zhao, Z.Q., Huang, D.S., Sun, B.Y.: Human face recognition based on multi-features using neural networks committee. Pattern Recogn. Lett. **25**, 1351–1358 (2004)

9. Zhao, Z.Q., Gao, J., Glotin, H., Wu, X.: A matrix modular neural network based on task decomposition with subspace division by adaptive affinity propagation clustering. Appl. Math. Modell. **34**, 3884–3895 (2010)

10. Lee, H., Grosse, R., Ranganath, R., Ng, A.Y.: Convolutional deep belief networks for scalable unsupervised learning of hierarchical representations. In: Proceedings of the 26th Annual International Conference on Machine Learning, pp. 609–616. ACM (2009)

11. LeCun, Y., Bottou, L., Bengio, Y., Haffner, P.: Gradient-based learning applied to document recognition. Proc. IEEE **86**, 2278–2324 (1998)

12. Lawrence, S., Giles, C.L., Tsoi, A.C., Back, A.D.: Face recognition: a convolutional neural-network approach. IEEE Trans. Neural Netw. **8**, 98–113 (1997)

13. Simard, P.Y., Steinkraus, D., Platt, J.C.: Best practices for convolutional neural networks applied to visual document analysis. In: 2013 12th International Conference on Document Analysis and Recognition, vol. 2, pp. 958–958. IEEE Computer Society (2003)

14. Hinton, G., Dong, L., Yu, D., Dahl, G.E., Mohamed, A., Jaitly, N., Senior, A., Vanhoucke, V., Nguyen, P., Sainath, T.N., et al.: Deep neural networks for acoustic modeling in speech recognition: the shared views of four research groups. IEEE Signal Process. Mag. **29**, 82–97 (2012)

15. Sermanet, P., Kavukcuoglu, K., Chintala, S., LeCun, Y.: Pedestrian detection with unsupervised multi-stage feature learning. In: 2013 IEEE Conference on Computer Vision and Pattern Recognition (CVPR), pp. 3626–3633. IEEE (2013)

16. Garcia, C., Delakis, M.: A neural architecture for fast and robust face detection. In: 2002 Proceedings of the 16th International Conference on Pattern Recognition, vol. 2, pp. 44–47. IEEE (2002)

17. Garcia, C., Delakis, M.: Convolutional face finder: a neural architecture for fast and robust face detection. IEEE Trans. Pattern Anal. Mach. Intell. **26**, 1408–1423 (2004)

18. Hinton, G.E., Srivastava, N., Krizhevsky, A., Sutskever, I., Salakhutdinov, R.R.: Improving neural networks by preventing co-adaptation of feature detectors (2012). arXiv preprint arXiv:1207.0580

19. Ranzato, M., Huang, F.J., Boureau, Y.L., LeCun, Y.: Unsupervised learning of invariant feature hierarchies with applications to object recognition. In: 2007 IEEE Conference on Computer Vision and Pattern Recognition. CVPR 2007, pp. 1–8. IEEE (2007)
20. Fei-Fei, L., Fergus, R., Perona, P.: Learning generative visual models from few training examples: an incremental bayesian approach tested on 101 object categories. Comput. Vis. Image Underst. **106**, 59–70 (2007)
21. Theunissen, F.E., Sen, K., Doupe, A.J.: Spectral-temporal receptive fields of nonlinear auditory neurons obtained using natural sounds. J. Neurosci. **20**, 2315–2331 (2000)
22. Zhang, J.R., Zhang, J., Lok, T.M., Lyu, M.R.: A hybrid particle swarm optimization-back-propagation algorithm for feedforward neural network training. Appl. Math. Comput. **185**, 1026–1037 (2007)
23. Bouvrie, J.: Notes on convolutional neural networks (2006)
24. Zheng, P., Zhao, Z.Q., Glotin, H.: Zhaohfut at imageclef 2012 plant identification task. In: CLEF (Online Working Notes/Labs/Workshop), Citeseer (2012)

Understanding Convolutional Neural Networks in Terms of Category-Level Attributes

Makoto Ozeki[(⊠)] and Takayuki Okatani

Tohoku University, Sendai, Japan
ozeki@vision.is.tohoku.ac.jp

Abstract. It has been recently reported that convolutional neural networks (CNNs) show good performances in many image recognition tasks. They significantly outperform the previous approaches that are not based on neural networks particularly for object category recognition. These performances are arguably owing to their ability of discovering better image features for recognition tasks through learning, resulting in the acquisition of better internal representations of the inputs. However, in spite of the good performances, it remains an open question why CNNs work so well and/or how they can learn such good representations. In this study, we conjecture that the learned representation can be interpreted as *category-level attributes* that have good properties. We conducted several experiments by using the dataset AwA (Animals with Attributes) and a CNN trained for ILSVRC-2012 in a fully supervised setting to examine this conjecture. We report that there exist units in the CNN that can predict some of the 85 semantic attributes fairly accurately, along with a detailed observation that this is true only for visual attributes and not for non-visual ones. It is more natural to think that the CNN may discover not only semantic attributes but non-semantic ones (or ones that are difficult to represent as a word). To explore this possibility, we perform zero-shot learning by regarding the activation pattern of upper layers as attributes describing the categories. The result shows that it outperforms the state-of-the-art with a significant margin.

1 Introduction

It has been recently reported in a number of literatures that convolutional neural networks (CNNs) show state-of-the-art performances in many benchmark tests, such as object category recognition, handwritten character recognition, medical image applications etc.; [9,13] to name a few. The main reason for such high performance of CNNs is arguably due to their ability of learning features. This ability is considered to be particularly advantageous for difficult problems, such as object category recognition, for which it is unclear what features should be extracted from images. Paying attention on how the inputs are represented internally in the networks as a result of learning, one may think that they learn the representations themselves [1].

© Springer International Publishing Switzerland 2015
D. Cremers et al. (Eds.): ACCV 2014, Part II, LNCS 9004, pp. 362–375, 2015.
DOI: 10.1007/978-3-319-16808-1_25

Despite their success, we lack understanding of why CNNs work so well. For example, it is unclear what in the images the learned networks actually look at and how the input image is represented in them.

This is in stark contrast with the recent accelerated improvements of methods for training deep networks [2,6,8,13]. This lack of understanding leads to real problems; for example, a lot of trial-and-errors are necessary when designing the network architecture for each problem.

There are only a few studies that have contributed to the understanding of convolutional and similar networks [11,12,15]. They share the same view that the features are extracted in a hierarchical manner, in order of simpler to more complex features, in their layers. Although it is interesting as it agrees with the findings of neuroscience, these results are merely "visualization" of the learned features and is far from the full understanding of convolutional networks.

In this paper, towards their better understanding, we consider a different approach, which is to attempt to understand them in terms of category-level attributes. Category-level attributes are various types of properties possessed by the categories to be recognized (e.g., general objects) such that they describe multiple categories in a distinguishable manner [5,10,14]. They are used as intermediate representations connecting the images and the categories to be recognized. A major application is zero-shot learning, i.e., learning to recognize new categories for which no sample is given.

Our approach is based on a conjecture that there should be some connection between the learned representation of CNNs and the category-level attributes. Good attributes which are useful for category recognition tasks such as zero-shot learning are required to describe the categories compactly as well as discriminatively. This requirement is almost the same as the requirement for good internal representations. Therefore, if CNNs can learn good internal representation, they should be good attributes, too.

In this study, we conducted a series of experiments to verify this conjecture by using AwA [10], one of the standard dataset for studying attributes; see Fig. 1. In the experiments, we use DeCAF (Deep Convolutional Activation Features) of Donahue et el. [4] to analyze a CNN trained for the $1,000$ object category recognition task of ILSVRC-2012. We show through experiments that some of theses attributes have a correlation with internal units of particularly higher layers. For example, there automatically emerges in the network a "stripe" neuron (i.e., a unit), which is highly responsive to categories possessing a "stripe" attribute. We also perform zero-shot learning by regarding the activation of a high layer as new attributes. The result shows that this approach outperforms the state-of-the-art method [14] that tailors attributes for the specific task of zero-shot learning.

2   Related Work

2.1   Visualization of Convolutional Networks

Lee et al. [12] propose convolutional DBNs (deep belief networks), which implements convolution and pooling in the framework of DBNs. Training them in an unsupervised manner, they visualize what features are learned by the networks.

They report that features are extracted in a hierarchical manner from lower to higher layers. Le et al. [11] consider a sparse deep autoencoder with a repeated structure of a local receptive field layer followed by a pooling layer. Training the autoencoder using a large number of images in an unsupervised manner, they report that there automatically emerge the units that selectively output a high response to specific objects such as cat faces, human faces, body shapes etc. automatically emerge. Zeiler et al. [15] have proposed a method for visualizing the features leaned by convolutional networks in a supervised fashion. For the network of Krizhevsky et al. [9] trained for object category recognition, they show that, similarly to the above studies, the features are extracted in a hierarchical manner corresponding to the layers.

The problem with these approaches is that although they can give us some insight into what features are learned and how they are extracted in the networks, they are merely visualization. It is difficult to use these results to immediately improve performances or to perform further analysis.

2.2   Transfer Learning by Deep Neural Networks

The recent advances in the study of deep neural networks are initiated by the study of Hinton et al. [7] on unsupervised pretraining of deep networks. Thus, it has been recognized that the deep neural networks are effective in semi-supervised learning settings, i.e., the case where there are a large number of unlabeled data and a few labeled data. Indeed, in the early studies of feature learning by deep networks [11,12], the main focus is on unsupervised learning of image features. It was discovered that the features learned by deep networks tend to be similar in lower layers even for different training data (e.g., faces, cars, etc.).

Recently, it is shown by Donahue et al. [4] that the CNN that is trained for ILSVRC-2012 in a fully supervised setting [9] can be repurposed to fairly different tasks of object recognition and achieve the state-of-the-art performances. The methodology is to train a simple classifier such as linear SVM using the activation patterns of a certain (usually higher-level) layer of the CNN for given training samples, which may be a small set of samples. Their study implies that the CNN trained for the specific task has acquired generic representation of objects that will be useful for all sorts of visual recognition tasks.

The methodology used in the present study is similar to Dohanue et al. [4], as we use the same CNN trained for ILSVRC-2012 and use the activation patterns of its certain layer to input images for other purposes. However, our study differs in that we focus on the analyses of the features and representations learned by the CNN. To be specific, we analyze the relation between the layer activation and category-level attributes.

2.3   Category-Level Attributes

Lampert et al. [10] point out that for object category recognition tasks, it becomes difficult to prepare a sufficient amount of training samples for each object category with a increasing number of the categories to be recognized. They show how this difficulty is mitigated by using attributes possessed by the object categories, and that it is possible to perform zero-shot learning, i.e., recognizing unknown categories for which no sample image is provided, by learning the intermediate relation between the images and their attributes instead of the direct relation between the images and their categories. They created the dataset AwA (Animals with Attributes), which contains fifty animal categories and their 85 attributes such as skin colors, textures, body shapes, and behaviors, as shown in Fig. 1.

The attributes defined in AwA, which are selected by human, are represented by words and have clear meaning. Thus, they are called *semantic attributes*. On the other hand, there is another type of attributes called *discriminative attributes* [5]. Discriminative attributes, which are usually discovered from data and thus need not be represented by words, are useful for some recognition tasks such as image description and zero-shot learning. Yu et al. [14] have recently proposed a method for designing such discriminative attributes that more directly helps zero-shot learning.

As it is closely related to the present study, we briefly summarize the method of Yu et al. here. Computing image features for the sample images of known categories, it first evaluates pairwise similarities among the known categories. It then determines attributes such that the image-based (dis)similarities among the categories are the best preserved in the (dis)similarities in their attribute values. Next, it determine a mapping from the image features to the attribute values such that it best reproduces their mapping for the known categories. Finally, zero-shot learning is performed using this mapping, which enables the computation of the attribute values from a test input image. There is no sample image for the unknown categories, and their relation to the attributes are unknown. Thus, they propose to use human-created pairwise similarities $\tilde{S}$ between the known categories and unknown ones, which enables the computation of the attributes of the unknown categories. This method achieves 46.94 % recognition rate for the task of zero-shot learning. They further propose an extended method that utilizes the known-unknown category similarity $\tilde{S}$ for the design of the attributes, which improves the performance to 48.30 %.

3   Relation of Learned Representation to Category-Level Attributes

We conducted several experiments to examine the conjecture that *the internal representations learned by CNNs can be interpreted as category-level attributes?*

3.1   Experimental Setup

As mentioned earlier, we used the dataset AwA [10] in our experiments. The dataset consists of fifty animal categories, to which 85 attributes are given. Example images with a few chosen attributes are shown in Fig. 1. All the attributes are listed in

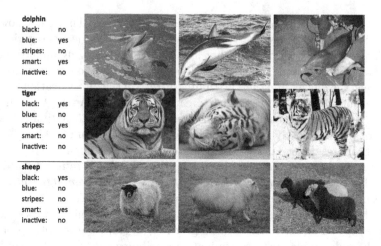

Fig. 1. Example of the images of animals and attributes given to them in the dataset of AwA (Animals with Attributes) [10].

Table 1. We analyze a CNN by using the responses of units in its single layer to input images. Although AwA only provides precomputed image features and not the original images because of the nature of the dataset, the authors kindly provide the original images at out request. For the experiment of predicting attributes by a linear SVM and that of zero-shot learning, the fifty categories are divided into forty and ten categories, and the former is used for training and the latter for testing, as is done in the earlier studies [10, 14].

We use DeCAF [4] to compute the responses of a CNN to input images; the CNN is trained for 1,000 object category recognition task of ILSVRC-2012. (Thus, the CNN analyzed here is the same as [4].) Following [9], we have also succeeded training a similar CNN for ILSVRC-2012 and duplicated a similar result of about 60 % top-1 recognition accuracy. As there was practically no difference between DeCAF and our CNN in the results of the analyses described below, we choose to show the results obtained by DeCAF for better repeatability of our results. In any case, the CNN we examined is trained for the object recognition task of ILSVRC-2012 using 1.2 million images of 1, 000 object categories. Note that the 1, 000 categories of ILSVRC-2012 and 50 animal categories in AwA share 17 categories.

However, there is a slight difference in our use of DeCAF from its standard usage. The features provided by DeCAF are usually the activation patterns of a layer to input images, or equivalently, the *output* of the rectified linear units in that layer. Instead of using these, we use the *inputs* to the same rectified linear units, which are merely the signals before applying the rectified linear function that discards all negative values by setting to zero.

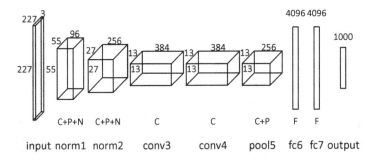

Fig. 2. The architecture of the CNN of DeCAF [4].

3.2   Predicting the Semantic Attributes of AwA

We first consider predicting the 85 attributes of AwA from the responses of the CNN to input images. These attributes, each of which is represented by a single word, are selected by human and describe the animal categories more or less in a distinguishable manner. Whether or not each category possesses an attribute is represented by a binary value (*yes/no*), as shown in Fig. 1. Some of them are concerned with visual properties of animals such as color, the number of legs, body shape etc., and others are with non-visual properties such as behaviors and food habits of animals.

Prediction by Fc7 Individual Units. We examined for individual units in the fc7 layer how its responses to input images relate to their attributes. To be specific, for each image of AwA and for each attribute, we pick the unit that best predicts the attribute and see its prediction accuracy. The accuracy is measured by the overlapped area s of the two histograms of the responses of that unit to the images with and without the attribute. They are normalized before the computation of s. Note that by the response of a unit, we mean the input to the rectified linear activation function, as mentioned above.

The resulting histograms for several selected attributes are shown in Fig. 3; the top row shows the top four attributes; the middle row shows attributes selected from the top 1/3 (but the top four); the bottom row shows attributes with the worst prediction accuracy. Note that the order of the two histograms (red for *yes* and blue for *no*) can be flipped horizontally, as we merely look at the separability of the attributes. Table 1 shows the results for all the attributes in the order of decreasing prediction accuracy.

It is observed from these results that some of the attributes can be predicted with very high accuracy by single unit responses, in spite of its simplicity. Moreover, the visual attributes, such as colors, textures, and body shapes, tend to be ranked high, whereas the non-visual attributes (shaded in the table), which describe the behaviors and other non-visual properties of the animals, tend to be ranked low. Although there are a few non-visual attributes that are ranked high, such as *swims* and *walks*, it might be possible to predict them from the

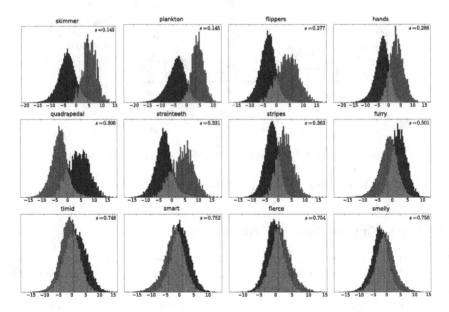

Fig. 3. Histograms of the responses of the fc7 unit that the best predicts each attribute. In each histogram, red bars indicate the images with the attribute and blue bars indicate those without the attribute. The two histograms are normalized. s is the area of their overlap, which measures the prediction (in)accuracy. Top row: the top four attributes with the highest accuracy. Middle row: selected other attributes from the top 1/3. Bottom row: selected four attributes of the worst ten.

surrounding environments of the animals. This might be true for the attributes with highest ranks, such as *skimmer* and *plankton*, which are solely given to animals living in water such as whale; they will be able to be predicted by simply detecting *blue* or *ocean*.

There are a few exceptions to the above observations, such as *black*, for which the prediction accuracy is low despite the fact that it is a visual attribute. This might be because of the way of determining the attributes in AwA that the attributes are given to each category, not to each image. For example, a category *sheep* is given an attribute *black*, which merely means that *some* sheep are in black; see Fig. 1 for such examples. In the above analysis, the unit associated with the attribute *black* is supposed to be activated for an input image of sheep that is not black at all.

Figure 4 shows examples of the prediction for the attributes *hands*, *stripes*, and *blue*.

For each attribute, the upper row shows the images randomly chosen from the top 0.5 % of the entire images sorted in the order of response of the unit; the lower row shows the bottom 0.5 % of the sorted images. (The 0.5 percentages correspond to a set of 150 images.) The unit is the same as the one in Fig. 3.

Table 1. Prediction accuracies of the 85 attributes of AwA by a single unit. Non-visual attributes such as animal's behaviors and natures are displayed in shaded boxes.

1st-22nd	s	23rd-44th	s	45th-66th	s	67th-85th	s
skimmer	0.145	furry	0.501	tail	0.604	vegetation	0.693
plankton	0.145	hairless	0.508	scavenger	0.626	meat	0.693
flippers	0.277	big	0.519	plains	0.631	fields	0.698
hands	0.286	longneck	0.524	pads	0.634	nocturnal	0.699
quadrapedal	0.306	tree	0.539	bulbous	0.640	muscle	0.700
strainteeth	0.331	hooves	0.542	nestspot	0.640	patches	0.703
ocean	0.352	arctic	0.542	fish	0.641	brown	0.703
stripes	0.363	toughskin	0.543	active	0.646	inactive	0.707
desert	0.364	horns	0.546	claws	0.649	meatteeth	0.717
swims	0.366	paws	0.546	grazer	0.649	solitary	0.718
water	0.366	strong	0.550	jungle	0.652	hunter	0.732
coastal	0.375	small	0.561	forager	0.654	chewteeth	0.741
ground	0.385	fast	0.563	lean	0.655	spots	0.742
blue	0.386	bipedal	0.568	bush	0.664	timid	0.748
red	0.401	stalker	0.572	slow	0.666	smart	0.752
walks	0.421	insects	0.572	white	0.675	fierce	0.754
tunnels	0.430	newworld	0.574	group	0.675	smelly	0.756
tusks	0.430	forest	0.576	mountains	0.677	gray	0.767
hops	0.451	domestic	0.577	longleg	0.678	black	0.774
orange	0.453	hibernate	0.594	oldworld	0.686		
yellow	0.454	weak	0.597	buckteeth	0.688		
flys	0.481	cave	0.599	agility	0.689		

Several observations can be made for the results. For the attribute *hands*, the unit seems to be tunĕd to detect primates. This is reasonable, as this attribute is solely given to the primates in AwA. Although this might not be so interesting because the unit is unlikely to actually search for hands in images, it will be rather rare that the concept automatically acquired by the CNN through learning happens to be the same as a manually given semantic attribute. However, the attribute *stripes* seems to be such a case; the top images contain zebras, raccoons, tigers, skunks, which do share this visual attribute and do not seem to have any other visual property in common. Thus, this unit is highly likely to detect the presence of stripe texture in the images. For the attribute *blue*, the unit also seems to actually detect this attribute in the images; interestingly, however, the "correct" prediction of the color for the images of *killer whales* are counted as incorrect predictions, since the animals are not given this attribute in AwA.

Differences Among Layers. In the above experiments we have considered only the units of the fc7 layer. To examine the differences among the layers, we computed s for the units of different layers. To be specific, for each of the fully-connected layers (i.e., fc6 and fc7), we pick a single unit with the maximum s in the layer, as in the same way as above. As mentioned above, the value s is the overlapped area of the two normalized histograms of the responses of a single unit to images *with and without* each attribute. For the lower layers (i.e., norm1, norm2, conv3, conv4, pool5), we pick a map instead of a single unit. By a map, we mean the outputs of a single filter in the convolutional layer.

370 M. Ozeki and T. Okatani

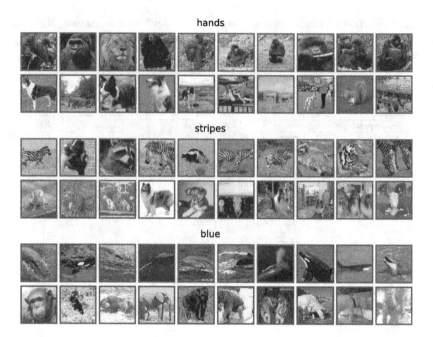

Fig. 4. Examples of the prediction of each attribute by a single unit. For each attribute, the upper row shows the images randomly chosen from the top 0.5 % of the images that the most activates the unit; the lower row shows those randomly chosen from the bottom 0.5 %. The images surrounded by red lines are *with* the attribute and those surrounded by blue lines are *without* the attributes. Best viewed in color (Colour figure online).

(For pooling layers (pool5) and contrast normalization layers (norm1, norm2), we use their pooled and normalized signals.) To be specific, we calculate the maximum response of the units in each map and use it to create the histograms. Thus, for these layers, each attribute is related not to a single unit but to a filter. This is because the units in these layers are considered not only to represent the presence of a feature but also to convey the positional information of the feature; thus, a single unit is not likely to represent an attribute. Using a map instead of a single unit indeed contributes to raise the prediction accuracies of these lower layers.

Figure 5 shows the prediction accuracies $(1 - s)$ of the different layers for several selected attributes. We have found from the results for all the attributes that the accuracy curves can be categorized into several types. The first type is that accuracy increases sharply with the height of layers, as seen in *hands* of Fig. 5. The second is that accuracy is already high at lower layers and continues to be high at higher layers, as shown in *blue*. Their difference is not necessarily clear and thus there are attributes of intermediate type, as seen in *stripes* of Fig. 5. The last is the type that accuracy tends to be low throughout entire layers, as in *smart* and *smelly* of Fig. 5. It should also be noted that there is no attribute such that accuracy decreases with the height of layers.

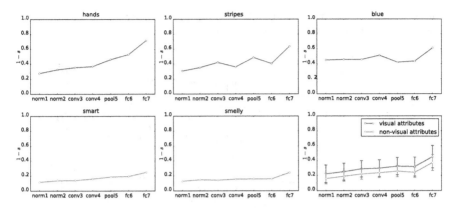

Fig. 5. Prediction accuracies of attributes by different layers. From top left to bottom right: *hands* (4), *stripes* (8), *blue* (14), *smart* (81), *smelly* (83), and the averaged accuracies for visual and non-visual attributes. The numbers in the parentheses indicate the rank in Table 1.

These differences among layers and attributes may be explained by how difficult it is to represent the attributes. Some attributes, such as colors, are easy to judge their presence in images. They are associated with low level features, which can be correctly extracted even by the lower layers. Some attributes, such as those related to body shapes like *hands*, are more difficult to judge their presence in images (even if it could be translated into *primates* in the CNN as mentioned earlier). They may need complicated feature extraction, which could only be performed at higher layers. Non-visual attributes, such as *smart* and *smelly*, cannot be correctly estimated even at higher layers.

Prediction by Linear SVM. In the above, we have considered the possibility that a single unit represents a particular attribute. It is more natural to think that each attribute is represented by a combination of multiple unit activations, e.g., a linear combination in the simplest case. Thus, we trained a linear SVM to predict each attribute from the responses of the entire fc7 units. We used the forty categories for training and the remaining ten categories for test, as in the standard procedure of the zero-shot learning. Table 2 shows the results, i.e., the prediction accuracies for the 85 attributes, sorted in their order. Apart from the the top ten attributes are predicted with more than 90 % accuracies, which is much better than the single unit results, the two results share the order of the attribute including the tendency that the visual attributes are easier to predict than non-visual ones.

3.3   Zero-Shot Learning

In the above experiments we consider the relation of layer activations to semantic attributes. These attributes are arbitrarily chosen by human. It could be possible

Table 2. Prediction accuracies of the 85 attributes of AwA by linear SVM using all the responses of the fc7 units. Non-visual attributes are in shaded boxes.

1st-22nd	s	23rd-44th	s	45th-66th	s	67th-85th	s
flys	0.999	bipedal	0.856	fast	0.737	bush	0.623
red	0.999	swims	0.855	hibernate	0.721	grazer	0.621
desert	0.999	water	0.855	gray	0.718	domestic	0.599
plankton	0.965	hooves	0.853	pads	0.713	hunter	0.598
hands	0.961	strainteeth	0.849	nocturnal	0.711	smelly	0.594
yellow	0.953	blue	0.847	tail	0.697	black	0.593
tunnels	0.947	longleg	0.844	mountains	0.697	slow	0.590
longneck	0.946	insects	0.837	muscle	0.691	meat	0.589
skimmer	0.941	hairless	0.833	forest	0.686	timid	0.582
tusks	0.926	weak	0.824	small	0.684	group	0.580
cave	0.926	paws	0.821	smart	0.675	patches	0.579
hops	0.918	scavenger	0.818	chewteeth	0.672	meatteeth	0.707
flippers	0.917	coastal	0.816	tree	0.672	brown	0.576
quadrapedal	0.914	plains	0.815	white	0.661	lean	0.573
ocean	0.896	furry	0.804	forager	0.660	active	0.572
horns	0.889	toughskin	0.789	agility	0.658	fierce	0.560
orange	0.886	strong	0.789	jungle	0.656	nestspot	0.544
stripes	0.881	big	0.781	solitary	0.653	fish	0.529
ground	0.881	fields	0.767	inactive	0.647	spots	0.527
oldworld	0.879	newworld	0.762	buckteeth	0.641		
walks	0.872	stalker	0.761	vegetation	0.634		
arctic	0.871	claws	0.740	bulbous	0.630		

that the CNN finds more general attributes than the 85 semantic attributes, some of which might not be even represented by words. To examine this possibility, we perform zero-shot learning by regarding the layer activation for an input image as its attributes. Based on the results in the last section, we choose the responses of the 4096 units in the fc7 layer.

Unlike the 85 semantic attributes, no relation is provided in advance between the discovered attributes and the unknown categories, and thus it is impossible to recognize the categories without additional information. To fulfill this missing link, Yu et al. [14] propose to use a similarity matrix between the 40 known categories and 10 unknown categories that are created by human subjects. (They used this matrix to perform zero-shot learning by their attributes, which are generated from the training data by their method.) Following their method, we borrow their similarity matrix that are publicly available at the authors' webpage[1]. Computing the similarities between an input image and the known 40 categories using its responses, we evaluate the correlation between them and the similarity matrix to classify the input image.

The details of the method is as follows. Before testing, we compute the responses of the fc7 units to each image of the known forty categories, which yields forty point sets in a 4096-dimensional space. At the time of testing, we compute the responses $[r_1, \ldots, r_{4096}]$ to the input image, and then evaluate its similarity to the j-th known category ($j = 1, \ldots, 40$) by the following distance metric:

---

[1] https://github.com/felixyu/category/tree/master/zero_shot_data.

Table 3. Results of zero-shot learning. The last row indicates the accuracy obtained when the output of the fc7 layer units are directly used for r_i's of (1). The accuracy one row above is obtained by using the inputs to the rectified linear function for r_i's.

Method	# Attributes	Accuracy
Lampert et al. [10]	85	40.5
Yu et al. [14]	200	46.94
Yu et al. (Adaptive) [14]	200	48.30
Our method	4096	**62.40**
Our method (after ReLU)	4096	59.14

$$d_j = \sum_{i=1}^{4096} \|r_i - \mathrm{NN}_j(r_i)\|^2, \tag{1}$$

where $\mathrm{NN}_j(r_i)$ is the response of the i-th unit that is the nearest to r_i among all the samples belonging to the j-th category. More rigorously, we use its inverse as a similarity. Finally, we compare the resulting similarity vector against the 10×40 similarity matrix $\tilde{\mathbf{S}}$ of Yu et al. [14] to determine into which of the ten categories the input image is classified. To be specific, the comparison is performed by the normalized correlation between the input similarity vector and each row vector of $\tilde{\mathbf{S}}'$:

$$\hat{c} = \underset{c}{\arg\max} \sum_j \frac{\tilde{S}_{cj} \cdot (1/d_j)}{(\sum_k \tilde{S}_{cj})(\sum_k (1/d_j))}. \tag{2}$$

The results are shown in Table 3. Our approach significantly outperforms[2] the accuracy reported in [10], where the 85 semantic attributes are used, and is even much better than the method of Yu et al., in which attributes are designed particularly for the purpose of zero-shot learning. Note that the accuracy of 48.30 % reported in [14] is achieved by utilizing $\tilde{\mathbf{S}}$ to design the attributes, meaning that the discovered attributes could be ineffective for other unknown categories. Thus, it is more appropriate to compare the accuracy of 46.94 % with the accuracy of 62.40 % achieved by our method. It should also be noted that our CNN is trained only for the purpose of the category recognition, not for zero-shot learning, and nevertheless this high performance is attained. This fact shows the goodness of the internal representation of CNNs as attributes for zero-shot learning. It is particularly important that CNNs can *automatically* discover attributes having good properties, as compared with the manually designed attributes and the ones discovered by a dedicated method.

---

[2] It should be noted that these comparisons might not be fair, as these studies [10,14] focused on how to use or how to generate attributes, given a set of image features. In other words, their method should work with the CNN activations used in our study, instead of the traditional hand-designed features.

4 Summary

Toward a better understanding of convolutional neural networks (CNNs), we conjecture that the internal representation learned by CNNs should have similarities to category-level attributes possessing good qualities. The experimental results support this conjecture. Despite the fact that the CNN is trained for a specific category recognition task, there automatically emerge units in the CNN that can predict some of the semantic attributes that are hand-designed. We also test zero-shot learning by treating the responses of units in a layer of the CNN as category-level attributes. The method shows much better performances than the state-of-the-art method that designs attributes particularly for the purpose of zero-shot learning based on traditional hand-designed image features.

Acknowledgement. This work was supported by JSPS KAKENHI Grant Numbers 25135701, 25280054.

References

1. Bengio, Y., Courville, A.C., Vincent, P.: Representation learning: a review and new perspectives, Computing Research Repository abs/1206.5538 (2012)
2. Cireşan, D., Meier, U., Schmidhuber, J.: Multi-column deep neural networks for image classification. In: CVPR (2012)
3. Deng, J., Dong, W., Socher, R., Li, L.-J., Li, K., Fei-Fei, L.: ImageNet: a large-scale hierarchical image database. In: CVPR (2009)
4. Donahue, J., Jia, Y., Vinyals, O., Hoffman, J., Zhang, N., Tzeng, E., Darrell, T.: DeCAF: a deep convolutional activation feature for generic visual recognition. In: ICML (2014)
5. Farhadi, A., Endres, I., Hoiem D., Forsyth, D.: Describing objects by their attributes. In: CVPR (2009)
6. Goodfellow, I.J., Warde-Farley, D., Mirza, M., Courville, A., Bengio, Y.: Maxout networks. In: ICML (2013)
7. Hinton, G.E., Salakhutdinov, R.R.: Reducing the dimensionality of data with neural networks. Science **313**, 504–507 (2006)
8. Hinton, G.E., Srivastava, N., Krizhevsky, A., Sutskever, I., Salakhutdinov, R.: Improving neural networks by preventing co-adaptation of feature detectors, Computing Research Repository abs/1207.0580 (2012)
9. Krizhevsky, A., Sutskever, I., Hinton, G.E.: ImageNet classification with deep convolutional neural networks. In: NIPS (2012)
10. Lampert, C.H., Nichisch, H., Harmeling, S.: Learning to detect unseen object classes by between-class attribute transfer. In: CVPR (2009)
11. Le, Q.V., Ranzato, M., Monga, R., Devin, M., Corrado, G.S., Dean, J., Ng A.Y.: Building high-level features using large scale unsupervised learning. In: ICML (2012)

12. Lee, H., Grosse, R., Ranganath, R., Ng, A.Y.: Convolutional deep belief networks for scalable unsupervised learning of hierarchical representations. In: ICML (2009)
13. Wan, L., Zeiler, M.D., Zhang, S., LeCun, Y., Fergus, R.: Regularization of neural networks using dropconnect. In: ICML (2013)
14. Yu, F.X., Cao, L., Feris, R.S., Smith, J.R., Chang S.-F.: Designing category-level attributes for discriminative visual recognition. In: CVPR (2013)
15. Zeiler, M.D., Fergus, R.: Visualizing and understanding convolutional networks. In: Fleet, D., Pajdla, T., Schiele, B., Tuytelaars, T. (eds.) ECCV 2014, Part I. LNCS, vol. 8689, pp. 818–833. Springer, Heidelberg (2014)

Robust Scene Classification with Cross-Level LLC Coding on CNN Features

Zequn Jie[1]([✉]) and Shuicheng Yan[2]

[1] Keio-NUS CUTE Center, National University of Singapore, Singapore, Singapore
jiezequn@nus.edu.sg
[2] Department of Electrical and Computer Engineering,
National University of Singapore, Singapore, Singapore

Abstract. Convolutional Neural Network (CNN) features have demonstrated outstanding performance as global representations for image classification, but they lack invariance to scale transformation, which makes it difficult to adapt to various complex tasks such as scene classification. To strengthen the scale invariance of CNN features and meanwhile retain their powerful discrimination in scene classification, we propose a framework where cross-level Locality-constrained Linear Coding and cascaded fine-tuned CNN features are combined, which is shorted as *cross-level LLC-CNN*. Specifically, this framework first fine-tunes multi-level CNNs in a cascaded way, then extracts multi-level CNN features to learn a cross-level universal codebook, and finally performs locality-constrained linear coding (LLC) and max-pooling on the patches of all levels to form the final representation. It is experimentally verified that the LLC responses on the universal codebook outperform the CNN features and achieve the state-of-the-art performance on the two currently largest scene classification benchmarks, MIT Indoor Scenes and SUN 397.

1 Introduction

Scene classification is a fundamental problem in computer vision. However, it is not an easy task due to the great diversity of image contents as well as the variations in illumination and scale conditions. Conventional approaches such as Bag-of-Features (BoF) model [1], Bag-of-Parts (BoP) [2], Object Bank [3], and their respective combinations with Spatial Pyramid Matching (SPM) [4], have achieved satisfactory performance in this task. These works [5,6] utilize hand-crafted features, e.g., SIFT [7] and HOG [8], which require designing lots of tricks and lack image representation power for different complex problems.

Recently, in contrast to hand-crafted features, image features learned from Convolutional Neural Network (CNN) [9] have achieved great success in vision recognition tasks [10–13]. Among these works, one of the greatest breakthroughs is that CNN has achieved an accuracy which is 10 % higher than all the hand-crafted feature based methods in ImageNet Large Scale Visual Recognition Challenge (ILSVRC) [14] which contains over 1 million images from 1000 categories. Inspired by the outstanding performance of CNN in large-scale image classification, many works [15–18] consider how to transfer CNN features pre-trained on

© Springer International Publishing Switzerland 2015
D. Cremers et al. (Eds.): ACCV 2014, Part II, LNCS 9004, pp. 376–390, 2015.
DOI: 10.1007/978-3-319-16808-1_26

ImageNet to small-scale computer vision tasks in which only a limited number of task-specific training samples are available. As generic global image representations, off-the-shelf CNN features pre-trained on ImageNet are successfully applied to various vision tasks, including object detection [18] and image retrieval [19]. Furthermore, to improve the adaptation and representation power of CNN features in specific tasks, the fine-tuned CNN features based on pre-trained ImageNet CNN features are also used and have achieved better performance in these transferred tasks [16,17,20].

Despite the great success of CNN in various vision tasks, as global image representations, CNN features retain too much global spatial information and lack invariance to scale transformation since raw pixels are filtered and pooled alternatively within their local neighborhoods in the network. Actually, as shown in [21], feature maps after each layer can be used to reconstruct the original image due to the high spatial order of CNN features. Although the max-pooling layer after each convolution layer provides a certain degree of invariance to local scale transformation, invariance to global scale transformation cannot be guaranteed. Based on the 4096-dimensional global CNN features, their variance to scale transformation will directly lead to the decrease of recognition accuracy when only scale transformed images are available for testing.

To improve the scale invariance of CNN features, a multi-level pooling framework has been proposed by [19]. Specifically, CNN features from patches with various sizes in different levels of the framework are extracted as mid-level image representations, followed by an intra-level pooling process over these patches. Within one level, densely distributed patch features cover the whole image and are pooled in an orderless way. By pooling the patch CNN features in each level, the final representation becomes patch-level orderless and scale invariant to a certain degree.

However, when the whole testing image is scaled, all the patches of its finer levels will be scaled by the same scaling ratio accordingly. In this case, CNN features of both the whole image and the patches of all levels will not work well since CNN features of each level are learned in a supervised manner from the training patches in the same level. To demonstrate this, we conduct an experiment on an image from SUN 397 [22] with the model trained on original training samples. Figure 1 shows the prediction of each patch in level 1 and level 2 of both the original image and its scaled version (10/6 ratio). As can be seen, both the whole image (level 1) and patches in level 2 obtain the correct predictions – "tent" by the fine-tuned CNN of their own level. In contrast, the scaled testing image obtains a wrong prediction – "mountain" using the fine-tuned CNN trained on the original non-scaled training images. A similar situation also happens in level 2, where 3 patches of the total 4 obtain wrong predictions. In this case, even if orderless pooling is performed on top of the CNN features of patches, no scale invariance can be guaranteed since the features to be pooled, i.e., CNN features of each patch have changed due to the scaling of the whole testing image.

In this paper, we present a simple but effective framework, which we refer to as cross-level LLC coding and cascaded fine-tuned CNN (*cross-level LLC-CNN*),

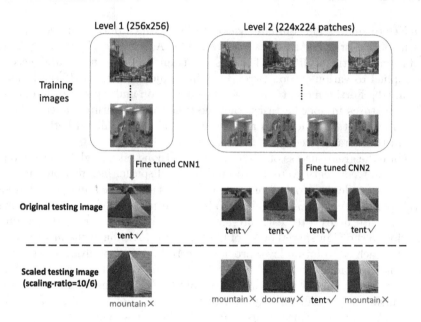

Fig. 1. Predictions of each patch in level 1 and level 2 of both the original image and its scaled version (10/6 ratio) with the CNN trained on original training samples. It is shown that predictions of the original testing image are all correct, while there are many wrong predictions for all levels of the scaled image.

to provide CNN features more robust to scale transformation. The pipeline is illustrated in Fig. 2. Details will be presented in Sect. 3. Our proposed framework first fine-tunes CNNs for each level in a cascaded way, which means the CNN parameters learned in the coarser level are utilized as the initialization of the finer level. Subsequently, CNN features of all the patches in multiple levels are extracted by their own fine-tuned CNNs. Then we learn a universal (cross-level) codebook on all the CNN features of multi-level patches by k-means. Based on this universal codebook, Locality-constrained Linear Coding (LLC) [23] is performed for all the CNN features. The locality-constrained nature of LLC ensures each patch to find its most similar patches among all the patches distributed in multiple levels, even if the image and its patches are scaled. This helps build a more robust representation to scale transformation. Finally, all the LLC features of patches in multiple levels are max-pooled together to build the final image representation.

Extensive experiments on two challenging scene classification datasets, i.e., MIT indoor scenes [24] and SUN 397 [22], verify the superiority of the cross-level LLC coding on the cascaded fine-tuned CNN features over other conventional methods. The rest of the paper is organized as follows. First, we give a survey of typical methods for scene classification in Sect. 2. Then we elaborate on our framework, cross-level Locality-constrained Linear Coding (LLC) of CNN features in Sect. 3. After showing experimental results in Sect. 4, we draw a conclusion in Sect. 5.

2   Related Work

Scene classification as a fundamental and challenging vision task has attracted much attention and great progress has been achieved in the past decades. Generally, methods which have been proposed to deal with this task can be categorized into two types: Bag-of-Features (BoF) and deep learning.

Conventional methods mostly belong to the Bag-of-Features framework type. Early methods of this type adopted K-means Vector Quantization (VQ) to encode local features [25]. Later, Sparse Coding (SC) [26] was proposed to relax the cardinality constraint of VQ, which requires that only one coefficient of the code words is 1 while the rest are all 0. To add spatial organization information to the orderless Bag-of-Features, Spatial Pyramid Matching (SPM) [4] partitions the entire image into multi-scale patches and performs VQ or SC on each patch. Also, Orientational Pyramid Matching (OPM) [27] was used to partition the image in a more discriminative way, with the consideration of the orientation information. In this type of framework, local scale invariant hand-crafted features are usually relied on, such as SIFT [7] and HOG [8]. The combination between low-level scale invariant features and mid-level orderless pooling builds a more robust representation to scale transformation. The main limitation of this type of framework lies in the designing of hand-crafted features, which needs lots of tricks and is not applicable to some specific complex problems.

The other type of framework, i.e., deep learning, tries to model high-level abstractions of visual data by using architectures containing multiple layers of non-linear transformations. Convolutional Neural Network (CNN), as a typical example of deep learning models, has achieved great success in image classification, including ILSVRC 2012, ILSVRC 2013, tiny image dataset CIFAR-10/100 [28] and hand-written digits recognition [29]. [21] later proved that CNN features do not have invariance to different kinds of geometric transformations, e.g., scale transformation and rotation transformation. To strengthen the representation power of CNN when scale transformation occurs, [19] proposed a multi-scale orderless pooling framework, which includes CNN feature extraction at multiple levels and VLAD [30] pooling over these features. Our approach differs from this work in the different CNN features extracted and the cross-level feature coding and pooling schemes.

3   Cross-Level LLC Coding on Multi-level CNN Features

3.1   Multi-level Cascaded Fine-Tuned CNNs

To capture the context information of various sizes of patches, similar to [19], we adopt a multi-level framework to extract fine-tuned CNN features in multiple levels. The patch sizes of level 1 to level 5 are chosen carefully as follows: 256*256, 224*224, 192*192, 160*160, 128*128. Intuitively, transferring the groundtruth label of the whole image to its patches requires the patches not to be too small. The reason is that in scene classification, the groundtruth label is the high-level semantic abstract on the whole image, and too small local patches usually cannot be summarized as the same abstract concept (groundtruth label) as that of the whole image. Actually, we have found that the single patch recognition accuracy of level 5 with patch size 128*128 only achieves 43.6 %, while the recognition accuracy of level 1 is 61.46 % on the MIT indoor scenes dataset. Fortunately, although in level 5, the single patch recognition accuracy is much lower than that of the whole image, the recognition accuracy using max-pooled features of this level can still obtain a satisfactory result of 64.97 %. Thus, we set the smallest patch size as 128*128. The stride of all the 5 levels is 32 pixels, thus we have 1, 4, 9, 16, 25 patches from level 1 to level 5 respectively.

To improve the discrimination and adaptation power of off-the-shelf CNN features on scene classification datasets, we fine-tune the CNN model pre-trained on ImageNet for each level in a cascaded way. We choose the same CNN architecture with [21] for its proven great performance in ILSVRC 2013. It contains five convolutional layers and three fully-connected layers with 60 million parameters. Since the numbers of categories in scene classification datasets differ from that in ImageNet, we change the number of the outputs of the last fully-connected layer, which represents the predicted probability of each target category, from 1000 in ImageNet to 67 and 397 in MIT indoor scenes and SUN 397 datasets respectively. Before fed into this CNN model, all the patches are resized to 256*256. During the stochastic gradient descent training process, the parameters of the first seven layers are initialized by the parameters pre-trained on ImageNet and the parameters of the last fully-connected layer are randomly initialized with a Gaussian distribution. The learning rates of the convolutional layers, the first two fully-connected layers and the last fully-connected layer are initialized as 0.001, 0.002 and 0.01, respectively and reduced to one tenth of the current rates after every 20 epochs (50 epochs in total). By setting the different learning rates for different layers, the parameters in different layers are updated by different rates. The main reasons for this setting are as follows: the first few convolution layers mainly extract low-level invariant features, such as texture and shape, thus the parameters are more consistent from the pre-trained dataset to the target dataset, whose learning rates are set as a relatively low value (i.e., 0.001); for the final few layers, especially the last fully-connected layer which is specifically adapted to the new target dataset, a higher learning rate is required to guarantee its fast convergence to the new optimum.

To strengthen the connections between the fine-tuned CNNs of different levels and reduce the convergence time, we adopt a cascaded fine-tuning strategy. Specifically, we use the model pre-trained on ImageNet as our initialization when training the CNN of level 1. When training on other finer levels, we always use the model trained on the last coarser level as our initialization. For example, the CNN trained on level 1 will be the initialization when training CNN on level 2. In Sect. 4, we will show the superiority of the cascaded fine-tuned CNN over off-the-shelf CNN and CNN fine-tuned with the pre-trained model on ImageNet in recognition accuracy.

3.2   Cross-Level LLC Coding and Pooling on CNN Features

Although separate fine-tuning of CNN for each level enhances the discrimination power of CNN features, it is still unstable for scale transformation, as fine-tuned CNNs are trained on the original non-scaled training images and patches, thus naturally characterize the image spatial organization of these non-scaled samples better.

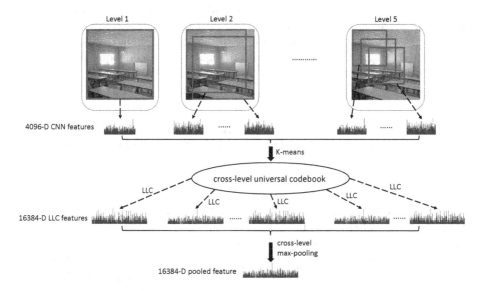

Fig. 2. Pipeline of cross-level LLC coding and max-pooling on CNN features. First, patch CNN features of all the 5 levels are clustered to learn a cross-level codebook. Next, all these CNN features are encoded based on this codebook via LLC coding. Finally, max-pooling is performed on all the encoded features to form a cross-level pooled feature, as the new image representation.

To solve this problem, we propose to use a cross-level feature coding and pooling scheme on the fine-tuned CNN features extracted from all patches of multiple levels. The pipeline is illustrated in Fig. 2. Firstly, a 4096-dimensional feature is extracted in each patch with the fine-tuned CNN of their own level. Subsequently, a cross-level codebook is learned by clustering all these multi-level patch CNN features into 16384 clusters (4 times as the 4096 dimensions) with the k-means algorithm. By doing this, different patch levels of CNN features can be found among the code words of this cross-level codebook such that the codebook gains multi-level representation power. Next, Locality-constrained Linear Coding (LLC) is performed on the multi-level CNN features based on the learned cross-level codebook. LLC coding enforces the corresponding encoding coefficients to be high if the code words are similar to the feature, and enforces the coefficients of other dissimilar code words to be zero [23]. The underlying hypothesis is that features approximately reside on a lower dimensional manifold in an ambient feature space [31]. Specifically, LLC coding uses the following criteria:

$$\min_C \sum_{i=1}^{N} ||x_i - Bc_i||^2 + \lambda ||d_i \odot c_i||^2 \tag{1}$$
$$\text{s.t. } \mathbf{1}^T c_i = 1, \forall i.$$

where N is the number of features to be encoded, x_i represents the ith encoded feature, B is the codebook matrix, c_i is the ith LLC coding result, $\odot$ denotes the element-wise multiplication, and $d_i \in R^M$ is the dissimilarity between the encoded feature and the code words with M denoting the codebook size. Specifically,

$$d_i = \exp\left(\frac{\text{dist}(x_i, B)}{\sigma}\right) \tag{2}$$

where $dist(x_i, B) = [dist(x_i, b_1), ..., dist(x_i, b_M)]^T$, and $dist(x_i, b_j)$ is the Euclidean distance between x_i and b_j. The analytical solution of LLC is as follows:

$$\tilde{c}_i = (C_i + \lambda \text{diag}(d)) \setminus \mathbf{1}$$
$$c_i = \tilde{c}_i \setminus \mathbf{1}^T \tilde{c}_i \tag{3}$$

where $C_i = (B - \mathbf{1}x_i^T)(B - \mathbf{1}x_i^T)^T$ denotes the data covariance matrix. Hence, LLC can be implemented very fast in practice.

By performing LLC on multi-level patch CNN features based on the cross-level codebook, different levels of CNN features extracted from patches of various sizes share a common codebook and can be encoded based on this codebook, regardless of their levels. This naturally enhances the scale invariance of the LLC features since no matter how the whole image and all of its patches are scaled, the CNN features can always find their similar code words in the cross-level codebook, either from the code words of their own levels or from other levels, and use these code words to represent them, leaving the reconstruction coefficients of all the rest dissimilar code words to be zero. As can be seen in Fig. 3, CNN features of the original image will probably be represented by the code words of their own level, while CNN features of the scaled image may be similar to the code words from other levels and represented by these code words.

After obtaining LLC features of all the patches from multiple levels, we max-pool these cross-level features together in a mid-level (patch-level) orderless manner to form the final image representation. Finally, a linear SVM is trained based on the cross-level pooled features to obtain the predictions. Experimental results on MIT indoor scenes and SUN 397 datasets shown in Sect. 4 verify the great discrimination and robustness to scale transformation of the proposed image representation.

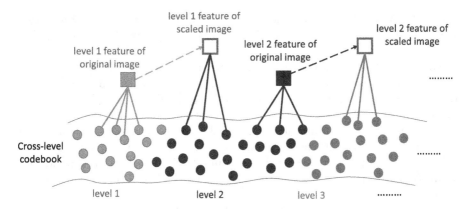

Fig. 3. Illustration of selected representation codewords of CNN features for original image and scaled image. Circles in different colors represent code words from different levels. Blue and red solid squares denote level 1 and level 2 CNN features of the original image, respectively, and blue and red hollow squares represent those of the scaled image respectively. (better viewed in color) (Color figure online)

4   Experiments

4.1   Datasets

We evaluate the proposed approach on the two currently largest scene classification datasets: MIT indoor scenes and SUN 397.

MIT Indoor Scenes. is the largest indoor scene dataset, which contains 67 categories and a total of 15620 images. The complex spatial layout of the indoor scene image makes the classification even more difficult than outdoor scene image classification. Therefore, this dataset is chosen as an important benchmark for the evaluation of our approach. The standard training/testing split for the MIT indoor scenes dataset consists of 80 training images and 20 testing images per category.

SUN 397. is the current largest scene classification dataset. It contains 397 scene categories, both indoor and outdoor, with at least 100 images per category. The 10 fixed splits for training and testing images are publicly available. For each category, there are 50 images for training and 50 images for testing. The accuracy is all averaged over all the 10 splits.

4.2   Multi-level Cascaded Fine-Tuning

Baselines. We compare our cascaded fine-tuned CNN with two baselines: (a) off-the-shelf CNN features extracted by the pre-trained model on ImageNet (here we choose DeCAF$_6$ [15] as our off-the-shelf CNN feature for its better performance than DeCAF$_7$); (b) fine-tuned CNN initialized by the pre-trained model on ImageNet.

We conduct the comparison experiments on both the MIT indoor scenes dataset and the SUN 397 dataset. To be fair, we test all these 3 CNN features by simple max-pooling within their own level and training a linear SVM, without cross-level LLC coding and pooling. Please note that for level 1, since the whole image yields only one feature, there is no need to do pooling, and since no coarser level exists, there are no cascaded fine-tuned results. All the fine-tuned CNN features are obtained after 50 epochs of training. L2 normalization is performed on all the CNN features before used to train the SVMs. The SVM parameter (C) is all set as 0.5.

The results on MIT indoor scenes and SUN 397 are shown in Tables 1 and 2 respectively for comparison. As can be seen, both on the MIT indoor scenes dataset and the SUN 397 dataset, fine-tuned CNN features, including those fine-tuned on ImageNet and cascaded fine-tuned ones on coarser levels of their own datasets, achieve higher accuracy than the off-the-shelf CNN features on all the levels. This is very natural since fine-tuned CNN features gain stronger discrimination power than generic off-the-shelf CNN features after the training on the specific datasets. The comparison between fine-tuned CNN on ImageNet and cascaded fine-tuned CNN shows that cascaded fine-tuned CNN features obtain higher accuracy than CNN fine-tuned on ImageNet by approximately 1 % on all levels. This demonstrates that initialization by the trained model on the coarser level of a specific dataset helps the finer level model to converge to a better optimum than initialization by the model pre-trained on ImageNet.

Table 1. Classification accuracy on MIT indoor scenes for off-the-shelf CNN features, fine-tuned CNN features on ImageNet and cascaded fine-tuned CNN features of each level.

	Level 1	Level 2	Level 3	Level 4	Level 5
off-the-shelf CNN	53.65	57.26	60.75	61.48	61.89
fine-tuned CNN on ImageNet	**61.46**	62.58	63.17	64.03	64.23
cascade fine-tuned CNN	—	**63.77**	**64.27**	**64.39**	**64.97**

Table 2. Classification accuracy on SUN 397 for off-the-shelf CNN features, fine-tuned CNN features on ImageNet and cascaded fine-tuned CNN features of each level.

	Level 1	Level 2	Level 3	Level 4	Level 5
off-the-shelf CNN	40.53	41.25	41.68	42.07	42.64
fine-tuned CNN on ImageNet	**43.75**	44.88	45.17	45.54	45.81
cascade fine-tuned CNN	—	**45.61**	**46.33**	**46.58**	**46.87**

4.3   Cross-Level LLC Coding and Pooling

Baselines. We compare our cross-level LLC and pooling approach (*cross-level LLC-CNN*) with multi-level pooled CNN features [19]. We choose multi-level max-pooling as the pooling method since we also perform max-pooling on our *cross-level LLC-CNN* features.

Classification Accuracy. We evaluate our cross-level LLC and pooling approach (*cross-level LLC-CNN*) on the MIT indoor scenes dataset and the SUN 397 dataset. The baseline method, multi-level pooled CNN is also tested for comparison with our *cross-level LLC-CNN*. The comparison results on each level and the combination of all levels are presented in Tables 3 and 4. Here, cross-level LLC coding and pooling on a single level means that max-pooling is only performed within this level, while a cross-level codebook is still learned over all the levels. For the combination from level 1 to level 5, the final output of multi-level pooled CNN is obtained by concatenating the pooled result of each level together. Before all coding and pooling procedures, all the CNN features are extracted by the cascaded fine-tuned models. All the fine-tuned CNN features are obtained after 50 epochs of training. L2 normalization is performed on all the CNN features after extraction. The SVM parameter (C) is all set as 0.5. For reference, we also include some typical state-of-the-art results to compare with our approach.

In Table 3, from the comparison results between the baseline method and our approach, we can observe that on some finer levels, i.e., level 3, 4 and 5, our *cross-level LLC-CNN* works better than multi-level pooled CNN. The reason may be that more patches are available on these 3 levels (9 patches in level 3, 16 patches in level 4 and 25 patches in level 5), and pooling over more LLC features covers more information compared with original CNN features. Moreover, on the combination of all the 5 levels, our *cross-level LLC-CNN* also achieves higher accuracy than the baseline method, i.e., multi-level pooled CNN, which is 68.96 % vs 67.87 %, with a lower-dimensional feature. Compared to other state-of-the-arts, *cross-level LLC-CNN* also obtains the highest performance. It is worth mentioning that, to our best knowledge, the former best performance on this dataset is achieved by Multi-scale VLAD pooling on off-the-shelf CNN features, proposed by [19]. Compared to this MOP-CNN framework, our *cross-level LLC-CNN* obtains higher accuracy. Actually, the patches they used, i.e., 25 patches in level 2 and 49 patches in level 3, are much more than ours. The larger number of patches brings higher time cost in codebook learning and VLAD pooling. In contrast, the smaller number of patches utilized in our approach and the fast LLC performing make our *cross-level LLC-CNN* work much faster than their MOP-CNN. Table 4 shows the experimental results on the SUN 397 dataset. Overall, the comparison results are similar with those on MIT indoor scenes dataset. On SUN 397, *cross-level LLC-CNN* outperforms multi-level pooled CNN on some finer levels (level 4 and level 5) and the combination of all the 5 levels. Compared to the state-of-the-arts, our approach achieves the best accuracy (50.87 %) on the combination of all the 5 levels with a relatively low feature dimension.

Table 3. Classification results on MIT indoor scenes for (a) baseline: multi-level pooled CNN; (b) *cross-level LLC-CNN*; (c) other state-of-the-arts.

Methods		Feature dimension	Accuracy
(a) multi-level pooled CNN (baseline)	level1	4096	61.46
	level2	4096	63.77
	level3	4096	64.27
	level4	4096	64.39
	level5	4096	64.97
	level1+level2+···+level5	20480	67.87
(b)*cross-level LLC-CNN* (Ours)	level1	16384	60.23
	level2	16384	62.47
	level3	16384	64.66
	level4	16384	65.48
	level5	16384	65.87
	level1+level2+···+level5	16384	**68.96**
(c) state-of-the-arts	SPM [4]	5000	34.40
	FV+Bag of Parts [2]	221550	63.18
	Mode Seeking [32]	60000	64.03
	SPM+OPM [27]	—	63.48
	MOP-CNN [19]	12288	68.88

Table 4. Classification results on SUN 397 dataset for (a) baseline: multi-level pooled CNN; (b) *cross-level LLC-CNN*; (c) other state-of-the-arts.

Methods		Feature dimension	Accuracy
(a) multi-level pooled CNN (baseline)	level1	4096	43.75
	level2	4096	45.61
	level3	4096	46.33
	level4	4096	46.58
	level5	4096	46.87
	level1+level2+···+level5	20480	49.23
(b)*cross-level LLC-CNN* (Ours)	level1	16384	40.48
	level2	16384	42.53
	level3	16384	45.80
	level4	16384	47.41
	level5	16384	48.53
	level1+level2+···+level5	16384	**50.87**
(c) state-of-the-arts	Xiao et al. [22]	—	38.00
	Decaf [15]	4096	40.94
	Fisher Vector [33]	256000	47.20
	SPM+OPM [27]	—	45.91

Scale Invariance. To evaluate the scale invariance of our approach, we randomly select 670 testing images (half of the total) in MIT indoor scenes testing set and scale them by different scaling ratios, i.e., 10/9, 10/8, 10/7, 10/6, 10/5. For SUN 397, we use a random training/testing split (we choose the first split in the experiment) to evaluate the scale invariance. In this split, 1000 testing images randomly selected from the testing set are scaled by the same scaling ratios with those for MIT indoor scenes. Specifically, when scaling by a factor of ρ, we crop the image around the center with $1/\rho$ times of the original size, as illustrated in Fig. 4. We compare the recognition accuracy over these scaled testing images of our *cross-level LLC-CNN* and the multi-level pooled CNN. Both methods are trained on non-scaled original training samples and the combination from level 1 to level 5 is adopted. Before all coding and pooling procedures, all the CNN features are extracted by the cascaded fine-tuned models. All the fine-tuned CNN features are obtained after 50 epochs of training. L2 normalization is performed on all the CNN features after extraction. The SVM parameter (C) is all set as 0.5.

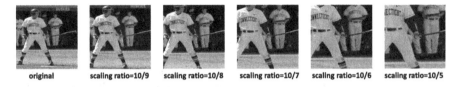

original   scaling ratio=10/9   scaling ratio=10/8   scaling ratio=10/7   scaling ratio=10/6   scaling ratio=10/5

Fig. 4. Illustration of the scaled testing image with different scaling ratios.

The curves of recognition accuracy vs scaling ratio on the MIT indoor scenes dataset and the SUN 397 dataset are shown in Figs. 5 and 6, respectively. Both figures reflect the trend that the recognition accuracy decreases with the increase of the scaling ratio, whatever method is used. This shows that CNN features do not have scale invariance, as mentioned by lots of works [19, 21]. However, with our *cross-level LLC-CNN*, the classification accuracy decreases much more slowly than multi-level pooled CNN as the scaling ratio increases. As can be seen, from the original image to the 10/5 ratio scaled image, the difference in accuracy between our approach and the baseline approach is becoming increasingly big as the scaling ratio increases. Specifically, recognition accuracy with our approach when the testing image is scaled by 10/5 can still remain 50.63 % and 34.32 % for MIT indoor scenes and SUN 397 respectively. In comparison, the accuracy when the scaling ratio reaches 10/5 drops to 35.42 % and 24.47 % for MIT indoor scenes and SUN 397 respectively. The accuracy differences are all over 10 %, showing the great superiority of our approach over the baseline approach. This superiority proves that LLC coding of CNN features on the cross-level codebook produces more robust features to the scale transformation, as LLC coding ensures that scaled CNN features can still be well represented by the cross-level codebook and their discrimination power is retained after scaling.

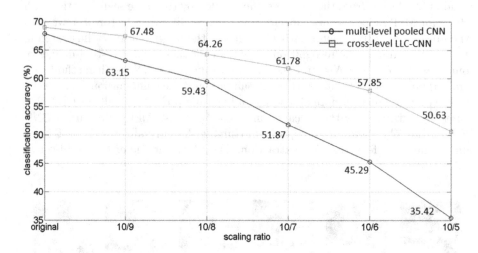

Fig. 5. Classification accuracy comparison between multi-level pooled CNN features and our *cross-level LLC-CNN* for scaled images with different scaling ratios on the MIT indoor scenes dataset.

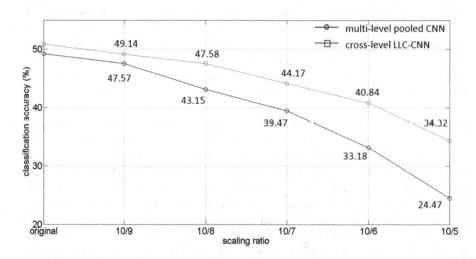

Fig. 6. Classification accuracy comparison between multi-level pooled CNN features and our *cross-level LLC-CNN* for scaled images with different scaling ratios on the SUN 397 dataset.

5   Conclusion

In this paper, we proposed a cross-level Locality-constrained Linear Coding and pooling framework (*cross-level LLC-CNN*) on multi-level CNN features to enhance the discrimination and scale invariance of the image representation for scene classification problems. Based on the cascaded fine-tuning scheme, the CNN features gain stronger discrimination in scene classification. In addition, with cross-level Locality-constrained Linear Coding and pooling on these multi-level fine-tuned CNN features, robustness to scale transformation is improved. We evaluated our approach on the MIT indoor scenes dataset and the SUN 397 dataset. Experimental results demonstrated that significant improvements in classification accuracy are achieved for both original and scaled testing images. In the future, we will explore how to improve the discrimination power and scale invariance of CNN in other vision tasks.

Acknowledgement. This research is supported by the National Research Foundation, Prime Ministers Office, Singapore under its International Research Centre @ Singapore Funding Initiative and administered by the Interactive &Digital Media Programme Office.

References

1. Csurka, G., Dance, C., Fan, L., Willamowski, J., Bray, C.: Visual categorization with bags of keypoints. In: Workshop on Statistical Learning in Computer vision, ECCV (2004)
2. Juneja, M., Vedaldi, A., Jawahar, C., Zisserman, A.: Blocks that shout: Distinctive parts for scene classification. In: IEEE CVPR, pp. 923–930 (2013)
3. Li, L.J., Su, H., Fei-Fei, L., Xing, E.P.: Object bank: A high-level image representation for scene classification & semantic feature sparsification. In: NIPS, pp. 1378–1386 (2010)
4. Lazebnik, S., Schmid, C., Ponce, J.: Beyond bags of features: Spatial pyramid matching for recognizing natural scene categories. In: IEEE CVPR, pp. 2169–2178 (2006)
5. Dong, J., Xia, W., Chen, Q., Feng, J., Huang, Z., Yan, S.: Subcategory-aware object classification. In: IEEE CVPR, pp. 827–834 (2013)
6. Dong, J., Chen, Q., Yan, S., Yuille, A.: Towards unified object detection and segmentation. In: Fleet, D., Pajdla, T., Schiele, B., Tuytelaars, T. (eds.) ECCV 2014, Part V. LNCS, vol. 8693, pp. 299–314. Springer, Heidelberg (2014)
7. Lowe, D.G.: Distinctive image features from scale-invariant keypoints. IJCV **60**, 91–110 (2004)
8. Dalal, N., Triggs, B.: Histograms of oriented gradients for human detection. In: IEEE CVPR, pp. 886–893 (2005)
9. LeCun, Y., Bengio, Y.: Convolutional networks for images, speech, and time series. In: The Handbook of Brain Theory and Neural Networks, vol. 3361 (1995)
10. Krizhevsky, A., Sutskever, I., Hinton, G.E.: Imagenet classification with deep convolutional neural networks. In: NIPS, pp. 1097–1105 (2012)
11. Jarrett, K., Kavukcuoglu, K., Ranzato, M., LeCun, Y.: What is the best multi-stage architecture for object recognition? In: IEEE ICCV, pp. 2146–2153 (2009)

12. Ouyang, W., Wang, X.: Joint deep learning for pedestrian detection. In: IEEE ICCV, pp. 2056–2063 (2013)
13. Sun, Y., Wang, X., Tang, X.: Hybrid deep learning for face verification. In: IEEE ICCV, pp. 1489–1496 (2013)
14. Deng, J., Dong, W., Socher, R., Li, L.J., Li, K., Fei-Fei, L.: Imagenet: A large-scale hierarchical image database. In: IEEE CVPR, pp. 248–255 (2009)
15. Donahue, J., Jia, Y., Vinyals, O., Hoffman, J., Zhang, N., Tzeng, E., Darrell, T.: Decaf: A deep convolutional activation feature for generic visual recognition. arXiv preprint arXiv:1310.1531 (2013)
16. Girshick, R., Donahue, J., Darrell, T., Malik, J.: Rich feature hierarchies for accurate object detection and semantic segmentation. arXiv preprint arXiv:1311.2524 (2013)
17. Oquab, M., Bottou, L., Laptev, I., Sivic, J., et al.: Learning and transferring mid-level image representations using convolutional neural networks. arXiv preprint (2013)
18. Sermanet, P., Eigen, D., Zhang, X., Mathieu, M., Fergus, R., LeCun, Y.: Overfeat: Integrated recognition, localization and detection using convolutional networks. arXiv preprint arXiv:1312.6229 (2013)
19. Gong, Y., Wang, L., Guo, R., Lazebnik, S.: Multi-scale orderless pooling of deep convolutional activation features. arXiv preprint arXiv:1403.1840 (2014)
20. Wei, Y., Xia, W., Huang, J., Ni, B., Dong, J., Zhao, Y., Yan, S.: Cnn: Single-label to multi-label. arXiv preprint arXiv:1406.5726 (2014)
21. Zeiler, M.D., Fergus, R.: Visualizing and understanding convolutional neural networks. arXiv preprint arXiv:1311.2901 (2013)
22. Xiao, J., Hays, J., Ehinger, K.A., Oliva, A., Torralba, A.: Sun database: Large-scale scene recognition from abbey to zoo. In: IEEE CVPR, pp. 3485–3492 (2010)
23. Wang, J., Yang, J., Yu, K., Lv, F., Huang, T., Gong, Y.: Locality-constrained linear coding for image classification. In: IEEE CVPR, pp. 3360–3367 (2010)
24. Quattoni, A., Torralba, A.: Recognizing indoor scenes. In: IEEE CVPR (2009)
25. Bosch, A., Zisserman, A., Muñoz, X.: Scene classification via pLSA. In: Leonardis, A., Bischof, H., Pinz, A. (eds.) ECCV 2006. LNCS, vol. 3954, pp. 517–530. Springer, Heidelberg (2006)
26. Yang, J., Yu, K., Gong, Y., Huang, T.: Linear spatial pyramid matching using sparse coding for image classification. In: IEEE CVPR, pp. 1794–1801 (2009)
27. Xie, L., Wang, J., Guo, B., Zhang, B., Tian, Q.: Orientational pyramid matching for recognizing indoor scenes. In: IEEE CVPR (2014)
28. Krizhevsky, A., Hinton, G.: Learning multiple layers of features from tiny images. Computer Science Department, University of Toronto, Tech. Rep. (2009)
29. LeCun, Y., Bottou, L., Bengio, Y., Haffner, P.: Gradient-based learning applied to document recognition. Proc. IEEE 86, 2278–2324 (1998)
30. Jégou, H., Douze, M., Schmid, C., Pérez, P.: Aggregating local descriptors into a compact image representation. In: IEEE CVPR, pp. 3304–3311 (2010)
31. Shabou, A., LeBorgne, H.: Locality-constrained and spatially regularized coding for scene categorization. In: IEEE CVPR, pp. 3618–3625 (2012)
32. Doersch, C., Gupta, A., Efros, A.A.: Mid-level visual element discovery as discriminative mode seeking. In: NIPS, pp. 494–502 (2013)
33. Sánchez, J., Perronnin, F., Mensink, T., Verbeek, J.: Image classification with the fisher vector: Theory and practice. IJCV 105, 222–245 (2013)

A Graphical Model for Rapid Obstacle Image-Map Estimation from Unmanned Surface Vehicles

Matej Kristan[1,2]($\boxtimes$), Janez Perš[1], Vildana Sulič[1], and Stanislav Kovačič[1]

[1] Faculty of Computer and Information Science, University of Ljubljana,
Slovenia, Ljubljana
{janez.pers,vildana.sulic,stanislav.kovacic}@fe.uni-lj.si
[2] Faculty of Electrical Engineering, University of Ljubljana, Slovenia, Ljubljana
matej.kristan@fri.uni-lj.si

Abstract. Obstacle detection plays an important role in unmanned surface vehicles (USV). Continuous detection from images taken onboard the vessel poses a particular challenge due to the diversity of the environment and the obstacle appearance. An obstacle may be a floating piece of wood, a scuba diver, a pier, or some other part of a shoreline. In this paper we tackle this problem by proposing a new graphical model that affords a fast and continuous obstacle image-map estimation from a single video stream captured onboard a USV. The model accounts for the semantic structure of marine environment as observed from USV by imposing weak structural constraints. A Markov random field framework is adopted and a highly efficient algorithm for simultaneous optimization of model parameters and segmentation mask estimation is derived. Our approach does not require computationally intensive extraction of texture features and runs faster than real-time. We also present a new, challenging, dataset for segmentation and obstacle detection in marine environments, which is the largest annotated dataset of its kind. Results on this dataset show that our model compares favorably in accuracy to the related approaches, requiring a fraction of computational effort.

1 Introduction

Obstacle detection is of central importance for lower-end small unmanned surface vehicles (USV) used for patrolling coastal waters (see Fig. 1). Such vehicles are typically used in perimeter surveillance, in which the USV travels along a pre-planned path. To quickly and efficiently respond to the challenges from highly dynamic environment, the USV requires an onboard logic to observe the surrounding, detect potentially dangerous situations, and apply proper route modifications. An important feature of such vessel is the ability to detect an obstacle at sufficient distance and react by replanning its path to avoid collision. The primary type of obstacle in this case is the shoreline itself, which can be avoided to some extent (although not fully) by the use of detailed maps and the satellite navigation. Indeed, [1] proposed an approach that utilizes an overhead

© Springer International Publishing Switzerland 2015
D. Cremers et al. (Eds.): ACCV 2014, Part II, LNCS 9004, pp. 391–406, 2015.
DOI: 10.1007/978-3-319-16808-1_27

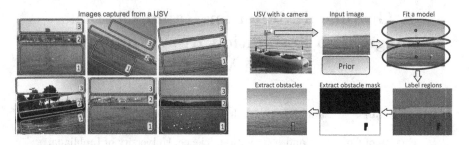

Fig. 1. Images captured from the USV split into three semantically different regions (left) and our approach for obstacle image-map estimation (right).

image of the area obtained from Google maps to construct a map of static obstacles. But such an approach cannot handle a more difficult class of dynamic obstacles that do not appear in the map (e.g., boats, buys and swimmers).

A small USV requires ability to detect near-by and distant obstacles. The detection should not be constrained to objects that stand out from the water, but should also detect flat objects, like debris or emerging scuba divers, etc. Operation in shallow waters and marinas constrains the size of USV and prevents the use of additional stabilizers. This puts further constraints on the weight, power consumption, types of sensors and their placement. Cameras are therefore becoming attractive sensors for use in low-end USVs due to their cost-, weight- and power-efficiency and a large field of view coverage. This presents a challenge for development of highly efficient computer vision algorithms tailored for obstacle detection in a challenging environments that the small USVs face. In this paper we address this challenge by proposing a segmentation-based algorithm for obstacle-map estimation that is derived from optimizing a new well-defined graphical model and runs at over 70 fps in Matlab on a single core machine.

1.1   Related Work

The problem of obstacle detection has been explicitly or implicitly addressed previously in the field of unmanned ground vehicles (UGV). In a trail-following application [2] use an omnidirectional camera to detect trail as a region that is most contrasted to its surrounding, however, dynamic obstacles are not addressed. Montemerlo et al. and Dahlkamp et al. [3,4] address the problem of low-proximity road detection of laser scanners by bootstrapping color segmentation with the laser output. The proximal road points are detected by laser, projected to camera and used to learn a Gaussian mixture model which is in turn used to segment the rest of the image captured by the camera. Combined with horizon detection [5], this approach significantly increases the distance at which the obstacles on the road can be detected. Alternatively, [6] casted the obstacle detection as a labelling task in which they employ a bank of pre-trained classifiers to 3D point clouds and a Markov random field to account for the spatial smoothness of the labelling.

Most UGV approaches for obstacle detection explicitly or implicitly rely on ground plane estimation from range sensors and are not directly applicable to aquatic environments encountered by USV. Scherer et al. [7] propose a water detection algorithm using a stereo bumblebee camera, IMU/GPS and rotating laser scanner for navigation on a river. Their system extracts color and texture features over blocks of pixels and eliminates the sky region using a pre-trained classifier. A horizon line, obtained from the onboard IMU, is then projected into the image to obtain samples for learning a color distribution of the regions below and above horizon, respectively. Using these distributions, the image is segmented and results of the segmentation are used in turn, after additional postprocessing steps, to train a classifier. The trained classifier is fused with a classifier from the previous frames and applied to the blocks of pixels to detect the water region. This system relies heavily on the quality of hardware-based horizon estimation, accuracy of pre-trained sky detector and the postprocessing steps. The authors report that the vision-based segmentation is not processed onboard, but requires special computing hardware, which makes it below a real-time segmentation at constrained processing power typical for small USVs.

Some of the standard range sensor modalities for autonomous navigation in maritime environments include radar [8], sonar [9] and ladar [10]. Range scanners are known to poorly discriminate between water and land in the far field [11], suffer from angular resolution and scanning rate limitations, and poorly perform when the beam's incidence angle is not oblique with respect to the water surface [12,13]. Several researchers have thus resorted to cameras [10,13–17] for obstacle and moving object detection instead. To detect dynamic objects in harbor, [14] assume a static camera and apply background subtraction combined with motion cues. However, background subtraction cannot be applied to a highly dynamic scenes encountered on a moving USV. Huntsberger et al. [17] attempt to address this issue using stereo systems, but require large baseline rigs that are less appropriate for small vessels due to increased instability and limit processing of near-field regions. Santana et al. [13] apply fusion of Lukas Kanade local trackers with color oversegmentation and a sequence of k-means clusterings on texture features to detect water regions in videos. Alternatively, [15,16] apply a low-power solution using a monocular camera for obstacle detection. They first detect the horizon line and then search for a potential obstacle in the region below the horizon. A fundamental drawback of [15,16] is that they approximate the edge of water by a horizon line and cannot handle situations in coastal waters, close to the shoreline or in marina. At that point, the edge of water does not correspond to the horizon anymore and can be no longer modeled as a straight line. Such cases call for more general segmentation approaches.

Many unsupervised segmentation approaches have been proposed in literature. Khan and Shah [18] use optical flow, color and spatial coordinates to construct features which are used in single Gaussians to segment a moving object in video. Felzenszwalb and Huttenlocher [19] have proposed a graph-theoretic clustering to perform segmentation of color images into visually-coherent regions. The assumption that the neighboring pixels likely belong to the same class is formally addressed in the context of Markov random fields (MRF) [20,21]. Wojek and Schiele [22] have extended the conditional random fields with dynamic models and perform the inference for object detection and labeling jointly in videos. The random field frameworks [23] have proven quite successful for addressing the semantic labeling tasks and recently [24] have shown that structural priors between classes further improve the labeling. The approaches like [22] use high-dimensional features composed of color and texture at multiple scales and object-class specific detectors to segment the images and detect the objects of interest. In our scenarios, the possible types of dynamic obstacles are unknown and vary significantly in appearance. Thus object-class specific detectors are not suitable. Recently, Alpert et al. [25] have proposed an approach that starts from a pixel level and gradually constructs visually-homogenous regions by agglomerative clustering. They achieved impressive results on a segmentation dataset in which an object was occupying a significant portion of an image. Unfortunately, since their algorithm incrementally merges regions, it is too slow for online application even at moderate image sizes. An alternative to starting the segmentation from pixel level is to start from an oversegmented image such that pixels are grouped into superpixels [26]. Li et al. [27] have proposed a segmentation algorithm that uses multiple superpixel oversegmentations and merges their result by a bipartite graph partitioning to achieve state-of-the-art results on a standard segmentation dataset. However, no prior information is provided to favor certain types of segmentations in specific scenes.

1.2   Our Approach and Contributions

We pursue a solution for obstacle detection that is based on concepts of image segmentation with weak semantic priors on the expected scene composition. Figure 1 shows typical images captured from a USV. While the images significantly vary in appearance, we observe that each image can be split into three semantic regions roughly stacked one above the other, implying a structural relation between the regions. The bottom region represents the water, while the top region represents the sky. The middle component can represent either land, parked boats a haze above horizon or a mixture of these.

Our **main contribution** is a graphical model for structurally-constrained semantic segmentation with application to USV obstacle-map estimation. The generative model assumes a mixture model with three Gaussian components for the dominant three image regions and a uniform component for explaining the outliers, which may constitute an obstacle in the water. We propose a graphical model with weak priors on the mixture parameters and a MRF over the prior as well as posterior pixel-class distributions to favor smooth segmentations. We derive an EM algorithm for the proposed model and show that the resulting optimization achieves a fast convergence at a low computational cost, without resorting to a specialized hardware. A similar segmentation model was proposed in [28], but their model requires a manually set variable, does not apply priors and is not derived from a single density function.

We apply this model to obstacle image-map estimation in USVs. The proposed model acts directly on color image and does not require expensive extraction of texture-based features. Combined with efficient optimization, this results in faster than realtime segmentation and obstacle-map estimation. Our approach is outlined in Fig. 1. The semantic model is fitted to the input image, after which each pixel is classified into one of the four classes. All the pixels that do not correspond to the water component are deemed to be a part of an obstacle. Figure 1 shows a detection of a dynamic obstacle (buoy) and of a static obstacle (shoreline).

Our **second contribution** is a marine dataset for semantic segmentation and obstacle detection, and the performance evaluation methodology. To our knowledge this will be the largest annotated publicly available marine dataset of its kind up to date. The remainder of the paper is structured as follows. In Sect. 2 we derive our semantic generative model, in Sect. 3 we present the obstacle detection algorithm, in Sect. 4 we experimentally analyze the algorithm on an extensive dataset and draw conclusions in Sect. 5.

2   The Semantic Generative Model

We consider the image as an array of measured values $\mathbf{Y} = \{\mathbf{y}_i\}_{i=1:M}$, in which $\mathbf{y}_i \in \mathcal{R}^d$ is a d dimensional measurement, a feature vector, at the i-th pixel in an image with M pixels. As we detail in the subsequent sections, the feature vector is composed of pixel's color and image coordinates. The probability of the i-th pixel feature vector is modelled as a mixture model with four components – three Gaussians and a single uniform component:

$$p(\mathbf{y}_i|\Theta) = \sum_{k=1}^{3} \phi(\mathbf{y}_i|\mu_k, \Sigma_k)\pi_{ik} + \mathcal{U}(\mathbf{y}_i)\pi_{i4}, \tag{1}$$

where $\Theta = \{\mu_k, \Sigma_k\}_{k=1:3}$ are the means and covariances of the Gaussian kernels $\phi(\cdot|\mu, \Sigma)$ and $\mathcal{U}(\cdot)$ is a uniform distribution. The i-th pixel label x_i is an unobserved random variable governed by the class prior distribution $\pi_i = [\pi_{i1}, \ldots, \pi_{i4}]$ with $\pi_{i1} = p(x_i = i1)$. The three Gaussian components represent the three dominant semantic regions in the image, while the uniform component represents the outliers, i.e., pixels that do not likely correspond to any of the three structures. To encourage segmentations into three approximately vertically aligned semantic structures, we define a set of priors $\varphi_0 = \{\mu_{\mu_k}, \Sigma_{\mu_k}\}_{k=1:3}$ for the mean values of the Gaussians, i.e., $p(\Theta|\varphi_0) = \prod_{k=1}^{3} \phi(\mu_k|\mu_{\mu_k}, \Sigma_{\mu_k})$. To encourage smooth segmentations, the priors π_i as well as posteriors over the pixel class labels, are treated as random variables, which form a Markov random field. Imposing the MRF on the priors and posteriors rather than pixel labels allows effectively integrating out the labels, which leads to a well-behaved class of MRFs [28] that avoid image reconstruction during parameter learning. The resulting graphical model with priors is shown in Fig. 2.

Let $\pi = \{\pi_i\}_{i=1:M}$ denote the set of priors for all pixels. Following [20] we approximate the joint distribution over the priors as $p(\pi) \approx \prod_i p(\pi_i|\pi_{N_i})$, and

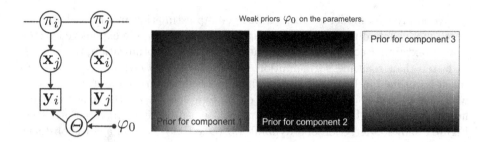

Fig. 2. The graphical model (left) with weak priors on three semantic components (right).

π_{N_i} is a mixture distribution over the priors of the i-th pixel's neighbors, i.e., $\pi_{N_i} = \sum_{j \in N_i, j \neq i} \lambda_{ij} \pi_j$, where λ_{ij} are fixed positive weights such that for each i-th pixel $\sum_j \lambda_{ij} = 1$. The potentials in the MRF are defined as $p(\pi_i | \pi_{N_i}) \propto \exp\left(-\frac{1}{2} E(\pi_i, \pi_{N_i})\right)$ with $E(\pi_i, \pi_{N_i}) = D(\pi_i \parallel \pi_{N_i}) + H(\pi_i)$. The term $D(\pi_i \parallel \pi_{N_i})$ is the Kullback-Leibler divergence which penalizes the differences between prior distributions over the neighboring pixels (π_i and π_{N_i}), while the term $H(\pi_i)$ is the entropy and penalizes uninformative priors π_i. The joint distribution for the graphical model in Fig. 2 can be written as

$$p(\mathbf{Y}, \Theta, \pi | \varphi_0) = \prod_{i=1}^{M} p(\mathbf{y}_i | \Theta, \varphi_0) p(\Theta | \varphi_0) p(\pi_i | \pi_{N_i}). \tag{2}$$

Diplaros et al. [28] argue that improved segmentations can be achieved by also considering an MRF directly on the pixel posterior distributions by treating the posteriors as random variables $\mathbf{P} = \{\mathbf{p}_i\}_{i=1:M}$, where the components of $\mathbf{p}_i$ are defined as $p_{ik} = p(x_i = k | \Theta, \mathbf{y}_i, \varphi_0)$, computed by Bayes rule from $p(y_i | x_i = k, \Theta)$ and $p(x_i = k)$. We can write the posterior over $\mathbf{P}$ as $p(\mathbf{P} | \mathbf{Y}, \Theta, \pi, \varphi_0) \propto \prod_{i=1}^{M} \exp(-\frac{1}{2} E(\mathbf{p}_i, \mathbf{p}_{N_i}))$, where $\mathbf{p}_{N_i}$ is a mixture defined in the same spirit as π_{N_i}. The joint distribution can now be written as

$$p(\mathbf{P}, \mathbf{Y}, \Theta, \pi | \varphi_0) \propto \exp[\sum_{i=1}^{M} \log p(\mathbf{y}_i, \Theta | \varphi_0) - \frac{1}{2}(E(\pi_i, \pi_{N_i}) + E(\mathbf{p}_i, \mathbf{p}_{N_i}))], \tag{3}$$

Due to coupling between π_i / π_{N_i} and $\mathbf{p}_i / \mathbf{p}_{N_i}$ the optimization of (3) is not straightforward. We therefore introduce auxiliary variables $\mathbf{q}_i$ and $\mathbf{s}_i$ and take the logarithm, which results in the following cost function

$$F = \sum_{i=1}^{M} [\log p(\mathbf{y}_i, \Theta | \varphi_0) - \frac{1}{2}(D(\mathbf{s}_i \| \pi_i \circ \pi_{N_i}) + D(\mathbf{q}_i \| \mathbf{p}_i \circ \mathbf{p}_{N_i}))], \tag{4}$$

where $\circ$ is the Hadamard (component-wise) product. Note that when $\mathbf{q}_i \equiv \mathbf{p}_i$ and $\mathbf{s}_i \equiv \pi_i$, (4) reduces to (3) (ignoring the constant terms). Maximization of F can now be achieved in an EM-like fashion. In the E-step we maximize F w.r.t.

$\mathbf{q}_i$, $\mathbf{s}_i$, while the M-step maximizes over the parameters Θ and π. We can see from (4) that the F is maximized w.r.t. $\mathbf{q}_i$ and $\mathbf{s}_i$ when the divergence terms vanish, therefore, $\mathbf{s}_i^{\text{opt}} = \xi_{s_i} \pi_i \circ \pi_{N_i}$, $\mathbf{q}_i^{\text{opt}} = \xi_{q_i} \mathbf{p}_i \circ \mathbf{p}_{N_i}$, where ξ_{s_i} and ξ_{q_i} are the normalization constants.

The M-step in not as straightforward, since direct optimization over Θ and π is intractable and we resort to maximizing its lower bound. We define $\hat{\mathbf{s}}_i = (\mathbf{s}_i + \mathbf{s}_{N_i})$ and $\hat{\mathbf{q}}_i = (\mathbf{q}_i + \mathbf{q}_{N_i})$ and by Jensen's inequality lower-bound the divergence terms as

$$- D(\mathbf{s}_i \| \pi_i \circ \pi_{N_i}) \geq \hat{\mathbf{s}}_i^T \log \pi_i \; ; \; - D(\mathbf{q}_i \| \mathbf{p}_i \circ \mathbf{p}_{N_i}) \geq \hat{\mathbf{q}}_i^T \log \mathbf{p}_i, \qquad (5)$$

where we have ignored the terms independent of π_i and $\mathbf{p}_i$. Substituting (5) into (4) and collecting the relevant terms yields the following lower bound on the cost function (4)

$$\hat{F} = \sum_{i=1}^{M} [\frac{1}{2}(\mathbf{q}_i + \mathbf{q}_{N_i})^T \log(\mathbf{p}_i p(\Theta|\varphi_0)) + \frac{1}{2}(\hat{\mathbf{s}}_i + \hat{\mathbf{q}}_i)^T \log \pi_i]. \qquad (6)$$

Differentiating (6) w.r.t., π_i and applying a Lagrange multiplier with the constraint $\sum_k \pi_{ik} = 1$, we see that $\hat{F}$ is maximized at $\pi_i^{\text{opt}} = \frac{1}{4}(\hat{\mathbf{s}}_i + \hat{\mathbf{q}}_i)$. Differentiating (6) w.r.t. the means and covariances of Gaussians, we obtain

$$\mu_k^{\text{opt}} = \beta_k^{-1} [\Lambda_k (\sum_{i=1}^{M} \hat{q}_{ik} \mathbf{y}_i^T) \Sigma_k^{-1} - \mu_{\mu_k}^T \Sigma_{\mu_k}^{-1}]^T, \qquad (7)$$

$$\Sigma_k^{\text{opt}} = \beta_k^{-1} \sum_{i=1}^{M} \hat{q}_{ik} (\mathbf{y}_i - \mu_k)(\mathbf{y}_i - \mu_k)^T, \qquad (8)$$

where we have defined $\beta_k = \sum_{i=1}^{M} \hat{q}_{ik}$ and $\Lambda_k = (\Sigma_k^{-1} + \Sigma_{\mu_k}^{-1})^{-1}$. An appealing property of the model (4) is that its E-step can be efficiently implemented through convolutions and Hadamard products. Recall that the calculation of the i-th pixel's neighborhood prior distribution π_{N_i} entails a weighted combination of the neighboring pixel priors π_j. Let $\pi_{.k}$ be the k-th component priors arranged in a matrix of image size. Then the neighborhood priors can be computed by the following convolution $\pi_{N_{.k}} = \pi_{.k} * \lambda$, where λ is a discrete kernel with its central element set to zero and its elements summing to one. Let $\hat{\mathbf{s}}_{.k}$, $\hat{\mathbf{q}}_{.k}$ and $\mathbf{p}_{.k}$ be the image-sized counterparts corresponding to sets of distributions $\{\hat{\mathbf{s}}_i\}_{i=1:M}$, $\{\hat{\mathbf{q}}_i\}_{i=1:M}$ and $\{\mathbf{p}_i\}_{i=1:M}$, respectively, and let λ_1 denote the kernel λ in which the central element is set to one. Then the calculation of the k-th component priors $\pi_{.k}^{\text{opt}}$ for all pixels in the E-step can be written as

$$\hat{\mathbf{s}}_{.k} = (\xi_{s.} \circ \pi_{.k} \circ (\pi_{.k} * \lambda)) * \lambda_1,$$
$$\hat{\mathbf{q}}_{.k} = (\xi_{q.} \circ \mathbf{p}_{.k} \circ (\mathbf{p}_{.k} * \lambda)) * \lambda_1,$$
$$\pi_{.k}^{\text{opt}} = (\hat{\mathbf{s}}_{.k} + \hat{\mathbf{q}}_{.k})/4. \qquad (9)$$

The EM procedure for fitting our generative model to the input image is summarized in Algorithm 1.

Algorithm 1. The EM algorithm for the segmentation model.

Require:
  Pixel features $\mathbf{Y} = \{\mathbf{y}_i\}_{i=1:M}$, priors φ_0, initial values for Θ and π.

Ensure:
  The estimated parameters π^{opt}, Θ^{opt} and the smoothed posterior $\{\hat{\mathbf{q}}_{\cdot k}\}_{k=1:4}$.

Procedure:
  1: Calculate the pixel posteriors $\mathbf{p}_{\cdot k}$ using the current estimates of π and Θ for all k (1).
  2: Calculate the new pixel priors $\pi_{\cdot k}^{\text{opt}}$ for all k using (9).
  3: Calculate the new parameter values Θ using (7) and (8).
  4: Iterate steps 1 to 3 until convergence.

---

3   Obstacle Detection

We formulate the obstacle detection as a problem of estimating an image obstacle map, i.e., determining the pixels in the image that correspond to the sea while all the remaining pixels represent the potential obstacles. We therefore first fit our semantic model from Sect. 2 to the input image and estimate the smoothed a posteriori probability distribution $\hat{\mathbf{q}}_{ik}$ across the four semantic components for each pixel. An $i - th$ pixel is classified as water if the corresponding posterior $\hat{\mathbf{q}}_{ik}$ reaches maximum for the water component among all four components. In our setting the component indexed by $k = 1$ corresponds to water region, which results in the labeled image B with the i-th pixel label b_i defined as

$$b_i = \begin{cases} 1 \; ; \; \arg\max_k \hat{\mathbf{q}}_{ik} = 1 \\ 0 \; ; \quad\quad otherwise \end{cases} . \tag{10}$$

Retaining only the largest connected region in the image B results in the current obstacle image map $\hat{B}_t$. All blobs of non-water pixels within the connected water region are proclaimed as potential *obstacles in the water*. This is followed by a nonmaxima suppression stage which merges detections that are located in close proximities (e.g., due to object fragmentation) to reduce multiple detections of the same obstacle. The water edge is extracted as the longest connected outer edge of the connected region corresponding to the water. Note also that the Algorithm 1 requires initial values for the parameters Θ and π. We exploit the continuity of sequential images in the videostream by taking the parameter values of the converged model from the previous time-step for initialization of the EM algorithm in the current time-step. The obstacle detection is summarized in Algorithm 2 and visualized in Fig. 1.

4   Experiments

4.1   Implementation Details

In our application, the measurement at each pixel is encoded by a five-dimensional feature vector $\mathbf{y}_i = [i_x, i_y, i_h, i_s, i_v]$, where (i_x, i_y) are the i-th pixel coordinates

---

Algorithm 2. The obstacle image map estimation and obstacle detection.

Require:

  Pixel features $\mathbf{Y} = \{\mathbf{y}_i\}_{i=1:M}$, priors φ_0, estimated model from previous time-step Θ_{t-1} and $\hat{\mathbf{q}}_{t-1}$.

Ensure:

  Obstacle image map $\hat{B}_t$, water edge $\mathbf{e}_t$, detected objects $\{\mathbf{o}_i\}_{i=1:N_{\text{obj}}}$, model parameters Θ_t and $\hat{\mathbf{q}}_t$.

Procedure:

  1: Initialize the parameters of Θ_t and π_t by Θ_{t-1} and $\hat{\mathbf{q}}_{t-1}$.

  2: Apply the Algorithm 1 and priors φ_0 to fit the model Θ_t and $\hat{\mathbf{q}}_t$ to the input data $\mathbf{Y}$.

  3: Calculate the new obstacle image map $\hat{B}_t$ and for interpretation also the water edge $\mathbf{e}_t$ and the obstacles in water $\{\mathbf{o}_i\}_{i=1:N_{obj}}$.

---

and the (i_h, i_s, i_v) are the pixel's HSV color channels. We have also determined that we achieve sufficiently good obstacle detection by performing detection on a reduced-size image of 50×50 pixels and then rescale the results to the original image size. This drastically speeds up the algorithm to approximately 14 ms per frame in our experiments. The uniform distribution component in (1) is defined over the image pixels domain and returns equal probability for each pixel. In our rescaled image this means that $\mathcal{U}(\mathbf{y}_i) = \frac{1}{50^2}$ at each pixel. The only constraint on the convolution kernel λ (9) is that the central element is set to zero and all elements sum to one. We use a Gaussian kernel with central element set to zero and set the size of the kernel to 2 % of image size, which results in a 3×3 pixels kernel. The spatial components in the feature vector play a dual role. On one hand they encode region texture through spatial correlation of colors. On the other hand they lend means to weakly constraining the Gaussian components such that they reflect the three dominant semantic image parts. This is achieved by the weak priors $p(\Theta|\varphi_0) = \prod_{k=1}^{3} \phi(\mu_k|\mu_{\mu_k}, \Sigma_{\mu_k})$ on the Gaussian means. The weak priors were estimated from a few typical images captured from the boat that highly varied in appearance and geometry and were not used for the testing phase. Figure 2 visualizes the spatial components of the weak priors. All parameters were kept constant in the experiments[1].

4.2   Marine Obstacle Detection Dataset (Modd)

The marine obstacle detection dataset consists of 12 video sequences, providing in total 4454 fully annotated 640×480 frames. The video sequences have been recorded from different platforms, but from a vantage point that is consistent with the limitations of the small (under 2 m) USV (see, e.g., Fig. 1). The Axis 207 W camera was placed approximately 0.7 m above the water surface, looking in front of the vehicle, with an approximately $55°$ field of view. Camera has been set up to automatically adjust to the variations in lighting conditions.

---

[1] For research purposes, we will provide the reference Matlab code of our approach, including the evaluation routines from the authors page.

Video sequences have been acquired on different times under different weather conditions. Each frame is annotated manually by a polygon denoting the edge of water and bounding boxes are placed on *large obstacles* (those that straddle the water edge) and *small obstacles* (those that are fully surrounded by water). See Fig. 3 for illustration.

4.3   Performance Evaluation

The performance evaluation methodology was designed to reflect the two distinct challenges that the USV faces: the water edge (shoreline or horizon) detection and obstacle detection. The former is measured as the root mean square error (RMSE) in water edge position (Edg), and the latter is measured via the efficiency of *small object* detection, expressed as precision ($Prec$), recall (Rec), F-score (F) and the average number of false positives per frame (aFP).

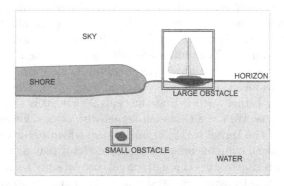

Fig. 3.   Scene representation in Modd dataset.

The following protocol is used to evaluate RMSE in water edge estimation. Areas where *large obstacles* intersect the ground truth water edge are removed. Note that, given the scene representation (Fig. 3), one cannot distinguish between large obstacles (e.g. large ships) and stationary elements of the shore (e.g. small piers). This way, a refined water edge was generated. For each pixel column in the full-sized image, a distance between water edge, as given by the ground truth and as determined by the algorithm is calculated. These values are averaged across all frames and videos and are shown in Table 1 as *Edg*.

The evaluation of object detection follows the recommendations from PAS-CAL VOC challenges [29], with small, application-specific modification: all small obstacles (provided as a ground truth or detected) that are closer to the annotated water line than 5 % of image height, are discarded prior to evaluation on each frame. This was done to ensure fair competition in situations where a detection may oscillate between fully water-enclosed obstacle, and the "dent" in the shoreline. This is also consistent with the problem of obstacle avoidance

– the USV is not concerned with avoiding small objects appearing right at the water edge. In counting false positives (FP), true positives (TP) and false negatives (FN), we followed the methodology of PASCAL VOC, with the minimum overlap set to 0.3. FP, TP and FN are used to calculate precision ($Prec$), recall (Rec), F-score (F) and average false positives per frame (aFP).

4.4 Results

In the following we denote our semantic-segmentation-based obstacle image-map estimation algorithm as SSM. To evaluate how much each part of our model contributes to performance, we have also implemented two variants of our approach, which we denote by UGM and UGM$_{col}$. In contrast to SSM, the UGM and UGM$_{col}$ do not use the MRF constraints and are in this respect only mixtures of a uniform pdf and three Gaussians with priors on their means. A further difference between UGM and UGM$_{col}$ was that UGM$_{col}$ ignored spatial information in visual features and relied only on color.

Note that SSM is conceptually similar to the Grab-cut algorithm [30], with two distinct differences. In contrast to the user-provided bounding box in [30], the SSM's weak supervision comes from the initialization of the parameters from the previous time-step and from the weak priors. The second distinction is that our approach does not explicitly calculate the segmentation mask to refine the mixture model. To further evaluate the MRF framework of our obstacle-map estimation algorithm, we have implemented a variant of our approach in which we apply a graph-cut [31] after each EM epoch to segment the image into a water/non-water mask. This mask is then used as in Grab-cut to refine the mixture model. We use exactly the same weakly-constrained mixture model as in SSM for fair comparison and denote this approach by GC. We have compared our approach also to the general segmentation approaches, namely the superpixel-based approach from Li et al. [27], SPX, and a graph-based segmentation algorithm from Felzenswalb and Huttenlocher [19], FZH. For fair comparison, all the algorithms were executed on the 50 × 50 images. We have experimented with the parameters of GC and FZH and have set them to optimal performance for our dataset. Since FZH was designed to run on larger images we have also performed the experiments for FZH on full-sized images – we denote this variant by FZH$_{full}$. All experiments were performed on a PC with 3.06 GHz Intel Xeon E5-1620 CPU in a single thread. The results are summarized in Table 1.

A Matlab implementation of SSM performed at rate higher 70 frames per second. Most of the processing was spent on fitting our semantic model and obstacle-map estimation (10 ms), while 4 ms was spent on the obstacle detection. For fair comparison of segmentation algorithms, we report in the Table 1 only the times required for the obstacle-map estimation. Although note that the obstacle detection part did require more processing time for the methods that delivered poor segmentation masks with more false positives. On average, our EM algorithm in SSM converged in three iterations. Note that the graph cut routine in GC SPX and the FZH were implemented in C and interfaced to Matlab, while all the other variants were entirely implemented in Matlab. Therefore,

Table 1. Performance evaluation on Modd. The table shows edge of water estimation error, precision, recall, F measure, average false positives and segmentation time, denoted by Edg, Prec, Rec, F, aFP, Time, respectively. The brackets show standard deviation where available.

	Edg [pix]	Prec	Rec	F	aFP	Time [ms]
SSM	10.8(8.9)	0.794	0.771	0.771	0.062	10(2)
GC	28.0(23.4)	0.555	0.736	0.606	0.348	15(3)
UGM	30.2(23.6)	0.524	0.738	0.575	0.525	11(2)
UGM$_{col}$	31.5(22.5)	0.118	0.490	0.177	2.692	11(3)
FZH	86.0(62.0)	0.728	0.525	0.554	0.043	16(1)
FZH$_{full}$	36.2(40.9)	0.440	0.802	0.529	0.621	200(3)
SPX	63.6(35.3)	0.007	0.001	0.001	0.079	55(1)

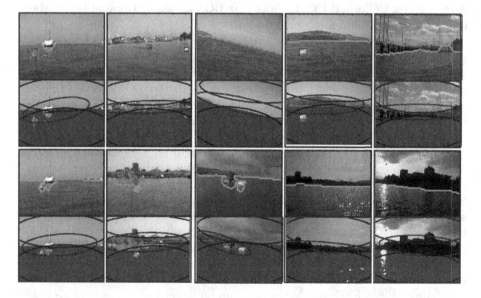

Fig. 4. Examples of water segmentation and obstacle detection. The detected edge-of-water is shown in green, while obstacles are shown as yellow rectangles. For each image we also show the spatial part of the three semantic components as three Gaussian ellipses and the portion of the image segmented as water in blue. Failure cases are shown in the bottom row with miss- and false detections (Color figure online).

the computational time results for segmentations are not directly comparable among the methods, but still offer a level of insight.

From the results in Table 1 we can observe that the SSM outperformed all competing approaches by all measures. When FZH$_{full}$ was run on full-sized images its recall improved compared to 50×50 image size version, but precision of object detection decreased, the false positive rate increased and the processing speed decreased by a factor of 10. Compared to GC, our approach delivered superior performance by all measures at comparable speed. This speaks of advantage of the continuos optimization in the MRF used in our model compared to the standard MRF on pixel labels that requires binarization by cuts. By far the worst performance was for the SPX, the reason being that the resulting segmentations were too general for the problem at hand.

The improved performance of SSM can be attributed exclusively to our carefully designed graphical model. This is evident from the results of UGM in which we have ignored the MRF constraints. We observe a significant drop in performance, especially precision. The performance further drops with UGM_{col}, which implies that spatial components in the feature vectors bear important information for proper segmentation. Figure 4 shows examples of segmentation maps from our approach, the spatial part of the Gaussian mixture and the detected objects in water. The appearance of water varies significantly between the various scenes, and the same is true for the other two semantic components. The images also vary in the scene composition in that the vertical position as well as the attitude of the water edge vary significantly. Nevertheless, the model is able to adapt well to these compositions and successfully decomposes the scene into obstacles and fairly well delineates the water edge. The bottom row shows failure cases. The first three images show failure when the object in water is detected as part of the above-water region. Note that in these cases the USV will still successfully avoid collision, but such detection represents a false negative in our performance evaluation. The rightmost two images show the performance when the boat is facing direct sunlight that causes significant glitters on the water surface. Even in these harsh conditions the model is able to interpret the scene well enough with few false obstacle detections.

5 Discussion and Conclusion

A graphical model for semantic segmentation of marine scenes was presented and applied to USV obstacle-map estimation. The model exploits the fact that scenes a USV encounters may be decomposed into three dominant visually- and semantically-distinctive components, one of which is the water. The appearance is modelled by a mixture of Gaussians and accounts for the outliers by a uniform component. The geometric structure is enforced by placing weak priors over the component means. A MRF model is applied on prior and posterior pixel-label distribution to account for the interactions across neighboring pixels. An EM algorithm is derived for fitting the model to image, which affords fast convergence and efficient implementation. The proposed model directly applies straight-forward features, i.e., color channels and pixel positions and avoids potentially slow extraction of more complex features. Nevertheless, the model is general enough to be directly applied without modifications to any other features. Results show excellent performance compared to related segmentation approaches and exhibits improved performance in terms of segmentation accuracy as well as speed.

Note that [32] have proposed an approach for inference in image segmentation that segments urban area images into three-strip segmentations by a dynamic program. In contrast to our approach, [32] only address the labeling part of the segmentation and require precomputed per-pixel label confidences. The resulting segmentation contains a homogenous bottom region, which prevents detection of obstacles without further re-processing the features of the bottom pixels. Our approach jointly learns the component appearance, estimates the per-pixel class probabilities, and estimates the segmentation within a single online framework, by optimizing a well-defined graphical model. Some related maritime segmentation approaches [7,15,16] rely on good horizon estimation to approximate the water edge, which makes them inapplicable to coastal regions. Note that in coastal regions, the water edge does not correspond to horizon and due to variety of shore line and piers takes shapes far from a straight line. Our graphical model does not make such a strict assumption which makes it applicable to off-shore as well as coastal regions. Nevertheless, the graphical model is still general enough to enable direct incorporation of externally measured horizon line along with its uncertainty if available.

As our second contribution, we have presented a new real-life marine segmentation dataset. This will be the largest publicly-available dataset of its kind to date. The experimental results show that the proposed algorithm performs favorably compared to the related solutions. While the algorithm provides high detection rates at low false positives it does so with a low processing time (our current C++ implementation of SSM runs close to 200 fps). Fast performance is of crucial importance for real-life implementations on USVs, as it allows the use in onboard embedded controllers and low-cost embedded, low-resolution cameras. In future work we will explore possibilities of porting our algorithm to such an embedded sensor. Since our optimization can be highly parallelized, we will explore this avenue in GPUs, which are becoming increasingly present in many modern embedded devices. Another avenue of further research will be analysis of additional low-level features for computation of better segmentation, addition of other modalities and extension to fast stereo systems, which may be feasible due to considerable computational speed of the proposed algorithm.

Acknowledgment. This work was supported in part by the Slovenian research agency programs P2-0214, P2-0094, and projects J2-4284, J2-3607, J2-2221. We also thank HarphaSea d.o.o. for their hardware used to capture the dataset.

References

1. Heidarsson, H., Sukhatme, G.: Obstacle detection from overhead imagery using self-supervised learning for autonomous surface vehicles. In: International Conference on Intelligent Robots and Systems, pp. 3160–3165 (2011)
2. Rasmussen, C., Lu, Y., Kocamaz, M.K.: Trail following with omnidirectional vision. In: International Conference on Intelligent Robots and Systems, pp. 829–836 (2010)

3. Montemerlo, M., Thrun, S., Dahlkamp, H., Stavens, D.: Winning the darpa grand challenge with an ai robot. In: AAAI National Conference on Artificial Intelligence, pp. 17–20 (2006)
4. Dahlkamp, H., Kaehler, A., Stavens, D., Thrun, S., Bradski, G.: Self-supervised monocular road detection in desert terrain. In: RSS, Philadelphia, USA (2006)
5. Ettinger, S.M., Nechyba, M.C., Ifju, P.G., Waszak, M.: Vision-guided flight stability and control for micro air vehicles. Adv. Rob. **17**, 617–640 (2003)
6. Lu, Y., Rasmussen, C.: Simplified markov random fields for efficient semantic labeling of 3D point clouds. In: IROS, pp. 2690–2697 (2012)
7. Scherer, S., Rehder, J., Achar, S., Cover, H., Chambers, A., Nuske, S., Singh, S.: River mapping from a flying robot: state estimation, river detection, and obstacle mapping. Auton. Rob. **33**, 189–214 (2012)
8. Onunka, C., Bright, G.: Autonomous marine craft navigation: on the study of radar obstacle detection. In: ICARCV, pp. 567–572 (2010)
9. Heidarsson, H., Sukhatme, G.: Obstacle detection and avoidance for an autonomous surface vehicle using a profiling sonar. In: ICRA, pp. 731–736 (2011)
10. Rankin, A., Matthies, L.: Daytime water detection based on color variation. In: International Conference on Intelligent Robots and Systems, pp. 215–221 (2010)
11. Elkins, L., Sellers, D., Reynolds, W.M.: The autonomous maritime navigation (amn) project: field tests, autonomous and cooperative behaviors, data fusion, sensors, and vehicles. J. Field Rob. **27**, 790–818 (2010)
12. Hong, T.H., Rasmussen, C., Chang, T., Shneier, M.: Fusing ladar and color image information for mobile robot feature detection and tracking. In: IAS, pp. 124–133 (2002)
13. Santana, P., Mendica, R., Barata, J.: Water detection with segmentation guided dynamic texture recognition. In: IEEE Robotics and Biomimetics (ROBIO), pp. 1836–1841 (2012)
14. Socek, D., Culibrk, D., Marques, O., Kalva, H., Furht, B.: A hybrid color-based foreground object detection method for automated marine surveillance. In: Blanc-Talon, J., Philips, W., Popescu, D.C., Scheunders, P. (eds.) ACIVS 2005. LNCS, vol. 3708, pp. 340–347. Springer, Heidelberg (2005)
15. Fefilatyev, S., Goldgof, D.: Detection and tracking of marine vehicles in video. In: Proceedings of the International Conference on Pattern Recognition, pp. 1–4 (2008)
16. Wang, H., Wei, Z., Wang, S., Ow, C., Ho, K., Feng, B.: A vision-based obstacle detection system for unmanned surface vehicle. In: International Conference on Robotics, Automation and Mechatronics, pp. 364–369 (2011)
17. Huntsberger, T., Aghazarian, H., Howard, A., Trotz, D.C.: Stereo visionbased navigation for autonomous surface vessels. JFR **28**, 3–18 (2011)
18. Khan, S., Shah, M.: Object based segmentation of video using color, motion and spatial information. In: Computer Vision Pattern Recognition, vol. 2, pp. 746–751 (2001)
19. Felzenszwalb, P., Huttenlocher, D.: Efficient graph-based image segmentation. Int. J. Comput. Vis. **59**, 167–181 (2004)
20. Besag, J.: On the statistical analysis of dirty pictures. J. Roy. Stat. Soc. **48**, 259–302 (1986)
21. Boykov, Y., Funka-Lea, G.: Graph cuts and efficient ND image segmentation. Int. J. Comput. Vis. **70**, 109–131 (2006)
22. Wojek, C., Schiele, B.: A dynamic conditional random field model for joint labeling of object and scene classes. In: Forsyth, D., Torr, P., Zisserman, A. (eds.) ECCV 2008, Part IV. LNCS, vol. 5305, pp. 733–747. Springer, Heidelberg (2008)

23. Lafferty, J., McCallum, A., Pereira, F.: Conditional random fields: probabilistic models for segmenting and labeling sequence data. In: Proceedings of the International Conference on Machine Learning, pp. 282–289 (2001)
24. Kontschieder, P., Bulo, S., Bischof, H., Pelillo, M.: Structured class-labels in random forests for semantic image labelling. In: ICCV, pp. 2190–2197 (2011)
25. Alpert., S.Galun, M., Basri, R., Brandt, A.: Image segmentation by probabilistic bottom-up aggregation and cue integration. In: CVPR, pp. 1–8 (2012)
26. Ren, X., Malik, J.: Learning a classification model for segmentation. In: ICCV, pp. 10–17 (2003)
27. Li, Z., Wu, X.M., Chang, S.F.: Segmentation using superpixels: a bipartite graph partitioning approach. In: CVPR, pp. 789–796 (2012)
28. Diplaros, A., Vlassis, N., Gevers, T.: A spatially constrained generative model and an EM algorithm for image segmentation. IEEETNN 18, 798–808 (2007)
29. Everingham, M., Van Gool, L., Williams, C.K.I., Winn, J., Zisserman, A.: The pascal visual object classes (VOC) challenge. IJCV 88, 303–338 (2010)
30. Rother, C., Kolmogorov, V., Blake, A.: GrabCut: interactive foreground extraction using iterated graph cuts. In: SIGGRAPH, vol. 23, pp. 309–314 (2004)
31. Bagon, S.: Matlab wrapper for graph cut (2006)
32. Felzenszwalb, P.F., Veksler, O.: Tiered scene labeling with dynamic programming. In: CVPR, pp. 3097–3104 (2010)

On the Performance of Pose-Based RGB-D Visual Navigation Systems

Dominik Belter, Michał Nowicki, and Piotr Skrzypczyński[(⊠)]

Institute of Control and Information Engineering, Poznań University of Technology,
ul. Piotrowo 3A, 60-965 Poznań, Poland
{dominik.belter,piotr.skrzypczynski}@put.poznan.pl,
michal.nowicki@cie.put.poznan.pl

Abstract. This paper presents a thorough performance analysis of several variants of the feature-based visual navigation system that uses RGB-D data to estimate in real-time the trajectory of a freely moving sensor. The evaluation focuses on the advantages and problems that are associated with choosing a particular structure of the sensor-tracking front-end, employing particular feature detectors/descriptors, and optimizing the resulting trajectory treated as a graph of sensor poses. Moreover, a novel yet simple graph pruning algorithm is introduced, which enables to remove spurious edges from the pose-graph. The experimental evaluation is performed on two publicly available RGB-D data sets to ensure that our results are scientifically verifiable.

1 Introduction

The introduction of compact and affordable RGB-D sensors, such like Microsoft Kinect and Asus Xtion Pro Live, triggered a new wave of research on visual SLAM (Simultaneous Localization and Mapping) [2,12,18] and VO (Visual Odometry) [33,38] systems that rely on the direct depth measurements. A RGB-D VO system computes the sensor motion between the consecutive keyframes (selected frames of the RGB-D data stream), and estimates the trajectory. It can be paired with a back-end for post-processing of a pose-graph, whose vertices correspond to the sensor poses, and whose edges represent constraints between these poses [9]. A pose-based RGB-D visual navigation system can be implemented in many different forms. However, the diversity of details in the published research on both VO and pose-based visual SLAM makes it hard, or even impossible to tell, which structure is the best one, and how the implementation of particular components influences the performance.

The computer vision literature is rich in papers concerning performance evaluation and comparison of various algorithms for feature detection/description [22,36], including comparative studies in the context of visual navigation [30]. Also authors of some papers on the RGB-D navigation methods or benchmarking, such like [12,13,17,24] demonstrate the performance of their systems on publicly available data, and in some cases include a comparison to other systems. However, to the extent of our knowledge, no study is available concerning

© Springer International Publishing Switzerland 2015
D. Cremers et al. (Eds.): ACCV 2014, Part II, LNCS 9004, pp. 407–423, 2015.
DOI: 10.1007/978-3-319-16808-1_28

the influence of the particular design choices made to a RGB-D navigation system on its performance. Among the few works that tackle this problem Endres *et al.* [12] evaluate only three different feature descriptors with their RGB-D SLAM, while Strasdat [34] shows several variants of a large-scale visual navigation system, being however concerned mostly with the passive vision sensors.

Hence, this paper attempts to experimentally evaluate several configurations of a pose-based RGB-D navigation system. We implemented a RGB-D VO/SLAM in two main configurations, which respectively are based on the visual tracking of point features, or on the frame-to-frame matching of salient visual features. These two front-ends are shown as pure frame-to-frame VO systems, then enhanced by local trajectory optimization, and finally, they are turned into the full pose-graph SLAM systems by adding the loop closure detection and global pose-graph optimization back-end. Moreover, we demonstrate how to improve the precision of the pose estimates by pruning the pose-graph from the edges that appear to be spurious. The experiments were performed using two publicly available data sets: the well-known TUM RGB-D benchmark [35], and the very recent ICL-NUIM dataset [17].

2   Pose-Based RGB-D Visual Navigation System

As the main idea of this paper is to demonstrate the performance of several configurations of the pose-based RGB-D navigation system, we divided our implementation into the separate front-end, which is an implementation of the VO concept, and the back-end implementing pose-graph optimization and the loop closure. The front-end and the back-end are implemented in separate Linux threads, and run asynchronous, exchanging only the necessary data: the pose-graph, and the data regarding the features and local descriptors for loop closure. Having the direct depth measurements from the Kinect or Xtion RGB-D sensor we consider the 3-D-to-3-D feature correspondences for frame-to-frame motion estimation [16]. Although combining the coordinates of the 2-D point features with the depth information we obtain 3-D positions of the point features, we do not keep these features in the system after computing the motion estimate. Optimization of a map structure containing potentially thousands of point features is time consuming, while advantages might be insignificant [13]. The lack of persistent 3-D features makes it impossible to use the sliding window bundle adjustment, implemented as in [11] or [23] to reduce the trajectory drift in the front-end. We took instead the approach suggested in [12]: we try to reduce locally the trajectory drift by constructing a pose-graph from m last sensor poses and estimate the motion constraints between the data frame attached to the current pose and the remaining m frames. Then, we apply the graph optimization provided by the back-end to this small pose-graph. This part of the approach, called Windowed Optimization (WO), should not be confused with the windowed bundle adjustment, because it is still purely pose-based and involves no features.

The front-end VO pipeline is proposed in two versions. The difference is in the approach to establish the correspondences between the 2-D features in the RGB

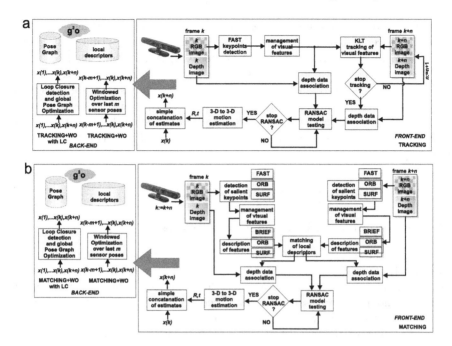

Fig. 1. Block diagram of the RGB-D visual navigation system in various configurations: the tracking-based version with optional Windowed Optimization and Loop Closure detection with pose-graph optimization (back-end) is depicted in (a), the matching-based version front-end with the same optional modules is shown in (b)

images. As we want to estimate the motion between the first image $I_{v(k)}$ and the last image $I_{v(k+n)}$ in a sequence of n images (n is considered to be small), we can detect the point features only in $I_{v(k)}$, and then track these points through the k images (Fig. 1a), or we can simply match the detected local descriptors of the features in $I_{v(k)}$ and $I_{v(k+n)}$ to obtain the correspondences (Fig. 1b). When the correspondences between $I_{v(k)}$ and $I_{v(k+n)}$ are established, the depth data are associated to the features resulting in two sets of matched 3-D points. The parameters of transformation between these two point patterns are estimated using a least squares estimation method [10,37]. To make the transformation estimation robust to the outliers resulting from imperfect tracking results or wrong feature matches, the estimation procedure is embedded in the RANSAC scheme [15].

The back-end for pose-graph optimization is based on the open-source g^2o software package for least square optimization [20]. This software takes a pose-graph produced by the front-end as input, and performs a minimization of a non-linear error function that is represented by this graph's constraints (see Sect. 4). Hence, the back-end can compute a globally consistent trajectory of the sensor, providing that all the constraints in the pose-graph (i.e. motion estimates) are correct [3]. We employ the g^2o back-end in two roles: to optimize small pose-graphs over a moving constant-length window in the Windowed Optimization procedure for local trajectory correction, and to optimize the global pose-graph, representing the whole recovered trajectory. The global optimization occurs whenever a loop closure is discovered. The loop closures are detected on RGB images by matching the frames belonging to poses that are positioned far enough along the trajectory. If a significant (visual) similarity between these frames is discovered on the basis of matching of the local descriptors a transformation is computed between the frames, and added as a constraint to the pose-graph.

3   Visual Odometry: The Front-End

3.1   Extraction and Management of Features

In the front-end we rely on feature-based methods for frame-to-frame motion estimation. Although the dense (appearance-based) methods are potentially more precise [19,33], as they use more data, this approach is more computation-intensive, and prone to failures due to occlusions and sudden scene changes. Thus, we focus exclusively on the feature-based approach, which is widely considered to be appropriate for real-time robotics applications [29]. The feature-based VO requires to detect a set of keypoints, which should be salient, repeatable, localized precisely in the image, and computed as fast as possible. We employ and test three point feature detectors: FAST [27], ORB [28], and SURF [5]. Using SURF we expected good results, but were concerned about the real-time performance of the system. On the other hand, FAST and ORB are more recent and more computation efficient algorithms, but they are less robust [30]. The SURF and ORB have their own feature descriptors, while the FAST detector is paired in our system with the low-complexity binary BRIEF [7] descriptor. To make the feature detection more robust we use two techniques that were proposed in [24]: unsupervised clustering of the keypoints, and detection of features in subimages. The detection of points in separate, slightly overlapping subimages is a heuristic that helps to distribute the keypoints evenly on the image. However, this heuristic cannot deal with situations where many features are detected on a small area in the image. To solve this problem the DBScan, a fast clustering algorithm [14] is employed. Clusters of features are formed, and then they are represented by maximum two points. This technique provides results similar to the quadtree-based point detection method described in [34], but is much faster.

3.2   Matching, Tracking, and Motion Estimation

The core part of the front-end is motion estimation based on two sets of corresponding point features, whose correspondences are determined either by matching or by tracking. The matching approach relies on the fact, that corresponding 2-D features on two images have similar neighborhood, thus they should have similar local descriptors, such like SURF, ORB, or BRIEF. The similarity of the investigated descriptors is determined using the Euclidean norm for SURF, or the Hamming distance for the binary descriptors BRIEF and ORB. The implementation of matching involves rejecting matches if multiple descriptors from the second image $I_{v(2)}$ correspond to the descriptor of the same feature from the first image $I_{v(1)}$, and accepting correspondences only if the j-th descriptor $I_{v(2)}^{j}$ from the second image is the best match for the i-th descriptor $I_{v(1)}^{i}$ from the first image, and at the same time the descriptor $I_{v(1)}^{i}$ is determined as the best match for descriptor $I_{v(2)}^{j}$.

In comparison to matching, the tracking does not need the description of features, and performs detection only on the subset of images. The idea of tracking is to detect features at the keyframe, and then looking for the position of this feature in the new image by searching locally. In our system, the tracking is performed using a pyramid implementation [6] of the Lucas-Kanade optical flow algorithm [4]. Tracking is initialized with points from the FAST detector, which is more efficient than the usual Shi-Tomasi from [31]. The maximum number of tracked features in our experiments was 500. Tracking is computationally less demanding than matching using classic descriptors, such like SIFT [21] or SURF. The VO front-end tracks features over a number of images of the RGB-D sequence between the two keyframes that are processed with depth images. When the number of successfully tracked features falls below a given threshold or the maximum allowed number of the RGB frames in tracking is reached (max. $n = 5$), the transformation between the keyframes is computed within the RANSAC scheme.

The RANSAC is used to randomly select 3 pairs of points from the set of tracked or matched features and to estimate the 3-D transformation using the Umeyama algorithm [37]. In every iteration, a model transformation is computed and evaluated. The number of RANSAC iterations is estimated using a simple probabilistic model [8] to improve speed. When the RANSAC-based model search is finished, the transformation is re-estimated from all inlier-pairs. Also, if the number of inliers is high, the iterative model correction is applied by rejecting the inliers that are the least probable within the model estimated so far [26].

4   Pose-Based Optimization: The Back-End

4.1   Pose-Graph Optimization

The back-end of our system is based on g^2o – a general framework for graph optimization [20]. We store each measurement between the robot/sensor poses in a graph (Fig. 2). Each vertex v_i in the graph represents a sensor pose. As motivated before, we do not keep point features in the graph structure. The edges in the graph represent measurements between two vertices. Measurement $\mathbf{M}_{ij}$ represents a 3-D transformation (translation and rotation) between poses v_i and v_j. The quality of the measurements is represented by an information matrix $\mathbf{\Omega}_{ij}$ (inverse of a covariance matrix), which can be obtained by propagating

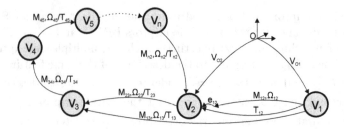

Fig. 2. Graph representation of the pose-based SLAM

uncertainty from the measurement model of the RGB-D sensor [25], or set as
identity matrix if equal uncertainty of all 3-D transformations is assumed.

The input variables, which are provided for the graph optimization are measurements (edges of the graph). The graph optimization returns poses of the
sensor (vertices of the graph) which correspond to the trajectory of the sensor.
The optimization is possible if at least one vertex has at least two incoming
edges. The Windowed Optimization procedure provides additional edges to the
graph. With this procedure we can add relations between more distant vertices
of the graph (edge M_{13} in Fig. 2). We can also add new measurements whenever
the robot returns to previously visited places. Loop closure procedure allows to
close the graph and improves the estimation of the sensor pose (edge M_{n2} in
Fig. 2). The graph optimization procedure minimizes the global error $\mathbf{E}$:

$$\mathbf{E} = \sum_{ij} \widetilde{\mathbf{e}}_{ij}^T \mathbf{\Omega}_{ij} \widetilde{\mathbf{e}}_{ij}, \tag{1}$$

where $\widetilde{\mathbf{e}}$ is a vector, which determines the discrepancy between the current vertex
pose and the measurements. Graphical representation of error computation for
each edge is presented in Fig. 2. The error $\mathbf{e}_{ij}$ is computed as:

$$\mathbf{e}_{ij} = \mathbf{M}_{ij}^{-1} \mathbf{T}_{ij}, \tag{2}$$

where $\mathbf{T}_{ij}$ is the estimated transformation between the considered vertices.
Defining the poses of the vertices v_i and v_j in the reference coordinate system
as $\mathbf{V}_{Oi}$ and $\mathbf{V}_{Oj}$, respectively, we can rewrite (2):

$$\mathbf{e}_{ij} = \mathbf{M}_{ij}^{-1} \mathbf{V}_{Oj}^{-1} \mathbf{V}_{Oi}. \tag{3}$$

Eventually, the homogeneous transformation $\mathbf{e}_{ij}$ is parametrised to the vector $\widetilde{\mathbf{e}}$
and used for optimization.

4.2   Graph Pruning

Despite of procedures in the front-end, which remove wrong matches and ensure
robust motion estimation, some wrong transformations might be added to the
graph. These outlier constraints (edges) influence the optimization results and

---

Algorithm 1. Local Adaptive Pruning procedure

Data: praph G

Result: pruned graph G_{pruned}

1 continue:=1;
2 **while** (continue=1) **do**
3 | OPTIMIZEGRAPH(); continue:=0;
4 | **for** i:=1:1:n **do**
5 | | edgeSet:= FINDINCOMINGEDGES(v_i);
6 | | outlier:= FINDOUTLIER(edgeSet);
7 | | **if** outlier != singleOutgoingEdge **then**
8 | | | REMOVEEDGE(outlier);
9 | | | continue = 1;
10 | | **end**
11 | **end**
12 **end**

---

output trajectory. While the recent results show that the back-end can be made robust to outlier constraints [1], we simply detect such edges and remove them from the pose-graph. For graph pruning we use the error value χ^2 (goodness of fit) provided by g^{2}o for each estimated edge: $\chi^2 = \widetilde{\mathbf{e}}_{ij}^T \mathbf{\Omega}_{ij} \widetilde{\mathbf{e}}_{ij}$.

We applied two approaches to remove outlier edges. In the simple approach we use the χ^2 test globally. The graph optimization and graph pruning stages are running alternately. After each optimization cycle we remove edges for which the χ^2 value is greater than a fixed threshold related to the χ^2 distribution (2.0 is used, which corresponds to 0.92 probability). If the vertex contains more than one incoming edge with χ^2 bigger than threshold we remove only the worst one in the single iteration. We repeat the pruning and optimization sequence until all remaining edges have the χ^2 value smaller than the selected threshold. The Local Adaptive Pruning procedure (Algorithm 1) exploits the locality of the pose-graph – we have observed that the incorrect constraints (edges) in the graph are usually the ones that "pull out" the given vertex in another direction than other edges incoming to the given vertex, having therefore a much worse χ^2 value. The adaptive pruning re-runs optimization until all outlier edges are removed. We search over the whole pose-graph. For each vertex v_i we find all incoming edges (FINDINCOMINGEDGES procedure). The procedure FINDOUTLIER detects an outlier within the set of edges incoming to the given node. To this end, this procedure computes the median value χ^2_{median} for all the incoming edges of the given node (edgeSet). The edge that has the biggest $\chi^2/\chi^2_{\mathrm{median}}$ value, and its χ^2 is at least p-times worse than the median is considered an outlier. We determined experimentally that $p = 10$ suits best for most of the analysed data sets and all the tested configurations of the system. The procedure REMOVEEDGE deletes the outlier edge only if its predecessor vertex in the pose-graph has more than one outgoing edge.

5   Experimental Results

5.1   Experiments and Data Sets

The aim of our experiments was to determine the properties of several configurations of the RGB-D visual navigation system. These configurations can be divided in two main groups: the VO systems, either frame-to-frame or using the Windowed Optimization (WO), and pose-based SLAM configurations, with the Loop Closure (LC) discovery and global optimization of the pose-graph. Note that the WO procedure always uses the same detector/descriptor pair as the main VO pipeline. The tracking-based variant was tested with the LC using three different detector/descriptor pairs, as in tracking there is no possibility to re-use the descriptors and they have to be computed for LC.

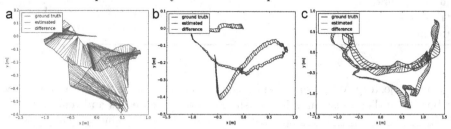

Fig. 3. Example recovered trajectories with the ATE error: trajectories ICL-NUIM living room/2 estimated using the Matching+WO FAST-BRIEF with LC variant (a), and the Matching+WO SURF with LC variant (b) show a dramatic difference in accuracy, simple Tracking VO performs well for the TUM fr1/room sequence (c)

The experiments were performed using the RGB-D data from two data sets: the TUM RGB-D data set [35], and the recent ICL-NUIM data set [17]. The TUM RGB-D data set, containing data acquired from either the Kinect or Xtion sensor in a scenario of indoor visual navigation, was used to evaluate a RGB-D SLAM system [12]. The ICL-NUIM data set contains RGB-D sequences from a synthetic environment with perfect ground-truth poses of the sensor. The rendored data is free from motion blur and artifacts, hence makes it easier to isolate the causes of failures. The perfect ground-truth is important when testing systems that achieve very small pose errors. The authors of [17] also tested several RGB-D visual navigation solutions on their data set, and their results can be directly compared to the performance of our systems. All experiments shown in this paper were conducted on a standard laptop computer with 2.5 GHz CPU and 8 GB RAM. We used the evaluation tools provided with the TUM RGB-D data set. The error metric mostly used is the Absolute Trajectory Errors (ATE), as it shows the difference between the recovered trajectory of the sensor and the ground truth trajectory (Fig. 3). The Relative Pose Error (RPE) is used to illustrate the local drift of the VO front-end.

5.2   Performance of the VO Front-End

From the results in Table 1, it can be observed that matching using the FAST-BRIEF (F-B) detector/descriptor pair definitively yields the biggest errors among

Table 1. Trajectory estimation results for various configurations of the visual navigation front-end for the TUM `fr1/room` dataset

Navigation system config.	Frame-to-frame				Windowed Optimization			
front-end type	ATE	RPE	Orient.	FPS	ATE	RPE	Orient.	FPS
detector & descriptor	RMSE	RMSE	RMSE		RMSE	RMSE	RMSE	
	[m]	[m]	[deg.]	[Hz]	[m]	[m]	[deg.]	[Hz]
Tracking	**0.191**	0.026	1.631	33.97	0.923	0.121	6.37	30.68
Matching FAST-BRIEF	1.194	0.052	5.179	50.17	1.042	0.056	4.755	29.57
Matching ORB	0.507	0.031	1.64	47.64	0.366	0.026	1.243	32.25
Matching SURF	0.201	0.017	1.42	20.76	0.206	0.019	0.864	17.16

the compared methods. When taking into account the RPE results, it is obvious that matching based of FAST-BRIEF performs so poorly not because of a single mismatch, but also due to the low precision of the motion estimation for each frame-to-frame increment.

The lowest ATE error (lowest errors are shown in bold in all tables) for the TUM `fr1/room` dataset (1362 frames, ground-truth trajectory 15.989 m) is obtained by pure tracking of FAST features, but this configuration results in bigger error when the WO is enabled. This is believed to be a result of the fact, that in the case of tracking the additional constraints introduced by WO are based on the features positions that have been already used when computing the regular frame-to-frame motion estimates. Therefore, the additional graph edges are redundant to the already existing edges in the simple tracking solution, and may only have a negative impact on the achieved results. The matching using SURF results in less motion drift when compared to matching with ORB, but both methods improve trajectory estimates when Windowed Optimization is used. What is worth noticing, are the framerates (FPS) of each variant The ORB presents similar, fast working speed to the FAST-BRIEF (even 30 Hz with the WO), with better results probably due to the ORB detection being performed on the image pyramid. The tracking has similar working speed (30 Hz) with and

Table 2. Trajectory estimation results for various configurations of the visual navigation front-end for the TUM `fr1/desk` dataset

Navigation system config.	Frame-to-frame				Windowed Optimization			
front-end type	ATE	RPE	Orient.	FPS	ATE	RPE	Orient.	FPS
detector & descriptor	RMSE	RMSE	RMSE		RMSE	RMSE	RMSE	
	[m]	[m]	[deg.]	[Hz]	[m]	[m]	[deg.]	[Hz]
Tracking	0.441	0.052	3.558	34.8	0.447	0.064	4.158	31.57
Matching FAST-BRIEF	0.659	0.131	9.425	49.35	0.693	0.11	8.249	29.14
Matching ORB	0.408	0.033	2.672	48.43	**0.073**	0.023	1.541	35.3
Matching SURF	**0.200**	0.027	1.882	20.38	**0.079**	0.022	1.378	18.46

without WO. The slowest of all the tested variants is matching based on SURF, which due to multiscale, complicated detection, floating point type descriptors and matching based on the Euclidean norm results in system operating with the maximal frequency of approx. 20 Hz.

Experiments evaluating the same variants were also performed for the TUM fr1/desk dataset (presented in Table 2) and for ICL-NUIM office/0 dataset (presented in Table 3). Similarly to the results presented in Table 1, the tracking results in lower error when local optimization is not used. Also, for the data sets in Tables 2 and 3, the matching based on FAST-BRIEF pair results in ATE and RPE errors that are much higher than the respective results for other variants. With the maximum frequency of FAST-BRIEF similar or worse than ORB, this proves that the FAST-BRIEF pair is unreliable, and should not be used in RGB-D visual odometry. The Windowed Optimization used with matching-based solutions with SURF or ORB results in slight improvements of the trajectory estimates. What is interesting, both solutions achieve similar ATE, which is below 8 cm for the TUM fr1/desk dataset (613 frames, ground-truth trajectory 9.263 m) and below 3.3 cm for the ICL-NUIM office/0 sequence (1510 frames, ground-truth trajectory 6.52 m) with the perfect ground-truth. These results compared to the results presented in [12,13,17] prove that even without the full SLAM optimization some variants of the proposed navigation system achieve similar or better results than the state-of-the-art solutions.

Table 3. Trajectory estimation results for various configurations of the visual navigation front-end for the ICL-NUIM office/0 dataset

Navigation system config. front-end type detector & descriptor	Frame-to-frame				Windowed Optimization			
	ATE RMSE [m]	RPE RMSE [m]	Orient. RMSE [deg.]	FPS [Hz]	ATE RMSE [m]	RPE RMSE [m]	Orient. RMSE [deg.]	FPS [Hz]
Tracking	0.167	0.012	1.904	22.55	0.629	0.076	1.664	20.5
Matching FAST-BRIEF	0.626	0.021	2.136	15.23	0.588	0.022	3.354	16.55
Matching ORB	0.047	0.009	0.469	25.27	0.033	0.007	0.408	24.05
Matching SURF	**0.030**	0.007	0.445	13.08	**0.030**	0.006	0.41	15.84

5.3 Influence of the Loop Closure

The trajectory recovered by the VO system using the frame-to-frame motion estimation has a drift, which can be decreased by the WO procedure, but will still grow with time, as there are no constraints on the trajectory that enforce the global consistency. A possibility to decrease drift estimation arises, whenever the robot/sensor re-visits already explored areas. To detect these situations a simple loop closure technique is used, which operates in the back-end. The results of evaluated versions with additional loop closure are presented in Tables 4 and 5. Due to the previously presented poor results for Tracking+WO, the loop closure module was added to the tracking solution without local optimization of the pose-graph. As expected, the addition of LC results in the decreased ATE and RPE.

Table 4. Trajectory estimation results for various configurations of the visual navigation front-end with the g^2o back-end optimization for the selected TUM datasets

Navigation system config.	TUM fr1/room				TUM fr1/desk			
front-end type	ATE	RPE	Orient.	FPS	ATE	RPE	Orient.	FPS
detector & descriptor	RMSE	RMSE	RMSE		RMSE	RMSE	RMSE	
all with g^2o back-end	[m]	[m]	[deg.]	[Hz]	[m]	[m]	[deg.]	[Hz]
Tracking with LC F-B	0.165	0.026	1.596	35.55	8.669	8.654	69.729	35.3
Tracking with LC ORB	**0.113**	0.024	1.383	35.64	**0.079**	0.033	2.54	33.62
Tracking with LC SURF	0.114	0.024	1.431	35.47	0.247	0.037	2.869	35.44
Matching+WO F-B with LC	1.042	0.056	4.755	29.57	5.802	5.027	56.019	29.31
Matching+WO ORB with LC	**0.107**	0.026	1.258	32.35	**0.055**	0.023	1.491	35.19
Matching+WO SURF with LC	**0.103**	0.019	0.837	16.75	**0.049**	0.021	1.356	18.47

In some cases, the loop closure makes these systems very precise with the ATE errors below 5 cm for the TUM fr1/desk and approx 10 cm for the bigger environment in the TUM fr1/room. For both of these data sets, the best results are obtained by the system variants based on matching with ORB and SURF, with the ORB-based version being however almost two times faster than the SURF-based one. A slightly higher error is observed for Tracking with LC, which has similar speed to the ORB-based matching. The variants based on the FAST-BRIEF perform poorly with an exception for Tracking with LC based on FAST-BRIEF for the TUM fr1/room, but even in that case the system achieves higher ATE than the similarly configured systems based on ORB or SURF.

On the synthetic ICL-NUIM data sets the lowest errors are for Tracking with LC based on SURF. Due to the fact, that the time allocated to the LC and global pose-graph optimization is constrained by the time of the frame-to-frame matching (the threads have to synchronize at each keyframe), the whole system operates faster (20 Hz), even with the relatively slow SURF detector/descriptor. The best ATE results equal to 2 cm for Tracking with the ORB-based LC for the ICL-NUIM office/0, and 2.1 cm for Tracking with SURF-based LC for the ICL-NUIM living room/2 (882 frames, ground-truth trajectory 8.42 m) demonstrate that in the absence of motion blur and image artifacts a simple, but carefully implemented RGB-D visual navigation system can achieve better results than most of the solutions compared in [17].

5.4 Pruning of the Pose-Graph

Unfortunately, there exist situations, where the constrains from loop closure have a negative influence on the performance of the pose-based SLAM. Even a single outlier constraint can have an arbitrary large impact on the graph optimization which is based on the least-squares principle. However, contrary to the situation in the filtration-based SLAM systems [32], such a wrong measurement can be removed, and then the pose-graph can be re-estimated in a correct form. Therefore, the influence of the proposed pose-graph pruning technique is demonstrated in Tables 6 and 7.

Table 5. Trajectory estimation results for various configurations of the visual navigation front-end with the g^{2}o back-end optimization for the selected ICL-NUIM datasets

Navigation system config.	ICL-NUIM office/0				ICL-NUIM living room/2			
front-end type	ATE	RPE	Orient.	FPS	ATE	RPE	Orient.	FPS
detector & descriptor	RMSE	RMSE	RMSE		RMSE	RMSE	RMSE	
all with g^{2}o back-end	[m]	[m]	[deg.]	[Hz]	[m]	[m]	[deg.]	[Hz]
Tracking with LC F-B	0.398	0.012	2.473	22.54	0.051	0.007	0.431	21.93
Tracking with LC ORB	**0.020**	0.009	0.671	22.45	0.067	0.013	0.518	20.04
Tracking with LC SURF	0.021	0.01	0.964	22.65	**0.021**	0.006	0.399	21.82
Matching+WO F-B with LC	0.588	0.022	3.354	16.55	0.912	0.035	2.901	15.1
Matching+WO ORB with LC	**0.015**	0.007	0.415	18.65	0.089	0.009	0.341	23.12
Matching+WO SURF with LC	0.062	0.057	1.174	12.12	0.036	0.006	0.303	14.35

Table 6. Pose graph pruning results for various configurations of the visual navigation front-end with or without back-end optimization for the TUM fr1/room dataset

Navigation system config.	Simple pruning – χ^2 test			Local adaptive pruning		
front-end type,	ATE	RPE	Orient.	ATE	RPE	Orient.
detector & descriptor,	RMSE	RMSE	RMSE	RMSE	RMSE	RMSE
back-end type	[m]	[m]	[deg.]	[m]	[m]	[deg.]
Tracking+WO	0.917	0.114	6.17	0.989	0.115	6.17
Matching+WO F-B	1.065	0.056	4.87	1.043	0.055	4.87
Matching+WO ORB	0.365	0.025	1.24	0.341	0.025	1.23
Matching+WO SURF	0.285	0.019	0.86	0.295	0.019	0.84
Tracking with LC F-B	0.164	0.025	1.59	0.165	0.025	1.59
Tracking with LC ORB	0.113	0.024	1.38	0.113	0.024	1.40
Tracking with LC SURF	0.113	0.024	1.43	0.113	0.024	1.43
Matching+WO F-B with LC	0.648	0.099	6.44	0.703	0.106	8.03
Matching+WO ORB with LC	0.055	0.022	1.49	0.048	0.022	1.49
Matching+WO SURF with LC	**0.048**	0.021	1.35	**0.039**	0.021	1.29

The back-end optimization (g^{2}o) improves the estimate of the trajectory by reducing the error (1) for the whole graph. Results obtained with one of the best variants of our navigation system (Matching+WO ORB with LC) for the ICL-NUIM office/0 are presented in Fig. 4. Before optimization the obtained trajectory is slightly distorted. After optimization and pruning the trajectory is smooth and very close to the ground truth trajectory.

In Fig. 5 we present some properties of the pruning method. Figure 5a presents the optimized trajectory for the ICL-NUIM office/0 data set, obtained with the Matching+WO SURF with LC variant of the system. (ATE RMSE error is about 6 cm). The same trajectory optimized with pruning is presented in Fig. 5b (ATE error is reduced to 1.5 cm). Incorrect matches introduced by the Loop Closure procedure moved the vertex indicated by the arrow no. 1 in Fig. 5a to a wrong

Table 7. Pose graph pruning results for various configurations of the visual navigation front-end with or without back-end optimization for the ICL-NUIM office/0 dataset

Navigation system config. front-end type, detector & descriptor, back-end type	Simple pruning – χ^2 test			Local adaptive pruning		
	ATE RMSE [m]	RPE RMSE [m]	Orient. RMSE [deg.]	ATE RMSE [m]	RPE RMSE [m]	Orient. RMSE [deg.]
Tracking+WO	0.527	0.048	1.26	0.715	0.090	1.80
Matching+WO F-B	0.584	0.021	2.11	0.586	0.020	2.15
Matching+WO ORB	0.032	0.006	0.40	0.028	0.006	0.40
Matching+WO SURF	0.030	0.006	0.41	0.029	0.006	0.40
Tracking with LC F-B	0.398	0.012	2.47	0.398	0.012	2.47
Tracking with LC ORB	0.020	0.009	0.67	0.021	0.008	0.46
Tracking with LC SURF	0.021	0.009	0.96	0.023	0.009	1.07
Matching+WO F-B with LC	0.588	0.022	3.35	0.583	0.020	3.10
Matching+WO ORB with LC	**0.015**	0.007	0.41	**0.014**	0.006	0.41
Matching+WO SURF with LC	0.061	0.057	1.17	**0.014**	0.006	0.41

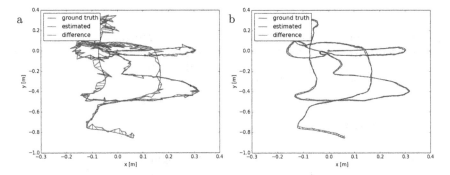

Fig. 4. Trajectory before (a) and after (b) g^2o optimization and pose-graph pruning. Matching+WO ORB with LC, ICL-NUIM office/0 data set

position. The erroneous measurement is detected by the pruning procedure and removed from the graph. This situation corresponds to the initial value of the RPE error presented in Fig. 5c. The RPE error is significantly reduced after pruning. The presented pruning procedure removes also incorrect edges introduced sporadically by the Windowed Optimization procedure (due to mismatching descriptors). The part of the trajectory indicated by arrow no. 2 in Fig. 5a is presented as details of the pose-graph in Fig. 5d. The procedure removes edges which do not fit to the obtained path and improves the final estimate of the poses.

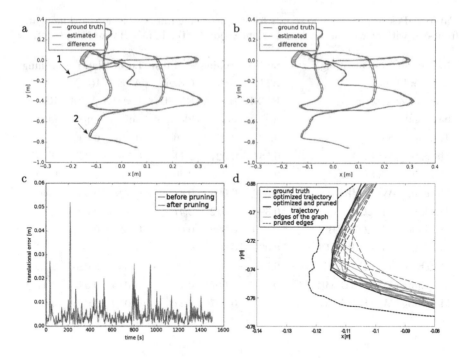

Fig. 5. Pruning properties presented for the Matching+WO SURF with LC on the ICL-NUIM `office/0` data set: trajectory obtained after g^2o optimization (a), trajectory obtained after g^2o optimization and pruning (b), RPE error before and after pruning (c), details of the pose-graph with removed edges (d)

6   Conclusions

This paper presents the comparison of several configurations of a relatively simple pose-based visual navigation system using the RGB-D data. The experimental results clearly show that there are significant differences in the performance of the considered variants of the visual navigation system, even though all these variants are based on the same general concept, and they share many critical components. Both structures of the VO, based on tracking and matching, respectively have proven to be suitable for the front-end of RGB-D SLAM system. The tracking-based VO pipeline is simple, fast and precise, but only if it is feed by good quality images at a high frame rate. On the other hand, the performance of the matching-based version critically depends on the used detector-descriptor pair. The performance of the ORB-based version was comparable or even slightly better than the performance of the tracking approach, with regard to both the precision and speed. An advantage of the matching-based version of the front-end is also the possibility to improve the trajectory by local pose-graph optimization, which turned out to be impossible with tracking. However, other variants based on matching did not perform so well, with the SURF-based version being the slowest one, and the FAST-BRIEF variant producing unacceptable trajectory errors. The ability to remove wrong loop closure constraints is very important to the pose-based RGB-D SLAM, as shown by our pose-graph pruning results. In the further research we plan to test robust estimation-based approaches to the outlier removal problem [1], and investigate how to efficiently include the point features in the optimization.

Acknowledgement. This research was financed by the Polish National Science Centre grant funded according to the decision DEC-2013/09/B/ST7/01583.

References

1. Agarwal, P., Grisetti, G., Tipaldi, G., Spinello, L., Burgard, W., Stachniss, C.: Experimental analysis of dynamic covariance scaling for robust map optimization under bad initial estimates. In: Proceedings of the IEEE International Conference on Robotics and Automation, Hong Kong, pp. 3626–3631 (2014)
2. Bachrach, A., Prentice, S., He, R., Henry, P., Huang, A., Krainin, M., Maturana, D., Fox, D., Roy, N.: Estimation, planning, and mapping for autonomous flight using an RGB-D camera in GPS-denied environments. Int. J. Robot. Res. **31**(11), 1320–1343 (2012)
3. Bailey, T., Durrant-Whyte, H.: Simultaneous localization and mapping: part II. IEEE Robot. Autom. Mag. **13**(3), 108–117 (2006)
4. Baker, S., Matthews, I.: Lucas-Kanade 20 years on: a unifying framework. Int. J. Comput. Vis. **56**(3), 221–255 (2004)
5. Bay, H., Ess, A., Tuytelaars, T., Van Gool, L.: Speeded-up robust features (SURF). Comput. Vis. Image Underst. **110**(3), 346–359 (2008)
6. Bouguet, J.Y.: Pyramidal implementation of the Lucas-Kanade feature tracker, description of the algorithm (2000)
7. Calonder, M., Lepetit, V., Ozuysal, M., Trzcinski, T., Strecha, C., Fua, P.: BRIEF: computing a local binary descriptor very fast. IEEE Trans. Pattern Anal. Mach. Intell. **34**(7), 1281–1298 (2012)
8. Choi, S., Kim, T., Yu, W.: Performance evaluation of RANSAC family. In: Proceedings of British Machine Vision Conference, London (2009)
9. Durrant-Whyte, H., Bailey, T.: Simultaneous localization and mapping: part I. IEEE Robot. Autom. Mag. **13**(2), 99–110 (2006)
10. Eggert, D.W., Lorusso, A., Fisher, R.B.: Estimating 3-D rigid body transformations: a comparison of four major algorithms. Mach. Vis. Appl. **9**(5–6), 272–290 (1997)
11. Engels, C., Stewenius, H., Nistér, D.: Bundle adjustment rules. In: Photogrammetric Computer Vision, September 2006
12. Endres, F., Hess, J., Engelhard, N., Sturm, J., Cremers, D., Burgard, W.: An evaluation of the RGB-D SLAM system. In: Proceedings of the IEEE International Conference on Robotics and Automation, St. Paul, pp. 1691–1696 (2012)
13. Endres, F., Hess, J., Sturm, J., Cremers, D., Burgard, W.: 3-D Mapping with an RGB-D camera. IEEE Trans. Robot. **30**(1), 177–187 (2014)
14. Ester, M., Kriegel, H.-P., Sander, J., Xu, X.: A density-based algorithm for discovering clusters in large spatial databases with noise. In: Proceedings of the International Conference on Knowledge Discovery and Data Mining, pp. 226–231 (1996)

15. Fischler, M., Bolles, R.: Random sample consensus: a paradigm for model fitting with applications to image analysis and automated cartography. Commun. ACM **24**(6), 381–395 (1981)

16. Fraundorfer, F., Scaramuzza, D.: Visual odometry: part II: matching, robustness, optimization, and applications. IEEE Robot. Autom. Mag. **19**(2), 78–90 (2012)

17. Handa, A., Whelan, T., McDonald, J., Davison, A.: A benchmark for RGB-D visual odometry, 3D reconstruction and SLAM. In: IEEE International Conference on Robotics and Automation, Hong Kong (2014)

18. Henry, P., Krainin, M., Herbst, E., Ren, X., Fox, D.: RGB-D mapping: using kinect-style depth cameras for dense 3D modeling of indoor environments. Int. J. Robot. Res. **31**(5), 647–663 (2012)

19. Kerl, C., Sturm, J., Cremers, D.: Robust odometry estimation for RGB-D cameras. In: Proceedings of the IEEE International Conference on Robotics and Automation, Karlsruhe, pp. 3748–3754 (2013)

20. Kümmerle, R., Grisetti, G., Strasdat, H., Konolige, K., Burgard, W.: g2o: a general framework for graph optimization. In: Proceedings of the IEEE International Conference on Robotics and Automation, Shanghai, pp. 3607–3613 (2011)

21. Lowe, D.G.: Distinctive image features from scale-invariant keypoints. Int. J. Comput. Vis. **60**(2), 91–110 (2004)

22. Mikolajczyk, K., Schmid, C.: A performance evaluation of local descriptors. IEEE Trans. Pattern Anal. Mach. Intell. **27**(10), 1615–1630 (2005)

23. Mouragnon, E., Lhuillier, M., Dhome, M., Dekeyser, F., Sayd, P.: Generic and real-time structure from motion using local bundle adjustment. Image Vis. Comput. **27**, 1178–1193 (2009)

24. Nowicki, M., Skrzypczyński, P.: Combining photometric and depth data for lightweight and robust visual odometry. In: European Conference on Mobile Robots, pp. 125–130 (2013)

25. Park, J.-H., Shin, Y.-D., Bae, J.-H., Baeg, M.-H.: Spatial uncertainty model for visual features using a Kinect sensor. Sensors **12**, 8640–8662 (2012)

26. Raguram, R., Chum, O., Pollefeys, M., Matas, J., Frahm, J.: USAC: a universal framework for random sample consensus. IEEE Trans. Pattern Anal. Mach. Intell. **35**(8), 2022–2038 (2013)

27. Rosten, E., Drummond, T.W.: Machine learning for high-speed corner detection. In: Leonardis, A., Bischof, H., Pinz, A. (eds.) ECCV 2006, Part I. LNCS, vol. 3951, pp. 430–443. Springer, Heidelberg (2006)

28. Rublee, E., Rabaud, V., Konolige, K., Bradski, G.: ORB: an efficient alternative to SIFT or SURF. In: IEEE International Conference on Computer Vision (ICCV), pp. 2564–2571 (2011)

29. Scaramuzza, D., Fraundorfer, F.: Visual odometry: part I the first 30 years and fundamentals. IEEE Robot. Autom. Mag. **18**(4), 80–92 (2011)

30. Schmidt, A., Kraft, M., Fularz, M., Domagala, Z.: Comparative assessment of point feature detectors and descriptors in the context of robot navigation. J. Autom. Mob. Robot. Intell. Syst. **7**(1), 11–20 (2013)

31. Shi, J., Tomasi, C.: Good features to track. In: IEEE Conference on Computer Vision and Pattern Recognition (CVPR 1994), pp. 593–600 (1994)

32. Skrzypczyński, P.: Simultaneous localization and mapping: a feature-based probabilistic approach. Int. J. Appl. Math. Comput. Sci. **19**(4), 575–588 (2009)

33. Steinbrücker, F., Sturm, J., Cremers, D.: Real-time visual odometry from dense RGB-D images, Workshop on Live Dense Reconstruction with Moving Cameras. In: IEEE International Conference on Computer Vision (ICCV), Barcelona (2011)

34. Strasdat, H.: Local accuracy and global consistency for efficient visual SLAM. Ph.D. dissertation, Imperial College, London (2012)
35. Sturm, J., Engelhard, N., Endres, F., Burgard, W., Cremers, D.: A benchmark for the evaluation of RGB-D SLAM systems. In: Proceedings of the IEEE/RSJ International Conference on Intelligent Robots and Systems, Vilamoura, pp. 573–580 (2012)
36. Tuytelaars, T., Mikolajczyk, K.: Local invariant feature detectors: a survey. Found. Trends Comput. Graph. Vis. **3**(3), 177–280 (2008)
37. Umeyama, S.: Least-squares estimation of transformation parameters between two point patterns. IEEE Trans. Pattern Anal. Mach. Intell. **13**(4), 376–380 (1991)
38. Whelan, T., Johannsson, H., Kaess, M., Leonard, J. J., McDonald, J. B.: Robust real-time visual odometry for dense RGB-D mapping. In: Proceedings of the IEEE International Conference on Robotics and Automation, Karlsruhe, pp. 5704–5711 (2013)

Elastic Shape Analysis of Boundaries of Planar Objects with Multiple Components and Arbitrary Topologies

Sebastian Kurtek[1], Hamid Laga[2,3]([⊠]), and Qian Xie[4]

[1] Department of Statistics, The Ohio State University, Columbus, USA
[2] Phenomics and Bioinformatics Research Centre, University of South Australia, Adelaide, Australia
[3] Australian Centre for Plant Functional Genomics, PtyLtd, Adelaide, Australia
hamid.laga@unisa.edu.au
[4] Department of Statistics, Florida State University, Tallahassee, Florida

Abstract. We consider boundaries of planar objects as level set distance functions and present a Riemannian metric for their comparison and analysis. The metric is based on a parameterization-invariant framework for shape analysis of quadrilateral surfaces. Most previous Riemannian formulations of 2D shape analysis are restricted to curves that can be parameterized with a single parameter domain. However, 2D shapes may contain multiple connected components and many internal details that cannot be captured with such parameterizations. In this paper we propose to register planar curves of arbitrary topologies by utilizing the re-parameterization group of quadrilateral surfaces. The criterion used for computing this registration is a proper distance, which can be used to quantify differences between the level set functions and is especially useful in classification. We demonstrate this framework with multiple examples using toy curves, medical imaging data, subsets of the TOSCA data set, 2D hand-drawn sketches, and a 2D version of the SHREC07 data set. We demonstrate that our method outperforms the state-of-the-art in the classification of 2D sketches and performs well compared to other state-of-the-art methods on complex planar shapes.

1 Introduction

Shape is an important feature for characterizing objects in various fields of science. Analyzing objects based on their shapes and modeling the variability they exhibit within and across classes are fundamental problems in computer vision and pattern recognition. There has been an increasing interest in using Riemannian frameworks for shape analysis of objects because of the breadth of tools that they offer. First, they allow one to remove all of the shape preserving

---

Electronic supplementary material The online version of this chapter (doi:10. 1007/978-3-319-16808-1_29) contains supplementary material, which is available to authorized users.

D. Cremers et al. (Eds.): ACCV 2014, Part II, LNCS 9004, pp. 424–439, 2015.
DOI: 10.1007/978-3-319-16808-1_29

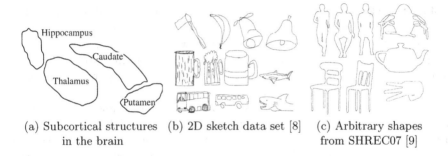

(a) Subcortical structures   (b) 2D sketch data set [8]   (c) Arbitrary shapes
   in the brain   from SHREC07 [9]

Fig. 1. Examples of planar shapes of arbitrary topology, which may contain multiple parts and complex internal features.

transformations from the representation space. Second, they allow for computing statistics (e.g. means, covariances, modes of variation) of shapes. However, most of this work is limited to shape analysis of the outer boundaries of objects, i.e. curves [1–3] and surfaces [4–6]. There are very few papers that study both shape boundaries and their interiors. Fuchs [7] considers such a case but their approach is not invariant to re-parameterization and also only considers shapes of the same topology.

In this paper, we propose a novel framework for analyzing shapes of planar objects of arbitrary topologies that can have multiple components as shown in Fig. 1. We propose to represent planar objects as level sets of their Euclidean distance functions. We consider each such function along with its smoothed gradient as an image $f : [0, 1]^2 \to \mathbb{R}^3$. We thus formulate the problem of analyzing curves as a problem in image analysis, and adapt a recently proposed Riemannian framework developed for statistical shape analysis of quadrilateral surfaces to the problem at hand. This framework is especially useful in registering multiple (non-intersecting) curves or curves with differing topologies. The registration step is very important in shape analysis as it allows one to generate meaningful comparisons of shape, where similar features are optimally matched across objects. Furthermore, the proposed registration criterion is a proper parameterization-invariant distance between images, and thus has nice mathematical properties. Such a framework, in principle, also allows one to perform subsequent statistical analysis of such objects such as computing their sample statistics. While at this stage we do not provide a setting for computing geodesic paths and proper statistics in this framework (future work), we display linear interpolations between registered shapes which can be used to asses the computed distances and registrations. We demonstrate this framework with multiple examples on toy shapes and real data from medical imaging and graphics. We also provide shape classification results on two very complex data sets: 2D sketches [8] and a 2D version of the SHREC07 data set [9]. We show that our framework performs well compared to state-of-the-art feature-based methods on the SHREC07 data set and significantly outperforms the state-of-the-art on the sketch data set. Note that feature-based methods are unable to perform subsequent statistical analysis such as computing shape means or covariances.

Related work. The concept of shape spaces with an associated metric was first proposed by Kendall [10] and then further developed by Dryden and Mardia [11]. In those frameworks, shapes were represented with a set of landmark points in the Euclidean space and compared using a Riemannian framework on the representation space of such objects. The main drawback of this approach is that the landmarks have to be detected and labeled before one can analyze the shapes. Alternatively, one can look at curves as continuous objects and represent them as elements of infinite-dimensional Riemannian manifolds. Zahn and Roskies [12] performed Fourier analysis on angle functions of arc-length parameterized curves. However, restricting the analysis to arc-length parameterized curves can be very limiting in practice. It is generally accepted that a better approach is to search for optimal parameterizations using a proper distance. Younes [1] and Younes et al. [2] defined parameterization-invariant Riemannian metrics on shape spaces of planar curves. Along this line of research, Klassen et al. [13] introduced a family of elastic metrics that quantify the relative amounts of bending and stretching needed to deform planar, closed curves into each other. Joshi et al. [14] extended this framework to curves in $\mathbb{R}^n$. Later on, Srivastava et al. [3] proposed a special representation of planar curves, called the square root velocity function (SRVF), which simplifies the computation of geodesics and geodesic distances between curves. The use of this representation chooses a specific instance of the elastic metric by fixing the parameters that control the bending and stretching energies.

The main limitation of these works is that they are based on a 1D parameterization of curves and thus only single boundaries of objects can be analyzed. There are few works that are able to analyze groups of curves simultaneously or curves of differing topologies. Fuchs et al. [7] handle the interior of the shapes instead of only the shape boundary. Thus, this framework is naturally defined for multiple components. However, it requires the topology to stay the same during the evolution, which can be limiting in real applications. In addition, this method is not invariant to re-parameterization. Kerr et al. [15] developed statistical models for multiple closed planar curves in a parameterization-invariant framework, but it cannot handle objects of differing topologies.

Another common representation of shape is using distance functions and their level sets [16], which can represent shapes of arbitrary topologies. For example, to register planar shapes, Paragios et al. [17] used Euclidean distance transforms while Munim and Farag [18] and Fahmi and Farag [19] used vector distance function-based representations. These three papers, however, assume that the global alignment between a pair of shapes can be solved by finding the optimal translation, rotation and anisotropic scaling between the shapes. Thus, these approaches are not applicable to shapes that undergo large articulated and elastic motions, such as the ones we consider in this paper. Although Yezzi and Saoto [20] used level sets, their approach is limited to planar shapes composed of a single closed curve. Also, while these methods are invariant to translation, rotation, and global scaling, none of them is invariant to re-parameterization.

There is a series of related work on Large Deformation Diffeomorphic Metric Mapping (LDDMM) [21] where planar objects of interest (curves, landmarks, etc.) are embedded in a 2D domain and the full domains are matched and compared.

This type of approach is similar in flavor to the proposed work, but the matching and comparison are performed differently. The LDDMM approach searches for a geodesic between the two images in the group of diffeomorphisms with an additional data matching term. In the proposed approach, the distance is computed on the space of level set functions modulo re-parameterization.

Another set of approaches represent complex shapes using point sets and compare them using the Hausdorff distance [22,23] or the symmetric area difference [24], which do not require a 1D parameterization of the objects. While these methods have proven very useful in a number of tasks including partial object matching, they often do not allow for elastic deformations between the objects of interest. Several other papers used shape descriptors to compare 2D and 3D objects [25–30]. The Inner Distance-based Shape Context (IDSC) of Ling and Jacobs [25] is robust to articulated motion and aware of inner holes in the shapes. This descriptor, however, works on closed planar shapes, with a single connected component and with clearly defined interior regions. Our approach does not have this restriction and can even handle stroke-based drawings, such as human-drawn sketches, as demonstrated in the experimental results section.

Overview and contributions. We propose to represent planar objects as level sets of distance functions. To compare these functions, we adapt a recent framework for shape analysis of quadrilateral surfaces proposed in [31], which provides a recipe for generating parameterization-invariant comparisons between shapes of surfaces. We utilize the same metric but adapt it to our problem. A similar approach was taken by Xie et al. [32] in the context of image registration. In addition to parameterization, we remove variability due to other shape preserving transformations such as translation, scale and rotation. Our contributions can be summarized as follows:

1. We formulate the problem of performing computations on the space of planar objects of arbitrary topology as the problem of analyzing their associated level set distance functions. For this purpose, we utilize the square root function transformation of surfaces. To the best of our knowledge, this is the first time that a parameterization-invariant framework (where optimal registrations are computed) is being proposed for the analysis of planar objects of arbitrary topology using the distance function representation.
2. We demonstrate this framework with several examples using toy shapes and real data such as medical images, 2D sketches, and 2D projections of natural and manmade 3D shapes. We consider examples involving multiple simple planar closed curves and planar curves with different topologies.
3. We demonstrate the utility of the proposed distance in two shape classification studies and show that it performs well compared to the feature-based state-of-the-art methods for analyzing such data. In particular, we show that the classification performance of the proposed framework outperforms, by more than 13 %, the state-of-the-art on the hand-drawn sketches of Eitz et al. [8], suggesting that the proposed framework is suitable for the analysis of complex shapes that do not have clearly-defined interior regions.

The rest of this paper is organized as follows. In Sect. 2, we provide details of the mathematical framework we will use to analyze shapes of complex planar contours with arbitrary topologies. In particular, we discuss how different shape preserving transformations are removed from the representation space. In Sect. 3, we present comparison and classification results on different types of data. We conclude in Sect. 4 and outline directions for future work.

2   Mathematical Framework

Several past papers have considered a planar object as a parameterized curve $\beta : D \to \mathbb{R}^2$, where D is a certain domain for the parameterization (e.g. $D = [0, 1]$ for open curves or $D = \mathbb{S}^1$ for closed curves). Unfortunately, using such a representation does not allow one to analyze shapes with interior details or multiple components as those shown in Fig. 1. For this purpose, we propose to utilize the level set function representation (e.g. Euclidean distance transform), which we will refer to as ψ. That is, in our framework $\psi : [0, 1]^2 \to \mathbb{R}$, and the object β is defined as its zero-level (isocontour) set. In this paper, we propose to adapt a recently developed framework for statistical shape analysis of parameterized quadrilateral surfaces to the problem of registering and comparing level set representations of planar shapes with arbitrary topologies and multiple components. To do this, we build on the Riemannian framework proposed by Kurtek et al. [31]. A major advantage of this framework is that it searches for optimal parameterizations of the given objects using a parameterization-invariant metric. We take advantage of this useful property in the proposed framework.

2.1   Translation, Scaling and Rotation Variability

The notion of shape is invariant to translation, scaling, rotation and re-parameterization. In this section, we provide details of how we remove some of these variabilities from the representation space. We assume that the data is originally given as a binary image, $I : [0, 1]^2 \to \{0, 1\}$. If the data is not given in this form, we begin by computing its binary image representation. For simplicity, we remove the translation and scaling variabilities at this stage using normalization. The area of an object present in a binary image can be computed using its zeroth moment, $A = \int_{[0,1]^2} I(s)ds$ where $s = (x, y)$ are the image coordinates. The centroid of a binary image can be computed using the first moments, $(\bar{x}, \bar{y}) = \frac{1}{A}(\int_{[0,1]^2} xI(s)ds, \int_{[0,1]^2} yI(s)ds)$. Thus, we first translate the object in the image such that its centroid has coordinates $(\bar{x}, \bar{y}) = (0.5, 0.5)$. Once centered, we normalize the scale of the object in the image by rescaling it to occupy a certain proportion of the area of the entire image. Note that this proportion is chosen based on the application of interest and affects the distance calculation. Thus, the computed distances are comparable within data sets but not across data sets. While, in principle, we could choose the same scale for all types of data (making all the distances comparable) this is not very practical when the objects of interest are very different across applications (see for example the 2D sketches vs. the medical imaging data). In both steps, we utilize nearest neighbor interpolation and a very high image resolution (1000×1000 pixels) to preserve all of the details of the given objects. These two steps ensure that our analysis is invariant to translation and rescaling of the objects present in the given images. While we could also normalize the orientation of the objects at this stage using the second moment, this approach can be unstable in practice. That is, for a small perturbation of the object the rotational alignment can change drastically. Thus, we take a different approach where we exhaustively search for the optimal rotation in a pairwise manner using the level set function representation.

Given two normalized binary images, I_1 and I_2, we are interested in computing the rotational alignment of the objects present within. We proceed as follows. First, we compute their corresponding signed distance function representations on the unit disk ($\mathbb{D}$) domain: $\tilde{\psi}_1, \tilde{\psi}_2 : \mathbb{D} \to \mathbb{R}$. Second, we generate a set of area preserving diffeomorphisms by rotating the initial disk parameterization by a set of angles $\theta \in [0, 2\pi)$. Call this set $\mathcal{H}$. In our implementation, we utilize 360 equally spaced angles. Thus, the set $\mathcal{H}$ contains 360 initial grid alignments. Next, we exhaustively search for the optimal rotation that best aligns the two signed distance functions using $\hat{h} = \arg\min_{h \in \mathcal{H}} \|\tilde{\psi}_1 - \tilde{\psi}_2 \circ h\|$, which corresponds to an angle of rotation $\hat{\theta}$. Finally, we apply this rotation to the second binary image to result in $\hat{I}_2$.

2.2   Square Root Representation of Level Set Functions

In order to optimally register two shapes with arbitrary topologies or multiple components and compute the distance between them, we adapt the framework of Kurtek et al. [31], which was defined and used for statistical shape analysis of quadrilateral surfaces. Let ψ be the distance transform of a binary image I. We first define a new function $f = (\nabla\psi, \psi)^T : [0, 1]^2 \to \mathbb{R}^3$, where $\nabla\psi$ is a smoothed gradient of the level set distance function ψ. With a slight abuse of notation we will refer to f as the level set function from now on. In our implementation, we smooth the gradient using a Gaussian filter. The gradient of the level set function provides important edge features of the objects of interest, which will be useful during the registration process. We let $\mathcal{F}$ represent the space of all such level set functions: $\mathcal{F} = \{f : [0, 1]^2 \to \mathbb{R}^3 | f \text{ is differentiable almost everywhere}\}$. Let Γ be the set of all diffeomorphisms of $[0, 1]^2$. Γ acts on $\mathcal{F}$ by composition: $(f, \gamma) \to f \circ \gamma$. One can define the standard $\mathbb{L}^2$ inner product on this space and utilize the resulting Riemannian structure for comparing level set functions. Unfortunately, the $\mathbb{L}^2$ Riemannian metric is not invariant to re-parameterizations (because $\|f_1 - f_2\| \neq \|f_1 \circ \gamma - f_2 \circ \gamma\|$) and thus cannot be used. Kurtek et al. [31] suggest an alternative approach based on a different representation termed the square root function. We present some details next.

Given a function f, its square root function (SRF) representation $q : [0, 1]^2 \to \mathbb{R}^3$ is defined as

$$q(s) = \sqrt{|n(s)|}f(s), \tag{1}$$

where $|\cdot|$ denotes the Euclidean norm in $\mathbb{R}^3$, and $n(s) = \frac{\partial f}{\partial x}(s) \times \frac{\partial f}{\partial y}(s)$. The resulting space of SRFs is a subset of $\mathbb{L}^2([0, 1]^2, \mathbb{R}^3)$, from now on simply referred

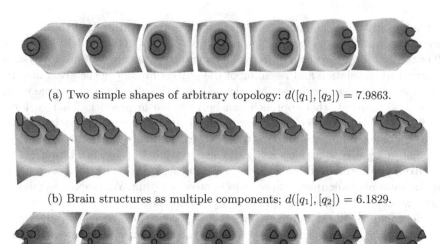

(a) Two simple shapes of arbitrary topology: $d([q_1], [q_2]) = 7.9863$.

(b) Brain structures as multiple components; $d([q_1], [q_2]) = 6.1829$.

(c) Synthetic human face. $d([q_1], [q_2]) = 6.645$.

Fig. 2. Linear deformation path between the most-left and the most-right level set functions. The zero-level set is highlighted in black. (The figure is best viewed in color.) (Color figure online)

to as $\mathbb{L}^2$. If a level set function f is re-parameterized to $f \circ \gamma$, its corresponding SRF changes to $(q, \gamma) = (q \circ \gamma)\sqrt{J_\gamma}$, where J_γ is the determinant of the Jacobian of γ. Given this new representation, it is easy to check that given two SRFs q_1 and q_2 we have $\|q_1 - q_2\| = \|(q_1 \circ \gamma)\sqrt{J_\gamma} - (q_2 \circ \gamma)\sqrt{J_\gamma}\|$. This property ensures that our framework is invariant to re-paramterizations of the level set functions. Thus, we will utilize the SRF representation and the natural $\mathbb{L}^2$ metric to register and compute distances between level set functions, which represent the complex planar objects of interest.

2.3   Registration and Distance Calculation

We have already removed the translation, scale, and rotation variabilities from the representation space by normalizing the given binary images and aligning them rotationally in a pairwise manner. Thus, we are left with removing the parameterization variability of the level set functions. This step can also be thought of as the registration process, where similar structures are matched together across the given objects. To do this, we will utilize the notion of equivalence classes. That is, we will define two level set functions, f_1 and f_2, as equivalent if they are within a re-parameterization of each other. This provides us with the following definition of an equivalence class: $[q] = \{(q \circ \gamma)\sqrt{J_\gamma} | q \in \mathbb{L}^2,\ \gamma \in \Gamma\}$. Thus, we can define a parameterization-invariant distance between level set functions by minimizing over the equivalence classes:

$$d([q_1], [q_2]) = \inf_{\gamma \in \Gamma} \|q_1 - (q_2, \gamma)\|. \tag{2}$$

$d([q_1], [q_2])$ defines the parameterization-invariant (extrinsic) geodesic distance between SRF representations of level set functions. We use it as a measure of similarity between planar objects that have arbitrary topologies and multiple components.

In addition to computing the distance, we would also like to display the path of deformation between the zero-levels of the registered level set functions. While the geodesic path under the pullback metric on $\mathcal{F}$ is a natural choice to do this, it is computationally expensive to compute [5]. Instead, we approximate these deformations using linear interpolation paths. As can be seen in the experimental results section, this does not seem to have any adverse effects. We note that the quality of the metric and registration is very closely related to how natural the deformations between the given objects are.

The computation of the distance in Eq. 2 requires solving an optimization problem over the re-parameterization group Γ. Kurtek et al. [31] outline a gradient descent approach to do this and we summarize it here for convenience. Begin by constructing a geodesic (straight line) between q_1 and the current element of $[q_2]$, call it r. If the geodesic is perpendicular to the equivalence class $[q_2]$, then r is the optimally registered (and closest) element of $[q_2]$ to q_1. If not, we update r in the direction of the projection of the geodesic while staying within $[q_2]$. This is accomplished in three steps. First, define an orthonormal basis for the tangent space $T_{\gamma_{id}}(\Gamma)$ using products of adapted Fourier bases. One cannot use the Fourier basis as given due to the fact that this vector field must be tangential to the boundary of $[0, 1]^2$. Then, use the differential of the mapping $\phi(\gamma) = (q \circ \gamma)\sqrt{J_\gamma}$ to find an update vector field b on $T_{\gamma_{id}}(\Gamma)$. Compute an infinitesimal update to the parameterization of r using $\gamma_{new} = \gamma_{id} + \epsilon b$, $\epsilon > 0$ and small, and compute the corresponding element of $[q_2]$ (a new version of r) using the mapping ϕ. Repeat these steps until the geodesic is perpendicular to $[q_2]$. This procedure reduces the distance at each iteration. It is computationally efficient but is not guaranteed to converge to the global solution. However, in practice we found that it produces natural correspondences and a measure of dissimilarity that outperforms the state-of-the-art.

Figure 2 shows three examples of deformation paths between synthetic shapes of arbitrary topology. For each example, we show the deformation field between the level set functions (plotted as surfaces) and between their corresponding zero-level set (highlighted in black), which corresponds to the boundaries of the 2D shapes of interest.

3   Experimental Results

We demonstrate the performance of the proposed framework using two types of results. First, we show several examples of computing deformation paths between 2D shapes that have fixed or varying topology and that may contain multiple parts (Sect. 3.1). The visual quality of the deformation paths is an indication of the quality of the computed correspondences. Next, we report experimental results on the classification and retrieval of 2D shapes (Sect. 3.2). We use three different data sets for evaluation, see Fig. 1:

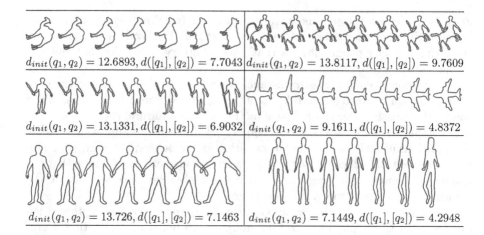

$d_{init}(q_1, q_2) = 12.6893, d([q_1], [q_2]) = 7.7043$ $d_{init}(q_1, q_2) = 13.8117, d([q_1], [q_2]) = 9.7609$

$d_{init}(q_1, q_2) = 13.1331, d([q_1], [q_2]) = 6.9032$ $d_{init}(q_1, q_2) = 9.1611, d([q_1], [q_2]) = 4.8372$

$d_{init}(q_1, q_2) = 13.726, d([q_1], [q_2]) = 7.1463$ $d_{init}(q_1, q_2) = 7.1449, d([q_1], [q_2]) = 4.2948$

Fig. 3. Deformation paths between shapes of the same topology, with no internal details.

Medical Imaging Data Set (Fig. 1(a)). We have manually extracted a set of four subcortical structures (putamen, hippocampus, thalamus and caudate) from 2D slices of 10 structural MRI images. Figure 1(a) displays an example with each of the subcortical structures labeled. There are two types of variation in this data. The first is topological because in some images the structures are represented by three closed curves while in others with four. The second type is in the shape and the relative locations, rotations and scales of the structures.

2D Human sketches (Fig. 1(b)). Eitz et al. [8] provide a data set of 20,000 objects sketched by humans. To demonstrate the performance of our approach, we use a subset of 100 sketches evenly distributed over 10 shape categories. Similar to the medical data set, the sketch data exhibit large topological variation as well as variations in the locations, scales and rotations of the different components of the objects. More importantly, most of the images in this data set are composed of strokes, with no clear definition of the interior and exterior regions of the sketched shapes.

SHREC07 watertight data set (Fig. 1(c)). This data set contains 400 three-dimensional objects evenly distributed into 20 classes [9]. For each of the 3D models, we generate a thumbnail image by rendering its frontal view into a binary image of size 450×600. Since the 3D data set contains complex shapes with arbitrary topology and pose, the resulting 2D images are of arbitrary topology. We use a subset of 100 images (the first five images of each class) in our analysis.

3.1 Shape Matching and Comparison

First, we focus on shapes that have the same topology as shown in Figs. 3, 4 and 5. In the first case, we compare shapes that can be represented by their outer boundaries only. Figure 3 shows several of such examples. Each row of the

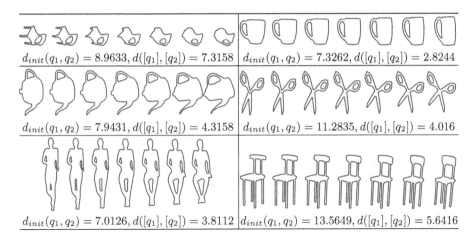

$d_{init}(q_1, q_2) = 8.9633, d([q_1], [q_2]) = 7.3158$ | $d_{init}(q_1, q_2) = 7.3262, d([q_1], [q_2]) = 2.8244$

$d_{init}(q_1, q_2) = 7.9431, d([q_1], [q_2]) = 4.3158$ | $d_{init}(q_1, q_2) = 11.2835, d([q_1], [q_2]) = 4.016$

$d_{init}(q_1, q_2) = 7.0126, d([q_1], [q_2]) = 3.8112$ | $d_{init}(q_1, q_2) = 13.5649, d([q_1], [q_2]) = 5.6416$

Fig. 4. Deformation paths between shapes of the same topology with internal details.

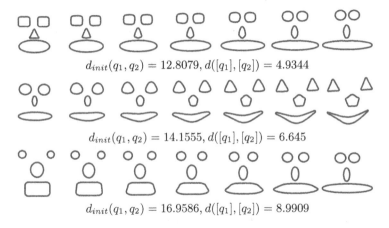

$d_{init}(q_1, q_2) = 12.8079, d([q_1], [q_2]) = 4.9344$

$d_{init}(q_1, q_2) = 14.1555, d([q_1], [q_2]) = 6.645$

$d_{init}(q_1, q_2) = 16.9586, d([q_1], [q_2]) = 8.9909$

Fig. 5. Deformation paths between shapes of the same topology with multiple components.

figure is a deformation path between the most-left and the most-right shapes. Note that the quality of the deformation is highly dependent on the quality of the computed correspondences between the level set functions; any error in the correspondences will result in distorted intermediate shapes. For each example, we also show the computed initial distance $d_{init} = \|q_1 - q_2\|$ (after rotational alignment, prior to optimization over Γ) and the computed parameterization-invariant distance d (after optimization over Γ) between the level set functions. In all of these examples, we used the same scale for each data set making the distances comparable.

Figure 4 shows examples of deformation paths between shapes with the same topology but of high genus, i.e. with internal details. Observe that the deformations are very natural. It is important to note that the topology is preserved along the deformation path.

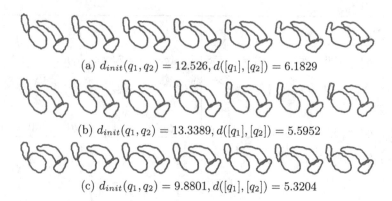

(a) $d_{init}(q_1, q_2) = 12.526, d([q_1], [q_2]) = 6.1829$

(b) $d_{init}(q_1, q_2) = 13.3389, d([q_1], [q_2]) = 5.5952$

(c) $d_{init}(q_1, q_2) = 9.8801, d([q_1], [q_2]) = 5.3204$

Fig. 6. Deformation paths between brain structures with multiple components and small topological changes.

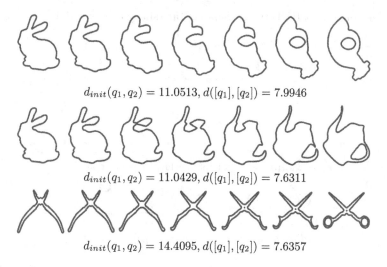

$d_{init}(q_1, q_2) = 11.0513, d([q_1], [q_2]) = 7.9946$

$d_{init}(q_1, q_2) = 11.0429, d([q_1], [q_2]) = 7.6311$

$d_{init}(q_1, q_2) = 14.4095, d([q_1], [q_2]) = 7.6357$

Fig. 7. Deformation paths between shapes of different topologies.

Figure 5 shows deformation paths between shapes of the same topology but that contain several components. In each of these examples, we compare two synthetic faces sketched by hand. Each face contains four components (corresponding to different face parts). Observe that our approach is able to match these shapes correctly and generate natural deformations. In all of the three examples, we observe a decrease in the distance between shapes of approximately 40 % due to the optimization over Γ.

In Fig. 6, we compare planar objects that have different topologies. Figures 6-(a) to (c) show a comparison between various brain structures. These shapes are naturally similar, but they exhibit two major types of variation. The first is topological because the structures are represented by two, three or four closed curves. The second type is in shape and the relative locations, rotations and

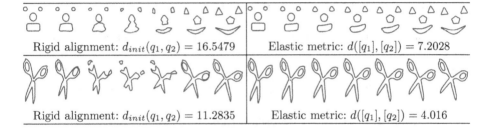

Rigid alignment: $d_{init}(q_1, q_2) = 16.5479$	Elastic metric: $d([q_1], [q_2]) = 7.2028$
Rigid alignment: $d_{init}(q_1, q_2) = 11.2835$	Elastic metric: $d([q_1], [q_2]) = 4.016$

Fig. 8. Comparison between deformation paths obtained with rigid alignment and with the elastic metric proposed in this paper. More examples are included in the supplementary materials.

scales of the structures. When we perform the optimization over Γ, the distance between the left-most and the right-most shapes reduces from 12.52 to 6.18, 13.33 to 5.59, and 9.88 to 5.32 for the cases (a), (b) and (c) respectively. In particular, observe how the topological change is carried in the intermediate shapes along the deformation paths. More examples of complex topological variations are shown in Fig. 7.

Finally, we compare in Fig. 8 the quality of the deformation paths that are generated without optimization over Γ vs. the deformation paths obtained using the full elastic metric, i.e. with optimization over Γ. We can clearly see that our elastic metric provides natural deformations and thus it finds correct correspondences. More examples are shown in the attached supplementary materials.

These examples show that our approach is able to handle shapes with arbitrary topology and with multiple structures. It is also able to compare shapes that have different topologies, which is a significant deviation from previous work [3,4]. Furthermore, the presented examples clearly demonstrate that the generated comparisons are natural and thus the computed distance is a good measure of differences between these shapes.

3.2 Classification Performance

To quantitatively evaluate the performance of the proposed metric, we consider the classification of hand-written sketches [8] and 2D projections of the 3D models in SHREC07 [9] data set described above. For each set, we computed the pairwise distances using the approach proposed in this paper and compared its classification performance against six algorithms in the literature, namely: (1) the rigid alignment defined as the Euclidean distance between rigidly-aligned pairs of shapes (unlike the proposed elastic metric, this metric does not search for the optimal re-parameterization of the level set functions), (2) The Hard and Soft Histogram of Oriented Gradients (HOG-hard and HOG-soft) of Eitz et al. [8], (3) the Modified Hausdorff distance [33], which is equivalent to the standard Hausdorff distance computed after normalizing the shapes for translation, scale and rotation, (4) the Inner Distance-based Shape Context (IDSC) [25],

Table 1. LOO 1,3,5-NN classification on the 2D human sketch data set [8].

	Hausdorff	D2	GEDT	HOG-hard	HOG-soft	Rigid align	IDSC	**Proposed**
LOO-1	65.0 %	49.0 %	68.0 %	65.0 %	72.0 %	70.0 %	25.0 %	**85.0 %**
LOO-3	57.0 %	46.0 %	54.0 %	56.0 %	64.0 %	73.0 %	17.0 %	**76.0 %**
LOO-5	49.0 %	38.0 %	44.0 %	48.0 %	54.0 %	67.0 %	5.0 %	**73.0 %**

Table 2. LOO 1,3,5-NN classification on the SHREC07 data set.

	Hausdorff	D2	GEDT	HOG-hard	Rigid align	IDSC	**Proposed**
LOO-1	74.0 %	40.0 %	75.0 %	61.0 %	68.0 %	83.0	**80.0 %**
LOO-3	57.0 %	24.0 %	64.0 %	37.0 %	47.0 %	79.0	**71.0 %**
LOO-5	40.0 %	12.0 %	45.0 %	20.0 %	31.0 %	69.0	**56.0 %**

which is a very popular descriptor used in the analysis of planar shapes undergoing articulated motion, (5) the D2 shape distribution [34], and (6) the Gaussian Euclidean Transform (GEDT) of the shape boundaries [34]. We use the leave-one-out 1,3,5-nearest neighbor (LOO 1,3,5-NN) classifiers in all examples, where the class is determined by a majority vote. Below, we discuss the classification performance on each data set.

2D sketch data set [8]. We use a subset of 100 sketches evenly distributed over 10 shape categories. Figure 1(b) shows a few examples from this data set. For these 100 objects, we first compute their Euclidean distance transforms and use the algorithm described in Sect. 2 to compute the pairwise distances. The resulting LOO 1-NN classification rate was 85 %, outperforming the best state-of-the-art descriptor by approximately 13 %, see Table 1. Note that HOG-hard achieved a 65 % LOO 1-NN classification rate while HOG-soft achieved a 72.0 % classification rate. These two methods use supervised learning to build the codebook. Our approach, which obtained 85.0 % LOO 1-NN performance, is completely unsupervised. The IDSC descriptor, which is extensively used for the analysis of planar shapes undergoing articulated motion, achieved 25 % LOO 1-NN classification rate, which is significantly below the proposed approach. Finally, note that the proposed elastic metric significantly outperforms all of the other methods when more neighbors are considered, and deteriorates much more slowly.

The SHREC07 data set. We performed a similar evaluation on the SHREC07 data set and report the performance in Table 2. Again, our metric outperforms the state-of-the-art by more than 5 % on LOO 1-NN classification, except the IDSC, which performed 3 % better.

Comparison with the Inner Distance-based Shape Context (IDSC) [25]. IDSC is a very popular descriptor that has been used for the registration of planar shapes in the presence of articulated motion. When used with shapes that have well defined interior regions, such as the SHREC07 data set, it slightly outperforms the metric proposed in this paper, see Table 2. IDSC, however, fails when used in the analysis of the 2D sketch data set as shown in Table 1. 2D sketches are composed of strokes with large topological variations and without clearly defined interior regions. Our approach outperformed all of the state-of-the-art methods on this data set. Note also that unlike the IDSC, our approach is invariant to all shape-preserving transformations including re-parameterization.

Computation time. The total computation time for comparing two objects is approximately 51s. This can be improved by optimally finding rotations without doing an exhaustive search as currently implemented.

4   Conclusions

We have proposed a novel framework for simultaneous registration and comparison of planar objects with multiple components and differing topologies. To accomplish this, we use the distance function representation and a parameterization-invariant framework for elastic shape analysis of surfaces. We validated our framework on different types of examples, which included objects of the same topology, high genus objects, objects with multiple components, and objects of different topologies. The resulting natural deformations show the strength of our method and the benefit of optimizing over the re-parameterization group when generating such comparisons. We also used the distance function for two classification experiments. The results show that we outperform the current state-of-the-art methods in the classification of 2D sketches as well as arbitrary planar shapes. There are many directions for future work. First, we would like to compute geodesics between distance functions using the metric proposed in [5]. This will enable us to generate means and covariances of shapes with different topologies. Second, we plan to extend this framework to the analysis of 3D objects that have arbitrary topology and multiple components.

Acknowledgement. This work is partially funded by the Australian Research Council (ARC) and the South Australian Government, Department of Further Education, Employment, Science and Technology.

References

1. Younes, L.: Computable elastic distance between shapes. SIAM J. Appl. Math. **58**, 565–586 (1998)
2. Younes, L., Michor, P.W., Shah, J., Mumford, D., Lincei, R.: A metric on shape space with explicit geodesics. Mat. E Applicazioni **19**, 25–57 (2008)
3. Srivastava, A., Klassen, E., Joshi, S.H., Jermyn, I.H.: Shape analysis of elastic curves in Euclidean spaces. IEEE Trans. Pattern Anal. Mach. Intell. **33**, 1415–1428 (2011)

4. Jermyn, I.H., Kurtek, S., Klassen, E., Srivastava, A.: Elastic shape matching of parameterized surfaces using square root normal fields. In: Fitzgibbon, A., Lazebnik, S., Perona, P., Sato, Y., Schmid, C. (eds.) Computer Vision – ECCV 2012. LNCS, vol. 7576, pp. 804–817. Springer, Berlin (2012)

5. Kurtek, S., Klassen, E., Gore, J.C., Ding, Z., Srivastava, A.: Elastic geodesic paths in shape space of parameterized surfaces. IEEE Trans. Pattern Anal. Mach. Intell. **34**, 1717–1730 (2012)

6. Kurtek, S., Srivastava, A., Klassen, E., Laga, H.: Landmark-guided elastic shape analysis of spherically-parameterized surfaces. Comput. Graph. Forum (Proc. Eurographics) **32**, 429–438 (2013)

7. Fuchs, M., Jüttler, B., Scherzer, O., Yang, H.: Shape metrics based on elastic deformations. J. Math. Imaging Vis. **35**, 86–102 (2009)

8. Eitz, M., Hays, J., Alexa, M.: How do humans sketch objects? ACM Trans. Graph. (Proc. SIGGRAPH) **31**, 44:1–44:10 (2012)

9. Giorgi, D., Biasotti, S., Paraboschi, L.: Shape retrieval contest 2007: Watertight models track. In: SHREC competition 8 (2007)

10. Kendall, D.G.: Shape manifolds, Procrustean metrics, and complex projective spaces. Bull. London Math. Soc. **16**, 81–121 (1984)

11. Dryden, I.L., Mardia, K.V.: Statistical Shape Analysis. John Wiley & Son, New York (1998)

12. Zahn, C.T., Roskies, R.Z.: Fourier descriptors for plane closed curves. IEEE Trans. Comput. **21**, 269–281 (1972)

13. Klassen, E., Srivastava, A., Mio, W., Joshi, S.H.: Analysis of planar shapes using geodesic paths on shape spaces. IEEE Trans. Pattern Anal. Mach. Intell. **26**, 372–383 (2004)

14. Joshi, S.H., Klassen, E., Srivastava, A., Jermyn, I.H.: Removing shape-preserving transformations in Square-Root Elastic (SRE) framework for shape analysis of curves. In: Yuille, A.L., Zhu, S.-C., Cremers, D., Wang, Y. (eds.) EMMCVPR 2007. LNCS, vol. 4679, pp. 387–398. Springer, Heidelberg (2007)

15. Kerr, G., Kurtek, S., Srivastava, A.: A joint model for boundaries of multiple anatomical parts. In: SPIE Medical Imaging (2011)

16. Osher, S., Fedkiw, R.: Level Set Methods and Dynamic Implicit Surfaces. Springer, New York (2003)

17. Paragios, N., Rousson, M., Ramesh, V.: Non-rigid registration using distance functions. Comput. Vis. Image Underst. **89**, 142–165 (2003)

18. Munim, H.A.E., Farag, A.: Shape representation and registration using vector distance functions. In: IEEE Conf. on Computer Vision and Pattern Recognition (2007)

19. Fahmi, R., Farag, A.A.: A global-to-local 2D shape registration in implicit spaces using level sets. In: IEEE International Conference on Image Processing. vol. 6, p. VI-237. IEEE (2007)

20. Yezzi, A.J., Soatto, S.: Deformotion: Deforming motion, shape average and the joint registration and approximation of structures in images. Int. J. Comput. Vis. **53**, 153–167 (2003)

21. Glaunes, J., Qiu, A., Miller, M.I., Younes, L.: Large deformation diffeomorphic metric curve mapping. Int. J. Comput. Vis. **80**, 317–336 (2008)

22. Huttenlocher, D.P., Klanderman, G.A., Kl, G.A., Rucklidge, W.J.: Comparing images using the Hausdorff distance. IEEE Trans. Pattern Anal. Mach. Intell. **15**, 850–863 (1993)

23. Davis, E.: Continuous shape transformation and metrics on regions. Fundamenta Informaticae **46**, 31–54 (2001)

24. Berkels, B., Linkmann, G., Rumpf, M.: Shape median based on symmetric area differences. In: Deussen, O., Keim, D.A., Saupe, D. (eds.) Vision, Modeling and Visualization, pp. 399–407 (2008)
25. Ling, H., Jacobs, D.W.: Shape classification using the inner-distance. IEEE Trans. Pattern Anal. Mach. Intell. **29**, 286–299 (2007)
26. Tabia, H., Laga, H., Picard, D., Gosselin, P.H., et al.: Covariance descriptors for 3D shape matching and retrieval. In: IEEE Conference on Computer Vision and Pattern Recognition (2014)
27. Wang, X., Feng, B., Bai, X., Liu, W., Jan Latecki, L.: Bag of contour fragments for robust shape classification. Pattern Recogn. **47**, 2116–2125 (2014)
28. Laga, H., Takahashi, H., Nakajima, M.: Spherical wavelet descriptors for content-based 3D model retrieval. In: IEEE International Conference on Shape Modeling and Applications, pp. 15–15. IEEE (2006)
29. Laga, H., Nakajima, M.: Supervised learning of salient 2D views of 3D models. J. Soc. Art Sci. **7**, 124–131 (2008)
30. Laga, H.: Semantics-driven approach for automatic selection of best views of 3D shapes. In: Proceedings of the 3rd Eurographics Workshop on 3D Object Retrieval, Eurographics Association, pp. 15–22 (2010)
31. Kurtek, S., Klassen, E., Ding, Z., Srivastava, A.: A novel Riemannian framework for shape analysis of 3D objects. In: IEEE Conference on Computer Vision Pattern Recognition, pp. 1625–1632 (2010)
32. Xie, Q., Kurtek, S., Christensen, G.E., Ding, Z., Klassen, E., Srivastava, A.: A novel framework for metric-based image registration. In: Dawant, B.M., Christensen, G.E., Fitzpatrick, J.M., Rueckert, D. (eds.) WBIR 2012. LNCS, vol. 7359, pp. 276–285. Springer, Heidelberg (2012)
33. Dubuisson, M.P., Jain, A.K.: A modified Hausdorff distance for object matching. Int. Conf. Pattern Recogn. **1**, 566–568 (1994)
34. Laga, H., Kurtek, S., Srivastava, A., Golzarian, M., Miklavcic, S.J.: A Riemannian elastic metric for shape-based plant leaf classification. In: DICTA, pp. 1–7 (2012)

3D Vision

A Minimal Solution to Relative Pose with Unknown Focal Length and Radial Distortion

Fangyuan Jiang[1]([envelope]), Yubin Kuang[2], Jan Erik Solem[1,2], and Kalle Åström[1]

[1] Centre for Mathematical Sciences, Lund University, Lund, Sweden
fangyuan@maths.lth.se
[2] Mapillary AB, Lund, Sweden

Abstract. In this paper, we study the minimal problem of estimating the essential matrix between two cameras with constant but unknown focal length and radial distortion. This problem is of both theoretical and practical interest and it has not been solved previously. We have derived a fast and stable polynomial solver based on Gröbner basis method. This solver enables simultaneous auto-calibration of focal length and radial distortion for cameras. For experiments, the numerical stability of the solver is demonstrated on synthetic data. We also evaluate on real images using either RANSAC or kernel voting. Compared with the standard minimal solver, which does not model the radial distortion, our proposed solver both finds a larger set of geometrically correct correspondences on distorted images and gives an accurate estimate of the radial distortion and focal length.

1 Introduction

Estimating the camera motions from the image matches is a fundamental problem in the geometric computer vision. It is also one of the essential components to the large-scale 3D reconstruction system, e.g. Photo Tourism [1]. However, as the wide-angle cameras, e.g. GoPro or the cameras with digital zoom become more common and popular, a lot of images captured are radially distorted. Without handling the distortion, it will have a non-negligible effect in the estimate of the essential matrix or fundamental matrix, since the epipolar constraints have to be set very loose in order to find enough correspondences, which might also increase the number of outliers. Besides, if the radially mis-aligned images are used in a Structure-from-Motion (SfM) pipeline, it can cause significant skewness [2]. So estimation of radial distortion is an important task in a reconstruction pipeline with images captured by distorted lens. See Fig. 1.

Early works on estimation of the radial distortion is usually done in an offline manner. One first calibrates the cameras, finds the focal length and the radial distortion parameter. The epipolar geometry is then estimated separately afterwards. This requires either the knowledge of the 3D points [3] or the extra calibration object or pattern [4]. However, these offline methods have a large drawback

© Springer International Publishing Switzerland 2015
D. Cremers et al. (Eds.): ACCV 2014, Part II, LNCS 9004, pp. 443–456, 2015.
DOI: 10.1007/978-3-319-16808-1_30

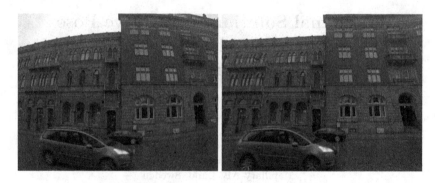

Fig. 1. An example of radially distorted image (Left) captured by a GoPro Hero3 camera and the undistorted image (right) using our method.

that one need to have the original camera lens at hand. If the images are from the archived collection, or downloaded from internet, then the offline calibration becomes impossible.

With the online estimation method, the calibration could be handled in a more general situations. The plumb line ideas [5–7] are based on the fact that a straight line is preserved under an ideal pinhole camera. Extra knowledge are required to tell which curves in the image are the projections of straight lines in the 3D scene. However, the real scene, e.g. natural scene does not always contain a straight lines. Even it does, recognition of such a line also needs some effort. Contrary to the plumb line methods, the other methods [2,8–14] requires nothing but only the rigidity assumption of the scene and the point correspondences between the views. Due to the simple assumption and off-the-shelf matching algorithms, e.g. SIFT [15], these methods become very popular.

The minimal problems, which are defined as using the minimal point correspondences to estimate the epipolar geometry as well as the camera calibration, e.g. focal length or radial distortion, plays an important role in these methods. The solver to the minimal problems are particularly useful when equipped with RANSAC [16], leading to a robust estimation method. However, to solve the minimal problems, one usually needs to handle some complex algebraic constraints. One example is when estimating the fundamental matrix F, the determinant constraint on F gives a cubic polynomial equation, which is difficult to cope with. This is why the early methods, such as [2,9] ignored this algebraic constraint, but solves a simpler system using more points than the minimal requirement. More specifically, in [2], a non-minimal algorithm is given to simultaneously estimate the fundamental matrix and the single radial distortion parameter. The division model it proposed for radial distortion is extensively used in the later works. In [9], the authors treated exactly the same problem as [2] but used a hidden-variable method on the polynomial equations. A kernel voting scheme is used instead of RANSAC to avoid the computation of undistorted image point in each iteration. Another work on non-minimal solver is [8], where a 4×4 radial fundamental matrix is proposed to model the bilinear relation between the lifted point in one view and the corresponding epipolar curve in the other view. A non-minimal 15 points algorithm is given. The drawback of these non-minimal methods is that it usually requires more RANSAC iterations to find an outlier-free set, which will increase the time complexity of the algorithms.

Thanks to the recent progress in the Gröbner basis method [17], solving a polynomial system becomes feasible, fast and stable. More focus are attracted to solving the minimal problems. All these works [11,13,14,18–20] are based on the minimal solvers. In [11], a minimal solver using eight point correspondences is given to estimate the fundamental matrix and the single radial distortion parameter for the uncalibrated case. In [18], two minimal problems are proposed. One is to estimate the essential matrix E and the same radial distortion assuming the two cameras are partially calibrated with known focal length f, the other is to estimate the fundamental matrix F and two different radial distortion parameters for two uncalibrated cameras. For the first problem, the trace constraint on E is used to reduce the problem to a minimal one. The exact rational arithmetic solvers are given for both problems in Maple, which is very slow and impractical. In [13], based on the efficient implementation of Gröbner basis computation in floating point arithmetic, two solvers, which are much faster, are proposed for the two minimal problems in [18]. In [14], the one-sided problems are studied, which is to estimate the radial distortion for one camera assuming the other is already known. Three minimal problems are solved regarding to the uncalibrated case using 8 points, the calibrated case with unknown focal length using 7 points and the calibrated case with known focal length using 6 points. In [19], absolute pose estimation problem with unknown focal length is considered by incorporating the radial distortion. A 4-point algorithm is given based on Gröbner basis. In [20], simple concepts from linear algebra, instead of Gröbner basis, are used that leads to a real-time solution to the same pose problem.

In this paper, we study the minimal problem of estimating the relative pose with both the focal length and the radial distortion unknown. This is a very general and useful setting when the images are captured by one camera model with distortion. Up to our knowledge, this still remains an unsolved problem in the area. Compared with the previous minimal problems, this is more difficult since when both focal length and radial distortion are unknown, the epipolar constraint on essential matrix E leads to a polynomial equation with higher degrees. Also estimating E generally requires more effort than estimating F as one need to incorporate extra constraint, e.g. trace constraint in the system. By using the division model in [2], we derive a parametrization and simplify the polynomial system using a linear elimination scheme. We then study the simplified polynomial system and verify the number of solutions. A fast and stable polynomial solver is developed to solve the system. With our solvers, one can use it with RANSAC or kernel voting, to find the estimate of camera motions, which could be served as the initialization for bundle adjustment.

2   Problem Formulation

In this section, we will first introduce the camera model and the model for radial distortion. We give a parametrization of the image point to incorporate the unknown radial distortion. A polynomial equation system is then formulated using all the constraints given by the epipolar geometry. By linearly eliminating several variables, one can obtain a more simplified and compact formulation with fewer unknowns.

2.1   Camera and Radial Distortion Model

In our formulation, we use the pinhole camera model and assume a one-parameter division model as in [2]. The intrinsic matrix K of the camera is defined as

$$
K = \begin{bmatrix} f & s & p_x \\ 0 & \gamma f & p_y \\ 0 & 0 & 1 \end{bmatrix}
\tag{1}
$$

where f is the focal length of the camera, For most cameras, the pixels are square and there is no skew, so we could safely assume the skew s is zero and the aspect ratio γ takes the unity. The principal point given by (p_x, p_y) is usually at the centre of the image, i.e. $(0,0)$. So by the above assumptions, we could reparametrize K using only one variable as

$$
K = \begin{bmatrix} 1 & 0 & 0 \\ 0 & 1 & 0 \\ 0 & 0 & w \end{bmatrix}
\tag{2}
$$

where $w = 1/f$. Note this can be done since K is only defined up to a scale. If we denote the inhomogeneous coordinates of undistorted image point as $\mathbf{x}_u = (x_u, y_u)^T$ and the radially distorted image point as $\mathbf{x}_d = (x_d, y_d)^T$, then the relation between $\mathbf{x}_d$ and $\mathbf{x}_p$ is given by the division model as

$$
\mathbf{x}_u = \frac{1}{1 + \lambda \|\mathbf{x}_d\|^2} \mathbf{x}_d
\tag{3}
$$

where λ is the distortion coefficient and $\|\mathbf{x}_d\|$ is the distance from $\mathbf{x}_d$ to the centre of distortion. Here we assume the center of distortion is known and at the center of the image.

If we use the homogeneous coordinates as $\mathbf{p}_u = (x_u, y_u, 1)^T$, $\mathbf{p}_d = (x_d, y_d, 1)^T$ and $r_d = \|\mathbf{x_d}\|$, then (3) can be written as

$$
\begin{bmatrix} x_u \\ y_u \\ 1 \end{bmatrix} \sim \begin{bmatrix} x_d \\ y_d \\ 1 + \lambda r_d^2 \end{bmatrix} = \begin{bmatrix} x_d \\ y_d \\ 1 \end{bmatrix} + \lambda \begin{bmatrix} 0 \\ 0 \\ r_d^2 \end{bmatrix}
\tag{4}
$$

which is equivalently

$$
\mathbf{p}_u \sim \mathbf{p}_d + \lambda \mathbf{z}
\tag{5}
$$

where $\mathbf{z} = (0, 0, r_d^2)^T$ is known since $\mathbf{x}_d$ is given. In some cases, we need the normalized image point $\mathbf{p}_n$, which can be represented as

$$
\mathbf{p}_n \sim K^{-1} \mathbf{p}_u
\tag{6}
$$

It is well known [21] that for two calibrated cameras, the essential matrix E has 5 degrees of freedom. For two cameras with constant but unknown focal length f and radial distortion λ, the degree of freedom is in total 7. In two-view geometry, each point correspondence gives one constraint. Thus, the minimal problem of auto-calibration with unknown focal length and radial distortion needs 7 correspondences.

2.2   Parametrization and Formulation

We present in the following the parameterization and the problem formulation based the epipolar constraints and the constraints on essential matrix E.

Given n point correspondences $\{(\mathbf{p}_{u_i}, \mathbf{p}'_{u_i}), i = 1, 2, ..., n\}$ of the undistorted image points, the epipolar constraints using fundamental matrix F are given by

$$\mathbf{p}_{u_i}^T(\lambda) \, \mathbf{F} \, \mathbf{p}'_{u_i}(\lambda) = 0, \quad i = 1, \dots, n. \tag{7}$$

where $\mathbf{p}_u(\lambda)$ is parametrized using (5). Using the normalized image points $\mathbf{p}_{n_i} \sim \mathbf{K}\mathbf{p}_{u_i}$, the epipolar constraint can also be expressed using the essential matrix E as

$$\mathbf{p}_{n_i}^T(\lambda, w) \, \mathbf{E} \, \mathbf{p}'_{n_i}(\lambda, w) = 0, \quad i = 1, \dots, n. \tag{8}$$

In our method, instead of directly parametrizing the essential matrix E, here we parametrize on F and solve for E implicitly. The reason is that using the constraint in (7) instead of (8) will get rid of the parameter w of the focal length, this gives much simpler equations and will lead to a linear elimination strategy as we will show in next section. The fundamental matrix F is parametrized as

$$\mathbf{F} = \begin{bmatrix} f_1 & f_4 & f_7 \\ f_2 & f_5 & f_8 \\ f_3 & f_6 & f_9 \end{bmatrix}. \tag{9}$$

where the last element f_9 is set to be one to fix the scale. Then from the relation $\mathbf{E} = \mathbf{K}^T \mathbf{F} \mathbf{K}'$ where $\mathbf{K}' = \mathbf{K}$ in our case, the essential matrix E is parametrized using calibration matrix K in (2) as

$$\mathbf{E} = \mathbf{K}^T \mathbf{F} \mathbf{K}' = \begin{bmatrix} 1 & 0 & 0 \\ 0 & 1 & 0 \\ 0 & 0 & w \end{bmatrix}^T \begin{bmatrix} f_1 & f_4 & f_7 \\ f_2 & f_5 & f_8 \\ f_3 & f_6 & 1 \end{bmatrix} \begin{bmatrix} 1 & 0 & 0 \\ 0 & 1 & 0 \\ 0 & 0 & w \end{bmatrix} = \begin{bmatrix} f_1 & f_4 & wf_7 \\ f_2 & f_5 & wf_8 \\ wf_3 & wf_6 & w^2 \end{bmatrix}. \tag{10}$$

On the other hand, the singularity of the essential matrix E is enforced as:

$$\det(\mathbf{E}) = 0. \tag{11}$$

along with the trace condition such that the two singular values are equal:

$$2(\mathbf{E}\mathbf{E}^T)\mathbf{E} - \text{trace}(\mathbf{E}\mathbf{E}^T)\mathbf{E} = 0. \tag{12}$$

Inserting (10) into (11) and (12), together with the point equations (7), we formulate the problem as solving a polynomial equation system. The polynomial system contains 17 equations in 9 unknowns, namely, $\{f_1, f_2, ..., f_8, \lambda, w\}$.

2.3 Eliminating Variables

Let us look at the first seven equations given by the point correspondences in (7), or equivalently

$$\begin{bmatrix} x_d \\ y_d \\ 1+\lambda r_d^2 \end{bmatrix}^T \begin{bmatrix} f_1 & f_4 & f_7 \\ f_2 & f_5 & f_8 \\ f_3 & f_6 & 1 \end{bmatrix} \begin{bmatrix} x_d' \\ y_d' \\ 1+\lambda r_d^2 \end{bmatrix} = 0, \tag{13}$$

by expanding the above multiplication and stack all the seven equations, one can reach the following linear system

$$\mathbf{Ax} = 0, \tag{14}$$

where $\mathbf{A}$ is a 7×15 coefficient matrix and $\mathbf{x} = (\lambda^2, \lambda f_3, \lambda f_6, \lambda f_7, \lambda f_8, f_1, \ldots, f_8, \lambda, 1)$ is a vector containing the unknown monomials. After applying the Gaussian elimination on (14), one can linearly eliminate 7 unknown monomials by expressing those in terms of the remaining 8 unknown monomials (include the constant 1). Since f_1, f_2, f_4, f_5 appear only in the linear terms in (13), so it is natural to eliminate those four variables. Besides, we also choose to eliminate $f_3, \lambda f_3$ and λ^2. This choice of eliminating variable will simplify the system as we will show. Now the eliminating monomials $\{f_1, f_2, f_3, f_4, f_5, \lambda f_3, \lambda^2\}$ can be represented as a linear combination of the remaining monomials, namely $\{\lambda f_6, \lambda f_7, \lambda f_8, f_6, f_7, f_8, \lambda\}$, or equivalently, each can are expressed as a quadratic function on unknown variables $\{f_6, f_7, f_8, \lambda\}$. For $f_1, f_2, \ldots, f_5$, we have

$$f_i = h_i(f_6, f_7, f_8, \lambda), \quad i = 1, 2, 3, 4, 5 \tag{15}$$

For λf_3 and λ^2, we have

$$\lambda f_3 = h_6(f_6, f_7, f_8, \lambda) \tag{16}$$

$$\lambda^2 = h_7(f_6, f_7, f_8, \lambda) \tag{17}$$

One can further eliminate f_3 in (16) by replacing it with $h_3(f_6, f_7, f_8, \lambda)$ as

$$\lambda h_3(f_6, f_7, f_8, \lambda) - h_6(f_6, f_7, f_8, \lambda) = 0 \tag{18}$$

So now one can substitute f_i in (10) with $h_i(f_6, f_7, f_8, \lambda)$ for $i = 1, 2, \ldots, 5$ and insert it into (11) and (12). Together with (17) and (18), we would obtain a well-defined system of 12 polynomial equations (Note the trace constraint (12) leads to 9 equations) with 5 unknowns $\{f_6, f_7, f_8, \lambda, w\}$. The equations are of degree at most 9.

Solving such a polynomial system is certainly a non-trivial task. It is a more complicated system compared with the previous work. The formulation in [11] for uncalibrated case gives 3 equations with 3 unknowns, the degree of which is 5. The polynomial system in [14] for calibrated case, assuming the radial distortion and focal length for one view is already known, contains 11 equations with 4 unknowns, the degree of which is 5 or 6. With the recent progress in Gröbner basis method, we will show in the next section that it is possible to find a fast and stable solver for our minimal problem.

3   Polynomial Solvers

In this section, we will focus on the polynomial system we derived in the previous section and aims at finding a fast and stable solver based on the Gröbner Basis method. We will first give a brief review of the Gröbner Basis method.

3.1   Review of Gröbner Basis Method

We are aiming at solving a polynomial equation system in the following form

$$h_1(x) = 0, h_2(x) = 0, \ldots, h_m(x) = 0 \tag{19}$$

where $H = \{h_1(x), \ldots, h_m(x) \mid h_i \in \mathbb{C}[x_1, \ldots, x_n]\}$ are polynomials in n variables over the field $\mathbb{C}$ of the complex numbers. Using the notation in the algebraic geometry [22,23], we consider the ideal I generated by the the polynomials $H = \{h_1(x), \ldots, h_m(x)\}$ defined by

$$I = \{\sum_{i=1}^{m} p_i h_i \mid p_i \in \mathbb{C}[x_1, \ldots, x_n],\ h_i \in H\} \tag{20}$$

In general, an ideal could be generated by different finite set of generators. However, all sets of generators share the same solutions. The idea of the Gröbner basis method for solving a polynomial equation system given by $\{h_i(x) = 0 | i = 1, \ldots, m\}$ is to find another set of generator $\{g_i(x) | i = 1, 2, \ldots, m\}$ that generates exactly the same ideal as $\{h_i(x)\}$ does, but $\{g_i(x) = 0\}$ is a much simpler problem to solve. It turns out that reduced Gröbner basis w.r.t the lexicographic ordering is such a set of generator, which is usually simple or even trivial to solve.

However, to compute the complete set of Gröbner basis is usually very difficult due to the numerical stability. Also it requires a proper choice of the monomial order, e.g. lexicographic order. Recent progress [17] in the Gröbner basis method provides a new action matrix method, which does not rely on finding the complete set of Gröbner basis, yet leads to a more stable algorithm. The key idea is to consider the quotient space $\mathbf{C}[\mathbf{x}]/I$, which is the space of all possible remainders under the multivariate division by the ideal I. By the theorem in [22], if the equation system (19) has finite zeros, then $\mathbf{C}[\mathbf{x}]/I$ is finite-dimensional linear space, the dimension of which coincides with the number of zeros of (19).

Using this property, within the quotient space $\mathbf{C}[\mathbf{x}]/I$, the multiplication with a monomial x_k, known as action variable could be regarded as a linear map from $\mathbf{C}[\mathbf{x}]/I$ to itself. Due to the finite dimension of $\mathbf{C}[\mathbf{x}]/I$, this linear map can be represented using a matrix M_{x_k}, called the action matrix. The eigenvalue of M_{x_k} directly gives the value of action variable x_k. The eigenvectors corresponds to the vector of monomials which are evaluated at the zeros of (19). More details are referred to [17].

3.2   A Polynomial Solver to Our Problem

We first study and explore the structure of the polynomial system generated from (11), (12), (17) and (18), one observation is that among the 12 equations, there are 4 equations has w as the common multiplier. To avoid the trivial and false solution $w = 0$, we divide w from all the 4 equations. The other observation is that, after we remove the common multiplier w, all the equations that contain w only contain the terms of even degrees, e.g. w^2, w^4, w^6. So we could simply replace w^2 with a new variable $z = w^2$. With these observations, we managed to simplify the system by decreasing the degree of the system from 9 to 7. Now we obtain a polynomial system contains one equation of degree 2, one of degree 3, two of degree 5, three of degree 6 and five of degree 7.

We then verify the number of solutions using some algebraic geometry tools. By generating the polynomial system with coefficients in $\mathbb{Z}_p$, and using Macaulay2 [24], we find that there are in general 68 solutions for this problem. Although the number of solution is relatively large, but we will show later in the experiments that most solutions in our problem are complex and thus could be simply removed.

To solve the system, we follow the method based on Gröbner basis in [17]. A redundant set of higher order polynomials, called *eliminating template*, are systematically generated from our initial polynomial equations by multiplying them with a set of monomials. With this step, one aim is to find a sufficient large set of monomials from which we could find the *basis*, i.e. a set of monomials. All the other monomials that are not included in *basis* could be represented as a linear combination of *basis*. The *permissible* monomials, which stay in itself after multiplication with an action monomial x_k will give us direct clues to construct the action matrix and further find the solution. Empirically we found that the following choice of multiplication monomials will generate a numerically stable solver. (i) the highest degree of monomials in those equations are up to 9 after the multiplication. (ii) the highest degree of those multiplication monomials are $\{4, 4, 4, 2, 4\}$ respectively for unknowns $\{f_6, f_7, f_8, w, \lambda\}$. After this multiplication step, the resulting *elimination template* contains 886 equations with 1011 monomials. Further attempt to reduce the size of the elimination template by decreasing the highest degree of multiplication monomials will affect the numerical stability as we tried.

We use a column-pivoting scheme [17] to select the basis with the improved numerical stability. The last 120 monomials is selected as the *permissible* set to construct the action matrix of size 68×68. Using the eigen-decomposition on the transpose of the action matrix, we could extract the solutions to our system from the resulting eigenvectors. Once we found the value of $\{f_6, f_7, f_8, w, \lambda\}$, the other unknowns on the fundamental matrix $\mathbf{F}$ could be found using (15). The essential matrix $\mathbf{E}$ is then solved from (10) as well.

4   Experiments

We test and validate our minimal solver on both synthetically generated image data and the real images. For synthetic image data, we validate the number of real solutions in general. We also test the numerical stability and the sensitivity to the noise. For the real images, we use both RANSAC and the kernel voting to obtain an accurate estimation of the essential matrix $\mathbf{E}$, the radial distortion coefficient λ as well as the focal length f. We also compared with the standard 7-point algorithm of fundamental matrix estimation, which do not handle the radial distortion. As we will show later, taking the radial distortion into consideration, we will obtain more inliers using the RANSAC.

We implement the solvers in MATLAB. The average running time for our minimal solver is around 400ms(milliseconds). The timing are recorded on a Macbook Air with 8GB memory and 1.8 GHz i5 CPU. One could further reduce the running time by implementing the solver in C or C++. Other optimization strategy, e.g. [25, 26] is also a choice.

4.1 Synthetic Data

We generated random 3D points within a cube of width 1000 centered at the origin. Two cameras are placed to be around 1000 units away from the origin. The two cameras are roughly pointing to the origin with a random rotation. The translation between the two camera centers is around 300 units. The focal length for both cameras are randomly generated around 1000. The 2D image points are generated by projecting the 3D points into the image plane of size 1000×1000. Based on the division model in (3), we distort the image point with the distortion coefficient uniformly sampled from $[-0.5, 0]$. The radial distortion is specified w.r.t. the normalized image points in the range of $[-1, 1]$.

The first experiment is to test the numerical stability and validate the number of real solutions. For this experiment, we use the noise free image data. We randomly generated 1000 synthetic scenes in the way described above. For each scene, we run our minimal solver with 7 points and evaluate the relative error between the estimated value of radial distortion λ, the focal length f and their ground truth value. The relative errors for λ is defined as follows

$$e(\lambda_{est}) = \frac{|\lambda_{est} - \lambda_{gt}|}{|\lambda_{gt}|} \tag{21}$$

where λ_{est}, λ_{gt} are respectively the estimated and the ground truth value for the distortion. The relative error of f is defined in the similar way.

We plot the distribution of log_{10} of the relative error for λ and f in the left of Fig. 2, . We can see that our solver is generally very stable and give the accurate estimation of both λ and f. The medians of the log_{10} relative error are -7.49 for λ and -7.16 for f. The statistic of the number of valid solutions is also plotted in the right of Fig. 2. By valid solutions, we mean the real roots of the polynomial system. Although the system have in total 68 solutions, but most of them are of complex value and could be simply removed without the need of further validation. For most cases, there are 4 to 10 valid solutions.

The performance of our solver in the presence of noises is also tested. The image points are perturbed with Gaussian noise with different standard deviation $\tau = 0, 0.01, 0.1, 0.5, 1, 2$ respectively. We tried different radial distortion parameter $\lambda = -0.01, -0.1, -0.2, -0.5$ as well. In Fig. 3, we plot the box with the middle red line in the box as the median of the log_{10} relative error, the top

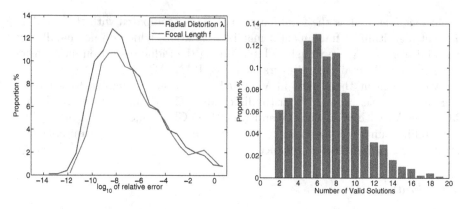

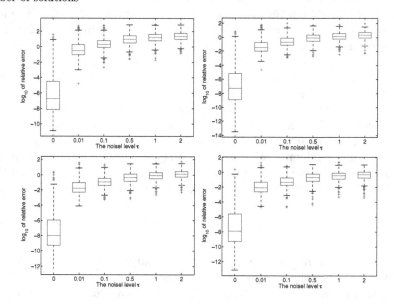

Fig. 2. Experiments on synthetic data without noise. Left: The distribution of log_{10} relative error of radial distortion λ and the focal length f. Right: The distribution of number of solutions

Fig. 3. Experiments on synthetic data with different noise levels. The log_{10} of relative error of λ for different radial distortion, where the ground truth are $\lambda = -0.01$ (Top left), $\lambda = -0.1$ (Top right), $\lambda = -0.2$ (Bottom left) and $\lambda = -0.5$ (Bottom right). See the text for detailed description.

and bottom edges of the box as the 25th and 75th percentiles. The red cross marks are the points lying beyond the 1.5 times the range. For noiseless data, our solver gives accurate estimates of radial distortion λ. We also noticed that the solver generally achieves more accurate estimates when the radial distortion is large. When noise level increases, the log_{10} relative errors also increase largely, to around 10^{-1}. This shows that one should use the solver on the repeatedly

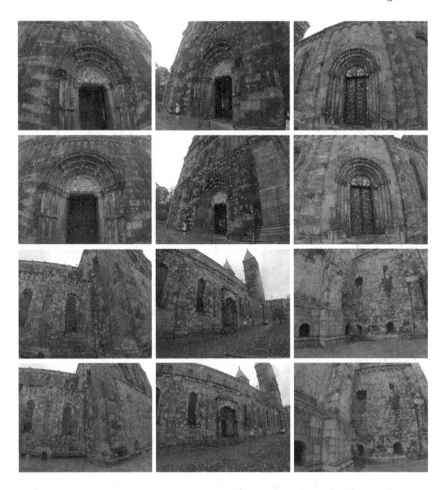

Fig. 4. Experiments on read data using RANSAC. The inlier set using different method are marked. The green star marks are inliers found by both methods. The red stars are the inliers only found using our method, The yellow starts are the inliers only found by standard 7 point solver. Note that the images are paired for the top two rows and bottom two rows (Color figure online).

drawn minimal samples and combine it with either the kernel voting scheme or the RANSAC when the real data are contaminated with noise or outliers. Note we also tested the noise sensitivity for the estimation of focal length f and obtained quite similar box plot. Due to the space limitation, we will omit the resulting plot here.

4.2 Real Data

We further evaluate the proposed solver on real images. A GoPro Hero3 camera is used to capture the images with a significant radial distortion. The camera is

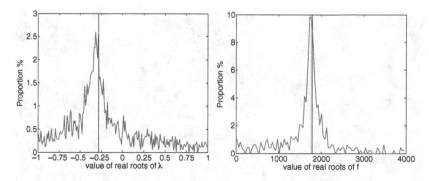

Fig. 5. Experiments on read data using kernel voting. The distribution of real roots (red curve) for radial distortion coefficient λ and focal length f are shown in the left and right figure respectively. The estimate of λ and f (blue line) as well as the ground truth of f (green line in the right figure) is also marked (Color figure online).

calibrated with the fixed focal length, which serves as the ground truth for the algorithm evaluation. A set of 36 images are paired and used to test our solver. The SIFT features are extracted from all the images and matched between each pair using method in [15]. This produce a set of tentative matches which also contains outliers.

We first use the RANSAC algorithm equipped with our minimal solver as a subroutine to estimate the essential matrix $\mathbf{E}$, the focal length f and the radial distortion λ. In each RANSAC iteration, different minimal sets of point correspondences are randomly drawn and are fed into our solver. With the estimated $\mathbf{E}$, λ and f, we compute the distance to the epipolar line for each point and obtain an inlier set containing all the points with distance smaller than a threshold. The solution with the maximum inlier set gives the final estimation of $\mathbf{E}$, λ and f. The standard 7 point algorithm, which does not consider the radial distortion, serves as a baseline in RANSAC to estimate the fundamental matrix. Note we set the RANSAC iterations to be 1000 and the threshold of inliers to be 3 pixels for both methods in the experiment. From Fig. 4, our minimal solver obtains a substantially larger inlier set due to the explicit modeling of the radial distortion. Quatitatively, our minimal solver gains average 49.37 % increase w.r.t. the number of inliers compared with the standard 7 point solver on the image set.

We also use a kernel voting scheme to estimate the $\mathbf{E}$, λ and f. To avoid the computation of the undistorted image point and the fundamental matrix in each iteration of RANSAC, the kernel voting finds the estimate by fitting a kernel, e.g. Gaussian kernel to all the solutions one obtained from different random minimal samples. The success of the method is based on the observation that the solved roots are all around the genuine root regardless of the noises. In this experiment, we randomly draw 1000 minimal set, solve them and keep all the real roots. Gaussian kernel with bandwidth $w = 0.02$ for radial distortion parameter λ and $w = 200$ for focal length f are fitted to all the solutions of λ and f. These bandwidths are reasonable choices considering that $\lambda \in [-1, 1]$ and $f \in [0, 2000]$.

Then the peak is picked out as the final solution for λ and f respectively. From the distribution of real roots of λ and f in Fig. 5, we could easily see the peak, around which are the genuine solutions. The kernel voting gives an estimate of -0.28 for λ and 1793.4 for f, which are plotted as blue lines in the Fig. 5. Note we also plot the ground truth value of f, which is 1765.6, in the right part of Fig. 5 as a green line. It shows the estimate of f is very close to the ground truth. Note the Fig. 5 is the plot for only one of the image pairs.

As we have tested, all the other image pair gives consistent estimate on λ and f and further validate the proposed solver.

5 Conclusion

In this paper, we have given a fast and numerically stable solver for the minimal problem of estimating the relative pose with unknown focal length and radial distortion. We use a division model for radial distortion and derive a parametrization and formulate a polynomial system. After studying the polynomial system, we simplify it by variable elimination and use Gröbner basis method to derive a solver. We evaluate our solver on both the synthetic data and real images. The solver is shown to be numerically stable on synthetic data. With the RANSAC or kernel voting, the solver could be applied to real image data with noises and outliers. It finds more point correspondences and gives accurate estimates on the relative pose, as well as focal length and radial distortion.

References

1. Snavely, N., Seitz, S.M., Szeliski, R.: Photo tourism: exploring photo collections in 3d. In: SIGGRAPH 2006: ACM SIGGRAPH 2006 Papers, pp. 835–846. ACM, New York (2006)
2. Fitzgibbon, A.W.: Simultaneous linear estimation of multiple view geometry and lens distortion. In: Proceedings of Computer Vision and Pattern Recognition Conference, pp. 125–132 (2001)
3. McGlone, J., Mikhail, E., Bethel, J., Mullen, R.: Manual of Photogrammetry. American Society for Photogrammetry and Remote Sensing, Maryland (2004)
4. Tsai, R.Y.: A versatile camera calibration technique for high-accuracy 3d machine vision metrology using off-the-shelf tv cameras and lenses. IEEE J. Rob. Autom. **3**, 323–344 (1987)
5. Devernay, F., Faugeras, O.D.: Straight lines have to be straight. Mach. Vis. Appl. **13**, 14–24 (2001)
6. Swaminathan, R., Nayar, S.K.: Nonmetric calibration of wide-angle lenses and polycameras. IEEE Trans. Pattern Anal. Mach. Intell. **22**, 1172–1178 (2000)
7. Kang, S.: Semiautomatic methods for recovering radial distortion parameters from a single image. Cambridge Research Laboratory technical report series. Digital, Cambridge Research Laboratory (1997)
8. Barreto, J., Daniilidis, K.: Fundamental matrix for cameras with radial distortion. In: IEEE International Conference on Computer Vision, Beijing, China (2005)
9. Li, H., Hartley, R.: A non-iterative method for correcting lens distortion from nine point correspondences. In: OMNIVIS 2005 (2005)

10. Stein, G.P.: Lens distortion calibration using point correspondences. In: CVPR, pp. 602–608 (1997)
11. Kukelova, Z., Pajdla, T.: A minimal solution to the autocalibration of radial distortion. In: Proceedings of the Conference on Computer Vision and Pattern Recognition (2007)
12. Kukelova, Z., Pajdla, T.: A minimal solution to radial distortion autocalibration. IEEE Trans. Pattern Anal. Mach. Intell. **33**, 2410–2422 (2011)
13. Kukelova, Z., Byröd, M., Josephson, K., Pajdla, T., Åström, K.: Fast and robust numerical solutions to minimal problems for cameras with radial distortion. Comput. Vis. Image Underst. **114**, 234–244 (2010)
14. Kuang, Y., Solem, J.E., Kahl, F., Åström, K.: Minimal solvers for relative pose with a single unknown radial distortion. In: Proceedings of the Conference on Computer Vision and Pattern Recognition (2014)
15. Lowe, D.G.: Distinctive image features from scale-invariant keypoints. Int. J. Comput. Vis. **60**, 91–110 (2004)
16. Fischler, M.A., Bolles, R.C.: Random sample consensus: a paradigm for model fitting with applications to image analysis and automated cartography. Commun. ACM **24**, 381–395 (1981)
17. Byröd, M., Josephson, K., Åström, K.: Fast and stable polynomial equation solving and its application to computer vision. Int. J. Comput. Vis. **84**, 237–255 (2009)
18. Kukelova, Z., Pajdla, T.: Two minimal problems for cameras with radial distortion. In: OMNIVIS (2007)
19. Josephson, K., Byröd, M.: Pose estimation with radial distortion and unknown focal length. In: Proceedings of the Conference on Computer Vision and Pattern Recognition, San Fransisco, USA (2009)
20. Kukelova, Z., Bujnak, M., Pajdla, T.: Real-time solution to the absolute pose problem with unknown radial distortion and focal length. In: IEEE International Conference on Computer Vision, ICCV 2013, Sydney, Australia, pp. 2816–2823, 1–8 December 2013 (2013)
21. Hartley, R.I., Zisserman, A.: Multiple View Geometry in Computer Vision. Cambridge University Press, Cambridge (2000)
22. Cox, D., Little, J., O'Shea, D.: Using Algebraic Geometry. Springer, New York (1998)
23. Cox, D., Little, J., O'Shea, D.: Ideals, Varieties, and Algorithms. Springer, New York (2007)
24. Grayson, D., Stillman, M.: Macaulay 2 (1993–2002). http://www.math.uiuc.edu/Macaulay2/ (An open source computer algebra software)
25. Kuang, Y., Åström, K.: Numerically Stable Optimization of Polynomial Solvers for Minimal Problems. In: Fitzgibbon, A., Lazebnik, S., Perona, P., Sato, Y., Schmid, C. (eds.) ECCV 2012, Part III. LNCS, vol. 7574, pp. 100–113. Springer, Heidelberg (2012)
26. Naroditsky, O., Daniilidis, K.: Optimizing polynomial solvers for minimal geometry problems. In: ICCV, pp. 975–982 (2011)

Simultaneous Entire Shape Registration of Multiple Depth Images Using Depth Difference and Shape Silhouette

Takuya Ushinohama, Yosuke Sawai, Satoshi Ono, and Hiroshi Kawasaki[✉]

Department of Information Science and Biomedical Engineering,
Graduate School of Science and Engineering,
Kagoshima University, Kagoshima, Japan
kawasaki@ibe.kagoshima-u.ac.jp

Abstract. This paper proposes a method for simultaneous global registration of multiple depth images which are obtained from multiple viewpoints. Unlike the previous method, the proposed method fully utilizes a silhouette-based cost function taking out-of-view and non-overlapping regions into account as well as depth differences at overlapping areas. With the combination of the above cost functions and a recent powerful meta-heuristics named self-adaptive Differential Evolution, it realizes the entire shape reconstruction from relatively small number (three or four) of depth images, which do not involve enough overlapping regions for Iterative Closest Point even if they are prealigned. In addition, to allow the technique to be applicable not only to time-of-flight sensors, but also projector-camera systems, which has deficient silhouette by occlusions, we propose a simple solution based on color-based silhouette. Experimental results show that the proposed method can reconstruct the entire shape only from three depth images of both synthetic and real data. The influence of noises and inaccurate silhouettes is also evaluated.

1 Introduction

3D shape measurement techniques have made significant progress, and have been widely used in various fields such as medical, education, digital archiving and entertainment fields. For such purposes, range scanners are used to acquire 3D shapes of real-world objects and scenes. Since the 3D scanners can capture only one side of the object, multiple depth images should be captured from different viewpoints and aligned to recover the entire shape of the object as shown in Fig. 1; such process is called *registration* in the paper.

Registration techniques can be divided into two classes: global (coarse) and local (fine) registration. The purpose of global registration is to align the relative

Electronic supplementary material The online version of this chapter (doi:10. 1007/978-3-319-16808-1_31) contains supplementary material, which is available to authorized users. Videos can also be accessed at http://www.springerimages.com/ videos/978-3-319-16807-4.

D. Cremers et al. (Eds.): ACCV 2014, Part II, LNCS 9004, pp. 457–472, 2015.
DOI: 10.1007/978-3-319-16808-1_31

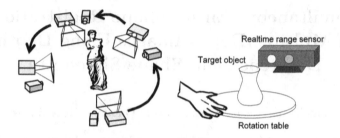

Fig. 1. Entire shape capturing system: (left) by moving projector and camera based 3D scanning systems and (right) by rotating the object.

positions without prior knowledge of the initial clues until being possible to perform a local registration. The local registration requires a good prealignment to converge to the optimum solution. Iterative Closest Point (ICP) [1] and Simultaneous ICP [2] are well known methods for local registration. On the other hand, although a large number of studies have been conducted on global registration, general and robust algorithm has not been established yet.

Global registration methods are mainly categorized into two approaches: matching-based [3–5] and parameter-based methods [6–9]. Matching-based methods estimate an approximated position by utilizing 3D shape features [10]. With the methods, not only different types of algorithms are required depending on type of 3D shape, *e.g.*, mesh, depth image or point clouds, but also an appropriate 3D shape feature should be selected. Since 3D features cannot be retrieved stably due to changes on view-direction and scale and noise, the method usually requires manual support in practical cases. To solve the problem of the matching-based methods, parameter-based methods that use meta-heuristics have been proposed [7]. Parameter-based methods enable registration of the object regardless of type of 3D shape by direct pose-space search approach and it is also reported that the methods are robust against measurement environments. One severe drawback of the parameter-based methods is that it is generally a difficult task to find the optimum solution, because of vast search space, and thus, usually special assumptions are not, *e.g.*, an angle of rotation is limited [11], etc.

In this paper, we propose a global registration method with parameter-based approach which does not have special assumptions. To realize robust and practical convergence even if there are only small number of input, *i.e.*, three or four, we introduce a new cost function and optimizing technique as follows.

- Silhouette-based cost function, which takes out-of-view and non-overlapping regions into account as well as depth differences at overlapping areas. With the function, it only requires few overlapping regions which is not enough for matching based approach [2].
- Simultaneous global registration method based on evolutionary computation algorithm named self-adaptive differential evolution (jDE) [12], which realizes registration of depth images without any prealignment.
- Silhouette refinement method using color information for projector-camera system to compensate deficient silhouettes of depth image, which inevitably occurs by occlusions of stereo pair.

2   Related Work

In order to improve the quality of registration which is prealigned, local registration method has been researched more then two decades. ICP and the extensions, which align the shape precisely by finding corresponding points as the closest point and minimizing the distance between them, are typical solutions [1,2]. However, if the initial alignment was not enough accurate, the algorithm will fail because it easily makes wrong matches or it makes the cost to be 0 for the point which has no corresponding points nearby.

To solve the problem of initial alignment of ICP, many researches have been conducted known as global registration. Typical solution is a matching based approach using feature point [3–5]. Sample Consensus Initial Alignment (SACIA) [13] is a well known prealignment method that extracts key-points based on Fast Point Feature Histograms (FPFH), which is a fast variant of Point Feature Histograms (PFH) [14], and aligns two depth images by the key-point correspondences. Since those techniques are based on feature matching, it cannot be used if there are only small overlapping areas. Recently, the method which realizes registration even if there are only small overlapping areas is proposed [5]. This method aligns two wide baseline range scans by maximizing their *contour coherence*, that is, minimizing a distance between corresponding contours extracted from the range images. However, the method still require a certain amount of overlaps and minimum four scans are required.

To solve the problem on matching based method, parameter-based methods have been proposed and those are summarized in [7]. Although previous methods have severe drawbacks on computational cost and vast local minima, our method overcomes the problem by using new cost functions as well as appropriate optimizing algorithm.

3   The Proposed Method

3.1   Overview

The proposed registration method first sets the specific viewpoint as the *source depth image*, transforms all the depth images to the viewpoint using the orientation and position parameters and merges them to make a *target depth image*. Then the target depth image is compared to the source depth image by calculating the cost based on silhouette and depth differences. Optimum parameters are found by minimizing the sum of the costs of different viewpoints.

As for the cost function of two depth images, usually depth differences of overlapping regions are used. With such method, if the number of images is small, size of overlapping region becomes small, which results in unstable registration. To overcome the problem, we propose a new cost function using non-overlapping region which is usually ignored for optimization. If all the depth images are transformed with the correct parameters, target depth image must be inside the silhouette of the source depth image. Based on the above standpoint, the proposed method simply puts cost on the part of the target depth image which is

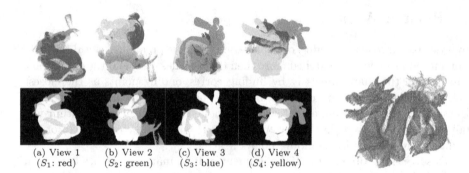

(a) View 1   (b) View 2   (c) View 3   (d) View 4
(S_1: red)   (S_2: green)   (S_3: blue)   (S_4: yellow)

Fig. 2. Example of the source and the transformed targets (upper) and their silhouettes (lower). In the upper images, four models are classified by color. In the lower images, white, blue, and light blue represent source, target, and overlapped regions, respectively (Color figure online).

Fig. 3. Example of locally optimum, but not globally. Each pair, red-blue and green-yellow, are well aligned, but not between them (Color figure online).

outside the source depth image. Figure 2 shows examples of the non-overlapping regions; white, blue and light blue regions denote the source image, the target image which is not overlapped with source image, and the source image which is overlapped with the target image. We put constant cost on blue regions.

3.2   Acquiring Multiple Depth Images Around the Object

In the method, we assume that the object is captured from multiple viewpoints to cover the entire shape. To achieve such scan, we assume either moving the scanner around the object or rotating the object with turn table, as shown in Fig. 1. Usually, to recover the entire shape using multiple scan data, it is required to scan the object from 8, 10 or more directions to have enough overlapping regions to stably run ICP or similar local registration methods. On the other hand, since our technique is based on silhouette of the object and we need almost no overlapping region in theory, just three or four scans are enough for entire shape registration, which greatly reduces the task of scanning process and cannot be realized by previous methods; this is an important advantage of our method.

In terms of scanning device, since either object or scanner moves during the scan, we assume realtime 3D scanner which can capture the shape only with a short period of time. There are two types of realtime scanner, such as stereo based one, *e.g.*, video-projector [15] or laser based system [16], and Time-Of-Flight (TOF) based one, *e.g.*, Kinect2 [16] and Swiss ranger [17]. Stereo based scanner inevitably produces occluded regions because of wide base-line, whereas TOF sensor does not have such drawbacks. Since our method is based on silhouette of the object and its accuracy is affected by the silhouette, TOF scanner is more suitable in theory. However, depth accuracy and spatial resolution of realtime TOF sensor is basically lower than that of stereo based one, and thus, stereo based scanner is considered main target in the paper. To compensate the occlusion problem, we propose an efficient method to refine the silhouette using color information which is captured by the camera of a projector-camera system.

4   Global Registration of Entire Shape Using Silhouette

4.1   Cost Function for Simultaneous Entire Registration

A problem of simultaneous entire shape registration involves variables corresponding to rigid transformation parameters of all N depth images except the last one which was fixed to common world coordinate system. Therefore, solution vector x consists of set of rotation angles represented by quaternion $(\theta_1, \phi_{x1}, \phi_{y1}, \phi_{z1}), (\theta_2, \phi_{x2}, \phi_{y2}, \phi_{z2}), \ldots, (\theta_{N-1}, \phi_{xN-1}, \phi_{yN-1}, \phi_{zN-1})$ and set of translation vectors $(x_1, y_1, z_1), (x_2, y_2, z_2), \ldots, (x_{N-1}, y_{N-1}, z_{N-1})$.

In each calculation of objective function (cost function) for optimization, first, the proposed method renders all the silhouette images with depth information of reconstructed objects using x from all the viewpoints of depth sensors which capture the input shapes. Here, depth images which corresponds to each depth sensor are called *source depth images* and denoted as $S_1, \ldots, S_N$ and the rest of the depth images are merged for each viewpoints and called *target depth images* and denoted as $T_1, \ldots, T_N$. Figure 2 shows examples of $S_1, \ldots, S_N$ (white) and $T_1, \ldots, T_N$ (blue and light blue) in the case of four scanned images.

The cost function proposed in this paper is calculated by comparing the target and source depth images. The cost function consists of the cost calculated by silhouettes and the cost calculated by depth differences. Since the proposed method does not depend entirely on the cost of overlapping region, the cost from silhouette is indispensable to prealignment. The cost from silhouette is based on the area size of the target regions stuck out from the silhouette of the source, and leads the target region to shrink into the view volume which is constructed by the source silhouette. It works efficiently to realize coarse, *i.e.*, globally consistent, registration at early stage of the optimization. The cost from depth difference at overlapping region works effectively on fine registration at the latter stage of the optimization; it makes the surface of source and the target close to each other. Based on the notation, objective function $F(x)$ is defined as follows:

$$F(x) = \frac{1}{N} \sum_{k=1}^{N} f(T_k, S_k) \tag{1}$$

$$f(t, s) = \frac{1}{p} \sum_{i=1}^{p} \delta(t_i, s_i) \tag{2}$$

$$\delta(t_i, s_i) = \begin{cases} C_1|s_i - t_i| & \text{(overlapping region)} \\ 1 & \text{(non-overlapping region)} \\ C_2 & \text{(outside of the view-field),} \end{cases} \tag{3}$$

where t and s denotes depth images of a target and a source, t_i and s_i denotes the depth values of pixel i in t and s, and p is the number of pixels in the depth images. The cost from silhouette corresponds to the cost of non-overlapping region and outside of the view-field is represented by $\delta(t_i, s_i)$, which returns high penalty value C_1 when i is outside of the view-field, moderate value C_2 when the pixel in s_i exists in non-overlapping region, and a value based on the distance between s_i and t_i in overlapping region. Here, C_1 and C_2 should be adjusted in order that the cost of overlapping region can be almost the same or smaller than the cost of non-overlapping region; higher C_2 enhances the force to bring the source and the target close to each other, however, if it is too high, it entraps to local optima in which the distance between them is minimum. Reasonable values for them are [1, 10] and [1, 50] with our experience, respectively.

4.2   Global Optimization by Self-adaptive Differential Evolution

As described in Sect. 4.1, the entire registration problem involves many variables in x and the cost function $F(x)$ to be minimized. The least number of scans to reconstruct the entire shape is three, and in this case the problem consists of 21 variables. This optimization problem seems partially separable; variables for each transformation vector can basically be optimized individually. However, to escape from local optima, many variables should be changed simultaneously. The most hard local optima are that more than one pair (or group) of shapes are registered in each local coordinate systems respectively and the pairs (or group) are not located appropriately in the global coordinate system as shown in Fig. 3. To escape from such local optima, changes of a few variables are not sufficient; variables for two transformation vectors of two shapes should be changed simultaneously.

Therefore, the proposed registration method adopts meta-heuristics for global optimization named self-adaptive Differential Evolution (jDE)[12]. Differential Evolution (DE) [18,19] is one of the most powerful stochastic real-parameter optimization algorithms. DE-variants and one other recent powerful EC algorithms named Evolution Strategy with Covariance Matrix Adaptation (CMA-ES) [20] occupied high ranks in the standard numerical benchmarks such as IEEE Int'l Conf. Evolutionary Computation (CEC) competition on real parameter optimization. DE is suited to multimodal, separable problems, whereas CMA-ES to unimodal, non-separable ones.

jDE is simple but powerful self-adaptive DE algorithms that successfully eliminate control parameter adjustment by letting individuals have their own control parameter values and statistically changing the values. jDE showed the best performance in the competition "Evolutionary Computation in Dynamic and Uncertain Environments" in CEC2009 [21].

Unlike Genetic Algorithm [22], DE employs difference of solution candidates to explore the search space. DE generates solution candidates (vectors) by mutation and crossover. First, a mutant vector is generated as follows:

$$v_{i,g+1} = x_{r_1,g} + F_{i,g}(x_{r_2,g} - x_{r_3,g}), \tag{4}$$

where g denotes the index of generation. $\boldsymbol{x}_{r_1,g}$, $\boldsymbol{x}_{r_2,g}$, and $\boldsymbol{x}_{r_3,g}$ are randomly chosen vectors from the interval $[1, NP]$ $(r_1 \neq r_2 \neq r_3 \neq i)$. Note that the notations in this section are based on previous work [12], and have different meanings from the other sections of this paper. The above mutant vector is recombined with the target vector by crossover to produce trial vector $\boldsymbol{u}_{i,g+1}$ as follows:

$$u_{j,i,g+1} = \begin{cases} v_{j,i,g+1} & \text{if } rand_{j,i} \leq CR_{i,g} \text{ or } j = j_{rand} \\ x_{j,i,g} & \text{otherwise} \end{cases} \tag{5}$$

Finally, the better one of $\boldsymbol{u}_{i,g+1}$ and $\boldsymbol{x}_{i,g}$ survives and become a member of generation $g+1$ as follows:

$$\boldsymbol{x}_{i,g+1} = \begin{cases} \boldsymbol{u}_{i,g+1} & \text{if } f(\boldsymbol{u}_{i,g+1}) \leq f(\boldsymbol{x}_{i,g}) \\ \boldsymbol{x}_{i,g} & \text{otherwise} \end{cases} \tag{6}$$

Scale factor $F_{i,g}$ and crossover rate $CR_{i,g}$ are control parameters which deeply influence the search performance; for instance, small scale factor urges a local search, and low values of crossover rate are recommended for separable problems. In jDE, $F_{i,g}$ and $CR_{i,g}$ associated with i-th solution are statistically changed as follows:

$$F_{i,g+1} = \begin{cases} F_l + rand_1 \times F_u & \text{if } rand_2 < \tau_1 \\ F_{i,g} & \text{otherwise} \end{cases} \tag{7}$$

$$CR_{i,g+1} = \begin{cases} rand_3 & \text{if } rand_4 < \tau_2 \\ CR_{i,g} & \text{otherwise} \end{cases} \tag{8}$$

where F_l and F_u determine the range of the scale factor. Letting F_l and F_u be 0 and 1 respectively frees a human developer to adjust the control parameters except the population size. The probabilities to change $F_{i,g}$ and $CR_{i,g}$ are τ_1 and τ_2 respectively. They does not affect the result by choosing $[0.05, 0.3]$, and are set to 0.1 according to the previous work [12]. By the above self adaptation process, adequate values of $F_{i,g}$ and $CR_{i,g}$ lead to better solution candidates that are more likely to survive, resulting in propagate those good parameter values.

4.3   Application to Projector-Camera System

When using a projector-camera system to obtain 3D shapes, self-occlusion causes deficiency of silhouette image due to stereo baseline. This silhouette deficiency may hamper the precise registration since the proposed method makes full use of silhouette for global optimization. Figure 4(a) and (b) show a missing silhouettes obtained by a projector-camera system and a failed example of reconstructed shape with deficient silhouette images, respectively. With these silhouette images, the accurate reconstruction result cannot be evaluated properly; the target are not completely be covered by the deficient silhouettes, and the value of the cost function increases. The targets are then biased to make themselves gather into the center of the shape. The larger stereo baseline for the projector-camera system is used, the larger deficient regions the silhouette involves.

To solve the problem, when using a projector-camera system, we propose the method which compensates the deficient regions on silhouette images by color information. To recover the deficient region of silhouette, we apply graph-cut algorithm using both color information and the silhouette of a depth image as the data cost. The extracted silhouette of the target object using graph-cut is shown in Fig. 4(c). The comparison between the original silhouette and the recovered one using color information is shown by red regions in Fig. 4(d). The above process is applied to each depth image. The cost function $\delta(t_i, s_i)$ in the recovered silhouette region in either source or target image is regarded as zero.

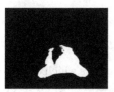   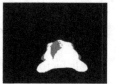

(a) Obtained silhouette image by projector-camera system. (b) Failed example reconstructed from (a) (c) Extracted region in color image. (d) Recovered silhouette.

Fig. 4. Example of silhouette recover with color image (Color figure online).

5   Evaluation

To verify the effectiveness of the proposed method, experiments were conducted with synthetic 3D model objects V_1, V_2, V_3, and V_4 shown in Fig. 5 and actual objects M_1, M_2, M_3, M_4, and M_5 measured by a projector-camera system. First, four experiments of different algorithm (Sect. 5.1), evaluation on influence of the size of the overlapped region (Sect. 5.2), comparison to previous work (Sect. 5.3), and noise influence (Sect. 5.4) were performed with the synthetic objects. Then, entire shape reconstructions using actual objects were demonstrated (Sect. 5.5). Finally, the influence of inaccurate silhouette (Sect. 5.6) and an ability on using multiple scans to recover a large object (Sect. 5.7) were examined.

In the experiments with the synthetic objects, depth images were synthesized by a virtual TOF camera by rotating the object around y-axis. The target position to decide a view-direction of virtual sensor was set to the center of the object. The sensor's position was set behind the object center to z direction with distance d_z:

$$d_z = \frac{L_{max} + m}{\tan(fov)}, \tag{9}$$

where L_{max} is the maximum value between the height and width of the synthetic object and m denotes the margin set to be 1. The field of view fov of the camera was set to 30 degrees. The number of created points is from 10,000 to 25,000. The object size are normalized to be settled in the box region $[-1.0, 1.0]$.

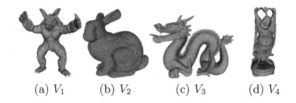

(a) V_1 (b) V_2 (c) V_3 (d) V_4

Fig. 5. Synthetic 3D model objects used in the experiments.

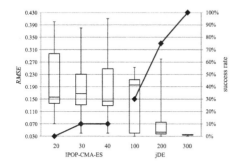

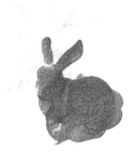

Fig. 6. Comparison on optimizers and their control parameters.

Fig. 7. Example local optimum from which IPOP-CMA-ES could not escape.

5.1   Comparison on Optimization Algorithms

In the first experiment, we compare the global optimization algorithm jDE with CMA-ES with restart (IPOP-CMA-ES) [23], that showed the best performance in Black Box Optimization Benchmarking 2012 [24]. Four depth images for each object V_1, V_2, V_3, and V_4 were used to reconstruct each model. According to the previous work [12,20], their control parameters, λ in IPOP-CMA-ES and population size NP in jDE, were changed $20, 30, 40$ and $100, 200, 300$, respectively. IPOP-CMA-ES restarted and doubled the value of λ when no improvement of the best solution occurred during last 50, 80, or 100 generations, and terminated after three restarts. jDE stopped when no improvement of the best solution could be seen during 200, 300, or 500 generations. 20 independent runs have been performed for each object and for each algorithm and its control parameter configuration. C_1 and C_2 were set to 2 and 4, respectively. Ranges of variables for translation and rotation were [-1.0, 1.0] and [-180°, 180°], respectively. In each run, the entire shape registration was regarded as success when $RMSE$ was less than 0.05.

Figure 6 demonstrates $RMSE$ (shown in box plots) and the success rates (shown by line graphs) of IPOP-CMA-ES and jDE in reconstructing V_2 from four images. The performance of jDE was better than IPOP-CMA-ES and improved in both the success rate and $RMSE$ as the population size increased, whereas the performance of IPOP-CMA-ES was worse than jDE and independent from λ. Since the fitness landscape of the registration problem based on the cost functions

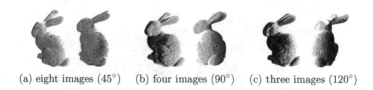

(a) eight images (45°)   (b) four images (90°)   (c) three images (120°)

Fig. 8. Difference of overlapped regions (red) on capturing angles (Color figure online).

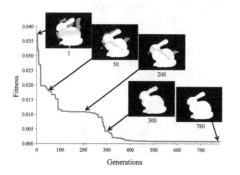

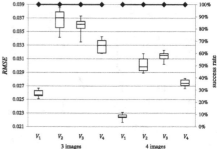

Fig. 9. Example transition of objective function value in reconstructing V_2 from three images.

Fig. 10. Results on the different number of captured images.

is globally multimodal in addition to local small perturbations, IPOP-CMA-ES was prone to fall into local optima as shown in Fig. 7. According to the above results, we basically set NP to 300 in the later experiments in this paper.

5.2 Influence on Size of Overlapping Region

Next, to show the advantage of the proposed method, we use only three or four images as the input to conduct registration; note that only little overlapped regions exist with such condition. We also test the registration with eight images which have enough overlapped region.

Input images were synthesized from virtual viewpoints with the interval of 120, 90 and 45 degrees, respectively. jDE stopped the search when no improvement of the best solution in the population could be seen in more than 1,000 generations. In the case reconstructing from eight images, NP was set to 1,600, a termination condition was extended to 4,000 generations, and only one run was performed due to the processing time. Figure 8 shows the overlapped region with red color for each dataset. As the number of captured images decreased, the overlapped region significantly reduced so that the pair-wised methods could hardly align the images.

Figure 9 shows an example transition of the objective function value of the best solution in reconstructing V_2 from three images. As the value decreased, the difference between the target and the source reduced. Figure 10 demonstrates

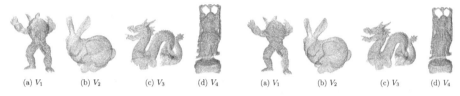

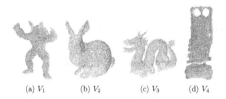

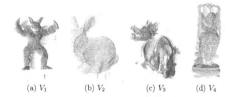

Fig. 11. Example results from three images by the proposed method.

Fig. 12. Example results from four images by the proposed method.

Fig. 13. Example results from eight images by the proposed method.

Fig. 14. Example pairwise registration results by SACIA.

RMSE shown in box plots and the success rates shown by line graphs, and Figs. 11, 12 and 13 show examples of the reconstructed 3D models. In the case reconstructing from eight images, the proposed method could succeed to align all images with RMSE of 4.55×10^{-2}, 6.63×10^{-2}, 6.40×10^{-2}, and 6.51×10^{-2} for V_1, V_2, V_3, and V_4, respectively. As shown in Fig. 10, the proposed method could reconstruct the entire shape from three or four images, despite the quite small overlapping regions.

5.3 Comparison with SACIA

The proposed method was compared with SACIA [13], a prealignment method based on key-point matching, in the case of using four images. Figure 14 shows the examples of the pair-wised registration results by SACIA. Due to less overlapping regions, it was difficult for SACIA to align two depth images. In contrast, the proposed method could align just with four depth images as shown in Figs. 10 and 12.

5.4 Robustness to Noise and Distortion

The robustness to noise of the proposed method was experimentally validated in this section with synthetic object V_2. First, the random uniform noise were added with the range of [-1.1, 1.1]. The amount of noise was 10 % and 15 % of the number of points of the tested objects [4]. Figure 15 shows the results. The proposed method successfully reconstructed the entire shapes in noise levels 10 %.

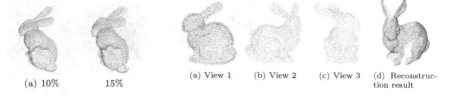

(a) 10%   15%

(a) View 1   (b) View 2   (c) View 3   (d) Reconstruction result

Fig. 15. Reconstruction result from noisy depth images

Fig. 16. Reconstruction result from distorted shape images

In the case with 15 % noise, the green target was a little off the other depth images, but being enough quality as prealignment.

Next, the influence of the measurement error and distortion was investigated by adding small perturbations to positions of all points with the radius of 0.001. Figure 16(a) to (c) show the object shapes whose points are perturbed, and Fig. 16(d) shows the reconstruction result with the obtained transformation parameters and with object shapes not involving the above point perturbations. From the results, we can confirm that the proposed method could avoid the influence of the small distortion and all depth images were successfully aligned.

5.5   Experiments with Real Data

We use a projector-camera system to scan real objects. The system consists of EPSON EMP-1715 as a projector and Point Grey GRAS-20S4C-C as a camera. The baseline between the projector and the camera was 30 cm, and the distance between the object and the camera was 70 cm. The real object M_1, M_2, M_3, M_4, and M_5 were used. Each object was shot three times with rotating 120 degrees and example scan results for each object are shown in Fig. 17.

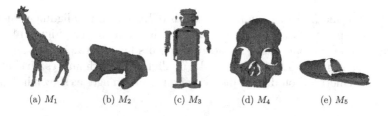

(a) M_1 (b) M_2 (c) M_3 (d) M_4 (e) M_5

Fig. 17. Real 3D model objects used in the experiments.

Figures 18 and 19 show the reconstruction results of the proposed method without and with silhouette recovery, respectively. Without silhouette recovery, although shapes are gathered into the center of the shape, all of them cannot be reconstructed properly. To the contrary, the proposed method with silhouette recovery successfully reconstructed the entire shapes of all tested objects.

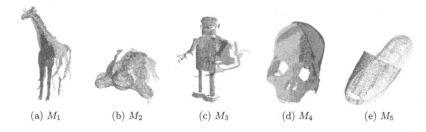

(a) M_1 (b) M_2 (c) M_3 (d) M_4 (e) M_5

Fig. 18. Reconstruction results without silhouette recovery.

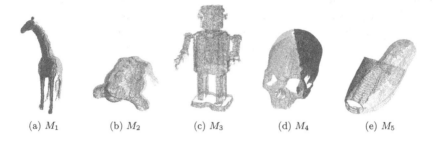

(a) M_1 (b) M_2 (c) M_3 (d) M_4 (e) M_5

Fig. 19. Reconstruction result with silhouette recovery.

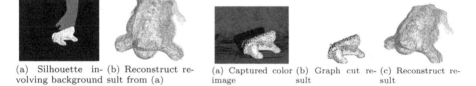

(a) Silhouette in- (b) Reconstruct re-   (a) Captured color (b) Graph cut re- (c) Reconstruct revolving background sult from (a)   image   sult   sult

Fig. 20. Result from over-   **Fig. 21.** Result from missing silhouette.
detected silhouette.

5.6   Influence of Graph Cut Error in Silhouette Recovery

The influence of the error in graph cut for the silhouette recovery was investigated
with M_2. The first case was the unexpected entering of the background to the
silhouette. We assumed that one of the silhouette image extracted by graph
cut involved the background region as shown in Fig. 20(a). The falsely detected
region in the silhouette (the upper red-colored area of the source in Fig. 20(a))
has sufficient size to involve the target shape. The second case tested is the
silhouette deficiency; a shaded area on the object was mistakenly recognized as
background even after graph cut as shown in Fig. 21(b).

Figures 20(b) and 21(c) show the reconstruction results by the proposed
method, demonstrating that the proposed method could reconstruct the entire
shape with enough accuracy without being affected by the silhouette recovery
failure.

5.7   Reconstruction of a Large Object from Partially Scanned Data

Reconstruction of a large object from partially scanned data, *e.g.*, face, hands, legs of statue, is practically important for wide applications [25]. Since our method basically assumes that the entire silhouette of object is available, pre-processing is necessary to apply our method, *i.e.*, constructing the entire silhouette of object by aligning multiple partial objects. To examine the proposed algorithm with the preprocessing, we conducted the experiment using synthetic data V_4. First, a virtual TOF camera scanned V_4 four times while moving the camera along y-axis in parallel. Then, as preprocessing, ICP was applied to the four images shown in Fig. 22(a), producing the depth image involving the entire silhouette of V_4 as shown in Fig. 22(b). Then, we do the same process by rotating the camera 120 degrees around y-axis. Finally, we apply the proposed method to the three preprocessed entire silhouettes and successfully reconstructed the entire shape as shown in Fig. 22(c).

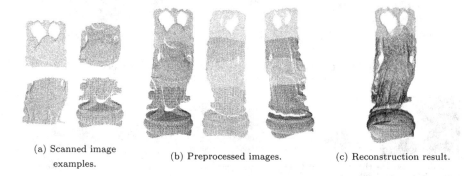

(a) Scanned image examples.   (b) Preprocessed images.   (c) Reconstruction result.

Fig. 22. Reconstruction result of large object with ICP-based preprocessing.

6   Conclusions

In this paper, we propose a simultaneous global registration method to achieve entire 3D shape reconstruction from relatively small number (three or four) of depth images. Even though input shapes do not involve enough overlapping regions, the proposed method reconstructs the entire shape without any initial positional information. This is realized by using the cost which is assigned on out-of-view and non-overlapped regions as well as overlapped ones with global optimization method by jDE. In addition, our method is applicable to not only TOF sensors, but also projector-camera systems with color-combined silhouette recovery method. Experimental results showed that the proposed method can reconstruct entire 3D models even from three images captured by 120 degrees intervals which have almost no overlapping regions. Results using real data captured by a projector-camera system showed that color-based silhouette technique allows accurate reconstruction even if deficient in the depth images. Speeding up for optimization is our important future research.

References

1. Besl, P.J., McKay, N.D.: A method for registration of 3-d shapes. IEEE Trans. Pattern Anal. Mach. Intell. **14**, 239–256 (1992)
2. NEUGEBAUER, P.: Geometrical cloning of 3d objects via simultaneous registration of multiple range image. In: Proceedings of the International Conference on Shape Modeling and Applications (1997)
3. Li, H., Hartley, R.: The 3d–3d registration problem revisited. In: Proceedings of the International Conference on Computer Vision, pp. 1–8 (2007)
4. Yang, J., Li, H., Jia, Y.: Go-icp: Solving 3d registration efficiently and globally optimally. In: IEEE International Conference on Computer Vision, pp. 1457–1464 (2013)
5. Wang, R., Choi, J., Medioni, G.: 3d modeling from wide baseline range scans using contour coherence. In: The IEEE Conference on Computer Vision and Pattern Recognition (CVPR), pp. 4018–4025 (2014)
6. Johnson, A., Hebert, M.: Using spin images for efficient object recognition in cluttered 3d scenes. IEEE Trans. Pattern Anal. Mach. Intell. **21**, 433–449 (1999)
7. Santamaría, J., Cordón, O., Damas, S.: A comparative study of state-of-the-art evolutionary image registration methods for 3d modeling. Comput. Vis. Image Underst. **115**, 1340–1354 (2011)
8. Silva, L., Bellon, O.R.P., Boyer, K.: Precision range image registration using a robust surface interpenetration measure and enhanced genetic algorithms. IEEE Trans. Pattern Anal. Mach. Intell. **27**, 762–776 (2005)
9. Brunnstrom, K., Stoddart, A.J.: Genetic algorithms for free-form surface matching. In: Proceedings of the International Conference on Pattern Recognition. vol. 4, pp. 689–693 (1996)
10. Salti, S., Tombari, F., Di Stefano, L.: A performance evaluation of 3d keypoint detectors. In: International Conference on 3D Imaging, Modeling, Processing, Visualization and Transmission, pp. 236–243 (2011)
11. He, R., Narayana, P.A.: Global optimization of mutual information: application to three-dimensional retrospective registration of magnetic resonance images. Comput. Med. Imaging Graph. **26**, 277–292 (2002)
12. Brest, J., Greiner, S., Boskovic, B., Mernik, M., Zumer, V.: Self-adapting control parameters in differential evolution: A comparative study on numerical benchmark problems. Trans. Evol. Comput. **10**, 646–657 (2006)
13. Rusu, R., Blodow, N., Beetz, M.: Fast point feature histograms (FPFH) for 3d registration. In: International Conference on Robotics and Automation, pp. 3212–3217 (2009)
14. Rusu, R., Blodow, N., Marton, Z., Beetz, M.: Aligning point cloud views using persistent feature histograms. In: International Conference on Intelligent Robots and Systems, pp. 3384–3391 (2008)
15. Furukawa, R., Kawasaki, H.: Uncalibrated multiple image stereo system with arbitrarily movable camera and projector for wide range scanning. In: IEEE Conference on 3DIM, pp. 302–309 (2005)
16. Zhang, Z.: Microsoft kinect sensor and its effect. MultiMedia **19**, 4–10 (2012)
17. Mesa Imaging AG.: SwissRanger SR-4000 (2011). http://www.swissranger.ch/index.php
18. Storn, R., Price, K.: Differential evolution a simple and efficient heuristic for global optimization over continuous spaces. J. Global Optim. **11**, 341–359 (1997)

19. Das, S., Suganthan, P.N.: Differential evolution: A survey of the state-of-the-art. IEEE Trans. Evol. Comput. **15**, 4–31 (2011)
20. Hansen, N., Ostermeier, A.: Completely derandomized self-adaptation in evolution strategies. Evol. Comput. **9**, 159–195 (2001)
21. Li, C., Yang, S., Nguyen, T.T., Yu, E.L., Yao, X., Jin, Y., Beyer, H.-G., Suganthan, P.N.: Benchmark generator for cec' 2009 competition on dynamic optimization (2008)
22. Goldberg, D.E.: Genetic Algorithms in Search, Optimization, and Machine Learning. Addison Wesley, Reading (1989)
23. Auger, A., Hansen, N.: A restart cma evolution strategy with increasing population size. Congr. Evolut. Comput. **2**, 1769–1776 (2005)
24. Brockhoff, D., Auger, A., Hansen, N.: On the effect of mirroring in the IPOP active CMA-ES on the noiseless BBOB testbed. In: Proceedings of the Annual Conference on Genetic and Evolutionary Computation, pp. 277–284 (2012)
25. Levoy, M., Pulli, K., Curless, B., Rusinkiewicz, S., Koller, D., Pereira, L., Ginzton, M., Anderson, S., Davis, J., Ginsberg, J., Shade, J., Fulk, D.: The Digital Michelangelo Project: 3D scanning of large statues. Proc. ACM SIGGRAPH **2000**, 131–144 (2000)

Joint Camera Pose Estimation and 3D Human Pose Estimation in a Multi-camera Setup

Jens Puwein[1]([✉]), Luca Ballan[1], Remo Ziegler[2], and Marc Pollefeys[1]

[1] Department of Computer Science, ETH Zurich, Zürich, Switzerland
puweinj@inf.ethz.ch
[2] Vizrt, Zürich, Switzerland

Abstract. In this paper we propose an approach to jointly perform camera pose estimation and human pose estimation from videos recorded by a set of cameras separated by wide baselines. Multi-camera pose estimation is very challenging in case of wide baselines or in general when patch-based feature correspondences are difficult to establish across images.

For this reason, we propose to exploit the motion of an articulated structure in the scene, such as a human, to relate these cameras. More precisely, we first run a part-based human pose estimation for each camera and each frame independently. Correctly detected joints are then used to compute an initial estimate of the epipolar geometry between pairs of cameras. In a combined optimization over all the recorded sequences, the multi-camera configuration and the 3D motion of the kinematic structure in the scene are inferred. The optimization accounts for time continuity, part-based detection scores, optical flow, and body part visibility.

Our approach was evaluated on 4 publicly available datasets, evaluating the accuracy of the camera poses and the human poses.

1 Introduction

Camera pose estimation is typically performed by establishing patch-based feature correspondences across images captured by the different cameras [1–4]. This task can be very challenging in case of cameras placed far apart from each other (wide baselines), or, in general, when no reliable correspondences can be found. This is the case, for instance, in Fig. 1, where, due to the homogenous background and the wide baselines, it is prohibitive to establish patch-based correspondences. In such scenarios, different features need to be used, namely features incorporating a higher level representation of the scene.

In this paper, we propose to exploit the motion of an actor in the scene to establish correspondences between static intrinsically calibrated cameras. Subsequently, the extrinsic parameters of the cameras and the pose of the actor at each time instant are inferred jointly based on image measurements. The goal is to find the camera disposition and the motion of a kinematic structure inside the scene which best explain the measured optical flow and the probabilities of each joint to be in specific locations in the images.

© Springer International Publishing Switzerland 2015
D. Cremers et al. (Eds.): ACCV 2014, Part II, LNCS 9004, pp. 473–487, 2015.
DOI: 10.1007/978-3-319-16808-1_32

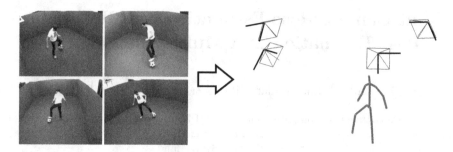

Fig. 1. Given the videos recorded by a set of fixed wide-baseline cameras, our approach recovers the extrinsic parameters of each camera in the scene together with the 3D pose of the moving person at each time instant.

Recent advances in human pose estimation allow for inference of the human pose even from a single image, without having to rely on any kind of foreground/background segmentation of the scene [5]. While these methods work very well for poses that are common in the training set, they often have shortcomings for others. Nevertheless, the results of these techniques can be leveraged to generate the high level correspondences necessary to provide an initial calibration of a static multi-camera setup. In this paper, we propose a method to identify the correctly detected joint positions in each frame of each camera. We then apply a standard structure-from-motion pipeline to these correspondences, taking pose ambiguities into account. Once an initial calibration and initial 3D joint positions are found, the 3D positions of the remaining joints are estimated using optical flow. The camera calibration and the 3D human poses are further optimized jointly leveraging the characteristic properties of multi-view videos, namely smooth 3D trajectories, consistency of 2D joint movements with respect to optical flow, and consistency with respect to discriminative scores of 2D joints. From the initialization to the final optimization, the method goes from single image 2D human pose estimation to the full joint estimation of 3D human poses and camera parameters in a multi-camera setup. Building only on a very general 2D human pose estimation approach, and starting with an extrinsically uncalibrated multi-camera sequence of a moving person, the camera calibration and the full 3D human poses at each time instant are computed.

2 Related Work

Human pose estimation has been tackled in various settings and with varying degrees of accuracy. At one end of the spectrum, there are the 2D human pose estimation approaches which aim at recovering the 2D position and orientation of the limbs or the positions of the joints of a human body from a single image [5,6]. These approaches first compute the probabilities of each limb or joint being at a particular position, orientation, and scale in the image. Subsequently, a kinematic structure is fit on top of these observations to maximize a posterior probability.

When multiple images of the same scene and at the same time instance are available, some methods infer the full 3D pose of the articulated object, provided that the intrinsic and extrinsic parameters of each input image are known [7–9].

At the other end of the spectrum, when video content is available, time continuity is leveraged to resolve pose ambiguities generated by missing observations or occlusions in single cameras [10–12] or multiple cameras [13–17]. These methods rely on a known pose of the actor in the first frame of the sequence to carry out tracking for all the subsequent frames.

Pose estimation in uncalibrated multi-camera setups has also been explored in the past. However, methods dealing with such a problem typically rely on structure-from-motion techniques, which are first applied to the input videos in order to recover the camera locations and orientations at each time instance. A 3D human pose tracking approach is then employed to recover the motion of the actor in the scene [18].

Structure-from-motion is in fact the standard approach to infer the camera calibration parameters from images. It is typically based on establishing patch-based correspondences between images taken from different cameras. When this kind of correspondences cannot be established, like in case of wide-baseline cameras, higher level features, such as people and object trajectories, have been used. For instance, walking people can be treated as moving vertical poles of constant height, and their motion trajectories are used to calibrate the cameras [19–21]. The main restriction of these methods resides in the assumption that each camera is capturing upright, walking people. This is too restrictive in a more general setting. In contrast, several existing methods match people trajectories between multiple views and use this additional information for camera calibration [22–26].

In this work, we propose to do something similar, but instead of using only the position of a person, we exploit the location of each body part, generating a higher number of reliable correspondences and a larger spread in the images.

Sinha and Pollefeys [27] propose to calibrate a camera network using silhouette frontier points by sampling epipoles in each pair of images. However, this method requires accurate segmentations of the actor.

Izo and Grimson [28] propose to perform camera calibration by matching silhouettes of a persons walking cycles across views. At every frame, silhouettes are compared to example silhouettes that are coupled to camera parameters. The final sequence is obtained by combining per frame observations in a Hidden Markov Model (HMM). This method also requires accurate segmentations and it is moreover restricted to specific motions of the actor, such as a walk.

Recently, Ye et al. presented a 3D human pose and camera calibration tracking approach using three kinect sensors [29]. Manual initialization of the camera poses and the human pose is necessary. Subsequently, camera poses and human models are optimized jointly using an iterative procedure.

Our approach can deal with very wide baselines, it does not rely on segmentation, it does not depend on manual initialization, and it does not require the scene to have textured regions to establish correspondences between images. It finds an initial setup by estimating the 2D poses of the actor in each camera independently and it tries to find a camera calibration and 3D human poses explaining the image observations.

3   Algorithm

The input to our method consists of a synchronized multi-view video sequence of a moving person. Cameras are assumed to be static, and their intrinsic parameters known a priori. Our goal is to estimate the full 3D pose of the person in the scene at each time instant together with the extrinsic parameters of each camera.

3.1   Initial Calibration

2D human pose estimation is first run on each camera and each frame independently. For this aim, we use the publicly available Matlab code for the Flexible Mixtures-of-parts (FMP) model [5]. FMP models humans as a tree-structured graphical model in which nodes correspond to joints and edges to body limbs. Unary terms model the appearance of each joint by means of HOG descriptors, and pairwise terms model the relative positioning of neighboring joints. Inference on this graphical model can be carried out very efficiently using dynamic programming and the generalized distance transform.

The resulting joint positions provide putative correspondences between cameras, which are then used for calibration. However, 2D human pose estimation usually does not differentiate between front and back facing people, or if it does, it does it very poorly. This is also the case for FMP. Hence, correspondences between symmetric body parts, like the arms and the legs, are ambiguous in the sense that it is not possible to differentiate between the left ones and right ones. To take this into account, both possibilities, front and back facing, have to be considered.

For each camera pair, the two-view geometry is estimated using RANSAC over the candidate joint correspondences [30]. During the sample selection, each view is chosen to be either front or back facing. When counting the inliers in each frame, the direction faced by the person which leads to the highest number of inliers is chosen.

Additionally, in order to avoid unstable configurations of minimal solutions when generating RANSAC hypotheses, correspondences are encouraged to be evenly distributed over the entire images. Therefore, when drawing the samples, sets of points originating from different joints and lying far apart temporally are assigned higher probabilities of being chosen. It is not necessary to consider all joints to establish correspondences. In fact, a wide spread of joint positions is obtained by using the head, the lower end of the spine, the wrists, and the ankles.

Cameras are added to a common world coordinate frame greedily, starting with a bundle adjustment of the camera pair with the most inlier correspondences [31]. Thereafter, in each step, the camera with the most inlier correspondences to the already included cameras is added, followed by a bundle adjustment. This process is repeated until all cameras are within a common world coordinate frame and refined using bundle adjustment.

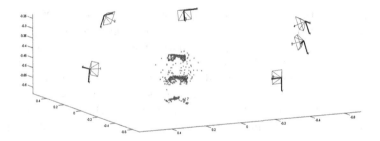

Fig. 2. Camera setup and joint positions used for the calibration of the INRA dancer dataset.

The result is an initial estimate of the poses of all cameras in the setup. An example of a camera setup and the joint positions used for its calibration is shown in Fig. 2.

3.2 Initial 3D Joint Positions

Body joints are triangulated using the initial camera calibration computed in the previous section. A triangulated joint position is considered valid if it can be triangulated by at least 3 cameras with a reprojection error below 5 pixels. In practice, triangulation is performed for each frame and each joint considering all the possible combinations of cameras that could verify that specific joint. The combination with the highest number of agreeing cameras is then kept.

For symmetric joints, like ankles and wrists, care has to be taken. For such pairs of joints, in a first step, the combination of cameras and front facing/back facing of the person that leads to the largest number of cameras verifying the joint is picked greedily. All remaining joint positions are used to potentially verify the second joint that is remaining. This leads to one 3D joint, two 3D joints, or no 3D joint of the same kind (e.g., left ankle and right ankle) per frame. Each joint might be either the left or right joint of the true 3D pose. In order to consistently label the 3D joints as left/right, an arbitrary left/right labeling is chosen for the first frame where both joints appear. This information is then propagated forward and backward through the whole sequence using optical flow.

Using the verified joints as anchors, the missing joint positions throughout the sequence can be inferred using optical flow.

3.3 Joint Optimization

The initial camera calibration and the initial 3D joint positions are refined in a combined optimization step, aiming at finding the correct camera configuration and a consistent kinematic structure evolving over time, explaining the observations.

Let $\boldsymbol{\theta}_c$ denote the extrinsic parameters of camera c, and let $\mathbf{X}_i^t$ denote the 3D coordinates of joint i at time t. $\mathbf{X}_i^t$ and $\boldsymbol{\theta}_c$ are unknowns of the problem.

Since the goal is to find a single kinematic structure for the whole recorded sequence, the length of each body limb needs to be constant over time. To achieve this, an additional set of unknowns is introduced, namely $e_{(i,j)}$, indicating the length of the limb $(i,j) \in \mathcal{E}$ connecting joint i and joint j. Here, $\mathcal{E}$ represents the edges of the kinematic structure to estimate. To enforce constant limb lengths, the kinematic structure has to minimize the following error functional

$$E_{limb}(\mathbf{X}, \mathbf{e}) = \sum_t \sum_{(i,j) \in \mathcal{E}} \left(\|\mathbf{X}_i^t - \mathbf{X}_j^t\| - e_{(i,j)} \right)^2. \tag{1}$$

To enforce time continuity, a constant velocity model for each joint in the structure is deployed by forcing the second derivative of $\mathbf{X}_i^t$ to be small. Formally, this is expressed by

$$E_{smooth}(\mathbf{X}) = \sum_{t,i} \|\ddot{\mathbf{X}}_i^t\|^2, \tag{2}$$

where $\ddot{\mathbf{X}}_i^t$ is approximated by central finite differences.

Concerning the image observations, both optical flow and part-based detection scores are used. It is assumed that the motion of the kinematic structure is coherent with the measured optical flow in each camera. Moreover the position of each joint in each frame should project to a 2D image position having a high detector score for the corresponding joint. To this aim, optical flow is computed for each video stream, and the detection scores are computed for each joint and each frame in each video.

Optical flow was computed using the OpenCV implementation of the algorithm introduced by Farnebäck [32, 33]. An example is shown in Fig. 3. Let $OF_{c,t}$ (x,y) denote the optical flow measured in camera c at time t for a generic pixel (x,y), and let $\pi(\boldsymbol{\theta}_c, \mathbf{X})$ be the projection function mapping 3D points $\mathbf{X}$ to 2D image coordinates in camera c, specified by the calibration parameter $\boldsymbol{\theta}_c$. In order to force the motion of the kinematic structure to be consistent with the measured optical flow in each image, the following functional should be minimized

$$E_{OF}(\mathbf{X}, \boldsymbol{\theta}) = \sum_{c,t,i} \|OF_{c,t}(\pi(\boldsymbol{\theta}_c, \mathbf{X}_i^t)) - (\pi(\boldsymbol{\theta}_c, \mathbf{X}_i^{t+1}) - \pi(\boldsymbol{\theta}_c, \mathbf{X}_i^t))\|^2. \tag{3}$$

Let $Det_{c,t,i}(x,y)$ denote the detection probability for joint i measured in camera c at time t for a generic pixel (x,y). Probabilities $Det_{c,t,i}$ are computed using the sigmoid function and an SVM model trained on the 2D joint locations that were used to initialize the 3D points in Sect. 3.2 [34]. The feature vectors are constructed by concatenating HOG feature vectors [35] and color histogram feature vectors. HOG features are computed using cell size 8, block size 4 and a block overlap of 3. The color feature vectors are obtained by binning the HSV values of 25×25 patches independently into 8 bins per channel. After training, the SVM model is evaluated for all cameras and all images to obtain $Det_{c,t,i}$.

By applying the negative logarithm, probabilities $Det_{c,t,i}$ are transformed to negative log-probabilities. An example of the resulting detection scores for

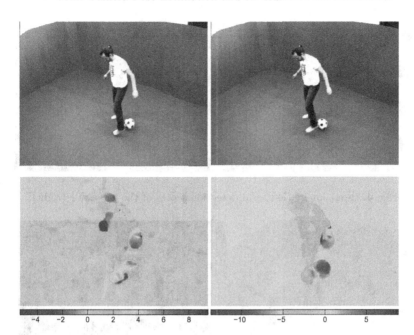

Fig. 3. Top row: two consecutive images from the Soccer Juggling sequence. Bottom row: optical flow in x-direction (left) and y-direction (right). The units of the color coding are given in pixels (Color figure online).

the left ankle is shown in Fig. 4. The values obtained by subsequently taking the square root are denoted as $\overline{Det}_{c,t,i}(x,y)$. To enforce the joint positions to be consistent with the trained detector, the following functional needs to be minimized:

$$E_{Det}(\mathbf{X},\boldsymbol{\theta}) = \sum_{c,t,i} \overline{Det}_{c,t,i}(\pi(\boldsymbol{\theta}_c,\mathbf{X}_i^t))^2. \tag{4}$$

In order to guide the optimization and in order not to digress too much from the initial solution, reprojected joints should be close to the joint positions that were used for initialization, if available. More formally,

$$E_{Rep}(\mathbf{X},\boldsymbol{\theta}) = \sum_{c,t,i} \nu_{c,i}^t L_\delta(\|\pi(\boldsymbol{\theta}_c,\mathbf{X}_i^t) - \mathbf{x}_{c,i}^t\|). \tag{5}$$

should be minimized. $\nu_{c,i}^t$ is a binary variable indicating whether joint i in camera c at time t was consistent with multiple cameras and hence used for initialization. To account for outliers, the robust Huber cost function L_δ is used [3]. The threshold δ was set to 5 pixels.

The final functional to minimize is a linear combination of the previously defined costs, i.e.,

$$\begin{aligned} E(\mathbf{X},\mathbf{e},\boldsymbol{\theta}) &= \lambda_1 E_{limb}(\mathbf{X},\mathbf{e}) + \lambda_2 E_{smooth}(\mathbf{X}) + \lambda_3 E_{OF}(\mathbf{X},\boldsymbol{\theta}) \\ &+ \lambda_4 E_{Det}(\mathbf{X},\boldsymbol{\theta}) + \lambda_5 E_{Rep}(\mathbf{X},\boldsymbol{\theta}) \end{aligned} \tag{6}$$

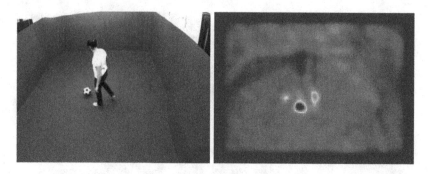

Fig. 4. Input image (left) and detection scores of the left ankle (right).

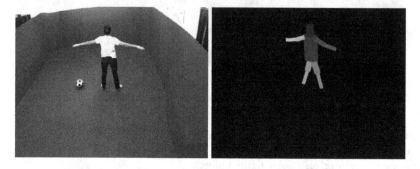

Fig. 5. The rendered 3D model of the human (right) and the corresponding image (left).

where the λ_i are constants defined to balance the influence of each term. For the experiments, the values λ_i were chosen in a grid search on the first 100 frames of the Soccer Juggling sequence [14] and kept constant for all experiments. Since the 3D reconstruction is only given up to scale, the torso of the person is set to a fixed length to ensure that $E(\mathbf{X}, \mathbf{e}, \boldsymbol{\theta})$ is not affected by scale changes of the 3D structure.

The optimization is carried out using the Levenberg-Marquardt algorithm. Taking advantage of the sparse structure of the Jacobian of E makes the optimization much more efficient. To account for occlusions in both Eqs. 3 and 4, a simple 3D model of a human is used, where every limb is modeled as a cylinder. By rendering the model in all images, it is easy to determine which joints are visible in which frames and in which cameras. Figure 5 shows an example of a rendered cylindrical model. Occluded joints are simply excluded from the sums in Eqs. 3 and 4.

The optimization iterates between the Levenberg-Marquardt algorithm and recomputing the visibility term. Figure 6 shows the final camera setup and an example pose for the INRIA dataset.

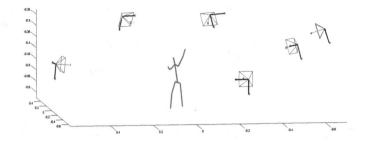

Fig. 6. Camera setup and 3D skeleton estimated for the INRA dancer dataset.

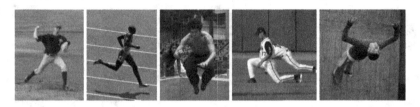

Fig. 7. Example training images of the LEEDS dataset.

4   Results

The presented approach was evaluated on 4 publicly available datasets, namely, the INRIA dancer dataset (201 frames, the first 6 cameras) [36], the HumanEva-II dataset (the first 500 frames, 4 cameras) [37], and the Soccer Juggling sequence (531 frames, 4 cameras) and the Sword Swing sequence (383 frames, 4 cameras), both from Ballan and Cortelazzo [14]. For all these datasets, a camera calibration is provided. The FMP model used in Sect. 3 was trained on the publicly available LEEDS sports dataset [38]. This model was then used for all experiments without any specific tuning. This shows that the presented method is general and applicable to a wide range of data. A few images from the LEEDS dataset are shown in Fig. 7.

The geometric verification of joints using the camera parameters provides a valuable confidence measure for estimated joint positions. Even though the 2D human pose estimates in the individual cameras are noisy and often incorrect, the presented method corrects many errors by using only joint positions verified by the geometry of the camera setup to create an initial guess of 3D joint positions. The final optimization further optimizes joint positions by fixing edge lengths, enforcing smooth motions and consistency with image measurements. A comparison of a few poses obtained from 2D human pose estimation and poses obtained by projecting optimized 3D poses can be found in Fig. 8.

Quantitative Evaluation. The presented approach was evaluated quantitatively in terms of camera pose estimation error and human pose estimation error. Table 1 illustrates the resulting positional distances between estimated

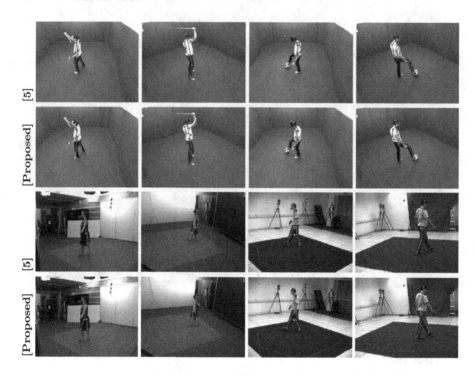

Fig. 8. Comparison with the baseline approach [5].

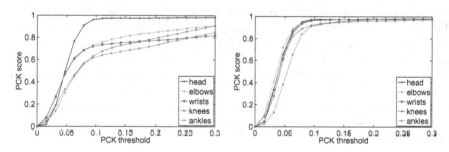

Fig. 9. PCK score obtained using the standard FMP model [5] (left), and the presented approach (right), on the Soccer Juggling dataset.

and groundtruth camera centers as well as the angular differences for the relative angles between all pairs of estimated cameras and all pairs of groundtruth cameras, respectively. The initial calibration obtained from Sect. 3 is compared with the calibration obtained from the final joint optimization of Sect. 3.

Since the presented method returns a 3D reconstruction up to a similarity transformation (rotation, translation and scale), the result needs to be aligned with the groundtruth for comparison. This was done by computing the global

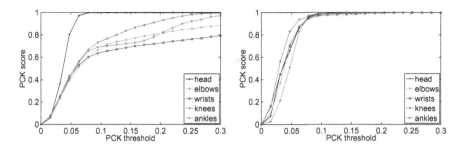

Fig. 10. PCK score obtained using the standard FMP model [5] (left), and the presented approach (right), on the Sword Swing dataset.

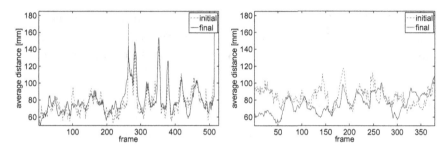

Fig. 11. Average per frame error of estimated 3D joint positions evaluated on the Soccer Juggling dataset (left), and on the Sword Swing dataset (right).

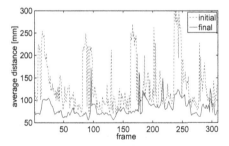

Fig. 12. Average per frame error of estimated 3D joint positions evaluated on the walking cycle of the HumanEva-II S4 dataset.

similarity transformation minimizing the squared distances between the ground-truth and the estimated camera centers.

Concerning the error in the human pose estimation, both 3D and 2D errors were evaluated for the Soccer Juggling and the Sword Swing dataset. The very good results obtained by Ballan and Cortelazzo were inspected visually and used as groundtruth [14]. In both cases, left/right flips of limbs were ignored

Table 1. Camera pose estimation error: average error ± standard deviation.

	Positional error [mm]		Angular error [deg]	
	initial	**final**	initial	**final**
Soccer Juggling	54 ± 11	**50 ± 13**	1.2 ± 0.7	**1.0 ± 0.5**
Sword Swing	71 ± 26	**58 ± 21**	0.9 ± 0.6	**1.0 ± 0.5**
INRIA	55 ± 13	**53 ± 13**	0.7 ± 0.5	**0.4 ± 0.3**
HumanEva-II	20 ± 7	**7 ± 2**	0.3 ± 0.2	**0.3 ± 0.3**

Table 2. 3D joint position estimation error: average error ± standard deviation [mm], on the Soccer Juggling dataset.

	Head	Elbows	Wrists	Knees	Ankles	Total
initial	68 ± 116	75 ± 119	87 ± 156	122 ± 129	115 ± 139	94 ± 127
final	**66 ± 115**	**79 ± 117**	**86 ± 154**	**123 ± 114**	**120 ± 144**	**96 ± 124**

Table 3. 3D joint position estimation error: average error ± standard deviation [mm], on the Sword Swing dataset.

	Head	Elbows	Wrists	Knees	Ankles	Total
initial	70 ± 19	93 ± 43	87 ± 51	69 ± 47	99 ± 43	84 ± 42
final	**34 ± 11**	**68 ± 38**	**64 ± 37**	**71 ± 34**	**94 ± 25**	**76 ± 41**

during the evaluation. The left arm was switched with the right arm, if the error decreased. The same holds for the legs.

To evaluate the 2D errors, 3D joint positions were projected into the images using the groundtruth camera calibration for the groundtruth 3D joint positions and the estimated camera calibration for the estimated 3D joint positions. To quantify the errors, the PCK measure introduced by Yang and Ramanan [5] was used. The PCK measure qualifies a detection as correct if the distance between the detected position and the groundtruth position is below $\alpha \max(w, h)$. w and h are the width and height of the axis-aligned bounding box containing all groundtruth joints in the respective image. Varying the PCK threshold α corresponds to varying the desired accuracy. PCK scores obtained by using the proposed approach are compared to the ones obtained by using the standard FMP approach [5]. The results for the Soccer Juggling dataset and the Sword Swing dataset are depicted in Figs. 9 and 10, respectively. While head positions are estimated accurately in both methods, the errors of the remaining body parts are decreased significantly by the presented method.

The average errors in 3D joint positions for the Soccer Juggling dataset and the Sword Swing dataset are given in Tables 2 and 3, respectively. A plot illustrating the average 3D joint position errors per frame is shown in Fig. 11. The aforementioned Tables 2 and 3 and Fig. 11 also compare the 3D joint positions obtained after the initialization with the ones obtained after the final optimization, described in Sects. 3.2 and 3.3. Especially for the Sword Swing dataset, the final optimization leads to a significant improvement of the 3D joint accuracy.

To evaluate the accuracy on the HumanEva-II dataset, the online evaluation tool has to be used [39]. For the S4 dataset, the walking cycle was evaluated (first 350 frames). The mean error over all joint positions after the final optimization was 82mm. To the best of knowledge, the state-of-the-art result for the walking cycle was obtained by Gall et al. By tracking a full 3D model of the person an error of 28mm was achieved [40]. A plot showing the average 3D joint position errors per frame is given in Fig. 12.

5 Conclusion

In this paper we presented a novel technique to calibrate a multi-camera setup by jointly estimating the extrinsic camera parameters and the 3D poses of a person in the scene, without relying on patch-based feature correspondences. 2D joint positions detected by 2D human pose estimation are used as higher level features to establish putative correspondences between cameras and to bootstrap the joint optimization of camera calibration and 3D poses. The final optimization takes advantage of the 3D articulated structure and temporal continuity and it enforces consistency with image measurements. The experimental evaluation on 4 publicly available datasets investigates the accuracy of the estimated camera poses and the 2D and 3D joint positions, showing the benefit of using the presented joint optimization.

Acknowledgements. This project is supported by a grant of CTI Switzerland, the 4DVideo ERC Starting Grant Nr. 210806 and the SNF Recording Studio Grant.

References

1. Lowe, D.G.: Distinctive image features from scale-invariant keypoints. Int. J. Comput. Vis. **60**(2), 91–110 (2004)
2. Bay, H., Ess, A., Tuytelaars, T., Gool, L.V.: Speeded-up robust features (surf). Comput. Vis. Image Underst. (CVIU) **110**, 356–359 (2008)
3. Hartley, R.I., Zisserman, A.: Multiple View Geometry in Computer Vision. Cambridge University Press, Cambridge (2000)
4. Ma, Y., Soatto, S., Kosecka, J., Sastry, S.S.: An Invitation to 3-D Vision. Springer, Heidelberg (2004)
5. Yang, Y., Ramanan, D.: Articulated human detection with flexible mixtures of parts. IEEE Trans. Pattern Anal. Mach. Intell. (PAMI) **35**, 2878–2890 (2013)
6. Andriluka, M., Roth, S., Schiele, B.: Pictorial structures revisited: people detection and articulated pose estimation. In: IEEE Conference on Computer Vision and Pattern Recognition (CVPR) (2009)
7. Amin, S., Andriluka, M., Rohrbach, M., Schiele, B.: Multi-view pictorial structures for 3D human pose estimation. In: Proceedings of the British Machine Vision Conference (BMVC) (2013)

8. Burenius, M., Sullivan, J., Carlsson, S.: 3D pictorial structures for multiple view articulated pose estimation. In: IEEE Conference on Computer Vision and Pattern Recognition (CVPR) (2013)
9. Belagiannis, V., Amin, S., Andriluka, M., Schiele, B., Navab, N., Ilic, S.: 3D pictorial structures for multiple human pose estimation. In: IEEE Conference on Computer Vision and Pattern Recognition (CVPR) (2014)
10. Ramanan, D., Forsyth, D.A., Zisserman, A.: Strike a pose: tracking people by finding stylized poses. In: IEEE Conference on Computer Vision and Pattern Recognition (CVPR) (2005)
11. Bregler, C., Malik, J.: Tracking people with twists and exponential maps. In: IEEE Conference on Computer Vision and Pattern Recognition (CVPR) (1998)
12. Salzmann, M., Urtasun, R.: Combining discriminative and generative methods for 3D deformable surface and articulated pose reconstruction. In: IEEE Conference on Computer Vision and Pattern Recognition (CVPR) (2010)
13. Sigal, L., Bhatia, S., Roth, S., Black, M., Isard, M.: Tracking loose-limbed people. In: IEEE Conference on Computer Vision and Pattern Recognition (CVPR) (2004)
14. Ballan, L., Cortelazzo, G.M.: Marker-less motion capture of skinned models in a four camera set-up using optical flow and silhouettes. In: International Symposium on 3D Data Processing, Visualization and Transmission (3DPVT) (2008)
15. Liu, Y., Stoll, C., Gall, J., Seidel, H.P., Theobalt, C.: Markerless motion capture of interacting characters using multi-view image segmentation. In: IEEE Conference on Computer Vision and Pattern Recognition (CVPR) (2011)
16. Ballan, L., Taneja, A., Gall, J., Van Gool, L., Pollefeys, M.: Motion capture of hands in action using discriminative salient points. In: Fitzgibbon, A., Lazebnik, S., Perona, P., Sato, Y., Schmid, C. (eds.) ECCV 2012, Part VI. LNCS, vol. 7577, pp. 640–653. Springer, Heidelberg (2012)
17. de La Gorce, M., Fleet, D., Paragios, N.: Model-based 3D hand pose estimation from monocular video. IEEE Trans. Pattern Anal. Mach. Intell. (PAMI) **76**, 231–243 (2011)
18. Hasler, N., Rosenhahn, B., Thormhlen, T., Wand, M., Gall, J., Seidel, H.P.: Markerless motion capture with unsynchronized moving cameras. In: IEEE Conference on Computer Vision and Pattern Recognition (CVPR) (2009)
19. Krahnstoever, N., Mendonca, P.: Bayesian autocalibration for surveillance. In: IEEE International Conference on Computer Vision (ICCV) (2005)
20. Lv, F., Zhao, T., Nevatia, R.: Camera calibration from video of a walking human. IEEE Trans. Pattern Anal. Mach. Intell. (PAMI) **28**, 1513–1518 (2006)
21. Chen, T., Del Bimbo, A., Pernici, F., Serra, G.: Accurate self-calibration of two cameras by observations of a moving person on a ground plane. In: IEEE Conference on Advanced Video and Signal Based Surveillance (AVSS) (2007)
22. Jaynes, C.: Multi-view calibration from planar motion for video surveillance. In: Second IEEE Workshop on Visual Surveillance (VS 1999) (1999)
23. Stein, G.P.: Tracking from multiple view points: Self-calibration of space and time. In: IEEE Conference on Computer Vision and Pattern Recognition (CVPR) (1999)
24. Bose, B., Grimson, E.: Ground plane rectification by tracking moving objects. In: IEEE International Workshop on Visual Surveillance and PETS (2004)
25. Meingast, M., Oh, S., Sastry, S.: Automatic camera network localization using object image tracks. In: IEEE International Conference on Computer Vision (ICCV) (2007)
26. Puwein, J., Ziegler, R., Ballan, L., Pollefeys, M.: PTZ camera network calibration from moving people in sports broadcasts. In: IEEE Workshop on Applications of Computer Vision (WACV) (2012)

27. Sinha, S., Pollefeys, M.: Camera network calibration and synchronization romsil-houettes in archived video. Int. J. Comput. Vis. **87**, 266–283 (2010)
28. Izo, T., Grimson, W.: Simultaneous pose estimation and camera calibration from multiple views. In: IEEE Conference on Computer Vision and Pattern Recognition Workshop (CVPRW) (2004)
29. Ye, G., Liu, Y., Hasler, N., Ji, X., Dai, Q., Theobalt, C.: Performance capture of interacting characters with handheld kinects. In: Fitzgibbon, A., Lazebnik, S., Perona, P., Sato, Y., Schmid, C. (eds.) ECCV 2012, Part II. LNCS, vol. 7573, pp. 828–841. Springer, Heidelberg (2012)
30. Fischler, M., Bolles, R.: Random sample consensus: a paradigm for model fitting with applications to image analysis and automated cartography. Commun. ACM **24**, 381–395 (1981)
31. Triggs, B., McLauchlan, P., Hartley, R., Fitzgibbon, A.: Bundle adjustment — a modern synthesis. In: Triggs, B., Zisserman, A., Szeliski, R. (eds.) Vision Algorithms 1999. LNCS, vol. 1883, pp. 298–372. Springer, Heidelberg (2000)
32. OpenCV. http://opencv.org/. Accessed 19 Aug 2014
33. Farnebäck, G.: Two-frame motion estimation based on polynomial expansion. In: Bigun, J., Gustavsson, T. (eds.) SCIA 2003. LNCS, vol. 2749, pp. 363–370. Springer, Heidelberg (2003)
34. Platt, J.C.: Probabilistic outputs for support vector machines and comparisons to regularized likelihood methods. In: Smola, A.J., Bartlett, P.L., Schölkopf, B., Schuurmans, D. (eds.) Advances in Large Margin Classifiers, pp. 61–74. MIT Press, Cambridge (2000)
35. Dalal, N., Triggs, B.: Histograms of oriented gradients for human detection. In: IEEE Conference on Computer Vision and Pattern Recognition (CVPR) (2005)
36. Inria: Inria dancer, 4D repository. http://4drepository.inrialpes.fr/public/datasets. Accessed 17 Jun 2014
37. Sigal, L., Balan, A., Black, M.: Humaneva: synchronized video and motion capture dataset and baseline algorithm for evaluation of articulated humanmotion. Int. J. Comput. Vis. **87**, 4–27 (2010)
38. Johnson, S., Everingham, M.: Clustered pose and nonlinear appearance models for human pose estimation. In: Proceedings of the British Machine Vision Conference (BMVC) (2010)
39. HumanEva. http://vision.cs.brown.edu/humaneva/. Accessed 19 Aug 2014
40. Gall, J., Rosenhahn, B., Brox, T., Seidel, H.P.: Optimization and filtering for human motion capture. Int. J. Comput. Vis. **87**, 75–92 (2010)

Singly-Bordered Block-Diagonal Form
for Minimal Problem Solvers

Zuzana Kukelova[1,2]([✉]), Martin Bujnak[3], Jan Heller[1], and Tomáš Pajdla[1]

[1] Czech Technical University in Prague, 166 27 Praha 6, Technická 2,
Prague, Czech Republic
a-zukuke@microsoft.com
[2] Microsoft Research Ltd., 21 Station Road, Cambridge CB1 2FB, UK
[3] Capturing Reality s.r.o., Bratislava, Slovakia

Abstract. The Gröbner basis method for solving systems of polynomial equations became very popular in the computer vision community as it helps to find fast and numerically stable solutions to difficult problems. In this paper, we present a method that potentially significantly speeds up Gröbner basis solvers. We show that the elimination template matrices used in these solvers are usually quite sparse and that by permuting the rows and columns they can be transformed into matrices with nice block-diagonal structure known as the singly-bordered block-diagonal (SBBD) form. The diagonal blocks of the SBBD matrices constitute independent subproblems and can therefore be solved, i.e. eliminated or factored, independently. The computational time can be further reduced on a parallel computer by distributing these blocks to different processors for parallel computation. The speedup is visible also for serial processing since we perform $O(n^3)$ Gauss-Jordan eliminations on smaller (usually two, approximately $\frac{n}{2} \times \frac{n}{2}$ and one $\frac{n}{3} \times \frac{n}{3}$) matrices. We propose to compute the SBBD form of the elimination template in the preprocessing offline phase using hypergraph partitioning. The final online Gröbner basis solver works directly with the permuted block-diagonal matrices and can be efficiently parallelized. We demonstrate the usefulness of the presented method by speeding up solvers of several important minimal computer vision problems.

1 Introduction

The Gröbner basis method for solving systems of polynomial equations was recently used to solve many important computer vision problems [2,3,7,19,24, 25]. This method became popular for creating efficient specific solvers to minimal problems and even an automatic generator for creating source codes of such minimal Gröbner basis solvers was proposed in [18].

Minimal solvers, such as the 5-point relative pose solver [22,25] or the P4Pf absolute pose solver [2], are often used inside a RANSAC [12] loop and are parts of large systems like SfM pipelines or recognition systems. Maximizing the efficiency of these solvers is therefore highly important.

© Springer International Publishing Switzerland 2015
D. Cremers et al. (Eds.): ACCV 2014, Part II, LNCS 9004, pp. 488–502, 2015.
DOI: 10.1007/978-3-319-16808-1_33

Gröbner basis solvers usually consist of two separate steps. In the first step Gauss-Jordan (G-J) elimination, QR, or LU decomposition of one or several matrices created using the so-called elimination templates [18] is performed. In the second step the solutions are extracted from the eigenvalues and eigenvectors of a multiplication (action) matrix [23].

Recently, several papers addressed the numerical stability and the speed of Gröbner basis solvers [4–6,8,18,21]. In [5,6,8], it has been shown that the numerical stability of Gröbner basis solvers can be improved by reordering columns in the elimination templates using QR or LU decompositions or by "basis extension". Several methods for reducing the size of the elimination templates in order to speed up the Gröbner basis solvers were presented in [18,21].

Most recently, two methods that speed up the second step of Gröbner basis solvers, i.e. the eigenvalue computations, were proposed in [4]. The first method is based on a modified matrix FGLM algorithm for transforming Gröbner bases and results in a single-variable polynomial which roots are efficiently computed only on a certain feasible interval using Sturm-sequences. The second method is based on fast calculation of the characteristic polynomial of an action matrix, again solved using Sturm-sequences. Both methods are in fact equivalent and can be used to significantly speed up the second step of Gröbner basis solvers.

In this paper, we present a method that can significantly speed up the first step of Gröbner basis solvers, i.e. G-J elimination, QR, or LU decomposition of matrices from the elimination templates. We observe that these elimination template matrices are usually quite sparse and by permuting the rows and the columns they can be transformed into matrices with an agreeable block-diagonal structure. The diagonal blocks of such permuted matrices constitute independent subproblems and as such can be solved, i.e. eliminated or factored, independently. The computational time can then be reduced on a parallel computer by distributing these blocks to different processors and by performing the computation in parallel. This speedup is also noticeable on single-threaded computers because $O(n^3)$ G-J eliminations on smaller (for the presented problems on two, approximately $\frac{n}{2} \times \frac{n}{2}$ and one $\frac{n}{3} \times \frac{n}{3}$) matrices is performed.

To obtain a reasonable speed-up, each block in the permuted matrix should contain comparable number of entries, i.e. some balance criterion should be maintained, and it should be as independent as possible from other blocks. For this purpose, we permute sparse rectangular matrices from the elimination templates into a singly-bordered block-diagonal (SBBD) form with minimum border size while maintaining a given balance criterion on the diagonal blocks.

The problem of permuting sparse matrices into SBBD form is usually formulated as hypergraph partitioning [1]. In this paper, we use state-of-the-art hypergraph partitioning tool PaToH [9] that uses multilevel hypergraph partitioning approaches based on Kernighan-Lin and Fiduccia-Mattheyses (KLFM) algorithms [11].

The use of row and column permutations to speed up computations is well-known in linear algebra and has been previously exploited in computer vision applications. For instance, in the bundle adjustment problem, one may transform the involved sparse matrices into arrowhead or block tridiagonal matrices [20,26]. However, such transformations are dependent on individual problem instances and therefore are not used widely in bundle adjustment.

On the other hand, in the proposed method the permutation of an elimination template matrix into SBBD form can be computed offline once for each type of minimal problem and applied to all instances. The final online Gröbner basis solvers work directly with the permuted block-diagonal matrices and can eliminate the diagonal blocks independently and perform the computations in parallel. Moreover, the proposed method can be used along with the methods from [4] that speed up the second step of Gröbner basis solvers.

We demonstrate the usefulness of the presented approach by speeding up solvers of several important minimal computer vision problems.

Next, we briefly describe the Gröbner basis method for solving systems of polynomial equations and the process of generating Gröbner basis solvers.

2   Gröbner Basis Method

Gröbner basis method for solving systems of polynomial equations became very popular in the computer vision community since it helps to find fast and numerically stable solutions to difficult problems.

Let

$$f_1(\mathbf{x}) = 0, \ldots, f_m(\mathbf{x}) = 0 \tag{1}$$

be a system of m polynomial equations in n unknowns $\mathbf{x} = (x_1, \ldots, x_n)$ that we want to solve and let this system have a finite number of solutions. The polynomials $f_1, \ldots, f_m$ define an *ideal* $I = \{\sum_{i=1}^{m} f_i \, h_i \mid h_i \in \mathbb{C}\,[x_1, \ldots, x_n]\}$, which is a set of all polynomials that can be generated as polynomial combinations of the initial polynomials $f_1, \ldots, f_m$. In general, an ideal can be generated by many different sets of generators which all share the same set of solutions. There is a special set of generators though, the reduced Gröbner basis w.r.t. the lexicographic ordering, which generates the ideal I but is easy (often trivial) to solve at the same time [10].

Unfortunately, computing the Gröbner basis w.r.t. the lexicographic ordering for larger systems of polynomial equations, and therefore for the most computer vision problems, is often not feasible.

Therefore, Gröbner basis solvers usually construct a Gröbner basis G under a different ordering, e.g. the graded reverse lexicographic (grevlex) ordering, which is often easier to compute. This Gröbner basis G is then used to construct a special multiplication matrix M_p [23], also called the "action matrix". Let A be the quotient ring $A = \mathbb{C}\,[x_1, \ldots, x_n]\,/I$ [10] and $B = \left\{\mathbf{x}^\alpha \mid \overline{\mathbf{x}^\alpha}^G = \mathbf{x}^\alpha\right\}$ its monomial basis, where $\mathbf{x}^\alpha = x_1^{\alpha_1} x_2^{\alpha_2} \ldots x_n^{\alpha_n}$ and $\overline{\mathbf{x}^\alpha}^G$ is the remainder of $\mathbf{x}^\alpha$ after the division by a Gröbner basis G. Then the action matrix M_p is the matrix of a linear operator $T_p \colon A \to A$ performing multiplication by a suitably chosen polynomial p in A w.r.t. the basis B.

The action matrix M_p can be viewed as a generalization of the companion matrix used in solving one polynomial equation in one unknown [10], since the solutions to our system of polynomial equations (1) can be obtained from the eigenvalues and eigenvectors of this action matrix.

3   Gröbner Basis Solvers

Many polynomial problems in computer vision share the convenient property that the monomials which appear in the set of initial polynomials (1) are, up to the concrete coefficients arising from non-degenerate image measurements, always identical. Thanks to this property, it is not necessary to use general algorithms [10] for computing Gröbner bases for solving these problems. Usually, specific Gröbner basis solvers that can efficiently solve all non-degenerate instances of a given problem are used in computer vision.

The process of creating these specific Gröbner basis solvers consist of two different phases. In the first "offline" phase, so-called "elimination templates" are found. These templates say which input polynomials should be multiplied with which monomials and then eliminated to obtain all polynomials from the grevlex Gröbner basis or at least all polynomials necessary for constructing an action matrix. For a one concrete problem, this phase is performed only once.

The second "online" phase consists of two steps. In the first step, the precomputed elimination templates are filled with specific coefficients arising from image measurements and eliminated using G-J elimination to construct the action matrix. Then, eigenvalues and eigenvectors of this action matrix are used to find solutions to the initial polynomial equations.

It was shown in [4], that the second step of the online solver can be sped up by replacing the eigenvalue computations with the computations of the characteristic polynomial of the action matrix and by efficiently finding roots of this polynomial using Sturm-sequences.

In this paper, we will show that at the cost of some preprocessing performed in the offline phase we can significantly speed up also the first step of online Gröbner basis solvers, i.e., G-J elimination, QR, or LU decomposition of matrices from the elimination templates.

Elimination templates are created in the offline phase by multiplying initial polynomials with monomials. Since we are multiplying polynomials by monomials only, the new generated polynomials have the same number of monomials as the polynomials from which they are created.

In the matrix representation of polynomials that is used in the elimination template, the rows of the matrix correspond to the individual polynomials and the columns to the monomials. This means that we are effectively only shifting the coefficients in this matrix when generating a new polynomial by multiplying some initial polynomial f_i by a monomial. A new row that corresponds to the new polynomial contains the same entries as the row corresponding to f_i, but in different columns. Therefore, the elimination template matrices are usually quite sparse. We will show that in these situations we can permute the rows and the columns of these matrices in the preprocessing offline phase and in this way create matrices that have a nice block-diagonal structure known as the singly-bordered block diagonal (SBBD) form. The diagonal blocks of such SBBD matrices can then be eliminated or factored using LU or QR decomposition independently. The computational time can be significantly reduced by distributing these blocks to different processors and by performing the computations in parallel. Moreover, there is speedup from approximately n^3 to $(k+1) \cdot \left(\frac{n}{k}\right)^3$, even for serial processing of an SBBD matrix with k well balanced blocks.

Since the permutation matrices that transform the elimination template matrix to the SBBD form are computed in the offline phase, the time spent computing these permutation matrices doesn't influence the speed of the final online solver. Moreover, the computational cost of finding the permutation matrices (for the presented solvers less than 0.1 s) is comparable or even lower than the computational time of the remaining steps of the offline phase.

4   Sparse Matrix Partitioning

In this section, we describe the singly-bordered block-diagonal form and the way how to transform a given matrix to this form.

4.1   Singly-Bordered Block-Diagonal Form

Our goal is to permute the rows and the columns of an $m \times n$ sparse matrix $\mathbf{A}$ into a k-way singly-bordered block-diagonal form

$$
\mathbf{A}_{SB} = \mathbf{P}_r \mathbf{A} \mathbf{P}_c^\top =
\begin{bmatrix}
\mathbf{A}_{11} & & & & \mathbf{B}_1 \\
& \mathbf{A}_{22} & & & \mathbf{B}_2 \\
& & \ddots & & \vdots \\
& & & \mathbf{A}_{kk} & \mathbf{B}_k
\end{bmatrix},
\tag{2}
$$

where $\mathbf{P}_r$ and $\mathbf{P}_c$ are, respectively, the row and the column permutation matrices to be determined, k is the pre-defined number of blocks, $\mathbf{A}_{11}, \dots, \mathbf{A}_{kk}$ are rectangular matrices and $\mathbf{B} = \left(\mathbf{B}_1^\top \dots \mathbf{B}_k^\top\right)^\top$ is $m \times n_c$ border submatrix. Columns of $\mathbf{B}$ are sometimes called the coupling columns.

In our case, we want to permute matrix $\mathbf{A}$ into an SBBD form $\mathbf{A}_{SB}$ (2) such that the number of coupling columns n_c is minimized while a given balanced criterion is satisfied, i.e. each block $\mathbf{A}_{jj}$, $j = 1, \dots, k$ of the permuted matrix $\mathbf{A}_{SB}$ contains comparable number of entries.

Using hypergraph model for sparse matrices, the problem of permuting a sparse matrix to SBBD form (2) reduces to the well-known hypergraph partitioning problem [1].

Next, we describe hypergraphs and hypergraph partitioning to a level pertinent to this work.

4.2 Hypergraph Partitioning

A hypergraph $\mathcal{H} = (\mathcal{V}, \mathcal{N})$ is defined as a set of vertices $\mathcal{V}$ and a set of nets (or hyperedges) $\mathcal{N}$, where every net $n_i \in \mathcal{N}$ is a subset of vertices, i.e. $n_i \subseteq \mathcal{V}$.

Definition 1. *Given a hypergraph $\mathcal{H} = (\mathcal{V}, \mathcal{N})$, $\Pi = \{\mathcal{V}_1, \ldots, \mathcal{V}_k\}$ is a k-way partition of $\mathcal{H}$, if the following holds:*

1. *$\mathcal{V}_j \neq \emptyset$, $\mathcal{V}_j \subseteq \mathcal{V}$, for $1 \leq j \leq k$, i.e. each part $\mathcal{V}_j$ is nonempty subset of $\mathcal{V}$,*
2. *$\mathcal{V}_i \cap \mathcal{V}_j = \emptyset$ for all $1 \leq i \leq j \leq k$, i.e. parts are pairwise disjoint,*
3. *$\bigcup_{j=1}^{k} \mathcal{V}_j = \mathcal{V}$, i.e. the union of all k parts is equal to $\mathcal{V}$.*

As in the case of graphs, we can associate weights with hypergraph vertices. Let us denote $w(v)$ the weight associated with a vertex v. Now, we can define the weight of a set of vertices $\mathcal{S}$ as

$$W(\mathcal{S}) = \sum_{v \in \mathcal{S}} w(v). \tag{3}$$

The partition $\Pi = \{\mathcal{V}_1, \ldots, \mathcal{V}_k\}$ is said to be *balanced* for a given $\epsilon \geq 0$, if each part $\mathcal{V}_j$ satisfies the balance criterion

$$\frac{W(\mathcal{V}_j)}{W_{avg}} \leq 1 + \epsilon, \; j = 1, \ldots, k, \tag{4}$$

where $W(\mathcal{V}_j)$ is the weight (3) of a part $\mathcal{V}_j$ and $W_{avg} = \frac{W(\mathcal{V})}{k}$.

Let $\mathcal{N}_S$ be the set of all nets (hyperedges) that connect more than one part of a partition Π in $\mathcal{H}$. This means that all nets $n_j \in \mathcal{N}_S$ have at least one vertex in more than one part $\mathcal{V}_i \in \Pi$. Such nets $n_j \in \mathcal{N}_S$ are called *cuts* or *external nets*.

Nets that connect only one part $\mathcal{V}_i \in \Pi$, i.e. they have all vertices in this part, are called *internal nets* of part $\mathcal{V}_i$. Let us denote the set of all internal nets of a part $\mathcal{V}_i$ as $\mathcal{N}_i$, $i = 1, \ldots, k$. Then, the k-way partition $\Pi = \{\mathcal{V}_1, \ldots, \mathcal{V}_k\}$ that is defined on the vertex set $\mathcal{V}$ can also be considered as a $(k+1)$-way partition $\Pi = \{\mathcal{N}_1, \ldots, \mathcal{N}_k; \mathcal{N}_S\}$ on the net set $\mathcal{N}$. The set $\mathcal{N}_S$ can be considered as a net separator whose removal gives k disconnected vetrex parts $\mathcal{V}_1, \ldots, \mathcal{V}_k$ as well as k disconnected net parts $\mathcal{N}_1, \ldots, \mathcal{N}_k$.

The goal of partitioning is to minimize a cost function called *cutsize* defined over the external nets $\mathcal{N}_S$. Let $c(n)$ denote the cost associated with the net $n \in \mathcal{N}$. Then a cost function can be defined as

$$\chi(\Pi) = \sum_{n_j \in \mathcal{N}_S} c(n_j). \tag{5}$$

In our problem of transforming a matrix to an SBBD form all nets have unit costs, i.e., $c(n) = 1$ for all $n \in \mathcal{N}$ and therefore the cost function has very simple form

$$\chi(\Pi) = \sum_{n_j \in \mathcal{N}_S} 1 = |\mathcal{N}_S|. \tag{6}$$

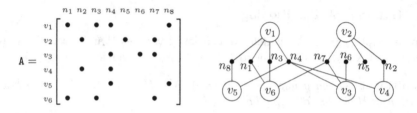

Fig. 1. A 6×8 matrix A (Left) and its column-net hypergraph representation (Right); symbol "•" represents a nonzero entry of the matrix A.

The hypergraph partitioning problem can be defined as a problem of dividing vertex set $\mathcal{V}$ of a hypergraph $\mathcal{H}$ into k parts, i.e. a problem of finding a k-way partition $\Pi = \{V_1, \ldots, V_k\}$, such that the cost (5) is minimized while the balance criterion (4) is fulfilled for a given ϵ:

$$\text{Given } \mathcal{H} = (\mathcal{V}, \mathcal{N}), \epsilon,$$
$$\text{find } \Pi = \arg\min \sum_{n_j \in \mathcal{N}_S} c(n_j),$$
$$\Pi = \{V_1, \ldots, V_k\} = \{\mathcal{N}_1, \ldots, \mathcal{N}_k; \mathcal{N}_S\}$$
$$\text{subject to } \frac{W(\cdot, \mathcal{V}_j)}{W_{avg}} \leq 1 + \epsilon, \ j = 1, \ldots, k.$$

Unfortunately, the hypergraph partitioning problem is known to be NP-hard [13].

4.3   Matrix Partitioning

An $m \times n$ matrix $A = (a_{ij})$ can be represented as a hypergraph $\mathcal{H}_A = (\mathcal{V}, \mathcal{N})$. In the column-net hypergraph model, $\mathcal{H}_A$ contains m vertices and n nets (hyperedges), i.e. there exists one vertex $v_i \in \mathcal{V}$ for each row i of A and one net $n_j \in \mathcal{N}$ for each column j of A. In this model, the net $n_j \subseteq V$ contains vertices corresponding to the rows that have nonzero entry in column j, i.e. $v_i \in n_j$ if and only if $a_{ij} \neq 0$. This means that the degree of the vertex v_i is equal to the number of nonzero entries in row i of A and the size of the net n_j is equal to the number of nonzero entries in column j of A.

Figure 1(Left) shows an example of a 6×8 matrix A and its column-net hypergraph representation (Right).

Using the hypergraph representation of the matrix A, the problem of transforming A to SBBD form A_{SB} (2) can be cast as a hypergraph partitioning problem in which the cost (6) is equal to the number of coupling columns n_c in A_{SB}. This claim can be formalized as theorem [1]:

Theorem 1. *Let $\mathcal{H}_A = (\mathcal{V}, \mathcal{N})$ be the hypergraph representation of the matrix A. A k-way partition $\Pi = \{V_1, \ldots, V_k\} = \{\mathcal{N}_1, \ldots, \mathcal{N}_k; \mathcal{N}_S\}$ of $\mathcal{H}_A$ gives a permutation of A to SBBD form A_{SB} (2), where vertices in $\mathcal{V}_i$ represent the rows and the internal nets in $\mathcal{N}_i$ the columns of the ith diagonal block of A_{SB}, and external nets in $\mathcal{N}_S$ represent the coupling columns of A_{SB}. Therefore,*

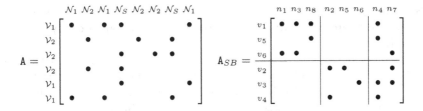

Fig. 2. (Left) 2-way partitioning $\Pi = \{\mathcal{V}_1, \mathcal{V}_2\} = \{\mathcal{N}_1, \mathcal{N}_2; \mathcal{N}_S\}$ of $\mathcal{H}_A$. (Right) SBBD form A_{SB} of A induced by Π.

– *minimizing the cutsize (6) minimizes the number of coupling columns, and*
– *if the criterion (4) is satisfied, then the diagonal submatrices are balanced.*

Figure 2(Left) shows a 2-way partitioning $\Pi = \{\mathcal{V}_1, \mathcal{V}_2\} = \{\mathcal{N}_1, \mathcal{N}_2; \mathcal{N}_S\}$ of the matrix $\mathcal{H}_A$ from Fig. 1 and its SBBD form A_{SB} induced by Π (Right).

5 Experiments

To demonstrate the usefulness of the presented approach, we used this method to speed up solvers of three important minimal relative and absolute pose problems. Even though these problems have been previously solved using the Gröbner basis method [18], the large elimination templates connected with these problems made the respective solvers relatively slow.

For each of these Gröbner basis solvers, we have precomputed the permutation matrices that transform the elimination template matrix into an SBBD form. We have formulated the problem of permuting the sparse matrix into an SBBD form as the hypergraph partitioning problem (see Sect. 4.3) and we have used the state-of-the-art hypergraph partitioning tool PaToH [9] to solve this problem. From PaToH, we have received the permutation matrices that we have used to permute the rows and the columns of the matrix from the elimination template.

Since PaToH uses heuristics for solving the hypergraph partitioning and each time returns a slightly different result, we have run this partitioning tool several times for every elimination template matrix. We have obtained reasonable and stable partitions from PaToH for all tested minimal solvers. In all PaToH runs, for the same elimination template matrix, PaToH returned very similar results with a similar number of coupling columns (± 5). We have selected the "best partitioning" as the partitioning with the smallest number of coupling columns (border) among all runs. For each problem, we have computed the permutation matrices only once in the preprocessing offline phase.

The difference between the new online Gröbner basis solvers and the original Gröbner basis solvers is that the new solvers work directly with the permuted block-diagonal matrices and therefore perform smaller G-J eliminations and moreover can be parallelized.

Since the numerical stability of the new solvers is similar to the numerical stability of the state-of-the-art solvers, in this section, we compare only the speed of the solvers.

Further, because all of the solvers are algebraically equivalent, we have evaluated them on synthetic noise free data only. In our experiments and performance tests, we executed each algorithm 10 K times on synthetically generated data. All scenes in these experiments were generated using 3D points randomly distributed in a 3D cube. Each 3D point was projected by cameras with random yet feasible orientations and positions and with random or fixed focal lengths. In the case of radial distortion problems, radial distortion generated by one-parameter division model was added to all image points to generate noiseless distorted points.

Next, we describe three minimal problems, the existing Gröbner basis solvers as well as the new SBBD solutions we based on these solvers, and the gained speed-up.

5.1   9-Point Relative Pose Different Radial Distortion Problem

Omnidirectional cameras and wide angle lenses are often used in computer vision applications. In fact, not only wide angle lenses but virtually all consumer camera lenses suffer from some amount of radial distortion. Ignoring this type of distortion, even for standard cameras, may lead to significant errors in 3D reconstruction, metric image measurements, or in camera calibration.

The first problem that we have studied is the problem of simultaneous estimation of the fundamental matrix and two radial distortion parameters for two uncalibrated cameras with different radial distortions from nine image point correspondences. This problem is useful in applications where images of one scene have been taken by two different cameras, for example by a standard digital camera and by a camera with a wide angle lens or by an omnidirectional camera.

This 9-point distortion problem can be after some manipulation of equations formulated as a system of four equations in four unknowns. Several Gröbner basis solutions to this problem exist [18,19]. The solution [18] which results in the smallest elimination template, performs G-J elimination of a 179×203 matrix and extracts 24 solutions from the eigenvalues and eigenvectors of a 24×24 action matrix.

The large 179×203 elimination template matrix makes the 9-point distortion solver [18] relatively slow and not very useful in real applications. However, we will show that this elimination template matrix can be transformed to a matrix in SBBD form and therefore the computational time of G-J elimination can be significantly reduced.

SBBD Form. For the 9-point distortion solver, as well as for the two remaining studied minimal solvers, we have obtained the best results, i.e. the smallest number of the coupling columns and a well balanced blocks in SBBD matrix (2), for two blocks.

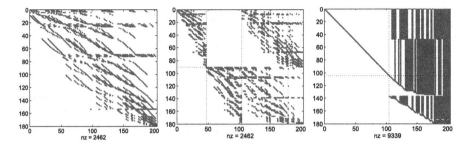

Fig. 3. 9-point radial distortion problem: (Left) the input 179×203 elimination template matrix. (Center) The SBBD form of this matrix found by PaToh for $k = 2$. The black dash-dot lines separate the independent blocks and the coupling columns with the red dash-dot line separating the last 24 basis columns. (Right) A matrix obtained after two independent G-J eliminations of the two blocks of A_{SB}.

First, we have removed the last 24 columns of the 179×203 elimination template matrix M from the state-of-the-art solver [18]. These columns correspond to the basis B of the quotient ring $A = \mathbb{C}\left[x_1, ..., x_n\right] / I$ and should not be permuted and eliminated. Then, we have used the square 179×179 matrix as the input to the hypergraph partitioning tool PaToH [9]. We set the weights to 1 and the PaToH imbalance ratio to 3 %. These are the deafult values for PaToH and worked well for all studied solvers.

Figure 3 shows the input 179×203 elimination template matrix (Left) and its SBBD form found by PaToh for $k = 2$ (Center). In this case, the size of the first block A_{11} in A_{SB} (2) is 90×47, the size of the second block A_{22} is 89×57 and the number of the coupling columns n_c together with the 24 basis columns is 99. The diagonal block matrices A_{11} and A_{22} are independent and can be therefore eliminated separately.

Figure 3(Right) shows the matrix M_r that we have obtained after two separate G-J eliminations of the rows of A_{SB} that correspond to A_{11} and A_{22}. In this case, we have permuted the eliminated rows such that the identity matrix is at the top left corner.

After performing these two separate eliminations, it is sufficient to perform G-J elimination of the bottom right 75×99 submatrix of M_r. It is not necessary to eliminate all rows of M_r above this bottom submatrix. To create the action matrix, we only need four from the first 104 rows and therefore it is sufficient to eliminate only these four rows from the top 104 rows of M_r.

5.2   P4P+f Problem

The second problem is the problem of estimating the absolute pose of a camera with unknown focal length from four 2D-3D point correspondences. This problem results in five equations in four unknowns and has ten solutions [2]. The P4P+f problem is very important in real Structure-from-Motion pipelines and therefore the efficiency of its solver is crucial.

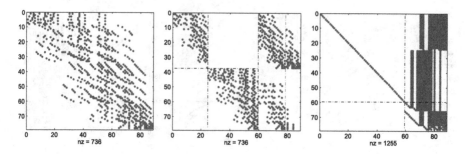

Fig. 4. P4P+f problem: (Left) the input 78×88 elimination template matrix. (Center) The SBBD form of this matrix found by PaToh for $k = 2$. The black dash-dot lines separate the independent blocks and the coupling columns and the red dash-dot line separate the last 10 basis columns. (Right) A matrix obtained after two independent G-J eliminations of the two blocks of A_{SB}.

As the basis of our method we have used the state-of-the art P4P+f solver downloaded from the webpage [16]. This solver performs G-J elimination of an 78×88 elimination template matrix and extracts solutions from a 10×10 action matrix.

SBBD Form. For the P4P+f solver, we have precomputed in the offline phase the 2-block SBBD form A_{SB} (2) of its 78×88 elimination template matrix. As for the 9-point distortion problem, we have fixed the last 10 columns that correspond to the basis B of the quotient ring A and run PaToH on a square 78×78 matrix.

Figure 4 shows the input 78×88 elimination template matrix of the P4P+f solver (Left) and its SBBD form A_{SB} found by PaToh for $k = 2$ (Center). In this case, we have obtained nice blocks of size 37×24 and 41×35, and a relatively small number of coupling columns $n_c = 19$. This means that together with 10 basis columns we have obtained a border of size 29.

Figure 4(Right) shows the matrix M_r which we have obtained after two separate G-J eliminations of the first 37 and the last 41 rows of the SBBD matrix A_{SB}. We have again permuted the eliminated rows such that the identity matrix is in the top left corner.

After performing the two independent eliminations, it is sufficient to perform G-J elimination of the bottom right 19×29 submatrix of M_r. Again, it is not necessary to eliminate all rows of M_r above this submatrix. To create the action matrix, it is sufficient to eliminate only four rows from the top 59 rows of M_r.

5.3   P4P+f+r problem

The last problem that we have solved is the problem of estimating the absolute pose of a camera with unknown focal length and unknown radial distortion from four 2D-3D point correspondences. As shown in [15], the consideration of radial

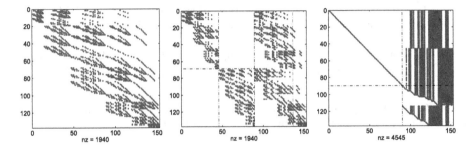

Fig. 5. P4P+f+r problem: (Left) the input 136 × 152 elimination template matrix. (Center) The SBBD form of this matrix found using PaToh for $k = 2$. The black dash-dot lines separate the independent blocks and the coupling columns, the red dash-dot line separates the last 16 basis columns. (Right) A matrix obtained after two independent G-J eliminations of the two blocks of A_{SB}.

distortion in absolute pose solvers may bring a significant improvement in many real world applications. The general formulation of this problem [15] results in five equations in five unknowns and in a quite large and impractical solver (a 1134 × 720 matrix) with 24 solutions. The final solver runs in about 70 ms.

A more practical solution to the P4P+f+r problem was proposed in [3]. By decomposing the problem into a nonplanar and planar cases, much simpler and efficient solvers were obtained. The planar solver is quite simple and performs G-J elimination of a 12 × 18 matrix. The solution to the non-planar case requires to perform G-J elimination of a 136×152 matrix and the eigenvalue computation of a 16 × 16 matrix. The non-planar solver from [3] was used as the input of our new method.

SBBD Form. The non-planar P4P+f+r solver [3] has 16 solutions. We have first reordered the columns of the 136 × 152 elimination template matrix of this solver, such that the columns corresponding to the 16 dimensional basis B of the quotient ring A were at the end of this matrix. Then, we have fixed these last 16 columns and executed the hypergraph partitioning tool PaToH [9] on the square 136 × 136 matrix. Again, we have set the weights to 1, the number of required blocks to 2, and the imbalance ratio to 3 %.

The input 136 × 152 elimination template matrix for the P4P+f+r solver can be seen in Fig. 5(Left) and its SBBD form A_{SB} found by PaToH for $k = 2$ in Fig. 5(Center). In this SBBD matrix A_{SB}, the size of the first block A_{11} is 68 × 45, the size of the second block A_{22} is 68 × 44, and the number of the coupling columns n_c together with the 16 fixed basis columns is 63.

Figure 5 (Right) shows the matrix M_r that has been obtained after two separate G-J eliminations of the first 68 and the last 68 rows of the SBBD matrix A_{SB} and after the permutation of the eliminated rows such that the identity matrix is at the top left corner. Again, these two blocks can be eliminated independently.

Table 1. Speed comparison of G-J eliminations of the original and the SBBD elimination template matrices for the three considered minimal problems.

9pt orig	9pt SBBD	P4P+f orig	P4P+f SBBD	P4P+f+r orig	P4P+f+r SBBD
932.9 μs	186.8 μs	58.7 μs	18.6 μs	320.8 μs	106.2 μs

Table 2. Speed comparison of sparse G-J eliminations of the original and the SBBD elimination template matrices for the three considered minimal problems.

9pt orig	9pt SBBD	P4P+f orig	P4P+f SBBD	P4P+f+r orig	P4P+f+r SBBD
362.8 μs	180.6 μs	23.1 μs	12.1 μs	116.2 μs	68.3 μs

After performing these two independent eliminations it is sufficient to perform G-J elimination of the bottom right 47×63 submatrix of M_r. In this case, we need the eight of the first 89 rows to create the action matrix. Therefore, in the final step it sufficient only to eliminate these eight rows from the top 89 rows of M_r.

5.4 Speedup

In our experiments we focused on the achieved speedup in the first step of the considered Gröbner basis solvers, i.e. the G-J elimination of the elimination template matrices. We reimplemented all state-of-the art solvers in C++ and used the same math libraries in all tests. In the second step of all Gröbner basis solvers, we used standard eigenvalue method [18] to find the solutions to the problem.

The second step of the Gröbner basis solvers can be sped up by replacing the eigenvalue computations with the characteristic polynomial method and Sturm sequences presented in [4]. However, the characteristic polynomial method [4] is independent from the method presented in this paper, i.e. the method from [18] speeds up a different part of Gröbner basis solvers, and therefore we didn't consider it in our experiments. The new SBBD method and the characteristic polynomial method [4] can be used concurrently to obtain final efficient solvers.

All tests were performed on an Intel i7-4700MQ 2.4 Ghz based laptop.

Table 1 shows the speed comparison of G-J eliminations of the original and the SBBD elimination template matrices for the three considered minimal problems. In this case we were not exploiting the sparsity of matrices in G-J elimination. We can see that for the 9pt radial distortion solver we have achieved almost 5× speed up, and for the P4P+f solver and the P4P+f+r solver more than 3× speed ups.

Table 2 shows the same speed comparison, however, in this case for sparse G-J eliminations. We can see that the speed ups are slightly smaller. This is caused by the fact that the original elimination template matrices have sparser structure than the submatrices used in the SBBD solvers.

Note that in the case of the 9pt SBBD solver there is almost no difference in running times between sparse and general G-J eliminations. This is caused by high fill-in of matrices that appear in this SBBD solver.

6 Conclusion

In this paper, we have shown that the elimination template matrices used in popular Gröbner basis solvers are usually quite sparse and that by permuting their rows and columns can be transformed into matrices with a nice block-diagonal structure known as the singly-bordered block-diagonal (SBBD) form. The permutation of an elimination template matrix into the SBBD form can be computed in the preprocessing offline phase using hypergraph partitioning. Therefore, the time for finding the permutation matrices doesn't influence the speed of the final online Gröbner basis solver.

The final online Gröbner basis solver works directly with the permuted SBBD matrices. The computational cost of the first step of these Gröbner basis solvers is significantly reduced since we perform $O(n^3)$ G-J eliminations on smaller (for the presented solvers usually two approximately $\frac{n}{2} \times \frac{n}{2}$ and one $\frac{n}{3} \times \frac{n}{3}$) matrices. Moreover, two of these three G-J eliminations can be performed independently and therefore parallelized. We have demonstrate the usefulness of the presented method by speeding up several important minimal computer vision solvers.

Acknowledgement. This work has been supported by the EC under project PRo-ViDE FP7-SPACE-2012-312377.

References

1. Aykanat, C., Pinar, A., Catalyurek, U.V.: Permuting sparse rectangular matrices into block-diagonal form. SIAM J. Scientific Comput. 12/2002 (2002)
2. Bujnak, M., Kukelova, Z., Pajdla, T.: A general solution to the P4P problem for camera with unknown focal length. In: CVPR (2008)
3. Bujnak, M., Kukelova, Z., Pajdla, T.: New efficient solution to the absolute pose problem for camera with unknown focal length and radial distortion. In: Kimmel, R., Klette, R., Sugimoto, A. (eds.) ACCV 2010, Part I. LNCS, vol. 6492, pp. 11–24. Springer, Heidelberg (2011)
4. Bujnak, M., Kukelova, Z., Pajdla, T.: Making minimal solvers fast. In: CVPR (2008)
5. Byröd, M., Josephson, K., Åström, K.: Improving numerical accuracy of Gröbner basis polynomial equation solver. In: ICCV (2007)
6. Byröd, M., Josephson, K., Åström, K.: A column-pivoting based strategy for monomial ordering in numerical Gröbner basis calculations. In: Forsyth, D., Torr, P., Zisserman, A. (eds.) ECCV 2008, Part IV. LNCS, vol. 5305, pp. 130–143. Springer, Heidelberg (2008)
7. Byröd, M., Brown, M., Åström, K.: Minimal solutions for panoramic stitching with radial distortion. In: BMVC (2009)

8. Byröd, M.: Numerical methods for geometric vision: From minimal to large scale problems. Ph.D. Thesis, Centre for Mathematical Sciences, Lund University (2010)
9. Catalyurek, U.V., Aykanat, C.: PaToH: Partitioning Tool for Hypergraphs, Version 3.1 (2011)
10. Cox, D., Little, J., O'Shea, D.: Using Algebraic Geometry, vol. 185, 2nd edn. Springer, Berlin, Heidelberg, New York (2005)
11. Fiduccia, C.M., Mattheyses, R.M.: A linear-time heuristic for improving network partitions. In: 19th ACM/IEEE Design Automation Conference (1982)
12. Fischler, M.A., Bolles, R.C.: Random Sample Consensus: A paradigm for model fitting with applications to image analysis and automated cartography. Comm. ACM **24**(6), 381–395 (1981)
13. Garey, M., Johnson, D., Stockmeyer, L.: Some simplified NP-complete graph problems. Theor. Comput. Sci. **1**, 237–267 (1976)
14. Hook, D., McAree, P.: Using sturm sequences to bracket real roots of polynomial equations. In: Graphic Gems I, pp. 416–423. Academic Press (1990)
15. Josephson, K., Byröd, M.: Pose estimation with radial distortion and unknown focal length. In: CVPR 2009 (2009)
16. http://cmp.felk.cvut.cz/minimal/
17. Kuehnle, K., Mayr, E.: Exponential space computation of Groebner bases. In: Proceedings of ISSAC. ACM (1996)
18. Kukelova, Z., Bujnak, M., Pajdla, T.: Automatic generator of minimal problem solvers. In: Forsyth, D., Torr, P., Zisserman, A. (eds.) ECCV 2008, Part III. LNCS, vol. 5304, pp. 302–315. Springer, Heidelberg (2008)
19. Kukelova, Z., Byröd, M., Josephson, K., Pajdla, T., Åström, K.: Fast and robust numerical solutions to minimal problems for cameras with radial distortion. Comput. Vis. Image Underst. **114**(2), 234–244 (2010)
20. Kushal, A., Agarwal, S.: Visibility based preconditioning for bundle adjustment. In: CVPR 2012
21. Naroditsky, O., Daniilidis, K.: Optimizing polynomial solvers for minimal geometry problems. In: ICCV 2011
22. Nister, D.: An efficient solution to the five-point relative pose. IEEE PAMI **26**(6), 756–770 (2004)
23. Stetter, H.J.: Numerical Polynomial Algebra. SIAM, Philadelphia (2004)
24. Stewenius, H., Nister, D., Kahl, F., Schaffalitzky, F.: A minimal solution for relative pose with unknown focal length. In: CVPR 2005
25. Stewenius, H., Engels, C., Nister, D.: Recent developments on direct relative orientation. ISPRS J. Photogrammetry Remote Sens. **60**, 284–294 (2006)
26. Triggs, B., McLauchlan, P.F., Hartley, R.I., Fitzgibbon, A.W.: Bundle adjustment – A modern synthesis. In: Triggs, B., Zisserman, A., Szeliski, R. (eds.) ICCV-WS 1999. LNCS, vol. 1883, pp. 298–375. Springer, Heidelberg (2000)

Stereo Fusion Using a Refractive Medium on a Binocular Base

Seung-Hwan Baek and Min H. Kim$^{(\boxtimes)}$

KAIST, Daejeon, Korea
{shwbaek,minhkim}@vclab.kaist.ac.kr

Abstract. The performance of depth reconstruction in binocular stereo relies on how adequate the predefined baseline for a target scene is. Wide-baseline stereo is capable of discriminating depth better than the narrow one, but it often suffers from spatial artifacts. Narrow-baseline stereo can provide a more elaborate depth map with less artifacts, while its depth resolution tends to be biased or coarse due to the short disparity. In this paper, we propose a novel optical design of heterogeneous stereo fusion on a binocular imaging system with a refractive medium, where the binocular stereo part operates as wide-baseline stereo; the refractive stereo module works as narrow-baseline stereo. We then introduce a stereo fusion workflow that combines the refractive and binocular stereo algorithms to estimate fine depth information through this fusion design. The quantitative and qualitative results validate the performance of our stereo fusion system in measuring depth, compared with homogeneous stereo approaches.

1 Introduction

Classical stereo matching algorithms employ a pair of binocular stereo images. Such stereo algorithms estimate depth by evaluating the distance of corresponding features, so-called disparity, via computing matching costs and aggregating the costs [1]. However, owing to the nature of triangulation in estimating depth, the depth accuracy strongly depends on its baseline between the stereo pair. For instance, a wide baseline elongates the range of the correspondence search so that the matching problem cannot be solved with high precision in typical locally-optimizing approaches [2]. On the contrary, a narrow baseline shortens the resolution of disparity; therefore, the accuracy of estimated depth could be degraded [3,4].

Recently, Gao and Ahuja [5,6] introduced a single depth camera based on refraction. Chen et al. [7] further extended this refractive mechanism. Such refractive stereo systems estimate depth from the change of light direction; therefore, the disparity in refractive stereo in general is smaller than that in binocular stereo, i.e., its performance is similar to that of binocular stereo with a narrow baseline. We take inspiration from refractive stereo to combine these two heterogeneous stereo systems, where a stereo fusion system is designed with a refractive medium placed on one of the binocular stereo cameras. In this paper, we introduce a novel

© Springer International Publishing Switzerland 2015
D. Cremers et al. (Eds.): ACCV 2014, Part II, LNCS 9004, pp. 503–518, 2015.
DOI: 10.1007/978-3-319-16808-1_34

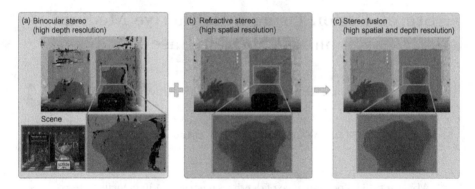

Fig. 1. (a) A binocular stereo detects depth accurately; whereas, it suffers from spatial artifacts caused by occlusions and featureless regions. (b) A refractive stereo improves the spatial resolution with less artifacts, but its depth resolution is coarse with fewer steps yet. (c) Our stereo fusion significantly improves the spatial and depth resolutions by combining these two heterogeneous stereo methods.

optical design that combines binocular and refractive stereo and its depth process workflow that allows us to fuse heterogeneous stereo inputs seamlessly to achieve fine depth estimates. Figure 1 shows a brief overview of our method.

2   Related Work

In this section, we briefly overview recent depth-from-stereo algorithms that are the most relevant to our work.

Multi-baseline Stereo. Okutomi and Kanade [3] proposed a multi-baseline stereo method. The proposed system consists of multiple cameras on a rail. Gallup et al. [8] estimated the depth of the scene by adjusting the baseline and resolution of images from multiple cameras so that the depth estimation becomes computationally efficient. Nakabo et al. [9] presented a variable-baseline stereo system on a linear slider. They controlled the baseline of the stereo system depending on the target scene for estimating the accurate depth map.

Zilly et al. [4] introduced a multi-baseline stereo system with various baselines. Four cameras are configured in multiple baselines on a rail. The two inner cameras establish a narrow-baseline stereo pair while two outer cameras form a wide-baseline stereo pair. We take inspiration from this work [4] to extend the multiple baseline idea, i.e., we extend the structure of traditional binocular stereo by adopting a refractive medium to one of the cameras. The camera viewpoints in the multi-baseline systems are secured mechanically at fixed locations in general. This design restricts the spatial resolution along the camera array while reconstructing the depth map. In contrast, our fusion system controls the baseline dynamically by rotating the medium. Our system requires a smaller space to operate consequently while acquiring input than the multi-baseline stereo systems.

Refractive Stereo. Nishimoto and Shirai [10] first introduced a refractive camera system by placing a refractive medium in front of a camera. Their method estimates depth using a pair of a direct image and a refracted one, assuming that the refracted image is equivalent to one of the binocular stereo images. Lee and Kweon [11] presented a single camera system that captures a stereo pair with a bi-prism. Gao and Ahuja [5,6] proposed a seminal refractive stereo method that captures multiple refractive images with a glass medium tilted at different angles. The rotation axis of the tilted medium is mechanically aligned to the optical axis of the camera. Shimizu and Okutomi [12,13] introduced a mixed approach that combines the refraction and the reflection phenomena. This method superposes a pair of reflection and refraction images via the surface of a transparent medium. Chen et al. [7,14] proposed a calibration method for refractive stereo. This method finds the pairs of matching points on refractive images with the SIFT algorithm [15] to estimate the pose of a transparent medium. In this paper, we adopt an optical hardware structure of refractive stereo [6] and combine it on a binocular stereo base.

3   Light Transport in Stereo

3.1   Baseline vs. Disparity

Binocular disparity describes pixel-wise displacement of parallax between corresponding points on a pair of stereo images taken from different positions. Therefore, it is natural that computing the disparity is accompanied with searching the corresponding points on an epipolar line. As disparity d depends on its depth, we can recover a depth z as:

$$z = fb/d, \tag{1}$$

where f is the focal length of the camera lens; b is the distance between the cameras, the so-called baseline. As shown here, the disparity is proportional to the baseline, i.e., when the baseline is wide, the range of disparity increases.

Wide-baseline stereo reserves more pixels for disparity than narrow-baseline stereo does. Therefore, wide-baseline systems can discriminate depth with a higher resolution. On the other hand, the search range of correspondences increases, and in turn, it increases the chances of false matching. Although the estimated disparity maps are plausible in terms of depth, but it contains many empty regions, where the depth values were not correctly estimated for occlusion and false matching. It is frequently observed in homogeneous regions and heavily-textured regions, where the corresponding point search fails.

Narrow-baseline stereo has a relatively short search range of correspondences. Hence, the false matching rarely happens so that we can achieve the accuracy and efficiency in the cost computation. In addition, the level of spatial noise in the disparity map is low, as the occluded area is small. However, narrow-baseline stereo reserves a small number of pixels to discriminate depth. The depth-discriminative power decreases accordingly. It trades off the discriminative power for the reduced spatial artifacts in the disparity map. Note that refractive stereo presents a smaller disparity than traditional binocular stereo because it creates the disparity from the change of the light direction by refraction. Therefore, we regard refractive stereo as being equivalent to narrow-baseline stereo in terms of disparity in this work.

3.2   Depth from Refraction

Our stereo fusion system includes a refractive stereo module on a binocular stereo architecture. Refractive stereo estimates depth using the refraction of light via a transparent medium. There has been several studies that tried to formulate the geometric relationship between refraction and depth [6,7]. Here we briefly formulate the foundations of general depth estimation from refractive stereo.

Suppose a 3D point p in a target scene is projected to p_d on an image plane through the optical center of an objective lens C directly without any transparent medium (Fig. 2a). Inserting a transparent medium in the light path changes the transport of the incident beam from p and reach at p_r on the image plane with a lateral displacement d (between w/ and w/o the medium). The displacement between p_d and p_r on the image plane is called *refractive disparity*.

Now we formulate the depth z of p using simple trigonometry: $z = fR/r$, where r is a refractive disparity, found by searching a pair of corresponding points; f is the focal length; $R = d/\sin(\theta_p)$ is the ratio of lateral displacement d to $\sin(\theta_p)$. Here θ_p is the angle between $\overrightarrow{p_rC}$ and the image plane. $\cos(\theta_p)$ can be computed by the normalized dot product of $\overrightarrow{p_re}$ and $\overrightarrow{p_rC}$ (Fig. 2b). Lateral displacement d, the parallel-shifted length of the light passing through the medium, is determined as [16]:

$$d = \left(1 - \sqrt{\frac{1 - \sin^2(\theta_i)}{n^2 - \sin^2(\theta_i)}}\right) t \sin(\theta_i), \qquad (2)$$

where t is the thickness of the medium; n is the refractive index of the medium; θ_i (the incident angle of the light) can be obtained by computing $\cos(\theta_i)$ as the normalized dot product of $\overrightarrow{Cp_r}$ and $\overrightarrow{Ce}$. The refracted point p_r lies on a line, the so-called *essential line*, passing through an *essential point* e (an intersecting

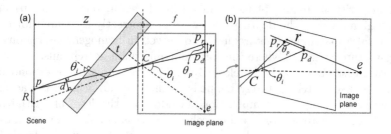

Fig. 2. (a) Cross-section view of the light path in refractive stereo. (b) A close-up view of the refractive light transport in 3D.

point of the normal vector of the transparent medium to the image plane) and
p_d (Fig. 2b). This property can be utilized to narrow down the search range of
correspondences onto the essential line, allowing us to compute matching costs
efficiently. It is worth noting that disparity in refractive stereo depends on not
only the depth z of p but also the projection position p_d of light and the position
of the essential point e, whereas the disparity in traditional stereo depends on
only the depth z of the point p. Prior to estimating a depth, we calibrate these
optical properties in refractive stereo in advance. See Sect. 4.2 for calibration.

4   System Implementation

4.1   Hardware Design

Our stereo fusion system consists of two cameras and a transparent medium on
a mechanical support structure. The focal length of the both camera lenses is
the same as 8 mm. The cameras are placed on a rail in parallel with a baseline of
10 cm to configure binocular stereo. We place a transparent medium on a rotary
stage for refractive stereo in front of one of the binocular stereo cameras. See
Fig. 3 for our hardware design. Note that this refractive stereo module is equivalent to narrow-baseline stereo while the binocular stereo structure is equivalent
to wide-baseline stereo in our system.

Our transparent medium is a block of clear glass. The measured refractive
index of the medium is 1.41 ($n = \sin(20°)/\sin(14.04°)$); the thickness of the
medium is 28 mm. We built a customized cylinder to hold the medium, cut in
45° from the axis of the cylinder. We spin the titled medium about the optical
axis from 0° to 360° in 10° intervals while capturing images. The binocular stereo
baseline and the tilted angle of the medium are fixed rigidly while capturing.

4.2   Calibration

Our stereo fusion system requires several stages of calibration prior to the depth
estimation. This section summarizes our calibration processes.

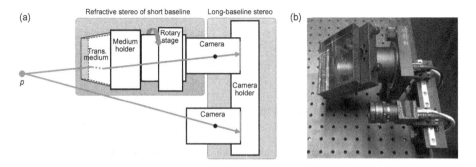

Fig. 3. (a) The schematic diagram of our stereo fusion system. A point p is captured by
both the refractive stereo and the binocular stereo module. (b) Our system prototype.

Geometric Calibration. We first calibrate the extrinsic/intrinsic parameters of the cameras, including the focal length of the objective lens, the center point of the image plane and the lens distortion in order to convert the image coordinates to the global coordinates. This allows us to derive an affine relationship between the two cameras and rectify the coordinates of these cameras with respect to the constraint epipolar line [17].

Refractive Calibration. Refractive stereo requires additional calibrations of the optical properties such as glass thickness, the refractive index and the essential point. Here we describe the calibration detail of the essential points. Analogous to the epipolar line in binocular stereo, refractive stereo forms an essential point e, where the essential lines forge to the essential point e outside the image plane, i.e., a refracted point p_r passes through a unrefracted pixel p_d and reaches the essential point e on the essential line (see Fig. 2b).

Gao and Ahuja [5,6] estimate the essential point by solving an optimization problem with a calibration target at a known distance. They precomputed the positions of the essential points for all angles by manually adjusting the normal axis of the glass, so that the accuracy of estimating the essential points does not depend on a target scene. Chen et al. [7] directly estimate the essential point on target scene images with a fact that the all essential lines meet at the essential point. They estimated the position of the essential point by computing intersection points of lines passing through each matching point on the superposed images with and without the medium. This method is considerably simpler than solving the optimization problem [5,6]; however, searching corresponding features with SIFT [7] is not consistent often such that the calibration accuracy is bound to the SIFT performance.

Our calibration method takes advantages of the both methods [6,7] to estimate the essential points with 36 poses of the refractive medium on the rotary

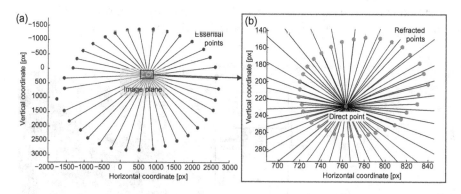

Fig. 4. (a) presents the calibrated results of the 36 essential points (blue dots) in our system. (b) shows an example of the locations of 36 refracted points (orange dots) from a direct point (w/o the medium, red point) in the coordinates of (763,229) at a distance of 30 cm. The location of the direct point has been refracted to 36 different positions per rotation due to refraction (Color figure online).

stage in advance. We take an image of a checkerboard without the medium once to compare it with other refracted images in different poses of the medium. Once we take a refracted image in a pose, we extract corner points from the both direct and refracted images following the proposed method in [6]. Note that the same feature points appear at different positions due to refraction. Superposing these two images, we draw lines by linking the corresponding points with all feature corners with the fact observed by Chen et al. [7]. We then compute the arithmetic mean of the coordinates of the intersection points to determine an essential point per rotation angle. We repeat this process with the 36 rotation poses of the medium predetermined in 10-degree intervals. See Fig. 4.

Color Calibration. Matching costs are calculated by comparing the intrinsic properties of color at the feature points. Since we introduce a transparent medium on a camera in binocular stereo, it is critical to achieve consistent camera responses with and without the medium. To do so, we employ a GretagMacbeth ColorChecker target of 24 color patches. Two sets of linear RGB colors, A and B (cameras with and without the medium with inverse gamma correction), are measured from the both cameras. We determine a 3×3 affine transformation M of A to B as a camera calibration function using least-squares [18]. We apply this color transform M for the linear colors through the medium, acquiring consistent colors through the medium.

5   Depth Reconstruction in Stereo Fusion

Our stereo fusion workflow consists of two main steps. We first estimate an intermediate depth map from a set of refractive stereo images (from the camera with the medium) and reconstruct a virtual direct image. Then, this virtual image and a direct image (from the other camera without the medium in a baseline) are used to estimate the final depth map referring to the intermediate depth map from refractive stereo. Figure 5 overviews the workflow of our stereo fusion method.

5.1   Depth from Refraction

Depth reconstruction from binocular stereo has been well-studied including matching cost computation, cost aggregation, disparity computation, and disparity refinement [1], whereas depth reconstruction from refraction has been relatively less discussed. In this section, we describe our approach for refractive stereo for reconstructing an intial depth map.

Matching Cost in Refractive Stereo. General binocular stereo algorithms define the *matching cost volumes* of every pixels per disparity [1], where a disparity implies a certain depth directly in binocular stereo. This relationship can be applied for all the pixels in the stereo image uniformly. In contrast to binocular stereo, the length of disparity in refractive stereo changes by not only the

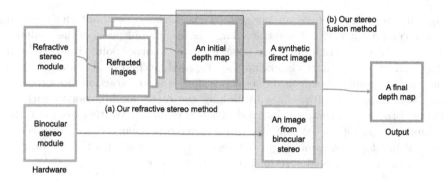

Fig. 5. Schematic diagram of our stereo fusion method. (a) Our refractive stereo method estimates an intermediate depth map from refractive stereo. (b) Our stereo fusion method reconstructs a final depth map from a pair of an image from binocular stereo and a synthetic direct image using the intermediate depth map.

depth but also the coordinates on the image plane and the pose of the medium. It means that the refracted points of a single direct point could have different refractive disparities depending on the coordinates on the image plane and the pose of the medium. We therefore define the matching cost volumes for our refractive stereo based on the depth, rather than the disparity. This allows us to apply a cost volume approach for refractive stereo.

Suppose we have a geometric position set P of the refracted points $p_r(p_d, z, e)$ of a direct point p_d at a depth z (see Fig. 2) with an essential point e ($e \in E$): $P(p_d, z) = \{p_r(p_d, z, e) | e \in E\}$. This set P can be derived analytically by refractive calibration (Sect. 3.2) so that we precompute this set P for computational efficiency.

We denote L as the set of colors observed at the refracted positions P, where l is a color vector in a linear RGB color space ($l \in L$). Assuming that the surface of the direct point p_d is Lambertian, the colors of the refracted points $L(p_d, z)$ would be the same. We use the similarity of $L(p_d, z)$ for the matching cost C of p_d with a hypothetical depth z [19].

$$C(p_d, z) = \frac{1}{|L(p_d, z)|} \sum_{l \in L(p_d, z)} K(l - \bar{l}), \tag{3}$$

where K is an Epanechnikov kernel [20]: $K(l) = 1 - \|l/h\|^2$ when $\|l/h\|$ is less than or equal to 1; otherwise, $K(l) = 0$; h is a normalization constant ($h = 0.01$); $\bar{l}$ is computed iteratively in $L(p_d, z)$ (for five iterations) using the mean shift method [21] as:

$$\bar{l} = \sum_{l \in L(p_d, z)} K(l - \bar{l})l \bigg/ \sum_{l \in L(p_d, z)} K(l - \bar{l}). \tag{4}$$

z in our refractive stereo is a discrete depth, of which range is set between 60 cm and 120 cm in 3 cm intervals. Note that we build a refractive cost volume per depth for all the pixels in the refractive image.

Cost Aggregation for Depth Estimation. In order to improve the spatial resolution of the intermediate depth map in refractive stereo, we aggregate the refractive matching cost using a window kernel G. An aggregated cost function C^A is defined as $C(p_d, z)$ convolved by a weighting factor G [22]:

$$C^A(p_d, z) = \sum_{q_d \in w} G(p_d, q_d) C(q_d, z), \tag{5}$$

where q_d is a pixel inside a squared window w, of which size is 7×7. We aggregate the refractive matching costs using a Gaussian kernel $G(p_d, q_d)$, defined as $(1/2\pi\sigma^2) \exp(-(\|p_d - q_d\|^2)/2\sigma^2)$, where σ is 9.6. Finally, we compute the optimal depth $Z(p_d)$ of the point p_d that maximizes the aggregated matching costs: $Z(p_d) = \arg\max_z C^A(p_d, z)$.

Depth and Direct Image Refinement. Even though the levels of the two cameras are the same on the rail as traditional binocular stereo, our stereo pair includes more than horizontal parallax due to the refraction effect. Prior to fusing the binocular stereo and the refractive depth input, we first reconstruct a synthetic image I_d (a direct image without the medium) by computing the mean radiance of the set $L(p_d, Z(p_d))$ using the mean shift method (Eq. (4)).

Reconstructing the direct image allows us to apply a depth refinement algorithm with a weighted median filter [23] by treating the direct image as guidance in order to fill in the holes of the estimated depth map. The weighted median filter replaces the depth $Z(p_d)$ using the median from the histogram $h(p_d, \cdot)$:

$$h(p_d, z) = \sum_{q_d \in w} W(p_d, q_d) f(q_d, z), \tag{6}$$

where $f(q_d, z)$ is defined as 1 when $Z(q_d) - z$ is 0; otherwise, $f()$ is 0. W is a weight function with a guided image filter [24], defined as $W(p_d, q_d) = \frac{1}{|w|^2} \sum_{k:(p_d,q_d) \in w_k} (1 + (l_d(p_d) - \mu_k)(\Sigma_k + \epsilon U)^{-1}(l_d(q_d) - \mu_k))$, where $l_d(p_d)$ is a linear RGB color of p_d on the direct image I_d; U is an identity matrix; k is the center pixel of window w_k including p_d and q_d; μ_k and Σ_k are the mean vector and covariance matrix of I_d in w_k. In our experiments, we set the size of w_k as 9×9, and ϵ as 0.001.

This median filter allows us to refine the hole artifacts in the depth map while preserving sound depth. After refining the depth map, the direct image is reconstructed again with the updated depth map. Figure 6 shows the result of the refinement, which are the updated depth map and the direct image.

Optimal Number of Refractive Images. The number of input refractive images is critical to the quality of depth estimation in refractive stereo. We were motivated to find out an optimal number of input refractive images so that we evaluated point-wise errors in estimating depth on a planar surface in a known distance. Figure 7b shows that the root-mean-square error decreases very fast while increasing the number of input up to six refractive images. Hence, we choose the optimal number of input refractive images as six. Note that we use six refractive images with 60° intervals for capturing results in this paper.

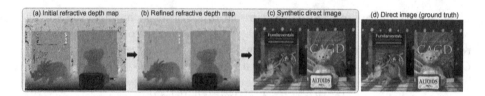

Fig. 6. (a) shows an initial depth map and (b) is the refined map with weighted median filtering. A refracted image is computed as a synthetic direct image (c), used for binocular stereo later. (c) is compared to a ground truth photograph (d).

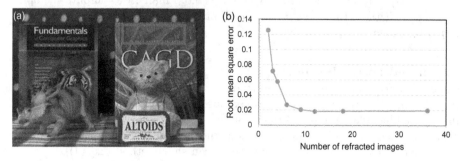

Fig. 7. (a) The red square indicates the area used for finding an optimal number of input refractive images. The book cover is a planar surface orthogonal to the camera optical axis with a constant depth. (b) The depth error drops down fast significantly up to six refractive inputs with different angles. No significant improvement is observed with more than six inputs (Color figure online).

5.2   Depth in Stereo Fusion

As described in Sect. 3.1, our binocular stereo with a wider baseline allows us to discriminate depth with a higher resolution than refractive stereo (equivalent to narrow-baseline stereo). We take inspiration from a coarse-to-fine stereo method [25, 26] to develop our stereo fusion method. Our refractive stereo yields an intermediate depth map with a high spatial resolution, which is on a par with narrow-baseline stereo. However, it is not surprising that the z-depth resolution of this depth map is discrete and coarse on the other hand. We utilize the fine depth map from refractive stereo in order to increase the z-depth resolution as high as possible with a high spatial resolution by limiting the search range of matching cost computation in binocular stereo using the refractive depth map (Fig. 8). To this end, we can significantly reduce the chances of false matching while estimating depth from binocular stereo between the direct and synthetic images. This enables us to achieve a fine depth map from binocular stereo, taking advantages of a high spatial resolution in refractive stereo.

Matching Cost in Stereo Fusion. Now we have a direct image I_b from the camera without the medium in the binocular module and the synthetic image

I_d reconstructed from the refractive stereo module (Sect. 5.1) with its depth map. Depth candidates with uniform intervals are not related linearly to the disparities with pixel-based intervals. We hence define a cost volume for stereo fusion on the disparity instead in order to fully utilize the image resolution. To fuse the depth from binocular and refractive stereo, we build a fusion matching cost volume $F(p_d, d)$ per disparity for all pixels as next. The fusion matching cost F is defined as a norm of the intensity difference: $F(p_d, d) = \|l_d(p_d) - l_b(p'_d)\|$, where p'_d is a shifted pixel by a disparity d from p_d; $l_b(p'_d)$ is a color vector of p'_d on image I_b.

Cost Aggregation in Stereo Fusion. The aggregated cost of the fusion matching costs is defined as:

$$F^A(p_d, d) = \sum_{q_d \in w} W(p_d, q_d) F(q_d, d). \tag{7}$$

Here W is the bilateral image filter [22] defined as $W(p_d, q_d) = exp(-(d(p_d, q_d)/\sigma_s^2 + c(p_d, q_d)/\sigma_c^2)$, where $d(p_d, q_d)$ is the Euclidean distance between p_d and q_d, $c(p_d, q_d)$ is the sum of differences of colors of RGB channels, σ_s and σ_c are the standard deviations for spatial distance and color difference. In our experiment, we select the window size, σ_s and σ_c as 9, 7 and 0.07.

Suppose the depth of point p_d is estimated as $Z(p_d)$ from refractive stereo. As we compute the refractive matching cost and aggregate the cost *per discrete depth interval* Δz in refractive stereo, let the actual depth of p_d be in between $(Z(p_d) - \Delta z)$ and $(Z(p_d) + \Delta z)$ as Z_{prev} and Z_{post}. The corresponding disparities of Z_{prev} and Z_{post} can be computed as d_{prev} and d_{post} using Eq. (1). Note that d_{post} is smaller than d_{prev}. We therefore estimate the optimal disparity $D(p_d)$ by searching the aggregated cost volume $F^A(p_d, d)$ within the range $[d_{post}, d_{prev}]$ as below:

$$D(p_d) = \arg\min_d F^A(p_d, d). \tag{8}$$

We compute Eq. (7) within the range of $[d_{post}, d_{prev}]$ exclusively for computational efficiency.

6   Results

We conducted several experiments to evaluate the performance of our stereo fusion method. We computed depth maps, of which resolution is 1280×960 with 140 depth steps, on a machine equipped with an Intel i7-3770 CPU and 16 GB RAM with CPU parallelization (GPU-based acceleration would be feasible as future work.) The computation times for estimating the depth map from six refractive inputs are ~77 s. for the first-half stage of refractive stereo and ~33 s. for the second-half stage of stereo fusion. The total computation time on runtime is ~110 s. We precomputed the refracted essential points per pixel in the image plane beforehand for computational efficiency.

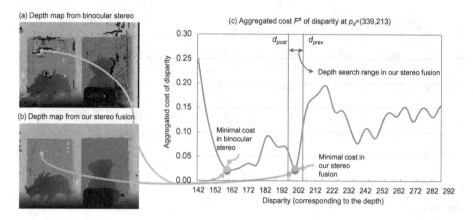

Fig. 8. The binocular depth map (a) includes artifacts due to false matching caused by occlusions, featureless regions and repeated patterns. Using the intermediate refractive depth map (b), we can limit the search range of a corresponding point p_d between d_{post} and d_{prev} for instance. This significantly reduces false matching frequency in estimating depth.

The first row in Fig. 9 compares three different depth maps by binocular only stereo (a), refractive only stereo (b) and our proposed stereo fusion method (c). Although the depth estimation of binocular only stereo (a) appears sound, (a) suffers from typical false matching artifacts around the edges of the front object due to occlusion. Refractive only stereo (b), obtained from the intermediate stage of our fusion method, presents depth without artifacts, but the depth resolution is significantly discretized and coarse. Our stereo fusion overcomes the shortcomings of the homogeneous stereo methods. It estimates depth as fine as binocular stereo without severe artifacts. In addition, we quantitatively evaluated the accuracy of our stereo fusion method compared with others in Fig. 9d. We measured three points in the scene using a laser distance meter (Bosch GLM 80) and compared the measurements by the three methods. The accuracy of our method is as high as the binocular only method (aver. distance error: ~2 mm), outperforming the refractive only method (aver. error: ~6 mm).

We compare our proposed method with a renowned graphcut-based algorithm [27] with an image of the same resolution. Global stereo methods in general allow for an accurate depth map, while requiring high computational cost. It is not surprising that this global method was about eight times slower than our method (see Fig. 10a). We also compare our method with a local binocular method [24], which computes the matching cost as the norm of intensity difference and aggregates the cost using the weight of the guided filter [24]. Its computing time was ~212 s. with the same scene (see Fig. 10b). This local method struggles with typical false matching artifacts. A refractive method using SIFT flow [7] is compared to ours (Fig. 10c and d). The same number of six refractive images were employed for both methods. While the refractive method suffers from wavy artifacts of SIFT flow and its depth resolution is very coarse, typical to refractive stereo, our method estimates depth accurately with less spatial artifacts in all test scenes.

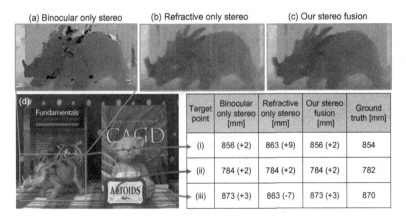

Target point	Binocular only stereo [mm]	Refractive only stereo [mm]	Our stereo fusion [mm]	Ground truth [mm]
(i)	856 (+2)	863 (+9)	856 (+2)	854
(ii)	784 (+2)	784 (+2)	784 (+2)	782
(iii)	873 (+3)	863 (-7)	873 (+3)	870

Fig. 9. The top row compares the three different depth maps of binocular only stereo (a), refractive only stereo (b) and our stereo fusion (c). (d) quantitatively compares the accuracy of three methods. Three points were measured by a Bosch laser distance meter. The accuracy of our stereo fusion is as high as binocular stereo; our depth map does not suffer from artifacts as refractive stereo.

Multi-baseline Stereo. Multi-baseline stereo methods such as trinocular stereo employ multiple views with various baselines. In this sense, multi-baseline approach is the most similar method to our approach, where the refractive stereo is equivalent to the short baseline stereo; the binocular stereo is equivalent to the long baseline stereo. We built a trinocular stereo setup, where the distance

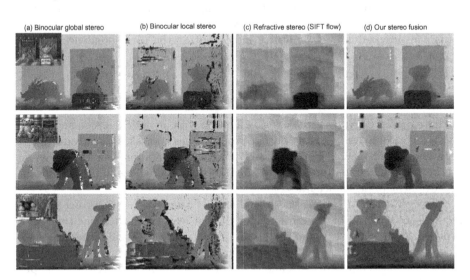

Fig. 10. The depth maps of three different scenes in each row were computed by four different methods. The first two columns (a) and (b) show global [27] and local binocular stereo [24] methods. The third column (c) presents a refractive stereo method [7]. Our method (d) estimates depth accurately without suffering from severe artifacts.

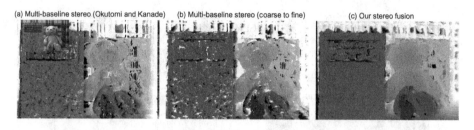

(a) Multi-baseline stereo (Okutomi and Kanade)   (b) Multi-baseline stereo (coarse to fine)   (c) Our stereo fusion

Fig. 11. Multi-baseline stereo methods are compared with our method. (a) is a depth map using a trinocular stereo method [3]. (b) is also a trinocular stereo method, implemented with the coarse-to-fine approach same as ours. (c) is the result of our stereo fusion method with the same number of input images.

between the right and the middle camera is set to 2 cm and the distance between the middle and the left one is set to 11 cm to yield multiple baselines. Figure 11a and b presents results of trinocular stereo. Figure 11a is the result of a multi-baseline method [3], where two pairs of matching costs are calculated from the short and the long baseline pairs, and these costs are combined as total matching cost to yield a depth map. Figure 11b is another implementation of trinocular stereo. Similar to our coarse-to-fine approach, we compute matching cost volumes from the short-baseline stereo pair and aggregate the volumes through the guided filter to yield an intermediate depth map. We then use this depth map to narrow the search range of correspondence same as ours. As shown in Fig. 11, our stereo fusion achieves an more elaborate depth map than the both trinocular stereo methods. We could speculate that our improvement is feasible as our refractive method utilizes the oval shape of corresponding points. This oval-shaped patterns can provide unique signatures in computing the correspondences in our system.

7   Conclusion

We have presented a novel stereo fusion method with an optical design and stereo fusion algorithm. We validate that our proposed method takes the advantages of both traditional binocular and refractive stereo. In addition, our fusion design can be easily integrated into any existing binocular stereo, yielding a significant improvement in depth accuracy.

However, there are some issues remained as future work. Our current method requires the rotation of the refractive module at least more than one time for a depth estimate. Therefore, our method is only allowed for static scenes. Suppose a depth map from refractive stereo contains errors, these errors remain from the stereo fusion stage, where we refine the depth resolution of the refractive depth map using binocular stereo.

Acknowledgement. Min H. Kim gratefully acknowledges Korea NRF grants (2013R1A1A1010165 and 2013M3A6A6073718) and additional support by Microsoft Research Asia and an ICT R&D program of MSIP/IITP (10041313).

References

1. Scharstein, D., Szeliski, R.: A taxonomy and evaluation of dense two-frame stereo correspondence algorithms. Int. J. Comput. Vis. (IJCV) **47**, 7–42 (2002)
2. Rhemann, C., Hosni, A., Bleyer, M., Rother, C., Gelautz, M.: Fast cost-volume filtering for visual correspondence and beyond. In: Proceedings of the Computer Vision and Pattern Recognition (CVPR), pp. 3017–3024. IEEE (2011)
3. Okutomi, M., Kanade, T.: A multiple-baseline stereo. IEEE Trans. Pattern Anal. Mach. Intell. (PAMI) **15**, 353–363 (1993)
4. Zilly, F., Riechert, C., Mller, M., Eisert, P., Sikora, T., Kauff, P.: Real-time generation of multi-view video plus depth content using mixed narrow and wide baseline. J. Vis. Commun. Image Represent. **25**, 632–648 (2013)
5. Gao, C., Ahuja, N.: Single camera stereo using planar parallel plate. In: Proceedings of the International Conference on Pattern Recognition (ICPR), vol. 4, pp. 108–111 (2004)
6. Gao, C., Ahuja, N.: A refractive camera for acquiring stereo and super-resolution images. In: Proceedings of the Computer Vision and Pattern Recognition (CVPR), pp. 2316–2323 (2006)
7. Chen, Z., Wong, K.Y.K., Matsushita, Y., Zhu, X.: Depth from refraction using a transparent medium with unknown pose and refractive index. Int. J. Comput. Vis. (ICJV) **102**, 1–15 (2013)
8. Gallup, D., Frahm, J.M., Mordohai, P., Pollefeys, M.: Variable baseline/resolution stereo. In: Proceedings of the Computer Vision and Pattern Recognition (CVPR), pp. 1–8 (2008)
9. Nakabo, Y., Mukai, T., Hattori, Y., Takeuchi, Y., Ohnishi, N.: Variable baseline stereo tracking vision system using high-speed linear slider. In: Proceedings of the International Conference on Robotics and Automation (ICRA), pp. 1567–1572 (2005)
10. Nishimoto, Y., Shirai, Y.: A feature-based stereo model using small disparities. In: Proceedings of the Computer Vision and Pattern Recognition (CVPR), pp. 192–196 (1987)
11. Lee, D., Kweon, I.: A novel stereo camera system by a biprism. IEEE Trans. Robot. Autom. **16**, 528–541 (2000)
12. Shimizu, M., Okutomi, M.: Reflection stereo-novel monocular stereo using a transparent plate. In: Proceedings of the Canadian Conference on Computer and Robot Vision (CRV), pp. 14–14. IEEE (2006)
13. Shimizu, M., Okutomi, M.: Monocular range estimation through a double-sided half-mirror plate. In: Proceedings of the Canadian Conference on Computer and Robot Vision (CRV), pp. 347–354. IEEE (2007)
14. Chen, Z., Wong, K., Matsushita, Y., Zhu, X., Liu, M.: Self-calibrating depth from refraction. In: Proceedings of the International Conference on Computer Vision (ICCV), pp. 635–642 (2011)
15. Lowe, D.G.: Distinctive image features from scale-invariant keypoints. Int. J. Comput. Vis. (IJCV) **60**, 91–110 (2004)
16. Hecht, E.: Optics. Addison-Wesley, Reading (1987)
17. Zhang, Z.: A flexible new technique for camera calibration. IEEE Trans. Pattern Anal. Mach. Intell. (PAMI) **22**, 1330–1334 (2000)
18. Kim, M.H., Kautz, J.: Characterization for high dynamic range imaging. Comput. Graph. Forum (Proc. EUROGRAPHICS 2008) **27**, 691–697 (2008)

19. Kim, C., Zimmer, H., Pritch, Y., Sorkine-Hornung, A., Gross, M.: Scene reconstruction from high spatio-angular resolution light fields. ACM Trans. Graph. (TOG) **32**(73), 1–12 (2013)

20. Duda, R.O., Hart, P.E.: Pattern Classification and Scene Analysis. Wiley, New York (1973)

21. Comaniciu, D., Meer, P.: Mean shift: a robust approach toward feature space analysis. IEEE Trans. Pattern Anal. Mach. Intell. (PAMI) **24**, 603–619 (2002)

22. Yoon, K.J., Kweon, I.S.: Adaptive support-weight approach for correspondence search. IEEE Trans. Pattern Anal. Mach. Intell. (PAMI) **28**, 650–656 (2006)

23. Ma, Z., He, K., Wei, Y., Sun, J., Wu, E.: Constant time weighted median filtering for stereo matching and beyond. In: Proceedings of the International Conference on Computer Vision (ICCV), pp. 1–8 (2013)

24. He, K., Sun, J., Tang, X.: Guided image filtering. In: Daniilidis, K., Maragos, P., Paragios, N. (eds.) ECCV 2010, Part I. LNCS, vol. 6311, pp. 1–14. Springer, Heidelberg (2010)

25. Barnard, S.T.: Stochastic stereo matching over scale. Int. J. Comput. Vis. (IJCV) **3**, 17–32 (1989)

26. Chen, J.S., Medioni, G.: Parallel multiscale stereo matching using adaptive smoothing. In: Faugeras, O. (ed.) ECCV 1990. LNCS, vol. 427, pp. 99–103. Springer, Heidelberg (1990)

27. Boykov, Y., Veksler, O., Zabih, R.: Fast approximate energy minimization via graph cuts. IEEE Trans. Pattern Anal. Mach. Intell. (PAMI) **23**, 1222–1239 (2001)

Low-Level Vision and Features

Saliency Detection via Nonlocal L_0 Minimization

Yiyang Wang[1], Risheng Liu[2], Xiaoliang Song[1], and Zhixun Su[1(✉)]

[1] School of Mathematical Sciences, Dalian University of Technology, Dalian, China
{yywerica,ericsong}@gmail.com
[2] School of Software Technology, Dalian University of Technology, Dalian, China
{rsliu,zxsu}@dlut.edu.cn

Abstract. In this paper, by observing the intrinsic sparsity of saliency map for the image, we propose a novel nonlocal L_0 minimization framework to extract the sparse geometric structure of the saliency maps for the natural images. Specifically, we first propose to use the k-nearest neighbors of superpixels to construct a graph in the feature space. The novel L_0-regularized nonlocal minimization model is then developed on the proposed graph to describe the sparsity of saliency maps. Finally, we develop a first order optimization scheme to solve the proposed nonconvex and discrete variational problem. Experimental results on four publicly available data sets validate that the proposed approach yields significant improvement compared with state-of-the-art saliency detection methods.

1 Introduction

The recent years have witnessed significant advances in saliency detection [1–6]. Visual saliency is making the most informative scene stand out from their neighbors and grabbing immediate attention. It is originally a task of eye fixation prediction [7–10], and recently has been extended to salient region detection [2,6,11–13]. Both of them can be categorized as either bottom-up [14] or top-down [15] approaches in general. The former is fast, pre-attentive, data-driven saliency extraction while the latter is slower, task dependent, goal driven saliency extraction [6]. In this paper, we focus on the bottom-up salient region detection.

Most bottom-up saliency methods rely on predefined assumptions about salient objects and backgrounds. One of the early bottom-up saliency detection methods is proposed by Itti et al. [8], which focuses on the role of color and orientation priors. Goferman et al. [1] propose a context-aware algorithm that represents the scene based on four assumptions of human visual attention. However, using the predefined assumptions only cannot generate maps that uniformly cover the whole object and suppress the background well. With the emergence of superpixels [16,17], an increasing number of image saliency detection approaches are proposed on region level to reduce calculation amount and receive uniform

Electronic supplementary material The online version of this chapter (doi:10.1007/978-3-319-16808-1_35) contains supplementary material, which is available to authorized users.

D. Cremers et al. (Eds.): ACCV 2014, Part II, LNCS 9004, pp. 521–535, 2015.
DOI: 10.1007/978-3-319-16808-1_35

foreground and suppressed background. One significant class among them is graph based approaches [7,18–24]. Yang et al. [19] propose to detect salient regions in images through manifold ranking on a graph which incorporates local grouping cues and boundary priors. Liu et al. [24] provide a diffusion viewpoint to model saliency detection which shows its well performance on salient region detection. However, all the previous work start from the perspective of improving the prior and achieving good results statistically on public benchmarks, but few of them take the characteristic of the ideal result into consideration.

We in this paper note that all of the ground truth saliency maps are binary images which contain a few intensity changes among neighboring pixels/superpixels. Namely, the intensity changes are very sparse. Due to the fact that the L_0 norm of a vector is the number of non-zero entries which directly measures sparsity, we propose a graph based nonlocal L_0 (NLL$_0$ for short) minimization for visual saliency detection. The proposed NLL$_0$ method is able to capture the sparse properties of saliency maps, thereby leading to reliable results. Furthermore, the graph construction plays a key role in graph based methods. Different from local graphs that connect neighbor regions in the spatial space (e.g. 1-ring and 2-ring graph), we construct a nonlocal graph based on the k-nearest neighbors (k-NN for short) in the feature space. This k-NN graph better extracts the structure of the image, and can generate a more uniform forward and suppressed background. Due to the discrete nature and the non-convexity of the proposed model, conventional convex optimization algorithm cannot be directly used to solve it. By extending alternating direction method (ADM) [25–27] to non-convex discrete optimization problem, this paper proposes an efficient numerical scheme to solve our NLL$_0$ saliency detection model. Overall, the main contributions in this paper are summarized as follows:

- We propose a novel NLL$_0$ model on image graph for saliency detection. As the L_0 norm is the naive metric used to describe sparsity of the gradients, the saliency maps of our proposed model can exactly highlight the foreground and suppress the background.
- A nonlocal graph is constructed in the feature space composed by color and spatial position features, and each vertex in this graph is connected to its k-NN.
- As a non-trivial by product, a first order numerical scheme is introduced to efficiently solve the non-convex discrete NLL$_0$ optimization model.

2   The Proposed Method

In this section, an L_0 norm based minimization is introduced on image graph to model saliency detection. For a given image, we first over segment it into superpixels by SLIC method [16] and construct a graph based on the k-NN of superpixels in the feature space. Then, our NLL$_0$ minimization is proposed on this graph incorporating with a saliency control map that is generated by contrast and object priors.

2.1 Graph Construction

It is worth mentioning that graph construction plays a key role in graph based methods [7,18–21], and the connected relationship is top priority. As two classic graphs, 1-ring and 2-ring graph are widely used in superpixel based saliency detection methods [18,19]. However, 1-ring and 2-ring graph are two typical graphs that connect neighbor elements in the spatial space (see Fig. 1(c) and (d) to have an intuitive sense), which is premised on the assumption that neighboring superpixels in the spatial space are likely to share similar saliency values. This assumption is absolutely incorrect near the edges between the salient and indistinctive regions thus may generate redundant regions. The example shown in Fig. 2 also shows that with these two graphs, the background and forward are not differentiated effectively. In this paper, we propose to construct graph in the feature space to take nonlocal relationship into consideration (Fig. 1(e)).

Given an image, we generate superpixels by SLIC method [16] to be the elements of saliency estimation, denoted as a vector of N elements with corresponding values $\mathbf{v} = (v_1, v_2, \cdots, v_N)$. It is not specific that any other edge preserving methods to generate superpixels can be used in this place. Then we construct an undirected, symmetric and weighted graph G. It consists a finite set E of edges and is associated with a weight function $\omega : E \to \mathbb{R}_+$ satisfying $\omega_{pq} = \omega_{qp}$, for all $pq \in E$.

The weight between superpixels p and q is expressed as:

$$\omega_{pq} = \exp(-\frac{\|\mathbf{f}_p - \mathbf{f}_q\|^2}{2\sigma^2}), \tag{1}$$

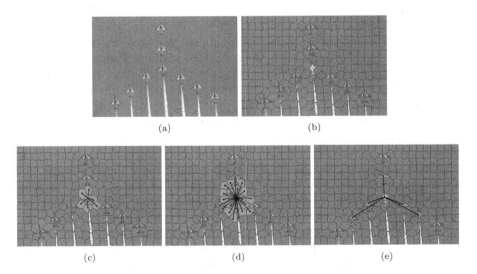

Fig. 1. The comparisons of 1-ring, 2-ring and k-NN graph. (a) The input image. (b) The superpixels of the input image, and a yellow patch is specified. (c) The connected relationship in 1-ring graph. (d) The connected relationship in 2-ring graph. (e) The connected relationship in k-NN graph (Color figure online).

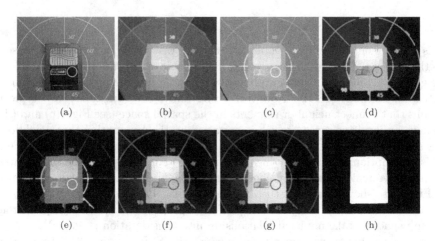

Fig. 2. Well performance of our graph from quality analysis. (a) Input image. (b) Result of 1-ring graph. (c) Result of 2-ring graph. (d) Result of k-NN graph. (e) Result of 2-ring graph with four boundaries of the image connected. (f) Result of k-NN graph with four boundaries of the image connected. (g) Result of our graph. (h) Ground truth.

where $\mathbf{f}_p = (\alpha \mathbf{c}_p, \mathbf{l}_p)$ is a feature vector at superpixel p comprising of its appearance $\mathbf{c}_p$ (i.e.,the mean of the superpixels in CIE LAB color space) and location $\mathbf{l}_p$ (i.e., the mean of the coordinates of superpixels in spatial space). Parameter α is used to control the balance between these two features, and $\| \cdot \|$ denotes the L_2 norm of a vector. For each superpixel p, we calculate its weight with every other q in image domain, and find its k-NN to exploit local relationships in the feature space. Keep these k values which indicate the most similar superpixels of p and set all the others to zero. The connected relationship between p and q is indicated by the nonzero ω_{pq}. Connecting neighbors in feature space performs well than other traditional graph construction methods from the results in the top line of Fig. 2.

With the purpose of reducing the geodesic distance of similar superpixels that have large spatial distance, Yang et al. [19] propose to connect the four boundaries of the image together in the 2-ring graph which performs well on generating suppressed background. We further enforce that the most indistinctive regions in saliency control map $\mathbf{v}^c$ (is discussed in Sect. 2.3) and the four boundaries of the image should be connected to each other to get a better performance. We choose the latter 25 % of the superpixels of $\mathbf{v}^c$ in descending order as the most indistinctive regions in our approach. The results shown in the second line of Fig. 2 indicate that the strategy of connecting boundaries and indistinctive regions together does improve the saliency result, and our proposed method have the best performance from both quality analysis (Fig. 2) and quantity analysis (Fig. 4(c)).

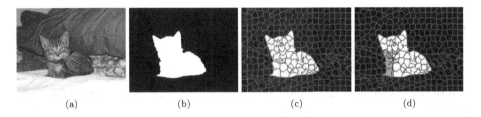

| (a) | (b) | (c) | (d) |

Fig. 3. The nonlocal gradient and its sparsity. (a) An input image. (b) The ground truth of the input image. (c) The superpixels of the ground truth, and a specified patch coloring in yellow. (d) The related patch (colored in cyan) when computing the nonlocal gradient of the specified yellow patch (Color figure online).

2.2 NLL$_0$ for Saliency Detection

As discussed before, the ideal result in salient region detection, i.e. the ground truth (Fig. 3(b)), has extremely sparse gradient on superpixels. To obtain the same property of our saliency result, we propose to minimize a variational formulation based on the L_0 norm of gradient. Though it is applied in many low-level image processing problems [28–30], we first extend it for graph based visual saliency detection. To begin with, we will introduce the basic definitions and notations which are borrowed from Bougleux et al. in [31] and Gilboa-Osher in [32], regarding local differential geometry operators that will be useful in the rest of the paper.

Different from the definition of gradient on a regular image grid, the gradient of each vertex p on the graph G is defined for pair points $pq \in E$ as:

$$\nabla_\omega \mathbf{v}_p = (\partial_q v_p : pq \in E). \tag{2}$$

Specifically, $\nabla_\omega \mathbf{v}_p$ is a vector of all partial derivatives, i.e. $\partial_q v_p = (v_q - v_p)\sqrt{\omega_{pq}}$, where ω_{pq} is the weight between p and q as discussed in Sect. 2.1.

A visual example is shown in Fig. 3(d) to explain the nonlocal gradient on graph. Suppose that p denotes the yellow region in Fig. 3(c). According to the definition of our k-NN graph, its k-NN are denoted by the cyan patches (see Fig. 3(d)). Regarding the definition of $\nabla_\omega \mathbf{v}_p$, we can conclude that most values of $\nabla_\omega \mathbf{v}_p$ are zero. Thus, a natural idea that depicts this property is to employ L_0 norm on $\nabla_\omega \mathbf{v}_p$. It can also be seen that only few superpixels has nonzero gradient in the ground truth, and that truly confirm the reliability of minimizing the L_0 norm of gradient.

Based on considerations above, the proposed NLL$_0$ model on image graph is defined as follows:

$$\min_{\mathbf{v}} \sum_p \|\nabla_\omega \mathbf{v}_p\|_0 + \frac{\lambda}{2}\|\mathbf{v} - \mathbf{v}^c\|^2, \tag{3}$$

where $\|\nabla_\omega \mathbf{v}_p\|_0$ is defined as $\|\nabla_\omega \mathbf{v}_p\|_0 = \sharp\{q|\partial_q v_p \neq 0; pq \in E\}^1$, λ is a positive constant that controls the trade-off between the sparsity and the fidelity term.

---

[1] The notation $'\sharp'$ is a mathematical representation which stands for the cardinality of a set.

The new symbol $\mathbf{v}^c$ in the fidelity term is the saliency control map which will be introduced in the next section.

2.3   Saliency Control Map

We in this paper use the contrast prior and object prior to compute the salient control map $\mathbf{v}^c$.

We use the contrast prior for the reason that research from perceptual analysis [33] and relative works [6,18,34] have indicated the effectiveness of the contrast measure. Given the mean color value $\mathbf{c}_p$ and the weight $\omega_{pq}^{(l)}$ between superpixel v_p and v_q in spatial space, the contrast measure of v_p is defined as:

$$v_p^{con} = \sum_{q \neq p} \omega_{pq}^{(l)} \|\mathbf{c}_p - \mathbf{c}_q\|^2, \tag{4}$$

where $\omega_{pq}^{(l)} = \exp(-\frac{1}{2\sigma_i^2}\|\mathbf{l}_p - \mathbf{l}_q\|^2)$ with normalized average coordinates $\mathbf{l}_p$ and $\mathbf{l}_q$.

On the other hand, object prior provides an assumption on the most likely location of salient region. Though there are many approaches on generating either high-level [5,23] or low level [1,13,18,35] object prior, we choose to use low-level object prior in this paper:

$$v_p^{obj} = \exp(-\frac{\|\mathbf{l}_p - \bar{\mathbf{l}}\|^2}{2\sigma_c^2}), \tag{5}$$

where $\bar{\mathbf{l}}$ is the central coordinate position of the interest.

Then we combine the above two priors together for each superpixel v_p to generate the saliency control map $\mathbf{v}^c$ in a simple way:

$$v_p^c = v_p^{con} \times v_p^{obj}. \tag{6}$$

Based on the experimental results, we use the convex-hull based center prior [35] as the object prior $\mathbf{v}^{obj}$ in this paper. More details and experimental analysis on the influence of the object prior are conducted in Sect. 4.3.

3   Optimization

Our NLL$_0$ minimization is indeed a very challenging problem due to its discreteness and non-convexity. For the failure of using the traditional gradient descent or other discrete optimization methods to optimize the problem, we propose a problem solving strategy based on ADM which is now very popular in solving large scale sparse representation problems [25–27].

By introducing an auxiliary variable $\mathbf{d}$, our graph based NLL$_0$ variational model can be written in an equivalent form:

$$\min_{\mathbf{d},\mathbf{v}} \quad \sum_p \|\mathbf{d}_p\|_0 + \frac{\lambda}{2}(v_p - v_p^c)^2,$$

$$\text{s.t.} \quad \mathbf{d}_p = \nabla_\omega \mathbf{v}_p, \qquad p = 1, \cdots, N. \tag{7}$$

We employ the ADM to solve problem (7). In each iteration, we alternatively solve

$$\mathbf{v}^{k+1} = \arg\min_{\mathbf{v}} \sum_p \frac{\lambda}{2}(v_p - v_p^c)^2 + \frac{\rho}{2}\|\mathbf{d}_p^k - \nabla_\omega \mathbf{v}_p + \frac{1}{\rho}\mathbf{y}_p^k\|^2,$$

$$\mathbf{d}^{k+1} = \arg\min_{\mathbf{d}} \sum_p \|\mathbf{d}_p\|_0 + \frac{\rho}{2}\|\mathbf{d}_p - \nabla_\omega \mathbf{v}_p^{k+1} + \frac{1}{\rho}\mathbf{y}_p^k\|^2, \qquad (8)$$

$$\mathbf{y}_p^{k+1} = \mathbf{y}_p^k + \rho(\mathbf{d}_p^{k+1} - \nabla_\omega \mathbf{v}_p^{k+1}).$$

The solution of the subproblem on v_p is characterized by its first order optimality condition:

$$\lambda(v_p - v_p^c) + \rho \operatorname{div}_\omega(\mathbf{d}_p^k - \nabla_\omega \mathbf{v}_p + \frac{1}{\rho}\mathbf{y}_p^k) = 0. \qquad (9)$$

Here, $\operatorname{div}_\omega \mathbf{u}$ is defined as the divergence of $\mathbf{u}$, and its discretization at p can be deduced

$$\operatorname{div}_\omega \mathbf{u}_p = \sum_q (u_{pq} - u_{qp})\sqrt{\omega_{pq}}, \quad pq \in E. \qquad (10)$$

where u_{pq} is the vector element corresponding to q [32].

According to Eq. (10), the solution v_p^{k+1} of the subproblem can be explicitly written as:

$$
\begin{aligned}
v_p^{k+1} = \frac{1}{\lambda + 2\rho\sum_q \omega_{pq}} (\lambda v_p^c \\
- \rho \sum_q \sqrt{\omega_{pq}}(d_{pq}^k - d_{qp}^k + \frac{1}{\rho}y_{pq}^k - \frac{1}{\rho}y_{qp}^k) \\
+ 2\rho \sum_q \omega_{pq} v_q^{k+1}).
\end{aligned}
\qquad (11)
$$

Though $\mathbf{v}^{k+1}$ can be directly solved by a linear system, a fast approximated solution $v_p^{k+1,n+1}$ is provided by a Gauss-Seidel iterative scheme, and 2 iterations ($n = 2$) are enough [36] to determine a good approximation of the minimizer in experiments:

$$
\begin{aligned}
v_p^{k+1,n+1} = \frac{1}{\lambda + 2\rho\sum_q \omega_{pq}} (\lambda v_p^c \\
- \rho \sum_q \sqrt{\omega_{pq}}(d_{pq}^k - d_{qp}^k + \frac{1}{\rho}y_{pq}^k - \frac{1}{\rho}y_{qp}^k) \\
+ 2\rho \sum_q \omega_{pq} v_q^{k+1,n}), \mathbf{v}^{k+1,n=0} = \mathbf{v}^k,
\end{aligned}
\qquad (12)
$$

The subproblem on $\mathbf{d}$ is apparently sophisticated subproblem due to the non-convexity and discontinuity of L_0 norm. We can obtain its solution by the following lemma which can be proved in the same way as [28].

Algorithm 1. Salient Region Detection via NLL_0

Input: Given image I and necessary parameters.
Postprocessing: Generate superpixels by SLIC [16].
Output: Saliency score $\mathbf{v}$ of the given image. $\mathbf{v} = \{v_p\}$.
1: Construct the k-NN graph on superpixels.
2: Calculate saliency control map $\mathbf{v}^c$ by (6).
3: Initialization: $v_p \leftarrow 0$, $\mathbf{d}_p \leftarrow \mathbf{0}$.
4: **repeat**
5:    **while** n < maxIter **do**
6:       Compute $v_p^{k+1,n+1}$ by (12).
7:    **end while**
8:    Compute $\mathbf{d}_p^{k+1}$ through the thresholding function (15).
9:    Update the Lagrangian multiplier $\mathbf{y}_p^{k+1}$ by (8).
10: **until** max iterations reached.

Lemma 1. *The optimal solution* $\mathbf{x}^\star$ *of the following problem:*

$$\min_{\mathbf{x}} \|\mathbf{x}\|_0 + \frac{\beta}{2}\|\mathbf{x} - \mathbf{z}\|^2, \tag{13}$$

is defined as: for every component x_i *of* $\mathbf{x}$,

$$x_i^\star = \begin{cases} 0, & |z_i| \leq \sqrt{\frac{2}{\beta}}, \\ z_i, & \text{otherwise,} \end{cases} \tag{14}$$

According to Lemma 1, the solution $\mathbf{d}_p^{k+1}$ of the subproblem on $\mathbf{d}$ is given as follows:

$$d_{pq}^{k+1} = \begin{cases} 0, & |\partial_q v_p^{k+1} - \frac{1}{\rho}y_{pq}^k| \leq \sqrt{\frac{2}{\rho}}, \\ \partial_q v_p^{k+1} - \frac{1}{\rho}y_{pq}^k, & \text{otherwise.} \end{cases} \tag{15}$$

Finally, the main steps of the proposed saliency detection method are summarized in Algorithm 1.

4   Experiments

Experiments taken in this paper can be divided into four parts: parameter evaluation in Sect. 4.1, comparison of graph in Sect. 4.2, analysis of object prior in Sect. 4.3 and comparison with state-of-the-art methods in Sect. 4.4.

4.1   Parameter Evaluation

We set the number of superpixels $N = 300$ in all the experiments. There are 5 parameters in our NLL_0 method: σ and α in Eq. (1), the number of nearest neighbors k, λ and ρ in Eq. (7). The parameters are empirically set to $\sigma^2 = 0.05$, $\alpha = 0.9$, $k = 5$, $\lambda = 0.001$ and $\rho = 0.0001$.

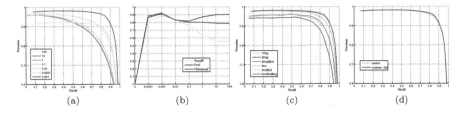

Fig. 4. (a) Precision and recall rate for the regularization parameter λ on the ASD data set. (b) Average precision, recall and F-measure curve with different λ parameter. (c) Effectiveness of our graph by PR-curve. (d) Comparison of using image center prior and convex-hull-based center prior as object control map respectively in our model.

The parameter λ is a weight directly controlling the balance between regularization and fidelity, which makes an important role in our approach. We assign λ as 0, 0.1, 0.01, 0.001, 0.0001, 1, 10 and 100 in our approach respectively. And draw the corresponding PR-curves (Fig. 4(a)) and the average precision, recall and F-measure curves (Fig. 4(b)) with different λ.

In particular, $\lambda = 0$ corresponds to an extreme case that only regular term is contained in the NLL$_0$ model. The gradient of each superpixel in the optimal solution of this case must be zero, which corresponds to an all-black color image. The PR-curve of $\lambda = 0$ is not drawn in Fig. 4(a) since it is a straight line from 0 to 0.2. With the increase of λ, the saliency control map $\mathbf{v}^c$ takes a bigger role in the NLL$_0$ model, and more edge information is remained. But it changes smoothly when $\lambda > 1$ (see Fig. 4(b)) and the PR-curves almost overlapped when $\lambda = 1, 10$ and 100.

Whether according to the PR-curves (Fig. 4(a)) or the average precision, recall and F-measure curves (Fig. 4(b)), $\lambda = 0.001$ is the best choice in our approach, which is fixed and applied in all the experiments in this paper.

4.2   Comparison of Graph

In Sect. 2.1, we give an example to illustrate the effectiveness of our k-NN graph. However, this is not sufficient. In this subsection we extensively test their validity by using public data set. We use the precision-recall curve to show the well performance of our graph.

Figure 4(c) shows the comparison result of 6 different strategies to construct graph. From the Fig. 4(c), the 2-ring graph is the worst choice for our NLL$_0$ method, the 1-ring graph and the 2-ring graph with boundaries connected (is used in [19]) perform almost the same. Leaving out the strategy of connecting the four boundaries and the most indistinctive regions together, the k-NN graph itself performs better than the graphs constructed in the spatial space, which furthermore indicates that the strategy of constructing graph in the feature space can contribute to the NLL$_0$ model. Also, the strategy that connects all the boundaries and background together does have a better effect.

4.3   Analysis of Object Prior

In this paper, we use low-level object prior $\mathbf{v}^{obj}$ in the saliency control map $\mathbf{v}^c$. Certainly, different coordinate positions $\bar{I}$ of the interest will generate different prior maps by Eq. (5). In this section, we conduct an experiment on two different strategies for obtaining $\bar{I}$, and the results show that our NLL_0 method is robust to these two low-level object priors.

Regarding the image center as $\bar{I}$ is a common assumption in saliency detection [1,13]. It hypothesizes that people taking photographs generally frame the focus and assign higher value to the image elements near the image center. But there always exist some special cases that image center assumption may bring wrong instruction. Xie et al. [35] propose a object prior which calculates the convex hull of the object and lets its center as $\bar{I}$, which obtains a more reasonable and robust object measure map. We use the two object priors in the saliency control map respectively, and the discrepancy between them is quite small through quantitative analysis (see Fig. 4(d)). An intuitive example is also given in Fig. 5. Though the prior maps generated by this two strategies are different (Fig. 5(b) and (d)), the final results (Fig. 5(c) and (e)) are nearly the same. The experimental results show the robustness of our NLL_0 method to the object prior.

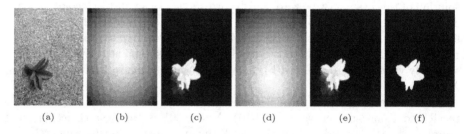

    (a)   (b)   (c)   (d)   (e)   (f)

Fig. 5. Robustness of the object prior. (a)Input image. (b) Object prior map based on image center [1,13,21]. (c) Result of using image center as the object prior. (d) Object prior map based on convex-hull [18]. (e) Result of using convex-hull center as the object prior. (f) Ground truth.

4.4   Comparison with State-of-the-Art Methods

Our experiments are conducted on ASD, MSRA, ECSSD and iCoseg data sets. The ASD data set contains 1000 images, is a subset of MSRA which contains a large variation among 5000 images of natural scenes, animals, people, etc. ASD is publicly available in salient object detection and is evaluated in almost every saliency paper. ECSSD is a data set with 1000 images, which includes many semantically meaningful but structurally complex images for evaluation. We use this data set to show the well-performance of difficult images with complex backgrounds. The iCoseg data set including 38 groups of 643 images, which is a publicly available co-segmentation data set. The images in iCoseg may contain

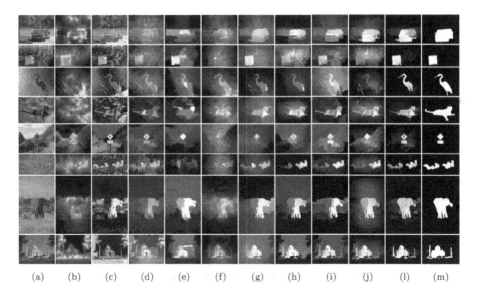

(a)   (b)   (c)   (d)   (e)   (f)   (g)   (h)   (i)   (j)   (l)   (m)

Fig. 6. Visual comparison on MSRA, ECSSD and iCoseg data sets. The top three rows are selected from MSRA data set, the middle three are from ECSSD data set, and the last two rows are chosen from iCoseg data set. We compare 9 state-of-the-art methods, from (b)–(j): CA [1], HC [6], RC [6], CB [13], LR [4], CH [18], MR [19], HS [37] and MC [20]. Saliency maps generated by our algorithm (l) is the closest to the ground truth (m).

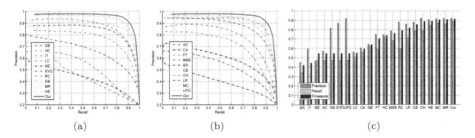

(a)   (b)   (c)

Fig. 7. Performance of the proposed algorithm compared with 20 state-of-the-art methods on the ASD database. (a), (b) Average precision recall curve by segmenting saliency maps using fixed thresholds. (c) Mean precision, recall, and F-measure values of the evaluated methods.

one or multiple salient objects. We use this data set to evaluate the performance of multiple salient object detection.

We compare our NLL_0 approach with 20 previous methods on ASD, including 12 earlier but classical algorithm: AC [11], FT [12], GB [7], HC [6], IT [8], LC [38], MSS [39], MZ [9], SR [10], SVO [2], CB [13], RC [6], and recent state-of-the-art algorithms: CA [1], CH [18], GS [3], HS [37], LR [4], MR [19], UFO [5], MC [20].

Visual comparison of selected 9 state-of-the-art approaches is shown in Fig. 6. As is shown in Fig. 6, our approach can deal with the challenging images with complex background and also works well on image contains multi-salient objects (the sixth row in Fig. 6).

Quantitative comparisons on ASD data set are shown in Fig. 7. Figure 7 (a) and (b) are the PR-curves of the 20 previous methods applied on ASD. All the methods are separated into two groups for the purpose of clear visual effect. It is shown that our approach favorable outperforms other methods, while achieves similar performance as HS, MR and MC in terms of PR-curve. However, as is discussed in [34], neither the precision nor recall measure considers the true negative counts. These measures respond the ability of assigning saliency to salient regions, but fail to react the ability of detecting the opposite. Our approach not only successfully assigns saliency to salient regions, but also successfully does the opposite. Comparison of the eighth to eleventh columns in Fig. 6 demonstrates the well performance of our approach on generating a well suppressed background. The time complexity of our algorithm mainly focuses on Gauss-Seidel iteration in the subproblem of u, and its running time is proportional to

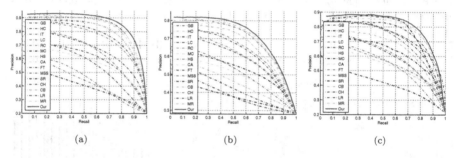

Fig. 8. Performance of the proposed algorithm compared with 15 state-of-the-art methods on the MSRA database through average precision recall curve. (a) Comparison on MSRA data set. (b) Comparison on ECSSD data set. (c) Comparison on iCoseg data set.

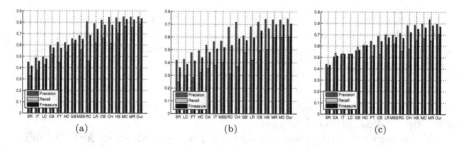

Fig. 9. Performance of the proposed algorithm compared with 15 state-of-the-art methods on the MSRA database through mean precision, recall, and F-measure values. (a) Comparison on MSRA data set. (b) Comparison on ECSSD data set. (c) Comparison on iCoseg data set.

the square of N at each iteration. Since few steps are enough for Gauss-Seidel strategy to get the desired result in our experiments, so the time complexity of our algorithm is totally $O(N^2)^2$.

We also compare 15 state-of-the-art approaches on MSRA, ECSSD and iCoseg data sets, for the reason that the relevant codes of some previous approaches are not publicly available. Figures 8 and 9 show the quantitative comparison through both PR-curve and F-measure. The difference between our method and others is clear, manifesting that our NLL_0 approach can be widely used in different types of images.

5   Conclusion and Future Work

This paper develops a energy minimization based on L_0 norm for salient region detection. We construct a graph based on the k-NN of superpixels in the feature space. Then, NLL_0 is proposed on this graph with saliency control map that is generated by contrast and object prior. We solve this non-convex minimization problem by an iterative strategy based on ADM. Our NLL_0 approach is evaluated on various challenging image sets with comparison to state-of-the-art techniques to show its superiority for saliency detection. In the future, we plan to focus on generating semantic features from the image that can better describe the characteristic of the salient region.

Acknowledgement. Risheng Liu is supported by the National Natural Science Foundation of China (No. 61300086), the China Postdoctoral Science Foundation (2013 M530917, 2014T70249), the Fundamental Research Funds for the Central Universities (No. DUT12RC(3)67) and the Open Project Program of the State Key Laboratory of CAD&CG, Zhejiang University, Zhejiang, China (No. A1404). Zhixun Su is supported by National Natural Science Foundation of China (Nos. 61173103, 91230103) and National Science and Technology Major Project (No. 2013ZX04005021).

References

1. Goferman, S., Zelnik-Manor, L., Tal, A.: Context-aware saliency detection. IEEE Trans. PAMI **34**, 1915–1926 (2012)
2. Chang, K.Y., Liu, T.L., Chen, H.T., Lai, S.H.: Fusing generic objectness and visual saliency for salient object detection. In: ICCV (2011)
3. Wei, Y., Wen, F., Zhu, W., Sun, J.: Geodesic saliency using background priors. In: Fitzgibbon, A., Lazebnik, S., Perona, P., Sato, Y., Schmid, C. (eds.) ECCV 2012, Part III. LNCS, vol. 7574, pp. 29–42. Springer, Heidelberg (2012)
4. Shen, X., Wu, Y.: A unified approach to salient object detection via low rank matrix recovery. In: CVPR (2012)

---

[2] We would like to list the running time (second per image) for the compared methods in our paper: Our 0.97s, CA 48.65s, CB 1.97s, LR 14.89s, CH 1.07s, MR 1.02s, MC 0.25s. It can be observed that our detector is comparable among all the MATLAB implementation based saliency detectors in our paper.

5. Jiang, P., Ling, H., Yu, J., Peng, J.: Salient region detection by ufo: Uniqueness, focusness and objectness. In: ICCV (2013)
6. Cheng, M.M., Zhang, G.X., Mitra, N.J., Huang, X., Hu, S.M.: Global contrast based salient region detection. In: CVPR (2011)
7. Harel, J., Koch, C., Perona, P.: Graph-based visual saliency. In: NIPS (2006)
8. Itti, L., Koch, C., Niebur, E.: A model of saliency-based visual attention for rapid scene analysis. IEEE Trans. PAMI **20**, 1254–1259 (1998)
9. Ma, Y.F., Zhang, H.J.: Contrast-based image attention analysis by using fuzzy growing. In: ACM Multimedia (2003)
10. Hou, X., Zhang, L.: Saliency detection: a spectral residual approach. In: CVPR (2007)
11. Achanta, R., Estrada, F.J., Wils, P., Süsstrunk, S.: Salient region detection and segmentation. In: Gasteratos, A., Vincze, M., Tsotsos, J.K. (eds.) ICVS 2008. LNCS, vol. 5008, pp. 66–75. Springer, Heidelberg (2008)
12. Achanta, R., Hemami, S., Estrada, F., Susstrunk, S.: Frequency-tuned salient region detection. In: CVPR (2009)
13. Jiang, H., Wang, J., Yuan, Z., Liu, T., Zheng, N., Li, S.: Automatic salient object segmentation based on context and shape prior. In: BMVC (2011)
14. Mai, L., Niu, Y., Liu, F.: Saliency aggregation: a data-driven approach. In: CVPR (2013)
15. Liu, T., Yuan, Z., Sun, J., Wang, J., Zheng, N., Tang, X., Shum, H.Y.: Learning to detect a salient object. IEEE Trans. PAMI **33**, 353–367 (2011)
16. Achanta, R., Shaji, A., Smith, K., Lucchi, A., Fua, P., Susstrunk, S.: SLIC superpixels compared to state-of-the-art superpixel methods. IEEE Trans. PAMI **34**, 2274–2282 (2012)
17. Shi, J., Malik, J.: Normalized cuts and image segmentation. IEEE Trans. PAMI **22**, 888–905 (2000)
18. Yang, C., Zhang, L., Lu, H.: Graph-regularized saliency detection with convex-hull-based center prior. IEEE Signal Process. Lett. **20**, 637–640 (2013)
19. Yang, C., Zhang, L., Lu, H., Ruan, X., Yang, M.H.: Saliency detection via graph-based manifold ranking. In: CVPR (2013)
20. Jiang, B., Zhang, L., Lu, H., Yang, C., Yang, M.H.: Saliency detection via absorbing markov chain. In: ICCV (2013)
21. Jiang, Z., Davis, L.S.: Submodular salient region detection. In: CVPR (2013)
22. Gopalakrishnan, V., Hu, Y., Rajan, D.: Random walks on graphs to model saliency in images. In: CVPR (2009)
23. Jia, Y., Han, M.: Category-independent object-level saliency detection. In: ICCV (2013)
24. Liu, R., Lin, Z., Shan, S.: Adaptive partial differential equation learning for visual saliency detection. In: CVPR (2014)
25. Boyd, S., Parikh, N., Chu, E., Peleato, B., Eckstein, J.: Distributed optimization and statistical learning via the alternating direction method of multipliers. Found. Trends Mach. Learn. **3**, 1–122 (2011)
26. Lin, Z., Liu, R., Su, Z.: Linearized alternating direction method with adaptive penalty for low-rank representation. In: NIPS (2011)
27. Liu, R., Lin, Z., Su, Z.: Linearized alternating direction method with parallel splitting and adaptive penalty for separable convex programs in machine learning. In: ACML (2013)
28. Xu, L., Lu, C., Xu, Y., Jia, J.: Image smoothing via l_0 gradient minimization. ACM TOG **30**, 174 (2011)

29. Xu, L., Zheng, S., Jia, J.: Unnatural l_0 sparse representation for natural image deblurring. In: CVPR (2013)
30. Pan, J., Su, Z.: Fast l_0-regularized kernel estimation for robust motion deblurring. IEEE Sig. Process. Lett. **20**, 841–844 (2013)
31. Bougleux, S., Elmoataz, A., Melkemi, M.: Discrete regularization on weighted graphs for image and mesh filtering. In: Sgallari, F., Murli, A., Paragios, N. (eds.) SSVM 2007. LNCS, vol. 4485, pp. 128–139. Springer, Heidelberg (2007)
32. Gilboa, G., Osher, S.: Nonlocal operators with applications to image processing. Multiscale Model. Simul. **7**, 1005–1028 (2008)
33. Einhäuser, W., König, P.: Does luminance-contrast contribute to a saliency map for overt visual attention? Eur. J. Neurosci. **17**, 1089–1097 (2003)
34. Perazzi, F., Krahenbuhl, P., Pritch, Y., Hornung, A.: Saliency filters: contrast based filtering for salient region detection. In: CVPR (2012)
35. Xie, Y., Lu, H.: Visual saliency detection based on bayesian model. In: ICIP (2011)
36. Bresson, X.: A short note for nonlocal tv minimization (2009)
37. Yan, Q., Xu, L., Shi, J., Jia, J.: Hierarchical saliency detection. In: CVPR (2013)
38. Zhai, Y., Shah, M.: Visual attention detection in video sequences using spatiotemporal cues. In: ACM Multimedia (2006)
39. Achanta, R., Susstrunk, S.: Saliency detection using maximum symmetric surround. In: ICIP (2010)

N^4-Fields: Neural Network Nearest Neighbor Fields for Image Transforms

Yaroslav Ganin$^{(\boxtimes)}$ and Victor Lempitsky

Skolkovo Institute of Science and Technology (Skoltech), Moscow, Russia
{ganin,lempitsky}@skoltech.ru

Abstract. We propose a new architecture for difficult image processing operations, such as natural edge detection or thin object segmentation. The architecture is based on a simple combination of convolutional neural networks with the nearest neighbor search.

We focus our attention on the situations when the desired image transformation is too hard for a neural network to learn explicitly. We show that in such situations the use of the nearest neighbor search on top of the network output allows to improve the results considerably and to account for the underfitting effect during the neural network training. The approach is validated on three challenging benchmarks, where the performance of the proposed architecture matches or exceeds the state-of-the-art.

1 Introduction

Deep convolutional neural networks (CNNs) [1] have recently achieved a breakthrough in a variety of computer vision benchmarks and are attracting a very strong interest within the computer vision community. The most impressive results have been attained for image [2] or pixel [3] classification results. The key to these results was the sheer size of the trained CNNs and the power of modern GPU used to train those architectures (Fig. 1).

In this work, we demonstrate that convolutional neural networks can achieve state-of-the-art results for sophisticated image processing tasks. The complexity of these tasks defies the straightforward application of CNNs, which perform reasonably well, but clearly below state-of-the-art. In particular, we show that by pairing convolutional networks with a simple non-parametric transform based on nearest-neighbor search state-of-the-art performance is achievable. This approach is evaluated on three challenging and competitive benchmarks (edge detection on Berkeley Segmentation dataset [4], edge detection on the NYU RGBD dataset [5], retina vessel segmentation on the DRIVE dataset [6]). All the results are obtained with the same meta-parameters, such as the configuration of a CNN, thus demonstrating the universality of the proposed approach.

The two approaches, namely convolutional **N**eural **N**etworks and **N**earest **N**eighbor search are applied sequentially and in a patch-by-patch manner, hence we call the architecture N^4 -*fields*. At test time, an N^4-field first passes each

D. Cremers et al. (Eds.): ACCV 2014, Part II, LNCS 9004, pp. 536–551, 2015.
DOI: 10.1007/978-3-319-16808-1_36

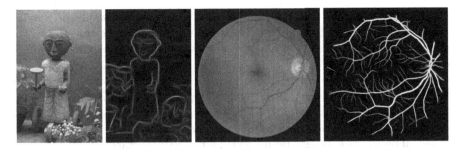

Fig. 1. N^4-Fields can be applied to a range of complex image processing tasks, such as natural edge detection (left) or vessel segmentation (right). The proposed architecture combines the convolutional neural networks with the nearest neighbor search and is generic. E.g. it achieves state-of-the-art performance on standard benchmarks for these two rather different applications with very little customization or parameter tuning.

patch through a CNN. For a given patch, the output of the first stage is a low-dimensional vector corresponding to the activations of the top layer in the CNN. At the second stage we use the nearest neighbor search within the CNN activations corresponding to patches sampled from the training data. Thus, we retrieve a patch with a known pixel-level annotation that has a similar CNN activation, and transfer its annotation to the output. By averaging the outputs of the overlapping patches, the transformation of the input image is obtained.

Below, we first review the related works (Sect. 2), describe the proposed architecture and the associated training procedures in detail (Sect. 3), and discuss the results of applying it on sample problems (Sect. 4). We conclude with a short discussion of the merits and the potential of the proposed approach (Sect. 5).

2   Related Work

There is a very large body of related approaches, as both neural networks and nearest neighbor methods have been used heavily as components within image processing systems. Here, we only review several works that are arguably most related to ours.

Neural Networks for Image Processing. The use of neural networks for image processing goes back for decades [7]. Several recent works have investigated large-scale training of deep architectures for complex edge detection and segmentation tasks. Thus, Mnih and Hinton [8] have used a cascade of two deep networks to segment roads in aerial images, while Shulz et al. [9] use CNNs to perform semantic segmentation on standard datasets. Kivinen et al. [10] proposed using unsupervised features extraction via deep belief net extension of mcRBM [11] followed by supervised neural net training for boundary prediction in natural images. State-of-the-art results on several semantic segmentation datasets were obtained by Farabet et al. [12] by using a combination of a CNN classifier and superpixelization-based smoothing. Finally, a large body of work, e.g. [3,13] simply frame the segmentation problem as patch classification, making generic CNN-based classification easily applicable and successful. Below, we compare N^4-fields against such baseline and find them to achieve better results for our applications.

Another series of works [14,15] investigate the use of convolutional neural networks for image denoising. In this specific application, CNNs benefit greatly from virtually unlimited training data that can be synthesized, while the gap between synthetic and real data for this application is small.

Neural networks have also been applied for descriptor learning, which resembles the way they are used within N^4-fields. Thus, Chopra et al. [16] introduced a general scheme for learning CNNs that map input images to multi-dimensional descriptors, suitable among other things for nearest neighbor retrieval or similarity verification. The learning in that case is performed on a large set of pairs of matching images. N^4-fields are different from this group of the approaches in terms of their purpose (image processing) and the type of the training data (annotated images).

Non-parametric Approaches to Image Processing. Nearest neighbor methods have been applied to image processing with a considerable success. Most methods use nearest neighbor relations within the same image, e.g. Dabov et al. [17] for denoising or Criminisi et al. [18] for inpainting. More related to our work, Freeman et al. [19] match patches in a given image to a large dataset of patches from different images, to infer the missing high-frequencies and to achieve super-resolution. All these works use the patches themselves or their band-passed versions to perform the matching.

Another popular non-parametric framework to perform operations with patches are random forests. Our work was in many ways inspired by the recent impressive results in Dollár et al. [20], where random forests are trained on patches with structured annotations. Their emphasis is on natural edge detection, and their system represent the state-of-the-art for this task. N^4-fields match the accuracy of [20] for natural edge detection, and perform considerably better for the task of vessel segmentation in micrographs, thus demonstrating the ability to adapt to new domains.

3 N^4-Fields

3.1   Architecture

We start by introducing the notation, and discussing the way our architecture is applied to images. The N^4-Fields transform images patch-by-patch. Given an image transform application, we wish to map a single or multi-channel (e.g. RGB) image patch $\mathcal{P}$ of size $M \times M$ to a segmentation, an edge map, or some other semantically-meaningful annotation $\mathbf{A}(\mathcal{P})$, which in itself is a single or multi-channel image patch of size $N \times N$. We take N to be smaller than M, so that $\mathbf{A}(\mathcal{P})$ represents a desired annotation for the central part of $\mathcal{P}$. For the

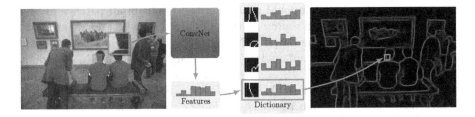

Fig. 2. The N^4 architecture for natural edge detection. The input image is processed patch-by-patch. An input patch is first passed through a pretrained convolutional neural network (CNN). Then, the output of the CNN is matched against the dictionary of sample CNN outputs that correspond to training patches with known annotations. The annotation corresponding to the nearest neighbor is transferred to the output. Overall, the output is obtained by averaging the overlapping transferred annotations.

simplicity of comparisons, in our experiments we use the sizes proposed in [20], in particular, $M = 34$ and $N = 16$.

Given the annotated data, we learn a mapping $\mathbf{F}$ that maps patches to the desired annotations. At test time, the mapping is applied to all image patches and their outputs are combined by averaging, thus resulting in an output image. The output of the processing for a pixel $p = (x, y)$ is the average of the outputs of N^2 patches that contain this pixel. More formally, the output of the mapping on the input image I is defined as:

$$\mathbf{F}(I)[x, y] = \frac{1}{N^2} \sum_{\substack{i,j:|i-x|\leq N/2 \\ |j-y|\leq N/2}} \mathbf{F}\left(I(i, j | M)\right)[x - i, y - i], \qquad (1)$$

where $\mathbf{F}(I)[x, y]$ denotes the value of image transform at pixel (x, y), $I(i, j | M)$ denotes the image patch of size $M \times M$ centered at (i, j), and $\mathbf{F}\left(I(i, j | M)\right)[x - i, y - i]$ is a pixel in the output patch at the position $(x - i, y - j)$ assuming the origin in the center of the patch.

Obviously, the accuracy of the transform depends on the way the transform $\mathbf{F}$ is defined and learned. Convolutional neural networks (CNNs) provide a generic architecture for learning functions of the multi-channel images and patches exploiting the translational invariance properties of natural images. The direct approach is then to learn a mapping $\mathcal{P} \rightarrow \mathbf{A}(\mathcal{P})$ in the form of a CNN. In practice, we found the flexibility of CNNs to be insufficient to learn the corresponding mapping even when a large number of layers with large number of parameters are considered. For complex transforms, e.g. natural edge detection, we observe a strong underfitting during the training, which results in a suboptimal performance at test time.

Convolutional neural network can be regarded as a parametric model, albeit with a very large number of parameters. A straightforward way to increase the fitting capacity of the mapping is to consider a non-parametric model. We thus combine a simple non-parametric mapping (nearest neighbor) and a complex parametric mapping (convolutional neural network). The input patch $\mathcal{P}$ is first mapped to an intermediate representation $\text{CNN}(\mathcal{P}; \Theta)$, where Θ denotes the parameters of the CNN. The output $\text{CNN}(\mathcal{P}; \Theta)$ of the CNN mapping (we call it a *neural code*) is then compared to a dictionary dataset of CNN outputs, computed for T patches $\mathcal{P}_1, \mathcal{P}_2, \ldots, \mathcal{P}_T$ taken from the training images, and thus having known annotations $\mathbf{A}(\mathcal{P}_1), \mathbf{A}(\mathcal{P}_2), \ldots, \mathbf{A}(\mathcal{P}_T)$. The input patch is then assigned the annotation from the dictionary patch with the closest CNN output, i.e. $\mathbf{A}(\mathcal{P}_k)$, where $k = \arg\min_{i=1}^{T} \|\text{CNN}(\mathcal{P}_i) - \text{CNN}(\mathcal{P})\|$ (Fig. 2). If we denote such nearest neighbor mapping as NNB, then the full two-stage mapping is defined as:

$$\mathbf{F}(\mathcal{P}) = \text{NNB}\left(\text{CNN}(\mathcal{P}; \Theta) \mid \{(\text{CNN}(\mathcal{P}_i; \Theta); \mathbf{A}(\mathcal{P}_i)) \mid i = 1..T\}\right), \qquad (2)$$

where $\text{NNB}(x \mid M = \{(a_i \mid b_i)\})$ denotes the nearest-neighbor transform that maps x to the value b_i corresponding to the key a_i that is closest to x over the dataset M. In our experiments, the dimensionality of the intermediate representation (i.e. the space of CNN outputs) is rather low (16 dimensions), which makes nearest neighbor search reasonably easy.

In the experiments, we observe that such a two-stage architecture can successfully rectify the underfitting effect of the CNN and result in better generalization and overall transform quality compared to single stage architectures that include either CNN alone or nearest neighbor search on hand-crafted features alone.

3.2   Training

The training procedure for an N^4-field requires learning the parameters Θ of the convolutional neural network. Note, that the second stage (nearest neighbor mapping) does not require any training apart from sampling T patches from the training images.

The CNN training is performed in a standard supervised way on the patches drawn from the training images $I_1, I_2, \ldots I_R$. For that, we define the surrogate target output for each input patch. Since for each training patch $\mathcal{P}$, the desired annotation $\mathbf{A}(\mathcal{P})$ is known, it is natural to take this annotation itself as such a target (although other variants are possible as described in Sect. 3.3), i.e. to train the network on the input-output pairs of the form $(\mathcal{P}, \mathbf{A}(\mathcal{P}))$. However, such output can be rather high-dimensional (when the output patch size is large) and vary non-smoothly w.r.t. small translations and jitter, in particular when our model applications of edge detection or thin object segmentations are considered. To address both problems, we perform dimensionality reduction of the output annotations using PCA. Experimentally, we found that the target dimensionality can be taken rather small, e.g. 16 dimensions for 16×16 patches.

Thus, the overall training process includes the following steps:

1. Learn the PCA projection on a subset of $N \times N$ patches extracted from the training image annotations.
2. Train the convolutional neural network on the input-output pairs $\{(\mathcal{P}, \text{PCA}(\mathbf{A}(\mathcal{P}))\}$ sampled from the training images.

3. Construct a dictionary $\{(\text{CNN}(\mathcal{P}_i;\Theta);\mathbf{A}(\mathcal{P}_i))|i = 1..T\}$ by drawing T random patches from the training images and passing them through the trained network.

After the training, the N^4-field can be applied to new images as discussed above.

3.3   Implementation Details

Training the CNN. We use the heavily modified cuda-convnet CNN toolbox[1]. The CNN architecture that was used in our experiments is loosely inspired by [2] (it comprises the layers shown in Fig. 3). We also tried a dozen of other CNN designs (deeper ones and wider ones) but the performance always stayed roughly the same, which suggests that our system is somewhat insensitive to the choice of the architecture given the sufficient number of free parameters.

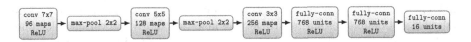

Fig. 3. The CNN architecture used in our experiments. See Sect. 3.3 for details.

The model was trained on 34×34 patches extracted at randomly sampled locations of the training images. Each patch is preprocessed by subtracting the per-channel mean (across all images). Those patches are packed into mini-batches of size 128 (due to the software/hardware restrictions) and presented to the network. The initial weights in the CNN are drawn from Gaussian distribution with zero mean and $\sigma = 10^{-2}$. They are then updated using stochastic gradient descent with momentum set to 0.9. The starting learning rate η is set to 10^{-1} (below in Sect. 4 we introduce an alternative target function which demands smaller initial $\eta = 10^{-3}$). As commonly done, we anneal η throughout training when the validation error reaches its plateau.

As the amount of the training data was rather limited, we observed overfitting (validation error increasing, while training error decreasing) alongside with underfitting (training error staying high). To reduce overfitting, we enrich the training set with various artificial transformations of input patches such as random rotations and horizontal reflections. Those transformations are computed on-the-fly during the training procedure (new batches are prepared in parallel with the network training).

Along with data augmentation we apply two regularization techniques which have become quite common for CNNs, namely dropout [21] (we randomly discard half of activations in the first two fully-connected layers) and ℓ_2-norm restriction of the filters in the first layer [21,22].

---

[1] https://code.google.com/p/cuda-convnet/.

Testing Procedure. At test time we want to calculate activations for patches centered at all possible locations within input images. A naive approach would be to apply a CNN in the sliding window fashion (separate invocation for each location). However this solution may be computationally expensive especially in case of deep architectures. Luckily it is rather easy to avoid redundant calculations and to make dense applications efficient by feeding the network with a sequence of shifted test images [23].

After neural codes for all patches are computed, nearest-neighbors search is done by means of k-d trees provided as a part of VLFeat package [24]. We use default settings except for maximum number of comparisons which we set to 30.

Our proof-of-concept implementation runs reasonably fast taking about 6 seconds to process an image of size 480×320, although we were not focusing on speed. Computational performance may be brought closer to the real-time by, for example, applying the system in a strided fashion [20] and/or finding a simpler design for the CNN.

Multi-scale Operation. Following the works [20,25] we apply our scheme at different scales. For each input image we combine detections produced for original, half and double resolutions to get the final output. While various blending strategies may be employed, in our case even simple averaging gave remarkably good results.

Committee of N^4-Fields. CNNs are shown [2,3,23] to perform better if outputs of multiple models are averaged. We found that this technique works quite well for our system too. One rationale would be that different instances of the neural network produce slightly different neural codes hence nearest-neighbor search may return different annotation patches for the same input patch. In practice we observe that averaging amplifies relevant edges and smooths the noisy regions. The latter is especially important for the natural edge detection benchmarks, as the output of N^4-fields is passed through the non-maximum suppression.

4   Experiments

We evaluate our approach on three datasets. Within two of them (BSDS500 and NYU RGBD), the processing task is to detect natural edges, and in the remaining case (DRIVE) the task is to segment thin vessels in retinal micrographs. Across the datasets, we provide comparison with baseline methods, with the state-of-the-art on those datasets, illustrate the operation of the method, and demonstrate characteristic results.

CNN Baselines. All three tasks correspond to binary labeling of pixels in the input photographs (boundary/not boundary, vessel/no vessel). It is therefore natural to compare our approach to CNNs that directly predict pixel labels. Given the input patch, a CNN can produce a decision either for the single central pixel or for multiple pixels (e.g. a central patch of size 16×16) hence we have two *CNN baselines*. We call them *CNN-central* and *CNN-patch* respectively. Each of

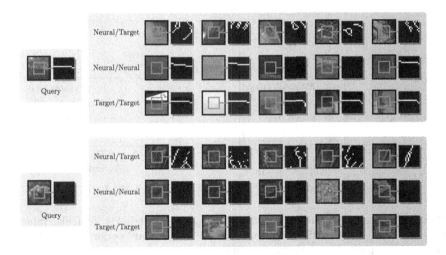

Fig. 4. Examples of nearest neighbor matchings of query patches to dictionary patches. For all patches, the ground truth annotations (edge sets) of the central parts are shown alongside. The righthand panels show the results of the nearest neighbor searches for different combinations of the query encoding and the dictionary patch encoding. *"Neural"* corresponds to the encoding with top-layer activations $CNN(\mathcal{P})$ of the CNN, while *"Target"* corresponds to the "ground truth" encoding $PCA(\mathbf{A}(\mathcal{P}))$ that the CNN is being trained to replicate. Matching neural codes to target codes (Neural/Target) works poorly thus highlighting the gap between the neural codes and the target PCA codes (which is the manifestation of the underfitting during the CNN training). By using neural codes for both the queries and the dictionary patches, our approach is able to overcome such underfitting and to match many patches to correct annotations (see Neural/Neural matching).

the CNNs has the same architecture as the CNN we use within N^4-fields, except that the size of the last layer is no longer 16 but equals the number of pixels we wish to produce predictions for (i.e. 1 for CNN-central and 256 for CNN-patch). At test time, we run the baseline on every patch and annotate chosen subsets of pixels with the output of the CNN classifier applying averaging in the overlapping regions. As with our main system, to assess the performance of the baseline, we use a committee of three CNN classifiers at three scales.

Nearest Neighbor Baseline. We have also evaluated a baseline that replaces the learned neural codes with "hand-crafted" features. For this, we used SIFT vectors computed over the input $M \times M$ patches as descriptors and use these vectors to perform the nearest-neighbor search in the training dataset. Since SIFT was designed mainly for natural RGB photographs, we evaluate this baseline for the BSDS500 edge detection only.

Alternative Encoding (AE). Given the impressive results of [20] on edge detection, we experimented with a variation of our method inspired by their method. We annotate each patch with a long binary vector that looks at the

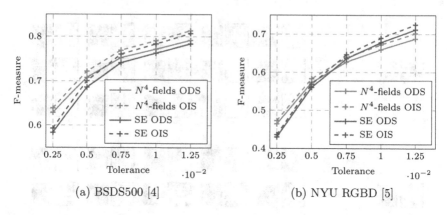

(a) BSDS500 [4]   (b) NYU RGBD [5]

Fig. 5. Performance scores for different tolerance thresholds (default value is $0.75 \cdot 10^{-2}$) used in the BSDS500 benchmark [4]. Algorithms' performance (ODS and OIS measures plotted as *dashed* and *solid* lines respectively) is going down as the tolerance threshold is decreased. N^4-fields (*blue* lines) handles more stringent thresholds better, which suggests that cleaner edges are produced, as is also evidenced by the qualitative results. See Sect. 4 for details (Color figure online).

pairs of pixels in the output $N \times N$ patch and assigns it 1 or 0 depending whether it belongs to the object segment. We then apply PCA dimensionality reduction to 16 components. More formally, we define the target annotation vector during the CNN training to be:

$$\mathbf{B}(P) = \mathrm{PCA}((v_1, v_2, \ldots, v_L)), \tag{3}$$

where $L = \binom{N^2}{2}$ and v_i is defined for i-th pair (p_l, p_m) of pixels in the ground truth segmentation $\mathbf{S}(\mathcal{P})$ and is equal to $\mathbf{1}\{\mathbf{S}(\mathcal{P})[p_l] = \mathbf{S}(\mathcal{P})[p_m]\}$. In the experiments, we observe a small improvement for such alternative encoding.

BSDS500 Experiments. The first dataset is Berkley Segmentation Dataset and Benchmark (BSDS500) [4]. It contains 500 color images divided into three subsets: 200 for training, 100 for validation and 200 for testing. Edge detection accuracy is measured using three scores: fixed contour threshold (ODS), per-image threshold (OIS), and average precision (AP) [4,20]. In order to be evaluated properly, test edges must be thinned to one pixel width before running the benchmark code. We use the non-maximum suppression algorithm from [20] for that (Fig. 7).

In general, N^4-fields perform similarly to the best previously published methods [10,20,26]. In particular, the full version of the system (the committee of three N^4-fields applied at three scales) matches the performance of the mentioned algorithms, with the alternative encoding performing marginally better (Table 1-a). Following [27] in order to account for the inherent problems of the dataset we also test our approach against the so-called "consensus" subset of the ground-truth labels. Within this setting our method significantly outperforms other algorithms in terms of ODS and AP (Table 1-b).

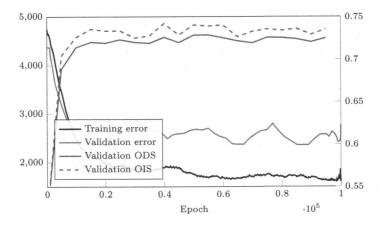

Fig. 6. The validation score (average precision) of the full N^4-fields and error rates (loss) of the underlying CNN measured throughout the training process. The strong correlation between the values suggests the importance of large-scale learning for the good performance of N^4-fields. This experiment was performed for the BSDS500 edge detection (hold out validation set included 20 images).

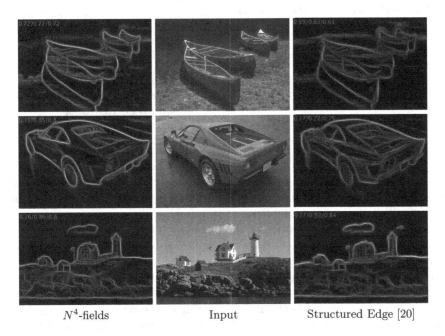

Fig. 7. Representative results on the BSDS500 dataset. For comparison, we give the results of the best previously published method [20]. The red numbers correspond to Recall/Precision/F-measure. We give two examples where N^4-fields perform better than [20], and one example (bottom row) where [20] performs markedly better according to the quantitative measure (Color figure online).

Table 1. Edge detection results on BSDS500 [4] (1both for the original ground-truth annotation and "consensus" labels) and NYU RGBD [5]. Our approach (N^4-fields) achieves performance which is better or comparable to the state-of-the-art. We also observe that the relative performance of the methods in terms of perceptual quality are not adequately reflected by the standard performance measures.

	ODS	OIS	AP
SE-MS, $T = 4$ [20]	.59	.62	.59
DeepNet [10]	.61	.64	.61
PMI + sPb, MS [26]	.61	**.68**	.56
N^4-fields, AE	**.64**	.67	**.64**

(b) BSDS500 [4] (Consensus)

	ODS	OIS	AP
SIFT + NNB	.59	.60	.60
CNN-central	.72	.74	.75
CNN-patch	.73	.75	.74
gPb-owt-ucm [4]	.73	.76	.73
SCG [25]	.74	.76	.77
SE-MS, $T = 4$ [20]	.74	.76	**.78**
DeepNet [10]	.74	.76	.76
PMI + sPb, MS [26]	.74	**.77**	**.78**
N^4-fields	**.75**	.76	.77
N^4-fields, AE	**.75**	**.77**	**.78**

(a) BSDS500 [4] (Any)

	ODS	OIS	AP
CNN, central	.60	.62	.55
CNN, patch	.58	.59	.49
gPb [4]	.53	.54	.40
SCG [25]	.62	.63	.54
SE-MS, $T = 4$ [20]	**.64**	**.65**	**.59**
N^4-fields	.61	.62	.56
N^4-fields, AE	.63	.64	.58

(c) NYU RGBD [5]

The benchmark evaluation procedure does not perform strict comparison of binary edge masks but rather tries to find the matching between pixels within certain tolerance level and then analyzes unmatched pixels [4]. We observed that the default distance matching tolerance threshold, while accounting for natural uncertainty in the exact position of the boundary, often ignores noticeable and unnatural segmentation mistakes such as spurious boundary pixels. Therefore, in addition to the accuracy evaluated for the default matching threshold, we report results for more stringent thresholds (Fig. 5a-left).

It is also useful to investigate how successful is the deep learning, and what is its role within the N^4-fields. It is insightful to see whether the outputs of the CNN within the N^4-fields, i.e. CNN($\mathcal{P}$) are reasonably close to the codes PCA($\mathbf{A}(\mathcal{P})$) that were used as target during the learning. To show this, in Fig. 4 we give several representative results of the nearest neighbor searches where different types of codes are used on the query and on the dictionary dataset sides (alongside the corresponding patches). It can be seen, that there are very accurate matches (in terms of similarity between true annotations) between PCA codes on both sides, and reasonably good matches between neural (CNN) codes on both sides. However, when matching the neural code of an input patch to PCA codes on the dataset side the results are poor. This is especially noticeable for patches without natural boundaries in them as we force our neural network to map all such patches into one point (empty annotation is always encoded with the same vector). This qualitative performance results in a notoriously bad quantitative performance of the system that uses such matching (from the neural codes in the test image to the PCA codes in the training dataset).

While CNN is clearly unable to learn to reproduce the target codes closely, there is still a strong correlation between the training error (the value of the loss function within the CNN) and the performance of the N^4-fields (Fig. 6). The efficiency of the learned codes and its importance for the good performance of N^4-fields is also highlighted by the fact that the nearest neighbor baseline using SIFT codes performs very poorly. Thus, optimizing the loss functions introduced above really makes edge maps produced by our algorithm agree with ground truth annotations.

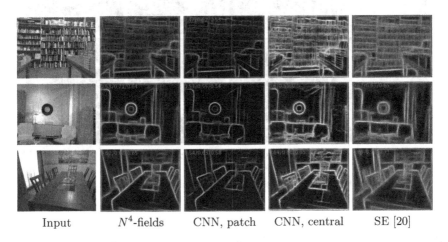

| Input | N^4-fields | CNN, patch | CNN, central | SE [20] |

Fig. 8. Results on the NYU RGBD dataset. For comparison, we give the results of the best previously published method [20] and the CNN baseline. We show a representative result where the N^4-fields perform better (top), similarly (middle), or worse (bottom) than the baseline, according to the numberic measures shown in red (recall/precision/F-measure format). We argue that the numerical measures do not adequately reflect the relative perceptual performance of the methods (Color figure online).

NYU RGBD Experiments. We also show results for the NYU Depth dataset (v2) [5]. It contains 1,449 RGBD images with corresponding semantic segmentations. We use Ren and Bo [25] script to translate the data into BSDS500 format and use the same evaluation procedure, following training/testing split proposed by [25]. The CNN architecture stays the same except for the number of input channels which is now equal to four (RGBD) instead of three (RGB).

The results are summarized in Table 1-c. Our approach almost ties the state-of-the-art method by [20] for the default matching threshold. However, just like in the case of the BSDS500 dataset this difference in scores may be due to the peculiarity of the benchmark. Indeed, Fig. 5b-right shows that for smaller values of matching thresholds, N^4-fields match or outperform the accuracy of Structured Edge detector [20].

Note on the Quantitative Performance. During the experiments, we observed a clear disconnect between the relative performance of the methods according to the quantitative measures, and according to the actual perceptual quality. This was especially noticeable for the NYU RGBD dataset (Fig. 8). We provide extended uniformly-sampled qualitative results at the project website[2] (Fig. 9).

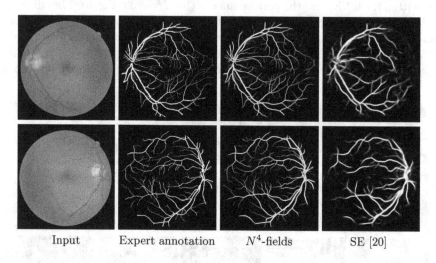

| Input | Expert annotation | N^4-fields | SE [20] |

Fig. 9. Representative results on the DRIVE dataset. A close match to the human expert annotation is observed.

DRIVE Dataset. In order to demonstrate wide applicability of our method, we evaluate it on the DRIVE dataset [6] of the micrographs obtained within the diabetic retinopathy screening program. It includes forty 768 × 584 images split evenly into a training and a test sets. Ground truth annotations include manually segmented vasculature as well as ROI masks.

We use exactly the same CNN architecture as in the BSDS500 experiment. Without any further tuning our system achieves state-of-the-art performance comparable to the algorithm proposed by Becker et al. [28]. Precision/recall curves for both approaches as well as for the baseline neural networks and [20] (obtained using the authors' code) are shown in Fig. 10. Notably, there is once again a clear advantage over the CNN baselines. Poor performance of [20] is likely to be due to the use of default features that are not suitable for this particular imaging modality. This provides an extra evidence for the benefits of fully data-driven approach.

---

[2] http://sites.skoltech.ru/compvision/projects/n4/ at the moment of publication.

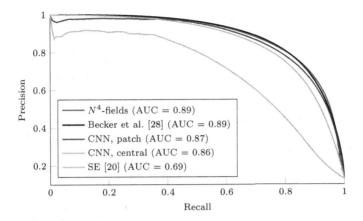

Fig. 10. Results for the DRIVE dataset [6] in the form of the recall/precision curves. Our approach matches the performance of the current state-of-the-art method by Becker et al. [28] and performs much better than baselines and [20].

5 Conclusion

We have presented a new approach to machine-learning based image processing. We have demonstrated how convolutional neural networks can be efficiently combined with the nearest neighbor search, and how such combination can improve the performance of standalone CNNs in the situation when CNN training underfits due to the complexity of a problem at hand. State-of-the-art results are demonstrated for natural edge detection in RGB and RGBD images, as well as for thin object (vessel) segmentation. Compared to the structured forests method [20], the proposed approach is slower, but can be adapted to new domains (e.g. micrographs) without retuning.

The future work may concern the fact that we use a PCA compression to define the target output during the CNN training. A natural idea is then to learn some non-linear transformation in the label space in parallel to the CNN training on the image patch input, so that the gap between the neural codes of the input patches and the target codes is minimized, and a closer match between the neural and the target codes is obtained. It remains to be seen whether this will bring the improvement to the overall performance of the system.

References

1. LeCun, Y., Boser, B.E., Denker, J.S., Henderson, D., Howard, R.E., Hubbard, W.E., Jackel, L.D.: Handwritten digit recognition with a back-propagation network. In: NIPS, pp. 396–404 (1989)
2. Krizhevsky, A., Sutskever, I., Hinton, G.E.: Imagenet classification with deep convolutional neural networks. In: NIPS (2012)

3. Ciresan, D.C., Giusti, A., Gambardella, L.M., Schmidhuber, J.: Deep neural networks segment neuronal membranes in electron microscopy images. In: NIPS, pp. 2852–2860 (2012)
4. Arbeláez, P., Maire, M., Fowlkes, C., Malik, J.: Contour detection and hierarchical image segmentation. IEEE Trans. Pattern Anal. Mach. Intell. 33(5), 898–916 (2011)
5. Silberman, N., Fergus, R.: Indoor scene segmentation using a structured light sensor. In: ICCV Workshops, pp. 601–608. IEEE (2011)
6. Staal, J., Abrmoff, M.D., Niemeijer, M., Viergever, M.A., van Ginneken, B.: Ridge-based vessel segmentation in color images of the retina. IEEE Trans. Med. Imaging 23(4), 501–509 (2004)
7. Egmont-Petersen, M., de Ridder, D., Handels, H.: Image processing with neural networks - a review. Pattern Recognit. 35(10), 2279–2301 (2002)
8. Mnih, V., Hinton, G.E.: Learning to detect roads in high-resolution aerial images. In: Daniilidis, K., Maragos, P., Paragios, N. (eds.) ECCV 2010, Part VI. LNCS, vol. 6316, pp. 210–223. Springer, Heidelberg (2010)
9. Schulz, H., Behnke, S.: Learning object-class segmentation with convolutional neural networks. In: ESANN, vol. 3 (2012)
10. Kivinen, J.J., Williams, C.K.I., Heess, N.: Visual boundary prediction: A deep neural prediction network and quality dissection. In: AISTATS, pp. 512–521 (2014)
11. Ranzato, M., Hinton, G.E.: Modeling pixel means and covariances using factorized third-order boltzmann machines. In: CVPR, pp. 2551–2558 (2010)
12. Farabet, C., Couprie, C., Najman, L., LeCun, Y.: Learning hierarchical features for scene labeling. IEEE Trans. Pattern Anal. Mach. Intell. 35(8), 1915–1929 (2013)
13. Jain, V., Murray, J.F., Roth, F., Turaga, S.C., Zhigulin, V.P., Briggman, K.L., Helmstaedter, M., Denk, W., Seung, H.S.: Supervised learning of image restoration with convolutional networks. In: ICCV, pp. 1–8 (2007)
14. Jain, V., Seung, H.S.: Natural image denoising with convolutional networks. In: NIPS, pp. 769–776 (2008)
15. Burger, H.C., Schuler, C.J., Harmeling, S.: Image denoising: can plain neural networks compete with bm3d? In: CVPR, pp. 2392–2399 (2012)
16. Chopra, S., Hadsell, R., LeCun, Y.: Learning a similarity metric discriminatively, with application to face verification.In: CVPR, vol. 1, pp. 539–546 (2005)
17. Dabov, K., Foi, A., Katkovnik, V., Egiazarian, K.: Image restoration by sparse 3d transform-domain collaborative filtering. In: Electronic Imaging 2008, International Society for Optics and Photonics, pp. 681207–681207 (2008)
18. Criminisi, A., Pérez, P., Toyama, K.: Region filling and object removal by exemplar-based image inpainting. IEEE Trans. Image Process. 13(9), 1200–1212 (2004)
19. Freeman, W.T., Pasztor, E.C., Carmichael, O.T.: Learning low-level vision. Int. J. Comput. Vis. 40(1), 25–47 (2000)
20. Dollár, P., Zitnick, C.L.: Structured forests for fast edge detection. In: ICCV (2013)
21. Hinton, G.E., Srivastava, N., Krizhevsky, A., Sutskever, I., Salakhutdinov, R.: Improving neural networks by preventing co-adaptation of feature detectors. CoRR abs/1207.0580 (2012)
22. Zeiler, M.D., Fergus, R.: Visualizing and understanding convolutional networks. CoRR abs/1311.2901 (2013)
23. Sermanet, P., Eigen, D., Zhang, X., Mathieu, M., Fergus, R., LeCun, Y.: Overfeat: Integrated recognition, localization and detection using convolutional networks. CoRR abs/1312.6229 (2013)
24. Vedaldi, A., Fulkerson, B.: VLFeat: An open and portable library of computer vision algorithms (2008). http://www.vlfeat.org/

25. Xiaofeng, R., Bo, L.: Discriminatively trained sparse code gradients for contour detection. In: NIPS, pp. 593–601 (2012)
26. Isola, P., Zoran, D., Krishnan, D., Adelson, E.H.: Crisp boundary detection using pointwise mutual information. In: Fleet, D., Pajdla, T., Schiele, B., Tuytelaars, T. (eds.) ECCV 2014, Part III. LNCS, vol. 8691, pp. 799–814. Springer, Heidelberg (2014)
27. Hou, X., Yuille, A., Koch, C.: Boundary detection benchmarking: Beyond f-measures. In: CVPR, vol. 2013, pp. 1–8. IEEE (2013)
28. Becker, C., Rigamonti, R., Lepetit, V., Fua, P.: Supervised feature learning for curvilinear structure segmentation. In: Mori, K., Sakuma, I., Sato, Y., Barillot, C., Navab, N. (eds.) MICCAI 2013, Part I. LNCS, vol. 8149, pp. 526–533. Springer, Heidelberg (2013)

Super-Resolution Using Sub-Band Self-Similarity

Abhishek Singh$^{(\boxtimes)}$ and Narendra Ahuja

University of Illinois at Urbana-Champaign, Champaign, USA
asingh18@illinois.edu

Abstract. A popular approach for single image super-resolution (SR) is to use scaled down versions of the given image to build an *internal* training dictionary of pairs of low resolution (LR) and high resolution (HR) image patches, which is then used to predict the HR image. This self-similarity approach has the advantage of not requiring a separate *external* training database. However, due to their limited size, internal dictionaries are often inadequate for finding good matches for patches containing complex structures such as textures. Furthermore, the quality of matches found are quite sensitive to factors like patch size (larger patches contain structures of greater complexity and may be difficult to match), and dimensions of the given image (smaller images yield smaller internal dictionaries). In this paper we propose a self-similarity based SR algorithm that addresses the abovementioned drawbacks. Instead of seeking similar patches directly in the image domain, we use the self-similarity principle independently on each of a set of different sub-band images, obtained using a bank of orientation selective band-pass filters. Therefore, we allow the different directional frequency components of a patch to find matches independently, which may be in different image locations. Essentially, we decompose local image structure into component patches defined by different sub-bands, with the following advantages: (1) The sub-band image patches are simpler and therefore easier to find matches, than for the more complex textural patches from the original image. (2) The size of the dictionary defined by patches from the sub-band images is exponential in the number of sub-bands used, thus increasing the effective size of the internal dictionary. (3) As a result, our algorithm exhibits a greater degree of invariance to parameters like patch size and the dimensions of the LR image. We demonstrate these advantages and show that our results are richer in textural content and appear more natural than several state-of-the-art methods.

1 Introduction

The single image super-resolution (SR) problem has received significant attention in recent years. Due to its ill-posed nature, this problem has fueled research in various statistical properties of natural images, which are used as priors for

Electronic supplementary material The online version of this chapter (doi:10. 1007/978-3-319-16808-1_37) contains supplementary material, which is available to authorized users.

D. Cremers et al. (Eds.): ACCV 2014, Part II, LNCS 9004, pp. 552–568, 2015.
DOI: 10.1007/978-3-319-16808-1_37

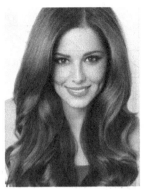 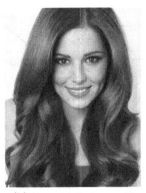 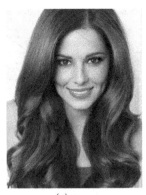

(a) Internal dictionary [6]   (b) External dictionary [2]   (c) Ours

Fig. 1. *Woman (2X):* Notice the hair. Methods based on internal dictionaries tend to smooth out fine details while preserving high contrast edges. External database driven methods can appear soft overall if the training patches are not relevant enough for super-resolving the given image. Our algorithm does not require external training images, and is designed to address the limitation of internal dictionaries. This helps enhance performance of internal dictionary based methods by better synthesizing complex image structures such as fine textures. Our results appear sharper, with more realistic details than those produced by the other schemes.

regularizing the SR problem. Learning based approaches, which attempt to predict high-resolution (HR) features corresponding to the low resolution (LR) features of the given image, have become the state-of-the-art in the field [1–5] (Fig. 1).

Many learning based methods first construct an *external* dictionary of LR-HR patch pairs using a database of several generic LR-HR image pairs. Given a test image to be super-resolved, this dictionary is used to predict the HR patch corresponding to each patch in the LR given image [2,3,5,7–9].

The quality of results of such methods, however, depends heavily on the construction of the external dictionary. The type and number of training images required for obtaining satisfactory SR quality is not clear. If a small database is used (for faster computations), then the results often have a strong dependence on the specific training images chosen. If a large training database is used (for better generalization), methods often have to rely on data reduction techniques such as sparsification [2] or clustering [9] of the training set for computational feasibility. This may cause a drop in performance due to loss of information in the compact representation. If a different scaling factor is desired, re-training is needed to learn new SR prediction functions for the new scaling factor.

To avoid external training databases and these problems associated with them, several methods have been proposed that exploit self-similarities within the *given* image. Similar patches are sought across scales of the given image to build an *internal* dictionary of LR-HR patch pairs. This dictionary is then used to predict the HR patch corresponding to each patch of the given image using nearest neighbor patch-matching, linear regression, etc. [6,10–14]. The general principle involved in such a self-similarity based SR algorithm is illustrated in

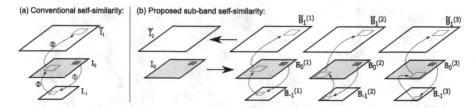

Fig. 2. (a) Conventional self-similarity based SR framework. Each patch of the given image I_0 is matched to a patch in I_{-1} in step 1. The corresponding patch (in the same location) in I_0 serves as the HR predictor (step 2). This patch is then pasted in the HR image $\tilde{I}_1$ (step 3). (b) The proposed sub-band self-similarity framework. Our method follows a series of similar steps as (a), but on each sub-band independently. Note that for super-resolving the patch shown in red, our algorithm allows for its various sub-bands to find matches in different spatial locations. See Sects. 3, 4, 5 for details (Color figure online).

Fig. 2(a). Self-similarity methods find their roots in fractal image coding from the 1990s [15,16], and are based on the idea that natural image patches tend to recur within and across scales in the same image [6,17]. It has been shown that internal dictionaries tend to contain more *relevant* training patches, and, in general, yield nearest-neighbor matches with lower error as compared to external dictionaries, with or without compact representation [17].

Internal dictionaries, however, have limitations while super-resolving textural regions. Indeed, [17] shows that the likelihood of finding a good internal match for a patch decreases as the gradient content of the patch increases. This suggests that textural details like hair, animal fur etc., often find suboptimal matches, using a self-similarity approach, and are thus averaged or smoothed out in the final SR result. The reason behind such a limitation is that the internal dictionary obtained from the given image generally has fewer number of LR-HR patch pairs than external dictionaries, which can potentially be as large as desired. Due to the limited size of the internal dictionary, textural patches (which contain complex structures) fail to find suitable representations. The size of the self-learned dictionary furthermore depends on the dimensions of the given image; smaller images consist of fewer patches and thereby yield fewer LR-HR patch pairs. Additionally, the quality of matches depends on the patch size chosen. For e.g., the complexity of structures in the patches increases with increase in patch size, making it difficult to find accurate matches.

Our Contributions: In this paper, we propose an SR algorithm that alleviates the abovementioned problems of self-similarity based approaches, *without* resorting to any external training database. We propose a self-similarity driven algorithm wherein, instead of seeking self-similar patches directly in the image domain, we use self-similarity based SR independently on images corresponding to different sub-bands. These sub-bands are the responses of the image to a bank of spatially localized, orientation selective band-pass filters. Effectively, we unravel the complexity of the structure by representing it in terms of simpler components, which, being simpler, are easier to find matches for. Unlike in the case of patch matching in the image domain, we allow the different directional frequency components of the patch to independently find their best matches in different locations in the image. Therefore, we synthesize HR patches by combining different frequency components from the best matches found at different locations. Such a combinatorial expansion of the internal dictionary allows for finding better (lower error) patch matches for a test image produces a better quality HR image. Our SR results appear richer in texture and more natural than those produced by state-of-the-art methods. We also show that our algorithm leads to improvements in two other important aspects of the SR problem that have not received much attention in the past. We show that our approach has greater degree of invariance to the choice of patch size, which can be a sensitive parameter, particularly for self-similarity methods. We also show that due to the ability of our algorithm to generate richer internal dictionaries, we are able to super-resolve extremely small images much better, thereby achieving greater invariance to the size of the input image, as compared to the existing self-similarity approach.

2   Previous Work

Among methods that rely on external dictionaries, Freeman et al. [7,18] propose an 'example-based' SR algorithm, wherein a Markov random field (MRF) model is used to learn the relationship between LR and HR patches. Reference [5] uses manifold learning to learn this relationship, by assuming the manifold of HR patches to be locally linear. Yang et al. [3] express image patches as sparse linear combinations of atoms from a fixed dictionary of image patches. Reference [9] proposes to cluster the patches in the dictionary to facilitate fast nearest neighbor searches. In [2,8,19], compact dictionaries are learnt from the raw patches, in order to support a sparse representation of the patches to be super-resolved. [20] uses an external database to learn first order regression functions to map 'in-place' (extremely localized neighborhood) patches to high resolution. Instead of learning LR-HR transformations using patches, several methods learn how edges transform across resolutions [21–23]. Primal sketches (ridges, corners, etc.) are used as primitives for super-resolution in [4]. External dictionaries are used to learn transform domain coefficients in [24,25]. Higher level features are used in [26,27] for learning the LR-HR mapping using external training databases.

Among internal dictionary based methods, Ebrahimi and Vrscay [10] combine ideas from fractal coding [15,16] and example-based algorithms (such as non-local means filtering [28]), to propose a self-similarity based SR algorithm. Glasner et al. [6] fuse together multiple matched patches from the internal dictionary of the image to generate HR patches, in a way similar to traditional multiframe SR. Freedman and Fattal [11] show that patches tend to recur across scales within local spatial neighborhoods, which they exploit for computational speed-up. In [13], transform domain matching criteria are used along with the traditional L_2 distance for patch-matching. A framework for super-resolving noisy images based on self-similarity principles in proposed in [14].

Our proposed algorithm retains the advantages of existing self-similarity based approaches, but also overcomes some of their limitations described in the previous section. In the next two sections, we describe the steps involved in our algorithm, which is conceptually quite straightforward and easy to implement. In Sect. 5, we discuss a number of important implications and corollaries resulting out of the proposed algorithm, and discuss the key advantages it brings over existing schemes. We demonstrate our performance vis-a-vis several other state-of-the-art methods, and corroborate our claims through a number of systematic experiments in Sect. 6.

3   Overview of Proposed Method

Notation: We denote the given image to be super-resolved as I_0. By I_1 we denote the HR version of I_0, whose linear dimension, or scale, is larger by a factor of s. Similarly, we denote by I_{-1}, the smaller version of I_0, by the scaling factor of $1/s$. We denote the super-resolved image(s) obtained using our algorithm using a *hat* (^) symbol. Therefore, our objective is to super-resolve I_0 to obtain an HR image $\hat{I}_1$, that best approximates the true HR image I_1. We use scripted letters to denote sets, we use lowercase boldface letters to denote image patches, and lowercase italicized letters to denote scalars and indices.

3.1   Algorithm Summary

To super-resolve the image I_0, our algorithm consists of the following steps, also summarized in Fig. 2(b):

1. We decompose the image I_0 into N sub-bands $\{B_0^{(j)}\}_{j=1}^N$, which are obtained as the responses of the image I_0 to a bank of spatially localized, orientation selective, bandpass filters. We use the steerable pyramid decomposition [29,30] for our work, although other schemes such as contourlet transform [31] may also be used.
2. We then apply a self-similarity based SR algorithm to each of the sub-bands $\{B_0^{(j)}\}_{j=1}^N$, independently, to yield the set of HR sub-bands $\{\tilde{B}_1^{(j)}\}_{j=1}^N$. We describe this step in detail in Sect. 4 and discuss the key advantages it brings in Sect. 5.
3. We then recombine the HR sub-bands $\{\tilde{B}_1^{(j)}\}_{j=1}^N$, by inverting the sub-band decomposition, to yield an HR image $\tilde{I}_1$.
4. Finally, in order to ensure that the downsampled version of our estimated HR image is close to the given LR image, we enforce the backprojection constraint [32] by minimizing,

$$J(\hat{I}_1) = |(\hat{I}_1 * f_{psf}) \downarrow -I_0|_2^2 \tag{1}$$

Starting with $\tilde{I}_1$ as initialization, we minimize the above cost function using a few iterations of gradient decent, to yield our final HR image $\hat{I}_1$.

4   Sub-band Self-Similarity

We independently super-resolve each sub-band $B_0^{(j)}$ of I_0, using a self-similarity approach adopted from previous work [6,17], summarized below:

For the sub-band $B_0^{(j)}$, we first obtain its downsampled version,

$$B_{-1}^{(j)} = \left(B_0^{(j)} * f_{psf} \right) \downarrow \tag{2}$$

where f_{psf} is an assumed point spread function. We then create internal dictionaries $\mathcal{L}^{(j)}$ and $\mathcal{H}^{(j)}$ that contain patches from $B_{-1}^{(j)}$ and their corresponding (higher resolution) patches from $B_0^{(j)}$, respectively. The sets $\mathcal{L}^{(j)}$ and $\mathcal{H}^{(j)}$ serve as our internal training database of LR-HR training patches, for super-resolving the sub-band $B_0^{(j)}$. To super-resolve $B_0^{(j)}$ to $\tilde{B}_1^{(j)}$, we do the following: For every patch $\mathbf{l}$ of $B_0^{(j)}$, we look for its $k = 5$ most similar patches $\{\mathbf{l}_i\}_{i=1}^k$ in the LR set $\mathcal{L}^{(j)}$, based on L_2 distances. Their corresponding HR patches $\{\mathbf{h}_i\}_{i=1}^k$ from the set $\mathcal{H}^{(j)}$ serve as individual predictors for the patch $\mathbf{l}$. We compute a weighted average of $\{\mathbf{h}_i\}_{i=1}^k$ to estimate the HR patch $\hat{\mathbf{h}}$ of $\mathbf{l}$ as follows,

$$\hat{\mathbf{h}} = \frac{\sum w_i \cdot \mathbf{h}_i}{\sum w_i}, \text{ where, } w_i = exp\left(\frac{-||\mathbf{l} - \mathbf{l}_i||_2^2}{2\sigma^2} \right). \tag{3}$$

Using a larger number of patch matches (k) tends to cause oversmoothing, whereas very small values such as $k = 1$ or 2 produces sharper images but with some artifacts. We repeat the above procedure for every patch $\mathbf{l}$ of $B_0^{(j)}$, to get the corresponding HR patches. These together constitute the super-resolved sub-band $\tilde{B}_1^{(j)}$.

5   Implications

Matching image patches based on intensity differences is often difficult if the patches contain complex structures such as textural detail [17]. Using sub-band decomposition, our algorithm essentially aims at decomposing complex textural structures into relatively simpler ones, that are easier to find matches for. For each image patch, our algorithm allows each of its sub-band components to find its optimal matches at *different* spatial locations in the image. This is illustrated in Fig. 2(b). The sub-bands of the red patch are allowed to find their optimal matches in different spatial locations in the LR sub-bands $B_{-1}^{(1)}, B_{-1}^{(2)}, B_{-1}^{(3)}$. This is in contrast to the conventional way of matching raw patches as shown in Fig. 2(a), where all frequency components of the matched patch are restricted to be from the same spatial location, since no sub-band decomposition is performed.

These properties of our algorithm have useful implications discussed below:

(1) Lower Matching Error: We expect our approach to find nearest neighbor (NN) matches with lower error, as compared to the traditional image domain patch matching. To verify this, we compute the NN error map for the image shown in Fig. 3. The error map is the error produced by a given LR image I_0 while reconstructing itself using its internal dictionary $\mathcal{L}$. In the SR algorithm, the NN error map therefore denotes the "training error" (in pattern recognition parlance). For the conventional self-similarity based SR, we obtain the error map as follows: Given the image I_0, we first obtain its reconstructed version $\tilde{I}_0$, by

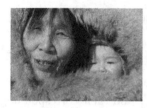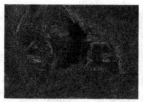

Fig. 3. *Left:* Input image. *Center:* Image indicating the errors obtained using conventional nearest neighbor search for each image patch, in the internal LR dictionary $\mathcal{L}$. *Right:* Corresponding error map obtained using the proposed sub-band based patch matching approach. Our approach yields lower matching errors, particularly around textural regions such as the fur around the faces.

replacing each patch of I_0 with its closest patch in the LR internal dictionary $\mathcal{L}$. We then compute the pixelwise difference between I_0 and $\tilde{I}_0$ to obtain the error map. To obtain the error map for our approach, instead of reconstructing $\tilde{I}_0$ directly, we reconstruct its sub-bands $\{\tilde{B}_0^{j)}\}_{j=1}^N$ using nearest neighbor searches in the internal sub-band dictionaries $\{\mathcal{L}^{(j)}\}_{j=1}^N$. We combine the reconstructed sub-bands $\{\tilde{B}_0^{j)}\}_{j=1}^N$ to obtain $\tilde{I}_0$ and compute its difference with the original image I_0 to obtain our error map.

Figure 3, *Center* and *Right* show the error maps obtained by the conventional approach and by our approach, respectively. Clearly, the errors are much lower for our algorithm, particularly in textured regions such as the fur surrounding the faces. We show in our results in Sect. 6 that this lower NN error translates to better reconstruction of textural details.

(2) Invariance to Patch Size: The choice of patch size has an important effect on the quality of the SR results, particularly for self-similarity based methods. Using larger patch sizes for conventional patch matching leads to greater difficulty in matching textural regions since the complexity of image structures is larger. On the other hand, using extremely small patch sizes is also not expected to improve results since very small patches may not contain enough structural information to learn their transformations across resolutions. For a given image, the optimal patch size to use is difficult to determine *a priori*. Using the proposed approach, complex patches are broken down into relatively simpler sub-bands. The simpler structure of the sub-bands decreases the variety of the sub-band patches and thus reduces the error of the best matching patch for a given dictionary size. Therefore, we expect our algorithm to suffer less if the patch size chosen is sub-optimal. Indeed, as compared to traditional self-similarity based SR, we find our results to be less sensitive to the choice of patch size. We show this in our experiments later in Sect. 6.

(3) Exponentially Larger Internal Dictionary: Allowing different sub-bands of the HR patch to come from different spatial locations of the LR image has an important corollary. Combining sub-bands from different locations effectively allows us to synthesize *new* patches, originally not present in the dictionary of raw image patches. This, in a sense, leads to a combinatorial expansion of the internal dictionaries $\mathcal{L}$ and $\mathcal{H}$, resulting in a dictionary whose size increases exponentially with the number of sub-bands. Further, this is achieved *without* the use of external databases. We illustrate this with a simple example in Fig. 4. We assume here that our raw patch dictionary $\mathcal{L}$ consists of only two patches as shown in the blue box. In this example we decompose these patches into $N = 3$ sub-bands as depicted in the black dotted box. Now, if using traditional image domain patch-matching, one is restricted to choosing among only two possible candidate matches while searching for a nearest neighbor match. However, if patch-matching is done independently for each sub-band, the number of unique combinations possible is $2^N = 8$. In Fig. 4 on the right, we show the patches resulting from each of the unique sub-band combinations. Clearly, in addition to the original two patches, several more new textural patches have been synthesized in this expanded dictionary. Note that one never has to explicitly obtain such an expanded dictionary. Such an expansion is an implicit consequence of independently finding best matches for the different sub-band patches.

(4) Invariance to Image Size: We have shown that super-resolving sub-bands independently has the overall effect of performing conventional patch-similarity based SR, but using a much larger internal dictionary, whose elements are generated by combining different sub-band patches from different locations in the scene. While the use of a larger dictionary is expected to be always beneficial in general, it becomes particularly useful in cases where the original internal dictionary is small, such as while super-resolving extremely small images. Indeed, as we show in Sect. 6, in such cases we observe a much greater improvement in our results over the conventional self-similarity approach. Our algorithm therefore yields relatively more consistent levels of performance across different image sizes. We corroborate this claim in Sect. 6.

6   Experiments and Results

Implementation Details: For the steerable pyramid, we use eight different orientation bands, and a single scale decomposition. Using more orientation bands

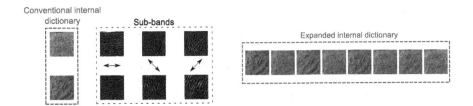

Fig. 4. An example showing a conventional self-similarity based training dictionary containing just two patches (blue box), along with their sub-band decompositions. Combining sub-bands of different patches effectively allows us to *synthesize* new patches, as shown in the expanded dictionary in the red box. Note that the size of the patches here is chosen to be quite large for illustration purposes (Color figure online).

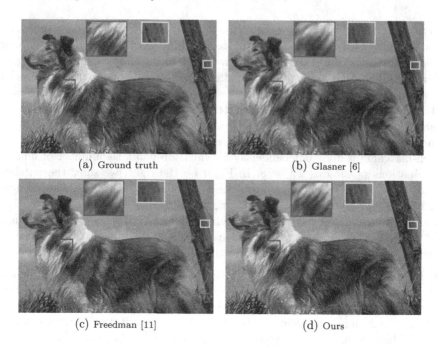

(a) Ground truth   (b) Glasner [6]

(c) Freedman [11]   (d) Ours

Fig. 5. *Dog (2X):* The dog fur, and the details on the wooden pole are better reconstructed using our method, and bear closer resemblance to the ground truth.

improved results in general, but the improvements became marginal beyond eight bands. We use only a single (highest) scale decomposition since the lower scale bands contain lower frequency information which does not pose much challenge for SR. We perform SR in two steps. Therefore, for 3X SR, we perform $\sqrt{3}$X SR twice. Our algorithm is used only on the luminance channel of color images. The chroma components are separately upscaled using bicubic interpolation and combined with our output to obtain the final color image.

We compare our results to eight popular single image SR methods[1] [2,6,9,11, 23,32–34], as described in the paragraphs below. Additional results are included as supplementary material.

Comparison with Self-Similarity Methods: Our most important comparison is with other self-similarity methods. We compare our results to [6,11], which are two very popular self-similarity based SR methods in the literature. Figure 5 shows results on the *Dog* image. Our result shows more detail and richer texture in the dog fur and the wooden pole. The self-similarity methods [6,11] in general are quite good at preserving sharpness of high contrast edges, but tend to smooth out finer details. Reference [11] tends to smooth details more than [6] since it performs only a very localized search for nearest neighbors, for computational reasons. Our result bears closer resemblance to the ground truth.

---

[1] The software for many of these methods were provided by the respective authors, while we implemented the others.

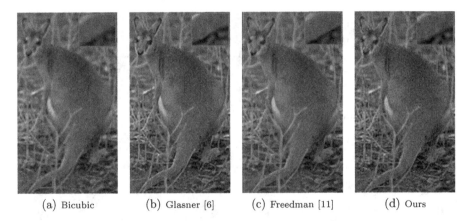

(a) Bicubic   (b) Glasner [6]   (c) Freedman [11]   (d) Ours

Fig. 6. *Kangaroo (3X):* Both Glasner [6] and Freedman [11] almost completely lose the textural details of the kangaroo's tail. Our algorithm is able to better synthesize this. Ground truth for this image is not available so absolute error cannot be obtained.

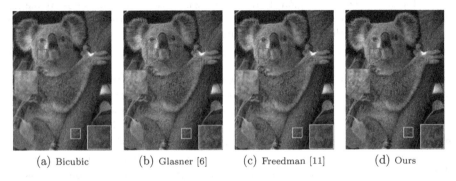

(a) Bicubic   (b) Glasner [6]   (c) Freedman [11]   (d) Ours

Fig. 7. *Koala (3X):* Our result shows richer texture in koala's fur and the tree trunk. Ground truth for this image is not available so absolute error cannot be obtained.

Figure 6 shows results on the *Kangaroo* image. Notice here that both [6] and [11] almost completely lose the textural details of the tail. Our algorithm is able to better preserve this texture.

Figure 7 shows results on the *Koala* image. Here as well, our algorithm is able to synthesize richer texture in the fur and the tree trunk, than both [6] and [11]. Note that the *Koala* and *Kangaroo* images do not have ground truth available.

Comparison with External Dictionary Based Methods: We now compare our results with methods that use external dictionaries for SR. Specifically, we consider [2] which is a popular method based on dictionary learning and sparse representations, the method in [33] that uses ridge regression for predicting HR patches, and the more recent method [9], which is based on using simple regression functions on a pre-clustered training dictionary. We also compare to the classic iterative backprojection algorithm [32] for reference.

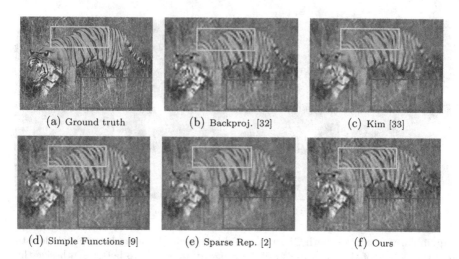

<table>
<tr><td>(a) Ground truth</td><td>(b) Backproj. [32]</td><td>(c) Kim [33]</td></tr>
<tr><td>(d) Simple Functions [9]</td><td>(e) Sparse Rep. [2]</td><td>(f) Ours</td></tr>
</table>

Fig. 8. *Tiger (4X):* Notice the grass above and below the tiger. Our result shows greater textural detail in the grass regions (red box), as compared to most methods. While [9] also seems to produce rich texture, it also produces ringing artifacts such as on the stripes of the tiger (yellow box) (Color figure online).

Figure 8 shows the results on the *Tiger* image. While Kim [33] reconstructs high contrast edges almost as sharp as ours, textural details appear highly washed out. The result of [2] also appears a little soft, both along high contrast edges as well as in textural regions such as the grass (red box). Reference [9] appears slightly more detailed than [2], but it shows excessive ringing artifacts such as along the stripes of the tiger (yellow box), much like the backprojection algorithm [32]. Overall, our result has richer textural details without excessive ringing artifacts.

Figure 9 shows results on the *Sunlight* image. Notice that the woman's hair appears most natural in our result. References [9,32] clearly show more ringing artifacts in the hair, whereas [2,33] are not able to reconstruct sufficient detail.

Comparison with Other Methods: We also compare our approach with two other methods popularly used in literature - the gradient profile prior (GPP) method [23], that is based on learning gradient profile transformations across resolutions, and the method in [34] that uses iterative feedback based upsampling, without any external databases. Figure 10 shows our results on the *Red hair* image. The fine strands of hair in the blue box are clearly visible in our result, but is lost in the results of [23,34]. Our result appears almost indistinguishable from the ground truth in this example.

Performance vs. Patch Size: The chosen patch size can have a significant effect on the quality of the SR results particularly for internal dictionary based methods. We have shown earlier that using the proposed approach, complex patches are broken down into simpler sub-bands, that can find closer (lower error) matches. Therefore, our algorithm should suffer less if patch size is increased. To verify this empirically, we do the following: We super-resolve 100 natural

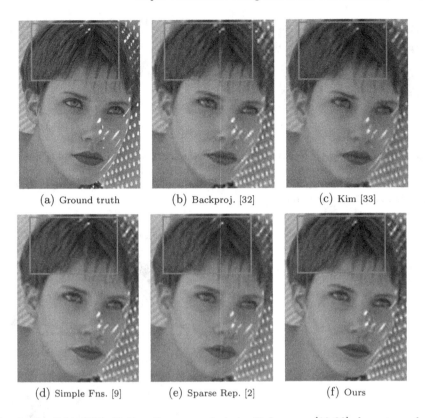

(a) Ground truth   (b) Backproj. [32]   (c) Kim [33]

(d) Simple Fns. [9]   (e) Sparse Rep. [2]   (f) Ours

Fig. 9. *Sunlight (4X):* Notice the woman's hair. References [19,33] do not produce sufficient detail in the hair, whereas [9,32] show excessive ringing artifacts. Our result appears more natural.

images (with known ground truth) using our method and also using the conventional self-similarity method of [6], with several different patch sizes, ranging from 2×2 to 11×11. We then plot the average output image quality (in terms of PSNR and SSIM [35]) as a function of the patch size used. The plots in Fig. 11 show our results. As expected, the performance of our algorithm not only remains higher throughout the tested range, but the loss of PSNR and SSIM is also much slower than the conventional self-similarity approach.

Performance vs. Image Size: Earlier, we showed that our algorithm has the effect of synthesizing a much larger internal dictionary, by combining sub-bands from different spatial locations in the image. We therefore expected our algorithm to perform significantly better than conventional self-similarity, if the input image size was very small. To verify this claim, we perform the following experiment: Consider super-resolving the set of images as shown in Fig. 12 on the left. Each image here is a cropped version of the image on its right. The leftmost (smallest) image, therefore, is a sub-image of all the other images, and appears in all of them, as marked by the red box. We now wish to see how well this

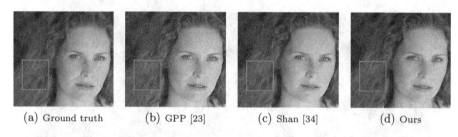

(a) Ground truth   (b) GPP [23]   (c) Shan [34]   (d) Ours

Fig. 10. *Red Hair (2X):* Notice the details of the hair as shown in the blue box. Fine strands of hair are discernible in our result, whereas they are smoothed out in the result of [23,34]. Our result seems almost indistinguishable from the ground truth in this example (Color figure online).

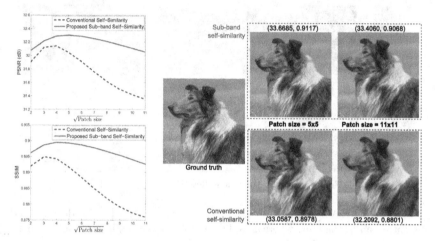

Fig. 11. *Left:* Plots of PSNR and SSIM as a function of the patch size used, for our algorithm as well as the conventional self-similarity method of [6]. *Right:* An example showing the effect of patch size on the results of both algorithms. Our result remains more consistent with patch size variation as compared to [6]. Numbers in brackets denote (PSNR in dB, SSIM [35]).

sub-image gets super-resolved in each of these images. Clearly, in the rightmost (largest) image, the sub-image has access to all the patches from its surrounding regions as well, which should therefore result in better SR. We compute SR quality (in terms of PSNR and SSIM [35]) of this sub-image, as a function of the size of the image containing it, and plot the result in Fig. 12 on the right. As expected, the conventional self-similarity approach [6] shows a more drastic reduction in performance for smaller image sizes, as compared to our method.

To visualize this effect of image size in a more practical SR problem, we perform the following experiment: We consider super-resolving two input images, as shown in the black dotted box in Fig. 13. The first image shows a group photograph, whereas the second is a cropped version containing just one of the faces, measuring only 20 × 25 pixels. We super-resolve both these images using the method of [6] as well as our proposed algorithm and show the results in the

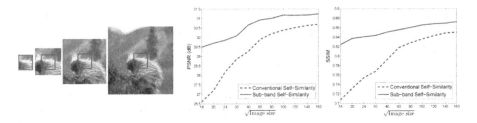

Fig. 12. *Left:* Data used for studying the performance of our algorithm as a function of the size of the input image. We use a series of cropped images as shown. We study how the common sub-image (red box) gets super-resolved in each of these images. *Right:* Plots showing the PSNR (in dB) and SSIM of the super-resolved sub-image as a function of the size of the image containing it. Our algorithm shows a much gradual decline in performance for smaller images, as compared to the conventional self-similarity method [6] (Color figure online).

blue and red dotted boxes respectively. We compare the quality of the super-resolved faces obtained using each method, in both the images. We make the following two observations: (1) In both images, the face is super-resolved better (visually) by our algorithm than the conventional internal dictionary based

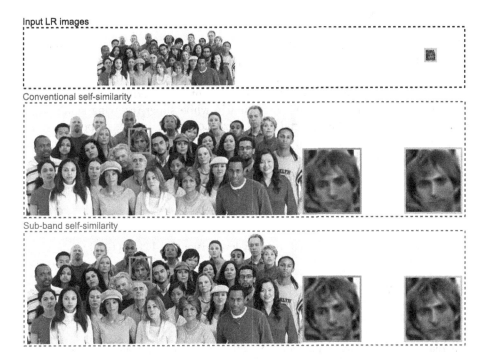

Fig. 13. An example showing the performance of our algorithm for very small input images. We super-resolve the two images shown in the black dotted box, the right one being a one face sub-image cropped from the left image. Our algorithm is able to super-resolve this small face image much better than the conventional self-similarity approach of [6] (Color figure online).

approach [6]. (2) There is a significant difference in the quality of the super-resolved faces from the bigger and the cropped images, using either method. Using our algorithm, however, this difference is smaller. Our algorithm is able to super-resolve the extremely small cropped image better than the conventional self-similarity approach.

In practice, small images are more commonly encountered as candidates for super-resolution than large ones. Our algorithm is therefore useful for practical applications like super-resolution of thumbnail images, detection/recognition of distant (small) faces in images/videos captured using surveillance cameras, etc. Like any self similarity based algorithm, our algorithm does not require manually chosen training images, which makes it all the more attractive in terms of portability and ease of implementation.

Computational Cost: Our algorithm applies a self-similarity SR algorithm (such as [6]) on R different sub-bands. A naive implementation would be R times slower than the corresponding self-similarity SR algorithm. But since each sub-band is super-resolved independently, they can be easily parallelized. Using such a parallelization, our algorithm is just around 1.5 times slower than the baseline self-similarity SR algorithm of [6].

7   Conclusion

While external dictionary based methods can produce good results in general, they are hindered by the problems associated with the choice and construction of the external training database. Internal dictionary based methods provide an attractive way to circumvent these issues, but also sacrifice some ability to reconstruct textural details well, particularly while super-resolving small sized images and/or when the optimal patch size not used. In this paper we have proposed a self-similarity based algorithm that overcomes these limitations. Our algorithm produces better SR results that remain fairly consistent across several scenarios commonly encountered in practice.

References

1. Freeman, W., Pasztor, E.: Learning low-level vision. In: ICCV (1999)
2. Yang, J., Wright, J., Huang, T., Ma, Y.: Image super-resolution via sparse representation. IEEE Trans. Image Proc. **98**, 1031–1044 (2010)
3. Yang, J., Wright, J., Huang, T., Ma, Y.: Image super-resolution as sparse representation of raw image patches. In: CVPR (2008)
4. Sun, J., Zheng, N.N., Tao, H., Shum, H.Y.: Image hallucination with primal sketch priors. In: CVPR (2003)
5. Yeung, D.Y., Yeung, D.Y., Xiong, Y.: Super-resolution through neighbor embedding. In: CVPR(2004)
6. Glasner, D., Bagon, S., Irani, M.: Super-resolution from a single image. In: ICCV (2009)
7. Freeman, W.T., Pasztor, E.C.: Learning low-level vision. IJCV **40**, 25–47 (2000)

8. Wang, S., Zhang, D., Liang, Y., Pan, Q.: Semi-coupled dictionary learning with applications to image super-resolution and photo-sketch synthesis. In: CVPR (2012)
9. Yang, C.Y., Yang, M.H.: Fast direct super-resolution by simple functions. In: ICCV (2013)
10. Ebrahimi, M., Vrscay, E.R.: Solving the inverse problem of image zooming using "Self-Examples". In: Kamel, M.S., Campilho, A. (eds.) ICIAR 2007. LNCS, vol. 4633, pp. 117–130. Springer, Heidelberg (2007)
11. Freedman, G., Fattal, R.: Image and video upscaling from local self-examples. ACM Trans. Graph. **28**, 1–10 (2010)
12. Yang, C.-Y., Huang, J.-B., Yang, M.-H.: Exploiting self-similarities for single frame super-resolution. In: Kimmel, R., Klette, R., Sugimoto, A. (eds.) ACCV 2010, Part III. LNCS, vol. 6494, pp. 497–510. Springer, Heidelberg (2011)
13. Singh, A., Ahuja, N.: Sub-band energy constraints for self-similarity based super-resolution. In: ICPR (2014)
14. Singh, A., Porikli, F., Ahuja, N.: Super-resolving noisy images. In: CVPR (2014)
15. Barnsley, M.: Fractals Everywhere. Academic Press Professional, Inc., San Diego (1988)
16. Polidori, E., luc Dugelay, J.: Zooming using iterated function systems (1995)
17. Zontak, M., Irani, M.: Internal statistics of a single natural image. In: CVPR (2011)
18. Freeman, W., Jones, T., Pasztor, E.: Example-based super-resolution. Comput. Graph. Appl. **22**, 56–65 (2002). IEEE
19. Yang, J., Wang, Z., Lin, Z., Cohen, S., Huang, T.: Coupled dictionary training for image super-resolution. IEEE Trans. Image Proc. **21**, 3467–3478 (2012)
20. Yang, J., Lin, Z., Cohen, S.: Fast image super-resolution based on in-place example regression. In: CVPR (2013)
21. Fattal, R.: Image upsampling via imposed edge statistics. ACM Trans. Graph. **26**(3), 95 (2007)
22. Sun, J., Sun, J., Xu, Z., Shum, H.Y.: Gradient profile prior and its applications in image super-resolution and enhancement. IEEE Trans. Image Proc. **20**, 1529–1542 (2011)
23. Sun, J., Sun, J., Xu, Z., Shum, H.Y.: Image super-resolution using gradient profile prior. In: CVPR (2008)
24. Jiji, C.V., Chaudhuri, S.: Single-frame image super-resolution through contourlet learning. EURASIP J. Appl. Signal Process. **2006**, 235 (2006)
25. Gajjar, P., Joshi, M.: New learning based super-resolution: Use of dwt and igmrf prior. IEEE Trans. Image Proc. **19**, 1201–1213 (2010)
26. Sun, J., Zhu, J., Tappen, M.: Context-constrained hallucination for image super-resolution. In: CVPR (2010)
27. HaCohen, Y., Fattal, R., Lischinski, D.: Image upsampling via texture hallucination. In: ICCP (2010)
28. Buades, A., Coll, B., Morel, J.M.: A non-local algorithm for image denoising. In: CVPR (2005)
29. Simoncelli, E., Freeman, W.: The steerable pyramid: a flexible architecture for multi-scale derivative computation. In: ICIP (1995)
30. Simoncelli, E., Freeman, W., Adelson, E., Heeger, D.: Shiftable multiscale transforms. IEEE Trans. Info. Theory **38**, 587–607 (1992)
31. Do, M., Vetterli, M.: The contourlet transform: an efficient directional multiresolution image representation. IEEE Trans. Image Proc. **14**, 2091–2106 (2005)
32. Irani, M., Peleg, S.: Improving resolution by image registration. CVGIP **53**, 231–239 (1991)

33. Kim, K., Kwon, Y.: Single-image super-resolution using sparse regression and natural image prior. IEEE TPAMI **32**, 1127–1133 (2010)
34. Shan, Q., Li, Z., Jia, J., Tang, C.K.: Fast image/video upsampling. ACM Trans. Graph. **27**, 1–7 (2008)
35. Wang, Z., Bovik, A., Sheikh, H., Simoncelli, E.: Image quality assessment: from error visibility to structural similarity. IEEE Trans. Image Proc. **13**, 600–612 (2004)

Raindrop Detection and Removal from Long Range Trajectories

Shaodi You[1]([✉]), Robby T. Tan[2], Rei Kawakami[1],
Yasuhiro Mukaigawa[3], and Katsushi Ikeuchi[1]

[1] The University of Tokyo, Tokyo, Japan
yousd@cvl.iis.u-tokyo.ac.jp
[2] SIM University, Singapore, Singapore
[3] Nara Institute of Science and Technology, Nara, Japan

Abstract. In rainy scenes, visibility can be degraded by raindrops which
have adhered to the windscreen or camera lens. In order to resolve
this degradation, we propose a method that automatically detects and
removes adherent raindrops. The idea is to use long range trajectories to
discover the motion and appearance features of raindrops locally along
the trajectories. These motion and appearance features are obtained
through our analysis of the trajectory behavior when encountering raindrops. These features are then transformed into a labeling problem,
which the cost function can be optimized efficiently. Having detected
raindrops, the removal is achieved by utilizing patches indicated, enabling
the motion consistency to be preserved. Our trajectory based video completion method not only removes the raindrops but also complete the
motion field, which benefits motion estimation algorithms to possibly
work in rainy scenes. Experimental results on real videos show the effectiveness of the proposed method.

1 Introduction

The performance of outdoor vision systems can be degraded due to bad weather
conditions such as rain, haze, fog and snow. On rainy days, it is inevitable that
raindrops will adhere to camera lenses, protecting shields or windscreens, causing
failure to many computer vision algorithms that assume clear visibility. One
of these algorithms is motion estimation using long range optical flow. In this
case the correct correspondence of pixels affected by adherent raindrops will be
erroneous, as shown in Fig. 1.b.

In this paper, our goal is to detect and remove adherent raindrops (or just
raindrops for simplicity) by employing long range trajectories. To accomplish
this goal, our idea is to first generate initial dense trajectories in the presence
of raindrops. Surely, these initial trajectories are significantly affected by raindrops, causing them to be terminated and drifted. We analyze the motion and

Electronic supplementary material The online version of this chapter (doi:10.
1007/978-3-319-16808-1_38) contains supplementary material, which is available to
authorized users. Videos can also be accessed at http://www.springerimages.com/
videos/978-3-319-16807-4.

D. Cremers et al. (Eds.): ACCV 2014, Part II, LNCS 9004, pp. 569–585, 2015.
DOI: 10.1007/978-3-319-16808-1_38

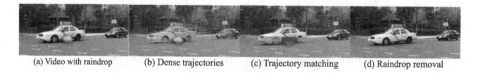

| (a) Video with raindrop | (b) Dense trajectories | (c) Trajectory matching | (d) Raindrop removal |

Fig. 1. An example of the results of our proposed detection and removal method. (a) Scene with raindrop. (b) Dense long trajectories. (c) Matching of trajectories occluded by raindrop. (d) Trajectory based video completion.

appearance behavior of the affected trajectories, and extract features from them. We formulate these features in a Markov-random-field energy function that can be optimized efficiently. Having detected raindrops, we use trajectory linking to repair the terminated or drifted trajectories. Finally, we remove the raindrops using the trajectory based video completion (Fig. 1.c and d). The overall pipeline is described in Fig. 2.

Unlike some existing methods, in this work, first we introduce a novel detection method applicable for both thick and thin raindrops as well as raindrops of any size, shape, glare, and level of blurring. We call a raindrop thick when we cannot see the objects behind it, and thin, when it is sufficiently blurred, but still allows us to partially see the objects behind it. Second, we perform a systematic analysis of the behavior of thick and thin raindrops along motion trajectories based on appearance consistency, sharpness, and raindrop mixture level. This analysis is novel, particularly when applied to raindrop detection. Third, we devise a method to detect and remove raindrops that allows us to recover the motion field. In addition, to our knowledge, our method is the first to address the problem of adherent raindrops in the framework of long range motion trajectories.

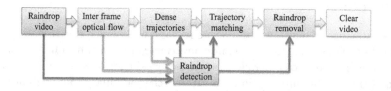

Fig. 2. The pipeline of our method.

2   Related Work

Bad weather has been explored in the past decades including: haze, mist, fog (e.g., [1–4]), falling rain and snow (e.g., [5–7]). For falling rain, Garg and Nayar study the physical model first [8], and later detect and remove it by adjusting camera parameters [6,9]. Barnum *et al.* [5] detect and remove both rain and snow. Recently, single image based methods are proposed by Kang *et al.* [10] and Chen *et al.* [7]. Unfortunately, applying these methods to handle adherent raindrops is infeasible, because of the significant physics and appearance differences between falling raindrops and adherent raindrops.

A number of methods have been proposed to detect thick adherent raindrops caused by sparse rain. Eigen et al. [11] and Kurihata et al. [12] proposed learning based methods, which are designed to handle raindrops, but not specifically to differentiate raindrops from opaque objects such as dirt. Both of the methods work only with small and clear (non-blurred) raindrops. Yamashita et al. utilize specific constraints from stereo and pan-tilt cameras [13,14], and thus is not directly applicable for a single camera. Roser et al. propose a ray-tracing based method for raindrops that are close to certain shapes [15,16], and thus can cover only a small portion of possible raindrops. You et al. [17] propose a video based detection method by using intensity change and optical flow. The method is generally useful to detect raindrops with arbitrary shapes, however the detection of thin raindrops are not addressed, and it requires about 100 frames to have good results. In comparison, our method only needs 24 frames, assuming the video frame rate is 24 *fps*.

As for raindrop removal, Roser and Geiger [15] utilize image registration, while Yamashita *et al.* [13,14] align images using the position and motion constraints from specific cameras. You *et al.* use temporal low-pass filtering and patch based video completion [18]. Generally, there are some artifacts in the repaired video because none of these methods consider motion consistency which is sensitive to human visual perception. Eigen *et al.* [11] replace raindrop image patches with clear patches through a neural-network learning technique, causing the method to be restricted on the raindrop appearance in the training data set. This method can only replace small and clear raindrops.

Sensor dust removal might be related to raindrop detections, [19–21], by considering raindrops as dust. Unlike dust however, raindrops could be large, not as blurred as dust, and affected by the water refraction as well environment reflection, making the sensor dust removal methods unsuitable for detecting raindrops.

For video based motion estimation, dense and temporally smooth motion estimation is desired. Sand *et al.* [22] propose particle video which generates motion denser than sparse tracking and longer than optical flow. Later, this idea is improved by Sundaram *et al.* [23] by utilizing GPU acceleration and large displacement optical flow [24]. Volz *et al.* [25] archive a pixel-level density by a new optical flow objective function, however their latency is limited to several frames. Rubinstein *et al.* [26] extend the temporal latency of methods [22,23] by linking the trajectories occluded by solid objects. This paper uses [23] for initial trajectory estimation but with different termination criteria, and utilizes trajectory linking as in [26] but with the features derived from our trajectory analysis over raindrops. As a result, the motion field estimation of degraded videos by raindrops can be much improved, compared to those that do not consider such degradation.

3   Trajectory Analysis

To find features that differentiate raindrops from other occlusions, as well as to identify thick and thin raindrops, we need to analyze the appearance of patches

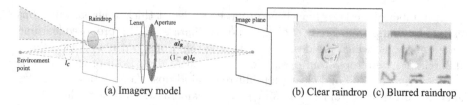

(a) Imagery model

(b) Clear raindrop (c) Blurred raindrop

Fig. 3. (a) Raindrop model. (b) Appearance of a clear raindrop. (c) Appearance of blurred raindrop observed on the image plane.

along individual trajectories and the consistency of forward/backward motion. For this, we first need to know the image formation model of raindrops, and the computation of long range trajectories.

Raindrop Model. Unlike opaque objects, raindrops can look different in different environments due to the focus of the camera on the environment. Figure 3 illustrates a raindrop physical model. Given a pixel located at (x, y), the appearance of the clear environment is denoted as $I_c(x, y)$ and the raindrop appearance as $I_r(x, y)$. For raindrops, the following mixture function models the intensity [17]:

$$I(x, y) = (1 - \alpha(x, y))I_c(x, y) + \alpha(x, y)I_r(x, y), \qquad (1)$$

where $\alpha(x, y)$ denotes the mixture level, which is dependent on the size and position of the raindrop as well as the camera aperture.

Dense Long Range Trajectories. Given a video sequence, we can form a $3D$ spatio-temporal space as illustrated in Fig. 4.a, where the spatial position of each pixel is indicated by (x, y) and the time of each frame i by t_i. The notation T in Fig. 4.b represents a trajectory consisting of a number of concatenated nodes $N(i)$, shown in Fig. 4.c, and can be expressed as:

$$T = \{N(i)\}, i_{start} \leq i \leq i_{end}$$
$$N(i) = (x(t_i), y(t_i)) = (x_i, y_i), t_{start} \leq t_i \leq t_{end}, \qquad (2)$$

where i is the index of the video frame, and (x_i, y_i) is the position of the node. The start and end of a trajectory are denoted by t_{start} and t_{end} respectively. Note

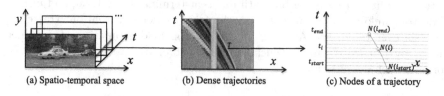

(a) Spatio-temporal space   (b) Dense trajectories   (c) Nodes of a trajectory

Fig. 4. Spatio-temporal space and dense trajectories. (a) 3D Spatio-temporal space; (b) A 2D slice visualizes the dense trajectories. (c) A trajectory consists of a number of concatenated nodes.

that the nodes are arranged in a temporal ascending order, where a trajectory has only one node at each frame.

We employ GPU-LDOF [23] to generate the initial dense trajectories. However, we ignore its trajectory termination criteria; since, [23] considers only solid occlusions, while in rainy scenes, there are thin raindrops, where the occluded scenes can still be seen. Another reason is that [23] considers occlusion boundaries to be sharp, while in our case, raindrop boundaries are usually soft due to the out-of-focus blur. We generate trajectories in a forward motion, from the first to the last frame. In this case occlusions by raindrops or other objects might cause some trajectories to stop, and consequently some areas in some frames will not have trajectories. To cover these areas, we also generate trajectories in a backward motion.

Figure 5 shows an example of the dense trajectories in a clear day scene and in a scene with a thick and in a scene with a thin raindrop. In our findings, with regard to occlusions, a trajectory can encounter the following events: (A) it is occluded by a solid non-raindrop object and drifted; (B) it is occluded by a thick raindrop and drifted; (C) it is occluded by a thin raindrop and drifted; and (D) it is occluded by a thin raindrop but not drifted.

These events encountered by trajectories allow us to identify the presence of raindrops. We consider that occlusions by thick raindrops or opaque objects will

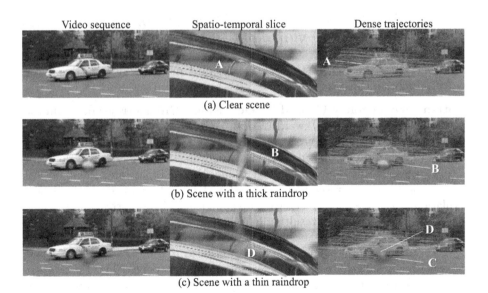

(a) Clear scene

(b) Scene with a thick raindrop

(c) Scene with a thin raindrop

Fig. 5. Video in rainy scenes and events on the trajectories. (a) A clear day scene. (b) A scene with a thick raindrop. (c) A scene with a thin raindrop. The clear scene data is from [22]. Four trajectory events are labeled as, A: Occluded by a solid non-raindrop object and drifted. B: Occluded by a thick raindrop and drifted. C: Occluded by a thin raindrop and drifted. D: Occluded by a thin raindrop but not drifted. The trajectory appearance of each event is shown in Fig. 6.

cause abrupt changes in both the appearance and the motion along trajectories, while occlusions by thin raindrops will mainly cause changes in the appearance, particularly the sharpness. The details of the analysis are as follows.

3.1   Motion Consistency Analysis

For a trajectory T generated by forward tracking, we consider a node $N(i)$ on frame t_i. Its succeeding $N(i+1)$ is found by referring to the forward optical flow $\boldsymbol{f}_i^+ = (u^+, v^+)_i$ from frame i to frame $i+1$:

$$N(i+1) = (x_i, y_i) + (u^+(x_i, y_i), v^+(x_i, y_i))_i = N(i) + \boldsymbol{f}_i^+(N(i)). \qquad (3)$$

Similarly, given a trajectory T' generated from backward tracking, nodes are related by the backward motion:

$$N'(i) = N'(i+1) + \boldsymbol{f}_{i+1}^-(N'(i+1)), \qquad (4)$$

where $\boldsymbol{f}_{i+1}^- = (u^-, v^-)_{i+1}$ is the backward optical flow from frame t_{i+1} to frame t_i.

If nodes along a trajectory are not occluded and the optical flow is correctly estimated, the following equation stands with negligible (sub-pixel) error:

$$
\begin{aligned}
m^+(N(i)) &= \| \boldsymbol{f}_i^+(N(i)) + \boldsymbol{f}_{i+1}^-(N(i) + \boldsymbol{f}_i^+(N(i))) \|_2 = 0 \\
m^-(N'(i)) &= \| \boldsymbol{f}_i^-(N'(i)) + \boldsymbol{f}_{i-1}^+(N'(i) + \boldsymbol{f}_i^-(N'(i))) \|_2 = 0
\end{aligned}
\qquad (5)
$$

where $m^+(N(i))$ and $m^-(N(i))$ are the forward motion consistency and the backward motion consistency of node $N(i)$, respectively.

Motion Inconsistency Caused by Occlusions. Given a trajectory from the forward tracking (or the backward tracking), the motion consistency $m^+(N(i))$ might not be zero if $N(i+1)$ is occluded. In events A and B, $N(i+1)$ is completely occluded by an opaque object or a thick raindrop. In this case, $N(i)$ does not have a corresponding node in the next frame. However, the inter-frame optical flow $\boldsymbol{f}_i^+$ still gives correspondence for $N(i)$. This is because the optical flow regulation forces every pixel to have correspondence. Thus, corresponding node $N(i) + \boldsymbol{f}_i^+(N(i))$ is wrong, resulting in a non-zero motion consistency.

In event C, $N(i+1)$ is occluded by a thin raindrop, which according to Eq. (1), can generate a partial occlusion. As illustrated in Fig. 6, in this event, the consistency is likely to be non-zero, since the pixel at $N(i+1)$ is the mixture of both the tracked node and the raindrop, where each of them has correspondence in the previous frame; causing both the forward and backward optical flow to likely generate wrong correspondence. Here, the mixture level α plays an important role for the wrong correspondence. Overall, the thicker the raindrop, the more likely the consistency is to be non-zero.

In event D, $N(i+1)$ is occluded by a considerably thin raindrop, where $N(i+1)$ is sufficiently visible such that both the forward and backward optical

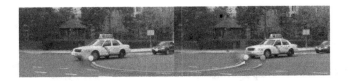

Fig. 6. When a point is covered by a thin raindrop, it has two correspondences in other frames: the raindrop and the covered object. The causes incorrect tracking for optical flow that assumes only one correspondence.

flow correctly match $N(i)$ with $N(i+1)$. In this event, the mixture level is close to zero, usually less than 0.2.

Motion Consistency Feature. Since events A, B and C might result in a non-zero motion consistency value, we can use the consistency, $m^+(N(i))$ and $m^-(N(i))$, as features to indicate the presence of occlusion, which in some cases, can be raindrops.

We calculate the motion consistency feature for each frame at t_i by collecting m^+ and m^- of all the nodes in the frame, denoted as M_i. Assuming the video frame rate is 24 fps[1] and raindrops are static in a short time period (one second), we sum up the features over 24 frames:

$$\mathcal{M}_i = \sum_{i-24 < j \leq i} M_j. \tag{6}$$

Some pixels might not have consistency values due to the failure of optical flow to track. In this case, we obtain the values from linear interpolation. Figure 8.a shows an example of $\mathcal{M}_i$.

As for event D, since possible occlusion can not be detected by the motion consistency, we detect it based on the appearance analysis, discussed in the subsequent section.

3.2 Appearance Analysis

Given a trajectory T, we crop a small image patch, denoted as $P(i)$, centered at each node $N(i)$ with length r, where r is set to 21 pixels by default (based on the resolution of our videos). Figure 7 shows an example of patches sequenced along trajectories for events A, B, C, and D.

---

[1] The 24fps framerate only for reference on how we can deal with raindrop dynamics since our method assumes static raindrops during the detection process, while in fact in the real world raindrops can move. Hence, assuming the widely adopted framerate, it means we assume raindrops at least do not move in 1-s period of time. Obviously, a higher framerate does not pose any problem (except for the computation time), however a much lower framerate will create a large displacement problem, which can affect the optical flow accuracy.

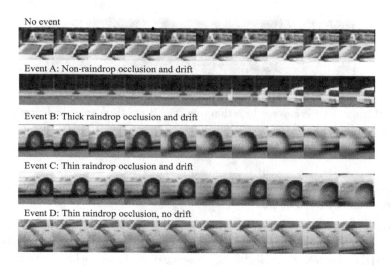

Fig. 7. Appearance of trajectories in Fig. 5. The patch size (21×21 pixels by default) is set to 41×41 pixels for better visualization.

Appearance Consistency. As can be seen in Fig. 7, all four events might generate appearance changes, particularly for events A, B and C. We calculate the appearance consistency for node $N(i)$ using:

$$a(N(i)) = \|SIFT(P(i+1)) - SIFT(P(i))\|_2, \tag{7}$$

where $SIFT(\ )$ is the SIFT descriptor [27], converts patch P to one feature array. For color images, RGB channels are converted separately and, later combined.

The reason of choosing SIFT is to achieve robustness against some degrees of affine deformation. Since even without occlusions, the appearance of an image patch might change. Note that within a few frames (i.e., fewer than 24 frames), these changes should be within the degrees where SIFT can still work, since they represent less than 1 s in real time.

Similar to the motion consistency, we compute the appearance consistency for frame t_i, denoted as A_i, by collecting the appearance consistency of all of the nodes in the frame. The integration of A_i over 24 frames is denoted as $\mathcal{A}_i$. Figure 8.b shows an example of $\mathcal{A}_i$.

The appearance consistency is able to detect all of the occlusion events (A, B, C, and D), however, it lacks the ability to distinguish a non-raindrop occlusion from a solid raindrop occlusion.

Sharpness Analysis. We define the sharpness of patch $P(i)$ as:

$$s(P(i)) = \sum_{(x,y) \in P(i)} \left\| \frac{\partial}{\partial x} I(x,y), \frac{\partial}{\partial y} I(x,y) \right\|_2 \tag{8}$$

where $I(x,y)$ is the intensity value of pixel (x,y). For color images, RGB channels are calculated separately and added up afterward.

Unlike blurred raindrops that have low sharpness in the area including the boundary, non-raindrop objects will have large sharpness at their boundary, or inside their area when they are textured. Therefore, by evaluating the sharpness, we can differentiate non-raindrop objects (Event A) from raindrops (Events B, C and D). The sharpness for frame t_i, denoted as S_i is the collection of the sharpness of all nodes in the frame. The integration of S_i over 24 frames is denoted as $\mathcal{S}_i$, Fig. 8.c shows an example of $\mathcal{S}_i$.

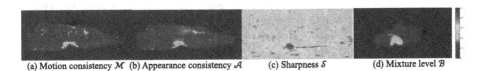

(a) Motion consistency $\mathcal{M}$ (b) Appearance consistency $\mathcal{A}$ (c) Sharpness $\mathcal{S}$ (d) Mixture level $\mathcal{B}$

Fig. 8. Raindrop features. (a) Accumulated motion consistency $\mathcal{M}$. (b) Accumulated appearance consistency $\mathcal{A}$. (c) Accumulated sharpness $\mathcal{S}$, colormap is inversed for visualization. (d) Mixture level estimation $\mathcal{B}$.

Raindrop Mixture Level. Analyzing the sharpness along trajectories does not only enable us to distinguish raindrops from non-raindrop objects, but it also allows us to estimate the raindrop mixture level, α. For a given patch $P(i)$, Eq. (1) can be rewritten as:

$$P(i) = (1 - \alpha(i))P_c + \alpha(i)P_r(i)$$
$$\alpha(i) = \alpha(N(i)) = \alpha(x(t_i), y(t_i)), \tag{9}$$

where P_c is the clear patch component and $P_r(i)$ is the raindrop component. $\alpha(i)$ is the mixture level of the patch. In the equation, we have made two approximations: First, the mixture level α inside a patch is constant. Second, the change of clear patch component P_c along the trajectory is negligible in a short time period (i.e., within 24 frames for a video with 24 fps).

From Eqs. (8) and (9), we can write the following:

$$\begin{aligned} s(P(i)) &= s[(1 - \alpha(i))P_c + \alpha(i)P_r(i)] \\ &\leq s[(1 - \alpha(i))P_c] + s[(\alpha(i)P_r(i)] \\ &= (1 - \alpha(i))s(P_c) + \alpha(i)s(P_r(i)). \end{aligned} \tag{10}$$

$$s((1 - \alpha(i))P_c) = s[P(i) - \alpha(i)P_r(i)] \leq s(P_c) + \alpha(i)s(P_r(i)). \tag{11}$$

Assuming the raindrop is sufficiently blurred, we have: $s(P_r(i)) = 0$. Substituting this in Eqs. (10) and (11) and comparing them, we have: $s(P(i)) = (1 - \alpha(i))s(P_c)$. Thus, we can estimate the mixture level of patch $P(i)$ by comparing the sharpness with a clear patch in the same trajectory as:

$$\alpha(i) = 1 - s(P(i))/s(P_c). \tag{12}$$

For a given patch $N(i)$, sharpness of a clear patch $sh(P_c)$ is obtained by evaluating the patch sharpness for m neighbor patches along the trajectory:

$$s(P_c) = \max s(P(i \pm j)), j \le m, \tag{13}$$

where $m = 10$ as default. When the clear patch has less texture, $s(P_c)$ is small and will result in a large error in Eq. (13). Hence, we only use textured patches to estimate the mixture level. Note that, if m is too small, the trajectory interval is too short, making us unable to have clear patches. On the contrary, if m is too large, the tracking drift will accumulate, causing the trajectories to be incorrect. In our observation for our test videos, $m = 10$ could avoid the problem.

Similarly, we can collect the mixture level for frame t_i, denoted as B_i. The integration of B_i is denoted as $\mathcal{B}_i$. Figure 8.d is an example of $\mathcal{B}_i$.

4   Raindrop Detection

The detection of raindrops can be described as a binary labeling problem, where for given a frame, the labels are raindrop and non-raindrop. Similarly, the mixture level can be described as a multiple labeling problem. The labeling can be done in the framework of Markov random fields (MRFs).

Raindrop Labeling. In the previous section, three features are shown for raindrop detection: motion consistency $\mathcal{M}$, appearance consistency $\mathcal{A}$ and sharpness $\mathcal{S}$. Thus, to detect raindrops, we combine these three features, after normalizing them, to form the following data term:

$$E_{data}(\boldsymbol{x}) = \|\mathcal{F}(\boldsymbol{x}) - (w_m + w_a)L(\boldsymbol{x})\|_1$$
$$\mathcal{F}(\boldsymbol{x}) = (w_m \mathcal{M}(\boldsymbol{x}) + w_a \mathcal{A}(\boldsymbol{x})) \max(0, 1 - w_s \mathcal{S}(\boldsymbol{x})) \tag{14}$$

where w_m, w_a and w_s are the weight coefficients for the three features. And $\mathcal{F}(\boldsymbol{x})$ is the combined feature. The weights were chosen empirically by considering the precision-recall curve, where a larger weight enabled more sensitive detection. We set $w_m = 16$, $w_a = 16$ and $w_s = 1$ by default. $L(\boldsymbol{x}) \in \{0, 1\}$ is the binary label, with 0 being non-raindrop. The normalization of the three features is done by setting the mean value to 0.5 and the variance to 0.5.

Since the boundaries of raindrops are significantly blurred, we can use a smoothness prior term for labeling neighboring pixels:

$$E_{prior}(\boldsymbol{x}) = \sum_{\boldsymbol{x}_j \in V(\boldsymbol{x})} |L(\boldsymbol{x}_j) - L(\boldsymbol{x})|, \tag{15}$$

where $V(\boldsymbol{x})$ is the neighbor of $\boldsymbol{x}$. We use graphcuts [28–31] to solve the optimization. Figure 9.a is an example of the labeling result.

Mixture Level Labeling. Having obtained the binary labeling of the raindrop areas, we further label the raindrop mixture level $\alpha(\boldsymbol{x})$ through multi-level labeling. We use the estimated mixture level $\mathcal{B}$ (Eq. (12)) as a clue. The data term is expressed as:

$$E'_{data}(\boldsymbol{x}) = w_b \|\mathcal{B}(\boldsymbol{x}) - \alpha(\boldsymbol{x})\|_1 + w_L \|\tilde{L}(\boldsymbol{x}) - \alpha(\boldsymbol{x})\|_1, \tag{16}$$

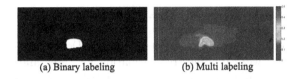

(a) Binary labeling   (b) Multi labeling

Fig. 9. Raindrop detection via labeling. (a) Binary labeling of the raindrop area. (b) Multiple labeling of the mixture level.

where $\tilde{L}(x)$ is the binary labeling result, w_b and w_L are the weight coefficients which are set to $w_b = 8$, $w_L = 2$ by default. $\alpha(x)$ has 21 uniform levels from 0 to 1. The prior term is set in a similar way to that of the binary labeling. Figure 9.b shows our estimated mixture level for all pixels.

5   Raindrop Removal

Having detected the raindrops, the next step is to remove them. The idea is that given a detected area of a raindrop, we collect the patches along the corresponding trajectories, and use these patches as a source of information to fill in the detected raindrop area.

Based on the binary labeling result, we first remove nodes in the trajectories that are labeled as raindrops, since these trajectories are likely to be incorrect or drifted. By this operation, some of the trajectories will be shortened, and the others will be broken into two trajectories.

To replace the removed nodes of trajectories, we match the corresponding existing trajectories based on [26], where the data term is based on SIFT, temporal order, and inter-frame motion. Figure 1.c is an example of matched trajectories. After matching, we interpolate the missing nodes. Given a matched trajectory pair T_i and T_j, the last node of T_i, denoted as $N^i(end) = (x(t^i_{end}), y(t^i_{end}))$, is matched to the first node of T_j, denoted as $N^j(1) = (x(t^j_{start}), y(t^j_{start}))$. Here, $t^i_{end} < t^j_{start}$ means for all matched pairs. We linearly interpolate the missing nodes between frames t^i_{end} and t^j_{start} based on:

$$N(k) = \frac{t^j_{start} - t_k}{t^j_{start} - t^i_{end}} N^i(end) + \frac{t_k - t^i_{end}}{t^j_{start} - t^i_{end}} N^j(1), \quad t^i_{end} < t_k < t^j_{start}. \quad (17)$$

5.1   Trajectory-Based Video Completion

Having obtained the trajectories for the raindrop areas, the raindrop completion is done by propagating the clear background pixels along a trajectory towards the raindrop area. Using the guidance of trajectories, we propose a removal strategy which preserves both spatial and temporal consistency.

The completion is done frame by frame. First, we start from the first frame and move forward until we find a frame t which contains interpolated nodes. For the frame t, inside a raindrop area, we denote the interpolated nodes as

$\{N_i(t)\}$, where i is the trajectory index. According to the trajectory, we find the corresponding nodes in the previous frame: $\{N_i(t-1)\}$. A transformation can be determined between the two sets of nodes. Depending on the number of nodes in the set, we use affine transformation for three and more matches, translation and rotation for two matches, and translation for one match. Then, the image patch from $t-1$ is transformed and placed at the raindrop area in t. By utilizing information from groups of nodes, we preserve both spatial consistency and temporal consistency. This process continues until it reaches the last frame. For the repaired patch, we denote its confidence as: $C(t) = C(t-1) - 1$. The confidence degrades by 1 every time it is propagated. And the non-interpolated patches have a confidence of 0.

Similarly, we do the backward process starting from the last frame. As a result, for each repaired area, there are two solutions: one from the forward process, and one from the backward process. We chose the one with the higher confidence. As for static or quasi-static areas where no linked trajectory exists, we use the video inpainting method by Wexler *et al.* [18] for repair. An example of the repaired video is shown in Fig. 1.d.

Thin Raindrops. For thin raindrops (event D, generally $\alpha < 0.2$), the trajectories inside the raindrop areas are already correct, therefore we do not need to propagate the appearance from other frames, since we can directly enhance the appearance. As discussed in Sec. 3.2, thin raindrops can be relatively blurred, hence to enhance them, for a node N with appearance P, we convert P to $\mathcal{P}$ using 2D-DCT and set the constant component $\mathcal{P}(0,0) = 0$. Then, we enhance the sharpness according to the mixture level: $\mathcal{P}' = \frac{1}{1-\alpha}\mathcal{P}$. We replace the constant component which is the one with a non-raindrop node along the trajectory. Finally, the enhanced patch P' is obtained using inverse-DCT.

6   Experiments

We conducted both quantitative and qualitative evaluation to measure the accuracy of our detection and removal method. Our video results are included in the supplementary material.

6.1   Raindrop Detection

Dataset. In our experiments, the video data were taken from different sources to avoid data bias and to demonstrate the general applicability of our method. Data 1 was from Sundarum *et al.* [23], data 3 was from KITTI Benchmark [32], data 5 and 7 were from You *et al.* [17] and the rest were downloaded from the Internet. In these data, the camera setups vary from a car mounted camera, a hand held camera to a surveillance camera.

Comparison with State-of-the-art. We used both synthetic and real raindrops, and compared our method with three state-of-the-art methods, Eigen *et al.*'s [11], You *et al.*'s [17] and Roser *et al.*'s [15]. The results are shown in

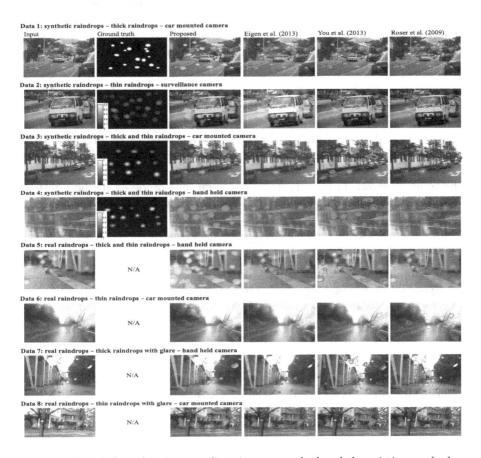

Fig. 10. The raindrop detection results using our method and the existing methods.

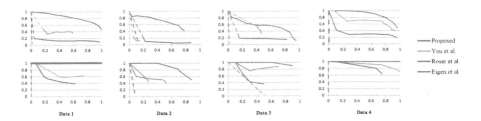

Fig. 11. Precision-recall curve on detection for the methods shown in Fig. 10. First row: evaluation at a pixel level. Second row: evaluation at number of raindrops level. Dashlines indicates the range where no data is available.

Fig. 10. As can be seen, Eigen *et al.*'s method failed to detect large and blurred raindrops, and mislabeled textured areas (such as trees) as raindrops. As for You *et al.*'s method, although it correctly detected thick raindrops, thin raindrops were simply neglected. Roser *et al.*'s method detected round raindrops and thin raindrops only when the background was textuerless.

Quantitative Evaluation. For the synthetic raindrops, data 1–4 in Fig. 10, we quantitatively evaluated using the precision-recall curve. In addition of number of raindrop level evalutation, we also performed pixel-level evaluation. The precision is defined as the number of the correctly labeled pixels divided by the number of all pixels labeled as raindrops. The recall is defined as the number of the correctly labeled pixels divided by the number of the actual raindrop pixels. The result is shown in Fig. 11. As can be seen, our proposed method outperformed some existing methods for both accuracy and recall. Our method have a low false alarm rate for both thick and thin raindrops. As for the real raindrops, data 5–8, our method successfully labeled thin raindrops as well as thick raindrops and achieved better precision.

False Alarm rate Evaluation. To test the robustness of our method, we ran our algorithm on the first four data shown in Fig. 10 with all the synthetic raindrop removed. Table 1 shows the number of raindrop spots detected, although there is no raindrop in the input videos. Our method shows a significantly low false alarm rate compared to the other methods.

Table 1. False alarms on Data 1–4 (Fig. 10) with all synthetic raindrops removed. Evaluated by number of spots erroneuously detected as raindrops.

	Proposed	Eigen et al.	You et al.	Roser et al.
Data 1	0	67	8	17
Data 2	1	48	16	12
Data 3	1	140	6	5
Data 4	0	12	4	2

Speed. On a 1.4 GHz notebook with Matlab and no parallelization, the interframe optical flow was about one minute per frame. The tracking and feature collecting together was about 0.2 s per frame. Graphcut was about 5 s for one detection phase. While our algorithm is not real time, we consider it to be still useful for offline applications, such as road accident analysis, Google-like street data collection, etc.

6.2   Raindrop Removal

Figure 12 shows the results of raindrop removal of a few methods, along with the groundtruth. The results include those of Eigen *et al.*'s [11] and You *et al.*'s [17]. Roser *et al.*'s method does not provide the implementation details for raindrop

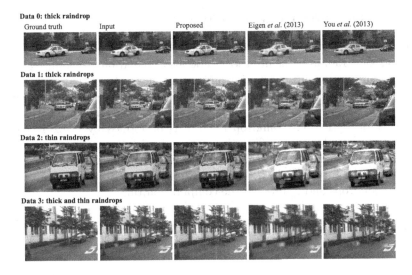

Fig. 12. The raindrop removal results.

removal, and thus it was not included. As can observed in the figure, our method removed both thin and thick raindrops. Eigen *et al.*'s method failed to remove large raindrops and it erroneously smoothed textured area. You *et al.*'s method failed to remove thin raindrops, and the quality is affected by the detection accuracy.

Repaired Motion Field. Figure 13 shows the results of the motion field estimation, before and after the raindrop removal. As shown in the figure, our method can improve the dense motion estimation, by removing the raindrops, and then repairing the motion fields.

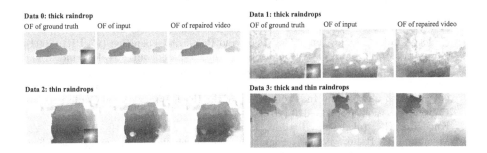

Fig. 13. Comparison on motion field estimation before and after raindrop removal.

7   Conclusion and Future Work

We have introduced a method that automatically detects and removes both thick and thin raindrops using a local operation based on the long trajectory analysis. Our idea is using the motion and appearance features that are extracted from analyzing the trajectories-raindrops encountering events. These features are transformed into a labeling problem which is efficiently optimized in the framework of MRFs. The raindrop removal is performed by utilizing patches indicated by trajectories, enabling the motion consistency to be preserved. We believe our algorithm can be extended to handle other similar occluders, such as dirt or dust. For future work, we consider exploring dense-trajectory analysis of dynamic raindrops and improving the computation time.

Acknowledgement. This work is supported by Next-generation Energies for Tohoku Recovery (NET), MEXT, Japan.

References

1. Tan, R.: Visibility in bad weather from a single image. In: IEEE Conference on Computer Vision and Pattern Recognition (CVPR) (2008)
2. Fattal, R.: Single image dehazing. In: SIGGRAPH (2008)
3. He, K., Sun, J., Tang, X.: Single image haze removal using dark channel prior. In: IEEE Computer Society Conference on Computer Vision and Pattern Recognition (CVPR) (2009)
4. Meng, G., Wang, Y., Duan, J., Xiang, S., Pan, C.: Efficient image dehazing with boundary constraint and contextual regularization. In: ICCV (2013)
5. Barnum, P., Narasimhan, S., Kanade, T.: Analysis of rain and snow in frequency space. Int. J. Comput. Vis. (IJCV) **86**, 256–274 (2010)
6. Garg, K., Nayar, S.: Vision and rain. Int. J. Comput. Vis. (IJCV) **75**, 3–27 (2007)
7. Chen, Y.L., Hsu, C.T.: A generalized low-rank appearance model for spatio-temporally correlated rain streaks. In: ICCV (2013)
8. Garg, K., Nayar, S.: Photometric model of a raindrop. CMU Technical report (2003)
9. Garg, K., Nayar, S.: Detection and removal of rain from video. In: IEEE Computer Society Conference on Computer Vision and Pattern Recognition (CVPR) (2004)
10. Kang, L., Lin, C., Fu, Y.: Automatic single-image-based rain streaks removal via image decomposition. IEEE Trans. Image Process. (TIP) **21**, 1742–1755 (2012)
11. Eigen, D., Krishnan, D., Fergus, R.: Restoring an image taken through a window covered with dirt or rain. In: Proceedings of the IEEE International Conference on Computer Vision, pp. 633–640 (2013)
12. Kurihata, H., Takahashi, T., Ide, I., Mekada, Y., Murase, H., Tamatsu, Y., Miyahara, T.: Rainy weather recognition from in-vehicle camera images for driver assistance. In: IEEE Intelligent Vehicles Symposium (2005)
13. Yamashita, A., Tanaka, Y., Kaneko, T.: Removal of adherent water-drops from images acquired with stereo camera. In: IROS (2005)
14. Yamashita, A., Fukuchi, I., Kaneko, T.: Noises removal from image sequences acquired with moving camera by estimating camera motion from spatio-temporal information. In: IEEE/RSJ International Conference on Intelligent Robots and Systems (IROS) (2009)

15. Roser, M., Geiger, A.: Video-based raindrop detection for improved image registration. In: Workshops of IEEE International Conference on Computer Vision (2009)
16. Roser, M., Kurz, J., Geiger, A.: Realistic modeling of water droplets for monocular adherent raindrop recognition using bezier curves. In: Asian Conference on Computer Vision (ACCV) (2010)
17. You, S., Tan, R.T., Kawakami, R., Ikeuchi, K.: Adherent raindrop detection and removal in video. In: IEEE Computer Society Conference on Computer Vision and Pattern Recognition (CVPR) (2013)
18. Wexler, Y., Shechtman, E., Irani, M.: Space-time video completion. In: IEEE Conference on Computer Vision and Pattern Recognition (CVPR) (2004)
19. Willson, R.G., Maimone, M., Johnson, A., Scherr, L.: An Optical Model for Image Artifacts Produced by Dust Particles on Lenses. Jet Propulsion Laboratory, National Aeronautics and Space Administration, Pasadena, CA (2005)
20. Zhou, C., Lin, S.: Removal of image artifacts due to sensor dust. In: IEEE Conference on Computer Vision and Pattern Recognition, CVPR 2007, pp. 1–8. IEEE (2007)
21. Gu, J., Ramamoorthi, R., Belhumeur, P., Nayar, S.: Removing image artifacts due to dirty camera lenses and thin occluders. ACM Trans. Graph. (TOG) **28**, 144 (2009)
22. Sand, P., Teller, S.: Particle video: Long-range motion estimation using point trajectories. Int. J. Comput. Vis. (IJCV) **80**, 72–91 (2008)
23. Sundaram, N., Brox, T., Keutzer, K.: Dense point trajectories by GPU-accelerated large displacement optical flow. In: Daniilidis, K., Maragos, P., Paragios, N. (eds.) ECCV 2010, Part I. LNCS, vol. 6311, pp. 438–451. Springer, Heidelberg (2010)
24. Brox, T., Malik, J.: Large displacement optical flow: descriptor matching in variational motion estimation. IEEE Trans. Pattern Anal. Mach. Intell. (TPAMI) **33**, 500–513 (2011)
25. Volz, S., Bruhn, A., Valgaerts, L., Zimmer, H.: Modeling temporal coherence for optical flow. In: 2011 IEEE International Conference on Computer Vision (ICCV), pp. 1116–1123. IEEE (2011)
26. Rubinstein, M., Liu, C., Freeman, W.T.: Towards longer long-range motion trajectories. In: British Machine Vision Conference (BMVC), pp. 1–11 (2012)
27. Lowe, D.G.: Distinctive image features from scale-invariant keypoints. Int. J. Comput. Vis. **60**, 91–110 (2004)
28. Fulkerson, B., Vedaldi, A., Soatto, S.: Class segmentation and object localization with superpixel neighborhoods. In: IEEE International Conference on Computer Vision (ICCV) (2009)
29. Boykov, Y., Kolmogorov, V.: An experimental comparison of min-cut/max-flow algorithms for energy minimization in vision. IEEE Trans. Pattern Anal. Mach. Intell. (TPAMI)s 26, 1124–1137 (2004)
30. Boykov, Y., Veksler, O., Zabih, R.: Efficient approximate energy minimization via graph cuts. IEEE Trans. Pattern Anal. Mach. Intell. (TPAMI) **20**, 1222–1239 (2001)
31. Kolmogorov, V., Zabih, R.: What energy functions can be minimized via graph cuts? IEEE Trans. Pattern Anal. Mach. Intell. (TPAMI) **26**, 147–159 (2004)
32. Geiger, A., Lenz, P., Urtasun, R.: Are we ready for autonomous driving? the kitti vision benchmark suite. In: Conference on Computer Vision and Pattern Recognition (CVPR) (2012)

Interest Points via Maximal Self-Dissimilarities

Federico Tombari[✉] and Luigi Di Stefano

DISI, University of Bologna, Bologna, Italy
{federico.tombari,luigi.distefano}@unibo.it
http://www.vision.deis.unibo.it

Abstract. We propose a novel interest point detector stemming from the intuition that image patches which are highly dissimilar over a relatively large extent of their surroundings hold the property of being repeatable and distinctive. This concept of *contextual self-dissimilarity* reverses the key paradigm of recent successful techniques such as the Local Self-Similarity descriptor and the Non-Local Means filter, which build upon the presence of similar - rather than dissimilar - patches. Moreover, our approach extends to contextual information the local self-dissimilarity notion embedded in established detectors of corner-like interest points, thereby achieving enhanced repeatability, distinctiveness and localization accuracy.

1 Introduction

The *self-similarity* of an image patch is a powerful computational tool that has been deployed in numerous and diverse image processing and analysis tasks. It can be defined as the set of distances of a patch to those located in its surroundings, with distances usually measured through the Sum of Squared Distances (SSD). Whenever the task mandates looking for large rather than small minima over such distances, we will use the term *self-dissimilarity*. Analogous to self-similarity is auto-correlation, which relies on the cross-correlation to compare the given to surrounding patches. An early example of deployment of self-dissimilarity in the computer vision literature is the Moravec operator [1], which detects interest points exhibiting a sufficiently large intensity variation along all directions by computing the minimum SSD between a patch and its 8 adjacent ones. The Harris Corner Detector [2] extends the Moravec operator by proposing Taylor's expansion of the directional intensity variation together with a saliency score which highlights corner-like interest points. Then, Mikolajczyk and Schmid developed the Harris-Laplace operator [3] to achieve scale-invariant detection of corner-like features.

More recently, the self-similarity concept has been used to develop the Local Self Similarity (LSS) region descriptor [4], which leverages on relative positions between nearby similar patches to provide invariant representations of a pixel's neighborhood. One of the main innovations introduced by this method with respect to previous approaches deploying self-similarities consists in the reference patch being spatially compared with a much larger neighborhood rather

D. Cremers et al. (Eds.): ACCV 2014, Part II, LNCS 9004, pp. 586–600, 2015.
DOI: 10.1007/978-3-319-16808-1_39

than with just its nearest vicinity. The LSS method computes a *self-similarity surface* associated with an image point, which is then quantized to build the descriptor. Notably, the inherent traits of self-similarity endow the descriptor with peculiar robustness with respect to diversity of the image acquisition modality [4,5]. As a further example, [6] exploits the concept of self-similarity to detect interest points associated with symmetrical regions in images. Specifically, auto-correlation based on Normalized Cross-Correlation among image patches is used as a saliency measure to highlight image regions exhibiting symmetries with respect to either a line (mirror symmetries) or a point (rotational symmetries). Interest points are successively detected as extrema of the saliency function over a scale-space. Though aimed at a different purpose such as denoising, the Non-Local Means (NLM) [7] and BM3D [8] filters exploit the presence of similar patches within an image to estimate the noiseless intensity of each pixel. In [7], this is done by computing the weighted average of measured intensities within a relatively large area surrounding each pixel, with weights proportional to the self-similarity between the patch centered at the given pixel and those around the other ones in the area. Instead, in [8] self-similarity allows for sifting-out sets of image patches grouped together to undergo a more complex computational process referred to as collaborative filtering.

In this paper we propose a novel interest point detector obtained by reverting the classical exploitation of self-similarity so as to highlight those image patches that are most *dissimilar* from nearby ones within a relatively large surrounding area. This concept, which will be referred to in the following as *contextual self-dissimilarity* (CSD), associates a patch's saliency with the absence of similar patches in its surroundings. Accordingly, CSD may be thought of as relying on the rarity of a patch, which, interestingly, is identified as the basic saliency cue also in the interest point detector by Kadir and Brady [9]. However, their work ascertains rarity in a strictly local rather than contextual approach, due to saliency consisting in the entropy of the gray-level distribution within a patch [9].

A peculiar trait with respect to several prominent feature detectors like [10–12] is that CSD endows our approach with the ability to withstand significant, possibly non-linear, tone mappings, such as e.g. due to light changes, as well as to cope effectively with diversity in the image sensing modality. A similar concept to CSD has been exploited in [13] for the purpose of detecting salient regions to create a visual summary of an image. In particular, the proposed saliency for a patch is directly proportional to the distance in the CIELab space to surrounding most similar patches and inversely proportional to their 2D spatial distance, the latter requirement due to the addressed task calling for spatially close rather than scattered salient pixels. Unlike [13], we aim here at exploiting self-dissimilarities for the task of interest point detection and propose a saliency measure which relies solely upon the CSD measured in the intensity domain.

Experiments demonstrate the effectiveness of the proposed detector in finding repeatable interest points. In particular, evaluation on the standard *Oxford* dataset as well as on the more recent *Robot* dataset vouches that our method attains state-of-the-art invariance with respect to illumination changes and remarkable performance with most other nuisances, such as blur, viewpoint changes and compression. Furthermore, we show the peculiar effectiveness of the proposed approach on a dataset of images acquired by different modalities.

2   Contextual Self Dissimilarity

The saliency concept used by our interest point detector relies on the computation of a patch's self-similarity over an extended neighborhood, which has already been exploited by popular techniques such as the LSS descriptor [4] and the NLM filter [7]. Unlike these methods though, we do not aim at detecting highly similar patches within the surroundings of a pixel, but instead at determining whether a pixel shows similar patches in its surroundings or not. Thus, the proposed technique relies on a saliency operator, λ, which measures the *Contextual Self-Dissimilarity* (CSD) of a point p, i.e. how much the patch around p is dissimilar from the most similar one in its surroundings:

$$\lambda\left(p, \rho_w, \rho_a\right) = \frac{1}{\rho_w^2} \min_{q \in \omega(p, \rho_a), q \neq p} \delta\left(\omega\left(p, \rho_w\right), \omega\left(q, \rho_w\right)\right) \tag{1}$$

As shown by (1), the proposed saliency operator is characterized by two parameters, ρ_w and ρ_a, defining respectively the size of the patches under comparison and the size of the area from which the patches to be compared are drawn. In addition, in the same equation, $\omega(p, \rho_w)$ denotes the operator defining a square image region centered at pixel p and having size equal to ρ_w pixels, while δ denotes the distance between the vectors collecting the intensities of two equally sized image patches, which in its simplest form can be the squared L_2 distance, or Sum of Squared Distances (SSD):

$$\delta\left(\omega\left(p, \rho_w\right), \omega\left(q, \rho_w\right)\right) = \| I\left(\omega\left(p, \rho_w\right)\right) - I\left(\omega\left(q, \rho_w\right)\right) \|_2^2 \tag{2}$$

Computing λ at all pixels determines a saliency map whose values are proportional to the rarity of the patch centered at each pixel with respect to the surrounding area. Normalization by means of the number of pixels involved in the computation of the self-dissimilarity helps rendering the saliency score independent of the patch size ρ_w. Parameter ρ_a establishes the spatial support of the saliency criterion. As a well-known trait in literature [14], certain saliency operators can be defined either locally or globally, depending on a patch's rarity being computed over small local neighborhoods or the whole image. By increasing ρ_a, the λ operator moves gradually from a local toward a contextual or even global saliency criterion. As mentioned in Sect. 1, we advocate replacing the local self-dissimilarity underpinning all the popular interest point detectors rooted in the Moravec operator with a contextual self-dissimilarity notion. To begin substantiating the claim, in the top-row of Fig. 1, we report results on a subset of the *Oxford* dataset that show how deployment of a contextual rather than local saliency criterion delivers dramatic improvements in terms of repeatability of the interest points[1].

---

[1] Interest point detection is run at multiple scales as described in Sect. 3.

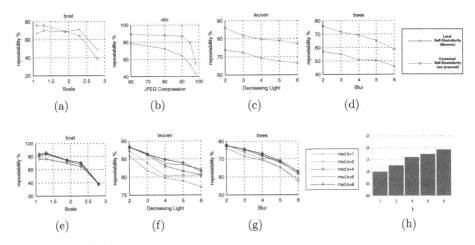

Fig. 1. Results on a subset of the *Oxford* dataset. Top row (*a–d*): Contextual vs. Local Self-Dissimilarity. Bottom row: repeatability (*e–g*) and relative execution times (*h*) for CSD interest points detected with different k values.

The saliency defined in (1) relies on estimating the minimum distance between the given and neighboring patches by simply picking one sample from observations, which is potentially prone to noise. Indeed, noise on both the central as well as the most dissimilar neighboring patch can induce notable variations in saliency scores, which may hinder repeatability and accurate localization of salient points. On the other hand, most existing operators grounded on self-similarity average out estimates over several samples. In the NLM filter, e.g., the noiseless value to be assigned to each pixel is averaged over all samples. Likewise, in the LSS descriptor, the discriminative trait associated to an image point is the union of the locations of similar patches in the neighborhood. A further operation which confers robustness to noise to the LSS descriptor is the binning operation carried out by quantizing into a spatial histogram the locations of most similar patches.

Therefore, we propose to modify (1) in the way the minimum of the distribution is estimated. Finding the most similar patch among a set of candidates can be interpreted as a 1-Nearest Neighbor (1-NN) search problem. We propose to modify the search task to a k-NN problem (with $k \geq 1$) and, accordingly, to estimate the minimum as the average across the k most similar patches:

$$\lambda^{(k)}\left(p, \rho_w, \rho_a\right) = \frac{1}{\rho_w^2 \cdot k} \sum_{i=1}^{k} \tilde{\delta}^i \left(\omega\left(p, \rho_w\right), \omega\left(q, \rho_w\right)\right) \tag{3}$$

where $\tilde{\delta}^1, \cdots, \tilde{\delta}^k$ are the k smallest value of the δ function found within the search area defined by ρ_a. Parameter k thus trades distinctiveness and computational efficiency for repeatability and accurate localization in noisy conditions. Figure 1, bottom row, highlights the impact of the chosen k on both performance as well as computational efficiency: a higher k yields generally improved repeatability at the expense of a higher computational cost. Although the optimal value may depend on the specific nuisances related to the addressed scenario, we found $k = 4$ to provide generally a good trade-off between performance and speed, and we thus suggest this as default setting in (3).

2.1   Computational Efficiency

Computing the CSD operator over an image with n pixels implies the operation in (3) to be repeated as many times as n, this yielding a complexity equal to $O(n \cdot \rho_w^2 \cdot \rho_a^2)$ which may turn out prohibitive for common image sizes. To reduce the computational burden inherent to the saliency operator presented thus far, we have devised an incremental scheme which can decrease the complexity to $O(n \cdot \rho_a^2)$, i.e. so as to render it independent on patch size.

The main intuition relies on the observation that, once the CSD operator has been computed at pixel p, most of the calculations associated with the next position, p', can be recycled. This is sketched in Fig. 2a, where the patches associated with p and q are depicted in blue, those associated with p' and q' highlighted in red. The figure intuitively shows that the distance between the patches at p' and q' can be computed as:

$$\delta\Big(\omega\,(p', \rho_w)\,, \omega\,(q', \rho_w)\Big) = \delta\Big(\omega\,(p, \rho_w)\,, \omega\,(q, \rho_w)\Big) +$$
$$-\delta\Big(\alpha(p'), \alpha(q')\Big) + \delta\Big(\beta(p'), \beta(q')\Big) \qquad (4)$$

where $\alpha(p')$, $\beta(p')$, $\alpha(q')$, $\beta(q')$ are the vectors collecting the intensities of the left and right vertical sides of the two patches, as highlighted in the Figure. In turn, as illustrated in Fig. 2b, the two distances between the corresponding sides of the patches appearing in (4) can be computed incrementally from the position just above p', denoted as p'' and highlighted in green, by adding and subtracting properly the squared differences between the intensities at the four

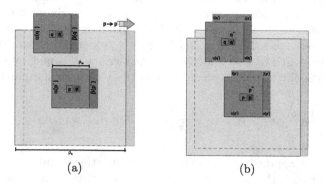

(a)   (b)

Fig. 2. Efficient computation of the distance between two patches: recursive scheme applied along columns (a) and along both columns and rows (b) (Color figure online).

corner positions of the patches, referred to as i, j, u, v. Accordingly, Eq. (4) can be further manipulated so to reach:

$$\delta\Big(\omega\left(p', \rho_w\right), \omega\left(q', \rho_w\right)\Big) = \delta\Big(\omega\left(p, \rho_w\right), \omega\left(q, \rho_w\right)\Big) - \delta\Big(\alpha(p''), \alpha(q'')\Big) +$$
$$+\delta\Big(\beta(p''), \beta(q'')\Big) - \big(I\left(i\left(p'\right)\right) - I\left(i\left(q'\right)\right)\big)^2 - \big(I\left(j\left(p'\right)\right) - I\left(j\left(q'\right)\right)\big)^2 +$$
$$+\big(I\left(u\left(p'\right)\right) - I\left(u\left(q'\right)\right)\big)^2 + \big(I\left(v\left(p'\right)\right) - I\left(v\left(q'\right)\right)\big)^2 \quad (5)$$

As it can be noticed from the above equation, the distance between the current pair p', q' needs not to be calculated from scratch but can instead be achieved incrementally from already available quantities by means of a few elementary operations. This approach, which can be regarded as a particular form of Box Filtering [15], allows calculating all distances between the central patch and those contained in the search area with a limited computational complexity and could be usefully deployed to reduce the complexity of self-similarity-based techniques too, such as [4,7].

The overall algorithm to compute the saliency operator λ is showcased in Algorithm 1, where for illustrative purposes only we consider the simplest case of Eq. (1), i.e. $k = 1$. In its practical implementation, δ_α and δ_β are assimilated to the same memory structure having size $w \cdot \rho_a^2$ elements, which is initialized by explicitly computing the column-wise squared difference within all search areas on the first image row. The δ_w data structure is instead as large as ρ_a^2 elements. Thus, the overhead in memory footprint required by incremental computation turns out as small as $(w+1) \cdot \rho_a^2$, which is favorably counterbalanced by a speed-up of about one order of magnitude with respect to the standard implementation.

3 Detection of Interest Points

Given its definition, the CSD operator yields a high score only when the current patch is highly dissimilar from all surrounding ones. This trait can be exploited to develop an interest point detector whereby interest points are given by the centers of those patches featuring a distinctive structure with respect to their surroundings, whatever such a structure may be. It is worth observing that, with the proposed approach, the self-similarity surface around interest points tends inherently to exhibit a sharp peak rather than a plateau, which is a desirable property as far as precise localization of extracted features is concerned. Indeed, given that the patch centered at an interest point must be highly dissimilar also to adjacent patches, it is unlikely for nearby points to exhibit a similar saliency as that of the interest point. Another benefit of relying on CSD to detect interest points concerns its potential effectiveness in presence of strong photometric distortions as well as multi-modal data, as vouched by the work related to the LSS descriptor [4]. Moreover, intuition suggest the approach to be robust to nuisances such as viewpoint variations and blur, given that the property of a patch to be somehow unique within its surroundings is likely to

---

Algorithm 1. Incremental computation of the λ operator

---

for $p \in$ first row **do**
  for $q \in \omega(p, \rho_a), \mathbf{q} \neq \mathbf{p}$ **do**
    $\delta_\alpha(p, q) = \delta\Big(\alpha(p), \alpha(q)\Big)$
    $\delta_\beta(p, q) = \delta\Big(\beta(p), \beta(q)\Big)$
  end for
end for
for $p \in$ all other rows **do**
  $\delta_{min} = inf$
  for $q \in \omega(p, \rho_a), \mathbf{q} \neq \mathbf{p}$ **do**
    if p is the first pixel of the row **then**
      $\delta_\omega(q) = \delta\Big(\omega(p, \rho_w), \omega(q, \rho_w)\Big)$
    else
      $\delta_\alpha(p, q) \ \ += \ \ \delta\Big(u(p), u(q)\Big) - \delta\Big(i(p), i(q)\Big)$
      $\delta_\beta(p, q) \ \ += \ \ \delta\Big(v(p), v(q)\Big) - \delta\Big((j(p), j(q)\Big)$
      $\delta_\omega(q) \ \ += \ \ \delta_\beta(p, q) - \delta_\alpha(p, q)$
    end if
    if $\delta_\omega(q) < \delta_{min}$ **then**
      $\delta_{min} = \delta_\omega(q)$
    end if
  end for
  $\lambda(p) = \frac{1}{\rho_a^2} \cdot \delta_{min}$
end for

---

hold even though the scene is seen from a (moderately) different vantage point and under some degree of blur.

However, ρ_w and ρ_a would set the scale of the structures of interest firing the detector. To endow the detector with scale invariance, as well as to associate a characteristic scale to extracted features, we build a simple image pyramid $I(l)$ comprising L levels, starting from level 1 (original image resolution) and rescaling, at each level l, the image of a factor f^l with respect to the base level. Denoting as w and h, respectively, the number of image columns and rows, once the scale factor f and the parameters ρ_a, ρ_w are chosen, the number of pyramid levels L can be automatically determined according to:

$$L = \left\lfloor log_f\left(\frac{min(w, h)}{(\rho_w + \rho_a) \cdot 2 + 1}\right)\right\rfloor \tag{6}$$

based on the constraint that the top level of the pyramid cannot be smaller than the area required to compute the saliency on one single point:

$$\frac{min(w, h)}{f^L} > (\rho_w + \rho_a) \cdot 2 + 1 \tag{7}$$

Once the saliency in (3) is computed at each point within the several layers of the image pyramid, for each level l the set of interest points, $\tilde{P}_l = \{\tilde{p}_1, \cdots, \tilde{p}_n\} \in$

$I(l)$, is extracted by means of a Non-Maxima Suppression (NMS) procedure. Specifically, an interest point $\tilde{p} \in I(l)$ is detected if it yields a saliency higher than all other saliency values within a window of size ρ_ν:

$$\tilde{p} \in I(l) s.t. \max_{p \in \omega(\tilde{p}, \rho_\nu), p \neq \tilde{p}} \lambda^{(k)}(p, \rho_w, \rho_a) < \lambda^{(k)}(\tilde{p}, \rho_w, \rho_a) \qquad (8)$$

As the features detected through the NMS stage are local maxima of the CSD operator, our proposal will be hereinafter also referred to as *Maximal Self-Dissimilarity* interest point detector (MSD). Afterwards, weak local maxima may be further pruned based on a saliency threshold τ_δ, which in our experiments is set to $\tau_\delta = 250$.

The search for local maxima throughout the image pyramid allows associating a characteristic scale to each detected interest point; given an interest point $\tilde{p}$ detected at coordinates (i_l, j_l) and pyramid level l, its associated i, j coordinates into the original image and characteristic scale size (or diameter) s are given by:

$$i(\tilde{p}) = i_l \cdot f^l \qquad j(\tilde{p}) = j_l \cdot f^l \qquad s(\tilde{p}) = (\rho_w \cdot 2 + 1) \cdot f^l \qquad (9)$$

For the purpose of successive feature description, a canonical orientation may also be associated to each interest point $\tilde{p}$ by accumulating into a histogram the angles between the interest point and the centers of the k most similar patches within $\omega(\tilde{p}, \rho_a)$ weighted by their dissimilarity, so as to then choose the direction corresponding to the highest bin in the histogram.

As already pointed-out, assessment of saliency based on the self-dissimilarity of a patch underpins both MSD as well as established detectors of corner-like structures, such as Moravec [1], Harris [2] and, more recently, the Harris-Laplace and Harris-affine detectors [3, 16], the key difference consisting in our proposal advocating assessment to occur across a larger surrounding area referred to as context rather than locally. It is also worth pointing out that, accordingly, our approach cannot deploy Taylor expansion of the dissimilarity function, as it is indeed the case of Harris-style detectors, due to Taylor expansion providing a correct approximation only locally, i.e. within a small neighborhood of the pixel under evaluation.

To further highlight the differences between the two approaches, in Fig. 3 we compare qualitatively the interest points extracted by MSD to those provided

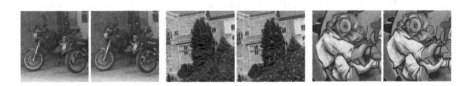

Fig. 3. Qualitative comparison between the interest points provided by MSD (green dots) and the Harris-Laplace detector [3] (red dots) on 3 image regions from the *Oxford* dataset. For clarity of visual comparison, only features of approximately the same medium-size scale are displayed for both methods (Color figure online).

by the Harris-Laplace (*harlap*) scale-invariant corner detector [3]. One of the most noticeable differences between the two approaches concerns *harlap* tending to yield multiple nearby responses around the most salient (and corner-like) structures, while this is not the case of MSD, as nearby corner-like structures tend to be similar and thus inhibit each other due to the requirement for interest points to be salient within the context. This is a favorable property as implies dealing with inherently fewer distinctive interest points in the successive feature matching stage. It can also be observed how, again due to the use of context, MSD features tend to be scattered over a more ample image area and in a more uniform way. Moreover, and unlike *harlap*, MSD can detect also a variety of salient structures quite different from corner-like ones, such as blob-like features, edge fragments and smoothly-textured distinctive patches.

As a final remark, the choice of parameters ρ_a, ρ_w is key to the performance of the proposed detector. In particular, too small a patch does not contain enough information to render the self-dissimilarity concept meaningful and effective due to dissimilarity tending to appear quite often small. Alike, this is the case of too big a patch, with dissimilarity getting now always high. Given the chosen patch size, as context is enlarged the detector tends to sift-out increasingly distinctive features, but this hinders both the quantity of extracted interest points, as it implies a high probability of finding similar structures around, as well as their repeatability, the latter issue occurring in cluttered scenes due to the likely inclusion into the context of similar patches belonging to nearby objects. Therefore, we have run several experiments to carefully select the key parameters of our method and found quite an effective trade-off pair to consist in $\rho_w = 7, \rho_a = 11$.

4   Experimental Results

To assess its performance, we compare here the proposed MSD algorithm to the state of the art in interest point detection. We consider first the standard *Oxford* benchmark dataset Sect. (4.1), then the more recent *Robot* dataset Sect. (4.2) and finally an additional dataset made out of image pairs acquired by different modalities Sect. (4.3). As anticipated, in all experiments we have ran MSD with the same set of parameters, i.e. $\rho_w = 7, \rho_a = \rho_\nu = 11, \tau_\delta = 250, f = 1.25$.

From the computational point of view, the incremental scheme outlined in Sect. 2.1 enables a quite efficient implementation even without advanced optimizations or deployment of the parallel multimedia-oriented instructions available in modern CPUs. Indeed, with the parameter settings used in the experiments, our implementation takes averagely 600 ms for image size 640 × 480 and 150 ms for image size 256 × 256 on a Intel i7 processor.

4.1   Evaluation on the *Oxford* Dataset

MSD has been tested on the *Oxford* dataset, a benchmark for keypoint detection evaluation introduced in [16]. The dataset includes 8 planar scenes and 5 nuisance factors: scale and rotation changes, viewpoint changes, decreasing illumination, blur and JPEG compression. Performance is measured according to two indicators: repeatability and quantity of correct correspondences, which account for, respectively, the relative and the absolute number of repeatable keypoints detected between the first - *reference* - image of a scene and each of the other five - *distorted* - images. Our proposal has been compared with state-of-the-art detectors including Difference-of-Gaussian (DoG) [10], Harris-Affine, Harris-Laplace, Hessian-Affine, Hessian-Laplace [3,16], MSER [11], FastHessian [12], and the recently introduced Wade algorithm [17]. All methods were tested using the binaries provided by the authors of [16], except for FastHessian, for which the original SURF code[2] was deployed, and Wade, for which the binaries provided by the authors[3] were used.

Figure 4 reports the performance of the evaluated detectors in terms of repeatability on the 8 image sets of the *Oxford* dataset, with each plot in both figures related to one image set. By looking at chart Fig. 4c we can see that MSD delivers the highest repeatability with respect to all other detectors in case of illumination changes. As vouched by charts Fig. 4d, e, MSD is also quite effective in withstanding viewpoint variations: it yields overall the best invariance on *Wall* and provides the best performance between similarity rather than affine-invariant detectors on the tougher *Graf* set. It is also worth pointing out that, on *Graf*, MSD features are significantly more repeatable up to 30° in-depth rotation than those provided by affine-invariant detectors such as MSER, Hessian-Affine and Harris-Affine. MSD is also remarkably robust to blur: charts Fig. 4g and h show that its repeatability is surpassed only by Wade, while also providing some moderate advantage at low blur levels on the *Trees* dataset. These experimental findings seem to substantiate the conjectured inherent effectiveness of the CSD operator to highlight patches remaining quite unique within their context under illumination variations, blur and moderate viewpoint changes. As far as the other nuisances addressed by the *Oxford* dataset are concerned, charts Fig. 4a, b show that MSD yields overall satisfactory scale invariance, turning out the second-best method in *Boat* and performing slightly worse than the best methods in *Bark*. Resilience to JPEG compression appears to be good alike, MSD ranking among the best methods in image set *ubc*. Considering again the comparison with established methods whose roots can be traced back to the self-dissimilarity concept, we wish to point out how MSD provides substantially better performance than the Harris-Laplace detector throughout all the experiments related to the *Oxford* dataset. Due to lack of space, we include the results dealing with the quantity of correct correspondences together with examples of detected features in the supplementary material. Yet, we wish to highlight here that also in terms of number of repeatable features MSD provides excellent performance, ranking among the best methods on this dataset together with Wade and Dog.

In addition to previous results, we have compared our method to the proposal in [6], which detects interest points driven by the concept of patch self-similarity (for better clarity, the results are displayed in a distinct figure, i.e. Fig. 5). As for

---

[2] http://www.vision.ee.ethz.ch/surf/.
[3] http://vision.deis.unibo.it/ssalti/Wave.

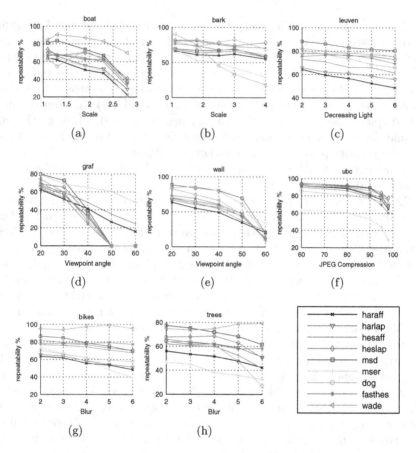

Fig. 4. Repeatability on the 8 sets of images of the Oxford dataset. The x axis denotes the level of difficulty of the considered nuisance.

this experiment, MSD is compared on the *Oxford* dataset to the 4 variants of the detector tested in [6]: as vouched by the charts, overall our proposal outperforms neatly all the variants proposed in [6], the margin appearing particularly substantial when it comes to nuisances such as illumination and view-point changes.

4.2 Evaluation on the *Robot* dataset

We have also evaluated MSD on the more recently introduced DTU *Robot* dataset [18]. This dataset contains 60 scenes of planar and non-planar objects, from different categories captured along four different paths by means of a robotic arm. As for this dataset, nuisances are represented mostly by scale and view-point changes as well as relighting. Due to space constraint, we could not include results on the whole dataset. Thus, as MSD already showed state-of-the-art performance with respect to illumination changes on the *Oxford* dataset, we have

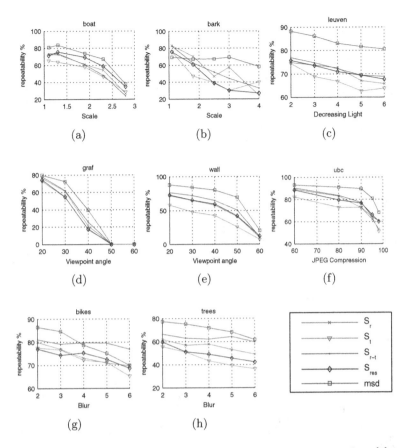

Fig. 5. Comparison between MSD and the 4 variants of the proposal in [6] on the Oxford dataset.

focused the evaluation on the scene subsets covering increasing scale variations (i.e., *linear path*) and different viewpoint changes (i.e., *first arc*, *second arc* and *third arc*, these last two also including scale variations since they were acquired at different distances from the reference image).

Results shown in Figs. 6a–d report the Average Recall Rate (analogous of the Repeatability) at increasing scale variations (Fig. 6a) and different viewpoint angles (Figs. 6b–d). To plot these charts, we added the MSD and Wade curves to those shown in [18] (whose data was kindly provided by their authors). These results show that MSD keypoints yield outstanding repeatability even when tested at high scale differences and notable viewpoint changes, remarkably outperforming all state-of-the-art methods on each evaluated scene subset. Also, the higher the scale variation, the higher the gap between MSD and the state of the art: this can be noticed especially in Fig. 6a and by considering that scale variations increase moving from the *first arc* through the *third arc*.

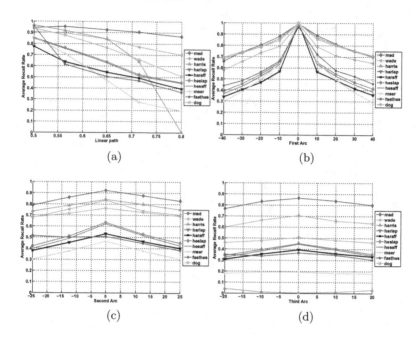

Fig. 6. Comparison of interest point detectors over the *Robot* dataset.

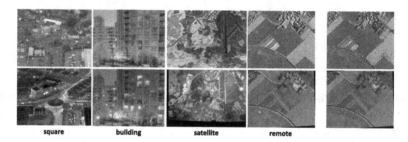

Fig. 7. The 4 considered multi-modal image pairs together with the features detected by MSD on the "remote" pair (rightmost column).

4.3   Evaluation on Multi-modal Images

Finally, MSD has been compared to the other considered detectors on a dataset containing 4 image pairs acquired with different modalities, kindly provided by the authors of [19]. This dataset includes an optical-infrared pair ("square"), a multi-temporal (day-night) pair ("building") and two SAR remote sensing pairs ("satellite" and "remote"). The dataset is shown in Fig. 7, together with qualitative results dealing with the interest points extracted by MSD on image pair "remote". Results are reported in terms of both repeatability and quantity (Fig. 8). Repeatability results (left chart) demonstrate that MSD yields remarkable performance on multi-modal images, so as to turn out, in particular, the best

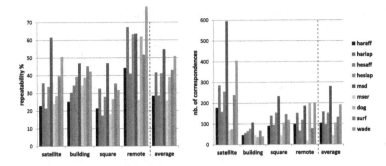

Fig. 8. Comparison of interest point detectors over 4 pairs of images related to different modalities in terms of repeatability and number of correct correspondences.

method in 3 out of the 4 pairs. As such, it provides the highest average repeatability. Moreover, MSD provides the largest quantity of repeatable features in 3 out of the 4 pairs, and just slightly less than the largest in the remaining pair (right chart). Accordingly, it turns out neatly the best method in terms of average quantity of repeatable features on the considered multi-modal dataset.

5   Conclusion and Future Work

The MSD detector is fired by image patches that look very dissimilar from their surroundings, whatever the structure of such patches may be (e.g. corners, edges, blobs, textures..). Despite its simplicity, such an approach inherently conveys remarkable invariance to nuisances such as illumination changes, viewpoint variations and blur. Likewise, it enables detection of repeatable features across multi-modal image pairs, as required, e.g., by remote sensing and medical imaging applications. Peculiarly, the MSD approach generalizes straightforwardly to detect interest points in any kind of multi-channel images, such as color images as well as the RGB-D images provided by consumer depth cameras like the Microsoft Kinect or the Asus Xtion, which are becoming more and more widespread in computer vision research and applications. Another direction for future investigation deals with the use of approximate k-NN techniques for dense patch matching, such as [20], to possibly further ameliorate the efficiency of the detector. Finally, pairing the MSD detector with an appropriate descriptor is another topic we plan to investigate next, LSS [4] likely representing a suitable starting point.

References

1. Moravec, H.: Towards automatic visual obstacle avoidance. In: Proceedings of the International Joint Conference on Artificial Intelligence (1977)
2. Harris, C., Stephens, M.: A combined corner and edge detector. In: Proceedings of the Alvey Vision Conference, pp. 147–151 (1988)

3. Mikolajczyk, K., Schmid, C.: Scale and affine invariant interest point detectors. Int. J. Comput. Vis. **60**, 63–86 (2004)
4. Shechtman, E., Irani, M.: Matching local self-similarities across images and videos. In: Proceedings of the Conference on Computer Vision and Pattern Recognition (CVPR 2007) (2007)
5. Huang, J., You, S., Zhao, J.: Multimodal image matching using self similarity. In: Proceedings of the Workshop on Applied Imagery Pattern Recognition (AIPR) (2011)
6. Maver, J.: Self-similarity and points of interest. Trans. Pattern Anal. Mach. Intell. (PAMI) **32**, 1211–1226 (2010)
7. Buades, A., Coll, B., Morel, J.: A review of image denoising methods, with a new one. Multiscale Model. Simul. **4**, 490–530 (2006)
8. Dabov, K., Foi, A., Katkovnik, V., Egiazarian, K.: Image denoising by sparse 3d transform-domain collaborative filtering. IEEE Tran. Image Process. **16**, 1395–1411 (2007)
9. Kadir, T., Brady, M.: Saliency, scale and image description. Int. J. Comput. Vis. **45**, 83–105 (2000)
10. Lowe, D.G.: Distinctive image features from scale-invariant keypoints. Int. J. Comput. Vis. **60**, 91–110 (2004)
11. Matas, J., Chum, O., Urban, M., Pajdla, T.: Robust wide baseline stereo from maximally stable extremal regions. In: Proceedings of the British Machine Vision Conference, BMVC 2002, vol. 1, pp. 384–393 (2002)
12. Bay, H., Ess, A., Tuytelaars, T., Van Gool, L.: Speeded-up robust features (surf). Comput. Vis. Image Underst. **110**, 346–359 (2008)
13. Goferman, S., Zelnik-Manor, L., Tal, A.: Context-aware saliency detection. In: Proceedings of the IEEE Conference on Computer Vision and Pattern Recognition (CVPR 2010) (2010)
14. Borji, A., Itti, L.: Exploiting local and global patch rarities for saliency detection. In: Proceedings of the Conference on Computer Vision and Pattern Recognition (CVPR 2012) (2012)
15. Mc Donnel, M.: Box-filtering techniques. Comput. Graph. Image Process. **17**, 65–70 (1981)
16. Mikolajczyk, K., Tuytelaars, T., Schmid, C., Zisserman, A., Matas, J., Schaffalitzky, F., Kadir, T., Gool, L.V.: A comparison of affine region detectors. Int. J. Comput. Vis. **65**, 43–72 (2005)
17. Salti, S., Lanza, A., Stefano, L.D.: Keypoints from symmetries by wave propagation. In: Proceedings of the International Conference on Computer Vision and Pattern Recognition (2013)
18. Aanæs, H., Dahl, A.L.: Steenstrup Pedersen, K.: Interesting interest points. Int. J. Comput. Vis. **97**, 18–35 (2012)
19. Hel-Or, Y., Hel-Or, H., David, E.: Fast template matching in non-linear tone-mapped images. In: Proceedings of the International Conference on Computer Vision (ICCV) (2011)
20. Barnes, C., Shechtman, E., Goldman, D.B., Finkelstein, A.: The generalized Patch-Match correspondence algorithm. In: Daniilidis, K., Maragos, P., Paragios, N. (eds.) ECCV 2010, Part III. LNCS, vol. 6313, pp. 29–43. Springer, Heidelberg (2010)

Improving Local Features by Dithering-Based Image Sampling

Christos Varytimidis$^{(\boxtimes)}$, Konstantinos Rapantzikos, Yannis Avrithis, and Stefanos Kollias

National Technical University of Athens, Athens, Greece
{chrisvar,rap,iavr}@image.ntua.gr,
stefanos@cs.ntua.gr

Abstract. The recent trend of structure-guided feature detectors, as opposed to blob and corner detectors, has led to a family of methods that exploit image edges to accurately capture local shape. Among them, the WαSH detector combines binary edge sampling with gradient strength and computational geometry representations towards distinctive and repeatable local features. In this work, we provide alternative, variable-density sampling schemes on smooth functions of image intensity based on dithering. These methods are parameter-free and more invariant to geometric transformations than uniform sampling. The resulting detectors compare well to the state-of-the-art, while achieving higher performance in a series of matching and retrieval experiments.

1 Introduction

Image representation based on local features is often used in many computer vision applications due to the balanced trade-off between sparsity and discriminative power. By ignoring non-salient image parts and focusing on distinctive regions, local features provide invariance, repeatability, compactness and computational efficiency.

Popular detectors like the Hessian-Affine [1] and SURF [2] are based on image gradients, while others like the MSER [3] are purely based on image intensity. All of them have been successfully applied to a variety of applications, but often the balance between quality and performance remains an issue. For example, the image coverage of the Hessian-Affine detector is limited, since—for a given threshold—multiple detections appear on nearby spatial locations at different scales. The MSER detector is fast, but often extracts sparse regular regions that are not representative enough. SURF is also fast, but detections are often not stable enough.

Although not so popular, another family of detectors is based on image edges, which are naturally more stable than gradient *e.g.* to lighting changes. The recently introduced WαSH detector [4] belongs to this family and is based on grouping edge samples using the weighted *α-shapes*, a well known representation in computational geometry. A weakness of WαSH is that edge sampling is roughly uniform along edges, with a fixed sampling interval s. In an attempt to overcome this limitation, we propose a different sampling scheme that relies

© Springer International Publishing Switzerland 2015
D. Cremers et al. (Eds.): ACCV 2014, Part II, LNCS 9004, pp. 601–613, 2015.
DOI: 10.1007/978-3-319-16808-1_40

directly upon image intensity. We demonstrate its efficiency by common statistics on image matching and retrieval experiments.

2   Related Work and Contribution

Edge-based local features have not become popular due to the lack of stable edges (*e.g.* under varying viewpoint) and computational inefficiency. One of the earliest attempts, the *edge-based region detector* (EBR), starts from corner points and exploits nearby edges by measuring photometric quantities across them. It is suitable for well-structured scenes (like *e.g.* buildings), but not for generic matching, as shown in [5]. Mikolajczyk *et al.* [6] propose an edge-based detector that starts from densely sampled edge points combined with automatic scale selection and use it for object recognition. Starting also from dense edge samples, Rapantzikos *et al.* [7] compute the binary distance transform and detect regions by grouping its local maxima, guided by the gradient strength of nearby edges.

Indirectly related to edges are the methods that exploit gradient strength across them by avoiding the thresholding step. Zitnick *et al.* [8] apply an oriented filter bank to the input image and detect *edge foci* (EF), *i.e.* points that are roughly equidistant from edgels with orientations perpendicular to the points. The idea is quite interesting, but computationally expensive. Avrithis and Rapantzikos [9] compute the weighted medial axis transform directly from image gradient, partition it and select associated regions as *medial features* (MFD) by taking both contrast and shape into account. Although those methods exploit richer image information compared to binary edges, gradient strength is often quite sensitive to lighting and scale variations.

The recently proposed WαSH detector [4] combines edge-sampling and grouping towards distinctive local features supported by shape-preserving regions. It is based on weighted α-shapes on uniformly sampled edges, *i.e.* a representation of triangulated edge samples parametrized by a single parameter α. WαSH uses a *regular triangulation*, where each sample is assigned a weight originating from the image domain. Despite this rich representation, WαSH is limited by its uniform sampling scheme, which is not stable under varying viewpoint.

In this work, we introduce two sampling methods that are based on the well known Floyd-Steinberg algorithm [10]. The latter was the first of the *error-diffusion* dithering approaches, where the idea is to produce a pattern of pixels such that the average intensity over regions in the output bitmap is approximately the same as the average over the same region in the original image. Error-diffusion algorithms compare the pixel intensity values with a fixed threshold and the resulting error between the output value and the original value is distributed to neighboring pixels according to pre-defined weights. The main advantages of these algorithms are the simplicity combined with fairly good overall visual quality of the produced binary images.

The Floyd-Steinberg algorithm has been extensively studied in the literature. Indicatively, Ostromoukhov [11] and Zhuand and Fang [12] have addressed the limitations of the initial algorithm, like the visual artifacts in highlights/dark areas and the appearance of visually unpleasant regular structures using intensity-dependent variable diffusion coefficients. Nevertheless, we use the initial algorithm because of its computational efficiency and the nature of our problem, which is sampling rather than halftoning.

Our work is also related to the work of Gu et al. [13], who detect local features as local minima and maxima of the β-stable Laplacian. They combine the local features in order to create a higher level representation, resembling the constellation model [13, 14]. However, we do not detect our sample points as features; we rather use them to initialize the WaSH feature detector.

The main contributions of this work are: (a) the introduction of two image sampling schemes of variable density, and (b) the application to local feature detection, evaluated on image matching and retrieval.

3   Background: The WαSH Detector

The WαSH feature detector [4] is based on α-*shapes*, a representation of a point set P in two dimensions, parametrized by scalar α. In fact, α-shapes are a generalization of the convex hull, which is not convex or even connected in general. In the simplest case, α-shapes use an underlying Delaunay triangulation, but *weighted* α-*shapes* in [4] use the *regular triangulation* instead. The latter is a generalization of Delaunay where each point in P is assigned a non-negative *weight*, hence it can capture more information from the image domain. In practice, weight is a function of image gradient in [4].

A particular *size* is assigned to every simplex (edge or triangle) in the triangulation, as a function of positions and weights of its vertices. Ordering simplices by decreasing size, a *component tree* is used to track the evolution of connected components as simplices are added to form larger regions. Connected components are potentially selected as features during evolution, according to a shape-driven strength measure. The resulting features correspond to blob-like regions that respect local image boundaries. Features are also extracted on cavities of image objects as well as regions that are not fully bounded by edges.

One important limitation of WαSH is that edge sampling is *uniform*, hence when sampling a contour, the representation scale is fixed. In a single image, objects of diverse scales have different representations: too dense on large objects, and too sparse on small ones. Though this may be partially compensated for by subsequent processes, a *sampling step* parameter is still needed to control the density of samples along edges. Further, uniform sampling naturally leads to severe undersampling of highly curved paths, so important details of object shape may be lost.

In Sect. 4 we introduce two alternative methods for sampling that apply on smooth functions of image input rather than binary edge maps and provide variable density samples. For the remaining process including triangulation, component tree and feature selection, we keep the same choices as in [4].

4   Dithering-Based Sampling

In this section we propose two image sampling methods based on error-diffusion. The goal is to adapt the spatial density of samples over the image and achieve a sparse representation without compromising structure preservation. Removing the limitation of samples belonging to binary edges, we expect to get a triangulated set of sparse samples that fits well with the underlying image structure.

For dithering, we use the Floyd–Steinberg algorithm [10], which is fast, requiring only one iteration over the image, and provides reasonable results. In our framework, the algorithm is not applied directly to the image intensity, but to a scalar function $s(x, y)$ over the image domain. The two methods we introduce are based on two different choices for $s(x, y)$. In both cases, the extracted samples are the nonzero points of the binary output of the Floyd-Steinberg algorithm. Each sample point (x, y) is assigned a weight that is proportional to the sampled function $s(x, y)$; these weights are needed for the remaining steps of the WαSH detector [4].

4.1   Gradient-Based Dithering

The gradient strength G of an image I is obtained by convolving with the gradient of a Gaussian kernel $g(\sigma)$ of standard deviation σ,

$$G = \|\nabla g(\sigma) * I\|. \tag{1}$$

Then, similar to [15], if $\hat{G}(x, y)$ is the gradient strength at point (x, y) normalized to $[0, 1]$, we use the non-linear function

$$s(x, y) = \hat{G}(x, y)^\gamma \tag{2}$$

to represent image boundaries, where γ is a positive constant. Error-diffusion is performed using the Floyd-Steinberg algorithm on $s(x, y)$ rather than image intensity $I(x, y)$. Increasing the value of γ results in sparser sampling.

In smooth regions of the image, e.g. in the interior of objects or on smooth background, G is low and samples are sparse, resulting in large triangles. Near image edges or corners on the other hand, G is high, samples are dense, and a finer tessellation is generated that captures important details. Variable sample density offers a computational advantage without compromising the descriptive power of the triangulation.

4.2   Hessian-Based Dithering

Instead of using the gradient strength as the input to error-diffusion, Yang *et al.* [15] use the largest eigenvalue of the Hessian matrix at each point. We also explore this option for our sampling.

If $H(x, y)$ is the Hessian matrix at point (x, y), again after filtering with Gaussian kernel $g(\sigma)$, let $\lambda_1(x, y)$ be its largest eigenvalue. It is known that λ_1 is the largest second order directional derivative of I. Similarly to (2), if $\hat{\lambda}_1(x,y)$ is the largest eigenvalue normalized to $[0,1]$, we use function

$$s(x,y) = \hat{\lambda}_1(x,y)^\gamma \qquad (3)$$

to represent image boundaries, again performing error-diffusion on $s(x,y)$.

The magnitude of the second order derivatives increases near image edges, so the error-diffusion algorithm will favour dense sampling at these regions. However, samples will now appear more scattered at both sides of an edge, making the triangulation more complex. At smooth areas, sampling is sparse, but since the Hessian is more sensitive to noise a grid-like sampling can occur (see Fig. 1f). Compared to the gradient-based sampling, the number of detected features is often lower (see Sect. 5).

4.3 Examples

A visual example of the sampling methods is shown in Fig. 1. Figure 1cd depict the normalized gradient strength $\hat{G}$ and the resulting gradient-based sampling. Notice the sparsity of the samples in smooth areas and the density in structured ones. Figure 1ef depict the Hessian response $\hat{\lambda}_1$ and the resulting sampling. Few weak edges are lost within the background noise in this case. For all examples we set $\gamma = 1$.

Figure 2 shows an example on a detail of an image along with different sampling methods and the resulting triangulations. The uniformly sampled edges are sparse and well distributed along the edges, but lose details at the corners and highly curved edge parts. On the other hand, the dithering-based methods are denser, but preserve the underlying structure better. In the Hessian-based approach, points are sampled on both sides of edges that—depending on the application—may prove useful at enforcing actual edge boundaries.

Examples of the features detected using either the baseline sampling of WαSH or the proposed sampling methods are depicted in Figs. 3, 4. In each example, the number of detected features for each method is approximately the same (around 200 for Fig. 3 and 50 for Fig. 4). In Fig. 3 we present the results on the first image of the *graffiti* dataset of [5]. Both dithering-based samplings detect more detailed regions of the image, and the gradient-based one better captures the correct boundaries of objects. In Fig. 4, the input image comes from the PASCAL VOC 2007 test set [16], a dataset heavily used for evaluating object recognition algorithms. Again the gradient-based variants capture finer details of the image that can boost the performance in recognition tasks (see the ceiling lamp and the chairs).

5   Experiments

We evaluate the proposed sampling methods and compare to the state-of-the-art, using two different experimental setups. The first is the matching experiment proposed by Mikolajczyk *et al.* [5], with the corresponding well-known dataset. We measure the *repeatability* and *matching score* of WαSH when using the proposed sampling methods, and also compare to other state-of-the-art detectors. The second experimental setup involves a large scale image retrieval application on the *Oxford 5K* [17] dataset. The performance is measured by the *mean average precision* (mAP) of the query results.

Following an initial brief evaluation of the proposed samplings, we set $\gamma = 1$ for all the experiments. For $\gamma > 1$ samplings were sparser and performance slightly dropped, while for $\gamma < 1$ the performance increased, but samplings were denser, increasing the computational cost of the feature detector.

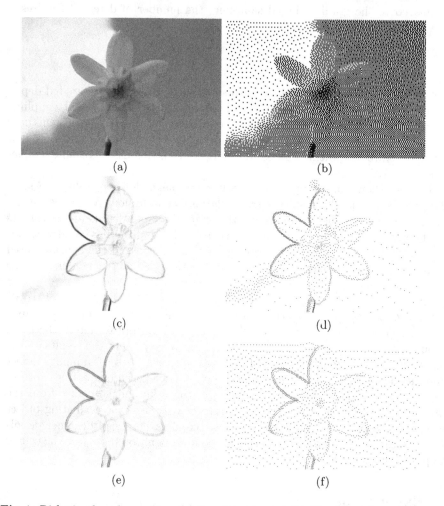

Fig. 1. Dithering-based sampling. (a) Input image and (b) Floyd-Steinberg dithering on (a). (c) Normalized gradient strength $\hat{G}$ and (d) sampling on $\hat{G}$. (e) Hessian response $\hat{\lambda}_1$ and (f) sampling on $\hat{\lambda}_1$. Figure is optimized for screen viewing.

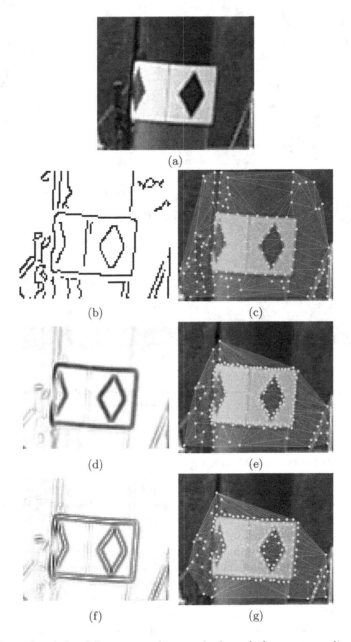

Fig. 2. Example of the different sampling methods and the corresponding triangulations. (a) Input image, a detail of the first image of the boat sequence of [5] (see Sect. 5.1). (b) Binary edge map and (c) uniform sampling on (b). (d) Normalized gradient strength and (e) error-diffusion on (d). (f) Hessian response and (g) error-diffusion on (f). (b,d,f) are shown in negative for better viewing and printing.

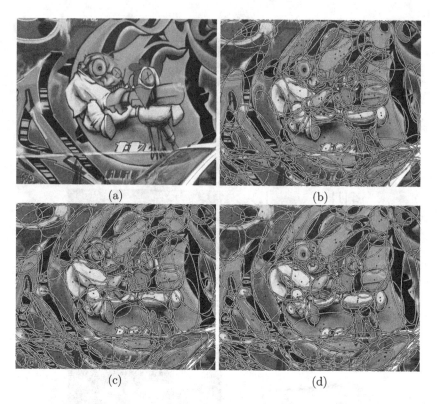

(a)   (b)

(c)   (d)

Fig. 3. Example of local features detection. (a) Input image and (b) baseline WαSH results using uniform sampling. (c) Results using the gradient-based sampling and (d) using the Hessian-based sampling.

5.1   Repeatability and Matching Score

In this experiment, we investigate the impact on performance of a matching application, when using the proposed sampling methods on WαSH. We also compare to the state-of-the-art detectors, Hessian-Affine and MSER, for which we use the executables provided by the corresponding authors and default parameters. The image sets used, evaluate the impact of changes in viewpoint, rotation, zoom, blur and illumination. For the matching score we use 128-dimensional SIFT descriptors for all detectors.

The results of the evaluation are depicted in Figs. 5 and 6. The last row of Fig. 6 shows the average scores for the 6 datasets. Along with the repeatability and matching score, we also provide the number of features detected. Overall, the gradient-based sampling performs best, followed by the Hessian-based one.

5.2   Image Retrieval

In this experiment, we evaluate the proposed variants of WαSH on an image retrieval application. The dataset is the *Oxford 5K*, consisting of images of

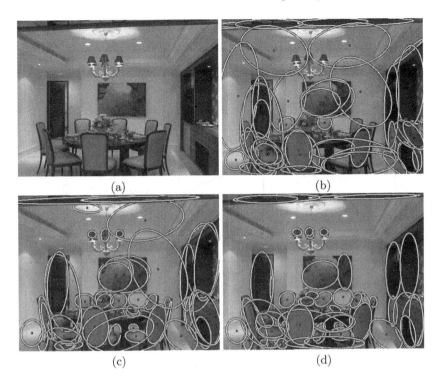

Fig. 4. Example of local features detection. (a) Input image and (b) baseline WαSH results using uniform sampling. (c) Results using the gradient-based sampling and (d) using the Hessian-based sampling.

buildings as queries, and other urban images as distractors. We compare against Hessian-affine, MSER, SIFT and SURF, using the corresponding executables and default values. For all detectors we extract SIFT descriptors, apart from SURF, which performs best using the corresponding descriptor.

For the different versions proposed, we adapt the selection threshold to extract approximately the same number of features as the baseline WαSH. For all detectors we create 3 different vocabularies of size 50K, 100K and 200 K visual words. We use the simple Bag-of-Words approach, as well as a spatial reranking of the results, using fastSM [17]. Performance is measured using the *mean Average Precision* (mAP) metric, and the results are shown in Table 1.

The number of features extracted by each detector is critical for the large scale retrieval applications, affecting the indexing time and memory needed to store the inverted files, while using a lower number of features typically drops performance. SURF extracted the least number of features, followed by the baseline WαSH and our variants. Despite the low number of features, SURF and baseline WαSH perform comparably to Hessian-affine. Increasing the size of the vocabulary boosted the performance of all detectors. The gradient-based variant we

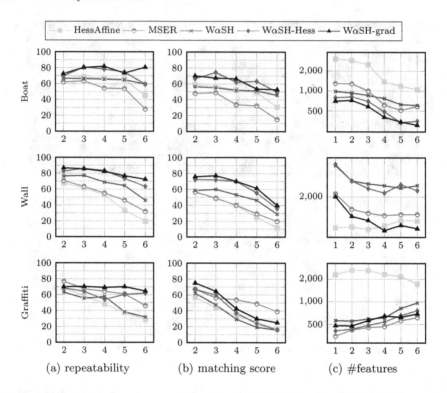

Fig. 5. Comparison of our proposed sampling methods to baseline WαSH and the state-of-the-art in sequences *boat, wall* and *graffiti*. #features: number of features detected per image. Hess: Hessian-based dithering; grad: gradient-based dithering.

propose outperformed all other detectors with and without the spatial verification step, a result that verifies the findings of Sect. 5.1.

Table 1. Results of the image retrieval experiment, using 3 different vocabularies, the Bag-of-Words model and spatial reranking of the results, measuring mean Average Precision.

Detector	Features ($\times 10^6$)	Bag-of-Words (mAP)			ReRanking (mAP)		
		50K	100K	200K	50K	100K	200K
HessAff	29.02	0.483	0.539	0.573	0.518	0.577	0.607
MSER	13.33	0.487	0.534	0.565	0.519	0.569	0.595
SIFT	11.13	0.422	0.465	0.495	0.441	0.486	0.517
SURF	**6.84**	0.465	0.526	0.574	0.509	0.573	0.603
WαSH	7.19	0.529	0.569	0.590	0.537	0.569	0.585
WαSH, grad	7.63	**0.531**	**0.580**	**0.605**	**0.543**	**0.578**	**0.609**
WαSH, Hess	7.29	0.518	0.553	0.582	0.511	0.557	0.584

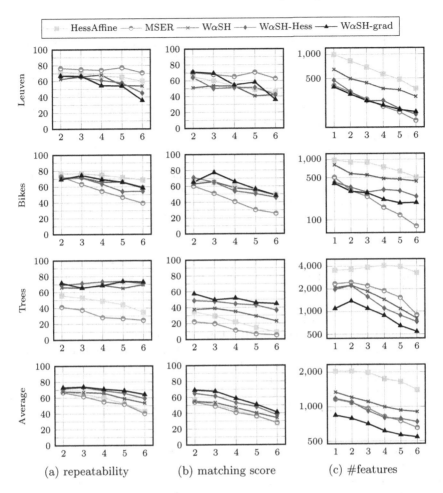

Fig. 6. Comparison of our proposed sampling methods to baseline WαSH and the state-of-the-art in sequences *leuven, bikes* and *trees*, together with the averaged values over the dataset.

6   Conclusions

In this paper we extend the recently introduced WαSH detector by proposing different image sampling methods. Image sampling is the first step of the algorithm and changes the qualities of the detected features, together with the overall performance of the detector. We propose two different image sampling methods that build on ideas from image halftoning. In that direction, we sample points based on error diffusion of smooth image functions. We thoroughly evaluate the performance of the proposed methods in a matching and an image retrieval experiment.

The proposed sampling methods, combined with the α-shapes grouping, result in a more accurate representation of the image structures. The detected features capture finer image structures, while keeping the high image coverage of the baseline method. Using the gradient-based scheme, the performance of WαSH increases in both applications, exceeding the state-of-the-art. In the future, we will further investigate the effect of the scaling factor γ applied on both proposed sampling methods, as well as evaluate the performance on different applications of the feature detector.

Acknowledgement. This work is supported by the National GSRT-funded project 09SYN-72-922 "IS-HELLEANA : Intelligent System for HELLEnic Audiovisual National Aggregator", http://www.helleana.gr, 2011-2014.

References

1. Mikolajczyk, K., Schmid, C.: An affine invariant interest point detector. In: Heyden, A., Sparr, G., Nielsen, M., Johansen, P. (eds.) ECCV 2002, Part I. LNCS, vol. 2350, pp. 128–142. Springer, Heidelberg (2002)
2. Bay, H., Ess, A., Tuytelaars, T., Van Gool, L.: Speeded-up robust features (SURF). Comput. Vis. Image Underst. (CVIU) **110**, 346–359 (2008)
3. Matas, J., Chum, O., Urban, M., Pajdla, T.: Robust wide-baseline stereo from maximally stable extremal regions. Image Vis. Comput. **22**, 761–767 (2004)
4. Varytimidis, C., Rapantzikos, K., Avrithis, Y.: WαSH: weighted α-shapes for local feature detection. In: Fitzgibbon, A., Lazebnik, S., Perona, P., Sato, Y., Schmid, C. (eds.) ECCV 2012, Part II. LNCS, vol. 7573, pp. 788–801. Springer, Heidelberg (2012)
5. Mikolajczyk, K., Tuytelaars, T., Schmid, C., Zisserman, A., Matas, J., Schaffalitzky, F., Kadir, T., Gool, L.: A comparison of affine region detectors. Int. J. Comput. Vis. (IJCV) **65**, 43–72 (2005)
6. Mikolajczyk, K., Zisserman, A., Schmid, C.: Shape recognition with edge-based features. Br. Mach. Vis. Conf. (BMVC) **2**, 779–788 (2003)
7. Rapantzikos, K., Avrithis, Y., Kollias, S.: Detecting regions from single scale edges. In: Kutulakos, K.N. (ed.) ECCV 2010 Workshops, Part I. LNCS, vol. 6553, pp. 298–311. Springer, Heidelberg (2012)
8. Zitnick, C., Ramnath, K.: Edge foci interest points. In: International Conference on Computer Vision (ICCV), pp. 359–366 (2011)
9. Avrithis, Y., Rapantzikos, K.: The medial feature detector: Stable regions from image boundaries. In: International Conference on Computer Vision (ICCV), pp. 1724–1731 (2011)
10. Floyd, R.W., Steinberg, L.: An adaptive algorithm for spatial gray-scale. Proc. Soc. Inf. Disp. **17**, 75–77 (1976)
11. Ostromoukhov, V.: A simple and efficient error-diffusion algorithm. In: Proceedings of the 28th Annual Conference on Computer Graphics and Interactive Techniques, pp. 567–572. ACM (2001)
12. Zhou, B., Fang, X.: Improving mid-tone quality of variable-coefficient error diffusion using threshold modulation. In: ACM Transactions on Graphics (TOG). vol. 22, pp. 437–444. ACM (2003)

13. Gu, S., Zheng, Y., Tomasi, C.: Critical nets and beta-stable features for image matching. In: Daniilidis, K., Maragos, P., Paragios, N. (eds.) Computer Vision – ECCV 2010. LNCS, vol. 6313, pp. 663–676. Springer, Berlin (2010)

14. Fergus, R., Perona, P., Zisserman, A.: Object class recognition by unsupervised scale-invariant learning. In: 2003 Proceedings of the IEEE Conference on Computer Society Computer Vision and Pattern Recognition, vol. 2, pp. Ii-264. IEEE (2003)

15. Yang, Y., Wernick, M., Brankov, J.: A fast approach for accurate content-adaptive mesh generation. IEEE Trans. Image Proc. **12**, 866–881 (2003)

16. Everingham, M., Van Gool, L., Williams, C.K.I., Winn, J., Zisserman, A.: The PASCAL Visual Object Classes Challenge 2007 (VOC2007) Results (2003). http://www.pascal-network.org/challenges/VOC/voc2007/workshop/index.html

17. Philbin, J., Chum, O., Isard, M., Sivic, J., Zisserman, A.: Object retrieval with large vocabularies and fast spatial matching. In: Computer Vision and Pattern Recognition (CVPR), pp. 1–8 (2007)

Poster Session 2

Sparse Kernel Learning for Image Set Classification

Muhammad Uzair$^{(\boxtimes)}$, Arif Mahmood, and Ajmal Mian

Computer Science and Software Engineering, The University of Western Australia,
35 Stirling Highway, Crawley, WA, Australia
muhammad.uzair@research.uwa.edu.au,
{arif.mahmood,ajmal.mian}@uwa.edu.au

Abstract. No single universal image set representation can efficiently encode all types of image set variations. In the absence of expensive validation data, automatically ranking representations with respect to performance is a challenging task. We propose a sparse kernel learning algorithm for automatic selection and integration of the most discriminative subset of kernels derived from different image set representations. By optimizing a sparse linear discriminant analysis criterion, we learn a unified kernel from the linear combination of the best kernels only. Kernel discriminant analysis is then performed on the unified kernel. Experiments on four standard datasets show that the proposed algorithm outperforms current state-of-the-art image set classification and kernel learning algorithms.

1 Introduction

In image-set classification, labelled training data consists of one or more sets per class where each set contains multiple images of the same class. The test set also contains multiple instances of the same class and is assigned the label of the nearest training set by maximizing some similarity measure [1–7]. Image set classification is useful in a wide range of applications including video-based face recognition, video surveillance, person re-identification in camera networks and object categorization.

Image-set classification is often performed in two steps. First, a representation is used to encode the intra-image as well as inter-image variations within a set based on some assumptions on the set structure. In the second step, the similarity between the image-set representations is measured, usually under certain constraints such as sparsity. Classification accuracy strongly depends on the specific set representation and the underlying assumptions and constraints. Most researchers focus on finding accurate image set representations. However, no single universal set representation can efficiently encode all types of image set variations. Image set representations make assumptions about the underlying data. Some assume that the underlying set data is single mode Gaussian [7–10] whereas it may be multi-modal or non-Gaussian. Others assume that an image set can be represented by linear subspace bases [5,11] whereas the actual

D. Cremers et al. (Eds.): ACCV 2014, Part II, LNCS 9004, pp. 617–631, 2015.
DOI: 10.1007/978-3-319-16808-1_41

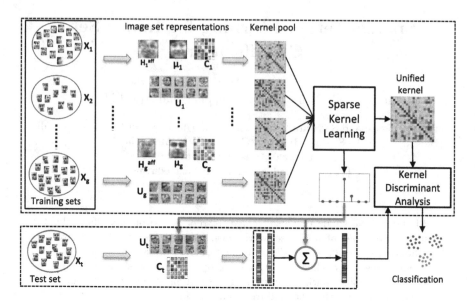

Fig. 1. Illustration of Sparse Kernel Learning. H_i^{aff}, μ_i, C_i and U_i are the affine hull, mean, covariance and subspace representations of image sets X_i. During training, SKL computes a pool of base kernels from different image set representations and automatically learns the best unified kernel from their sparse combination. In the test stage, only the kernels corresponding to the non-zero weights are computed.

data may lie on complex manifolds [2,6]. Moreover, in the presence of only few images per set, the estimation of subspace bases and manifold parameters may be inaccurate. Some image set classification algorithms [3,4] are variants of nearest neighbour whereas the image sets may overlap in some low dimensional space. Thus, no single representation performs good in all cases. In the absence of validation data, automatic selection of the most discriminative representations is a challenging problem. Moreover, there is a lack of systematic procedure for the selection and integration of efficient image set representations.

One solution to the above problem is along the lines of Multiple Kernel Learning (MKL) [12] where different types of features are expressed in terms of kernels and effectively integrated for improving classification. These have been applied to different computer vision tasks such as object categorization [13], object detection [14], multi-class object classification [15] and image set classification [1,16]. In the case of image set classification, a pool of base kernels can be derived using different image set representations and their associated distance measures. A unified kernel can then be learned from their combination. Recently, Lin et al. [17] proposed a multiple kernel learning algorithm for dimensionality reduction (MKLDR). In MKLDR algorithm, the image data is represented by different features from which a set of base kernels is derived. The weighted combination of these base kernels are then used to learn a discriminative low dimensional subspace for classification. In MKLDR, all features are considered important and the weights assigned to different kernels do not necessarily correspond to their exact performance ratios [17]. Thus, the kernel combination using this strategy can

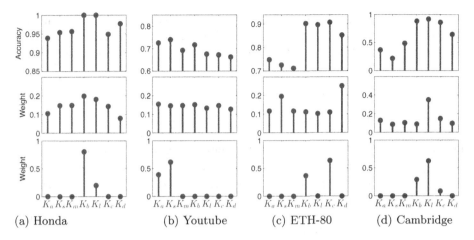

Fig. 2. Sparse kernel learning (SKL): **Top row** Individual accuracies of the kernels derived from each image set representation using their associated distance measures. Affine hull [3] (K_a), Affine hull [4] (SANP distance K_s), mean (K_m), subspace bases (K_b), Covariance (log-Euclidean kernel K_l), Covariance (Cholesky kernel K_c), Manifold [2] (MMD kernel K_d) (see Sect. 3) **Middle row** Weights learned by the MKLDR algorithm [17]. **Bottom row** Sparse weights learned by the proposed algorithm.

reduce the overall classification accuracy (see Table 2) because a higher weight assigned to a poor feature degrades the quality of the overall mixture.

We propose a sparse kernel learning (SKL) algorithm that automatically learns a subset of the most discriminative base kernels derived from a pool of image set representations and their associated distance measures (see Fig. 1). Given a large number of image set kernels, our goal is to learn sparse kernel weights, without using validation data, such that the sparse combination of these kernels minimize intra-set distances and maximize inter-set distance. To the best of our knowledge, sparse kernel learning has not been formulated previously for image set classification. We impose sparsity on the kernel learning such that poor performing kernels are discarded and the final mixture is more discriminative. An additional advantage of sparsity is that only a few kernels are required to be computed at runtime. Figure 2 shows the effectiveness of the proposed SKL algorithm. In the case of Youtube dataset, the MKLDR algorithm assigned weights to all the image set kernels which has degraded the overall accuracy. In the case of ETH-80 dataset, MKLDR assigned the highest weight to the MMD kernel K_d (derived from the manifold representation). However, the MMD kernel is not the best performer on this dataset. In contrast, MKL automatically learns a subset of the most discriminative kernels (subspace kernel K_b and Cholesky kernel K_c) while assigning zero weights to the others.

The SKL objective function is formulated as a graph embedding linear discriminant analysis criterion with ℓ_1 norm regularization. The enforcement of sparsity ensures that only the most discriminant image set kernels get non-zero weights. Once we obtain the unified kernel by the sparse linear combination of the most discriminative image set kernels, we perform Kernel Linear Discriminant

Analysis (KLDA) based classification. For experiments, we use four standard datasets and derive seven image set kernels. Our results outperform the MKLDR algorithm [17] as well as seven state-of-the-art image set classification algorithms.

2   Proposed Method

2.1   Problem Formulation

Let $G \equiv \{X_j\}_{j=1}^g \in \mathcal{R}^{d \times N}$ be the gallery containing g image sets and N images: $N = \sum_{j=1}^g n_j$, where n_j is the number of images in the j-th image set. Let $X_j = \{x_j^i\}_{i=1}^{n_j} \in \mathcal{R}^{d \times n_j}$ be the j-th image set, where $x_j^i \in \mathcal{R}^d$ is a d dimensional feature vector obtained by lexicographic ordering of the pixel elements of the i-th image in the j-th set. Instead of pixel values, the vector x_j^i may also contain feature values such as LBP or HoG features. The value of n_j may vary across image sets while the dimensionality of x_j^i remains fixed. Let c be the number of object classes and $Y = \{y_j\}_{j=1}^g$ be the class labels of the image sets in G. A distance matrix $d_r \in \mathcal{R}^{g \times g}$ is obtained for the gallery G such that $d_r(i, j) = d_r(X_i, X_j)$ is the distance between sets X_i and X_j using a distance measure r. Let R be the total number of distance measures each of which generating a distance matrix d_r. We convert each distance matrix d_r to a kernel matrix K_r using the Gaussian function as

$$K_r(i, j) = e^{\left(\frac{-d_r(i,j)}{\sigma_r^2}\right)}, \tag{1}$$

where σ_r is a Gaussian scale factor. The ith column of the kernel matrix K_r shows the relative position of the set X_i w.r.t. all other sets in the gallery. Therefore, we consider $K_r(i) \in \mathcal{R}^g$ a feature vector describing the set X_i. For R different distance measures, X_i has R different features descriptions. Our goal is to select a subset $L < R$ features such that when they are combined, their overall discrimination capability is maximized. For this purpose we propose to use the graph embedding linear discriminant analysis with sparsity constraints.

2.2   Sparse Kernel Learning

We represent X_i with a tensor $T_i = [K_1(i), ..., K_R(i)] \in \mathcal{R}^{g \times R}$ which is formed by concatenating all feature descriptors of X_i. For the gallery G we have g such matrices $G_t \equiv \{T_i\}_{i=1}^g$. For the graph embedding linear discriminant analysis the within class scatter matrix S_w and the between class scatter matrix S_b are formulated in a pairwise manner

$$S_w = \sum_{i,j=1}^g w_{ij}(T_i - T_j)^\top (T_i - T_j), \tag{2}$$

$$S_b = \sum_{i,j=1}^g \acute{w}_{ij}(T_i - T_j)^\top (T_i - T_j). \tag{3}$$

where $w_{ij} = \begin{cases} 1/n_k & \text{if } (T_i, T_j) \in c_k, \\ 0 & \text{otherwise,} \end{cases}$ and $\acute{w}_{ij} = 1/g$, n_k are the number of image sets in class c_k with label y_k.

In conventional graph embedding discriminant analysis [18], a projection matrix is learned such that the between-class similarity is minimized and the within-class similarity is maximized. In contrast, we formulate a sparse linear discriminant analysis criterion to learn an optimal linear combination of different features $K_r(i)$. We make the weight learning sparse so that the non-discriminative feature descriptors get zero weights while the more discriminative ones get high weights. Therefore, we formulate the following objective function for performing sparse discriminant analysis on S_w and S_b. The aim is to maximize the linear discriminant objective function with additional ℓ_1 and ℓ_2 norms regularizations:

$$\min_{Q} \ \left(\text{trace}(Q^\top (S_w - S_b)Q) + \sum_j \lambda_j \|q_j\|_1 + \alpha \|Q\|_2^2\right) \quad \text{s.t.} \quad Q^\top Q = I, \quad (4)$$

where q_j is the jth column of Q, α is a constant and λ_j are the coefficients of ℓ_1 norm. Minimizing the scatter difference term means that the optimal projections Q^* should be able to minimize the within-class scatter S_w and maximize the between-class scatter S_b. The scatter difference term of the above objective function (4) is similar to the Max Margin Criterion [19] whereas the ℓ_1 norm regularization is added to ensure sparse solutions and the term $\alpha \|Q\|_2^2$ is the positive ridge penalty. The approximate sparse solutions of (4) can be obtained by rewriting the objective function as a set of Sparse PCA criteria [20]:

$$\min_{Q} \ \|\Psi^\top D - UQ^\top D\|^2 + \sum_j \lambda_j \|q_j\|_1 + \alpha \|Q\|_2^2 \quad \text{s.t.} \quad U^\top U = I. \quad (5)$$

where Ψ and D are obtained from the SVD of $S_w - S_b$: $S_w - S_b = \Psi \Sigma \Psi^\top$ and $D = \Psi \sqrt{abs(\Sigma)} \Psi^\top$. Algorithm 1 shows the proposed method to solve the objective function in 5.

Once the termination criteria in the Algorithm 1 is met, we obtain a final sparse projection matrix Q which is computed by SVD. The weight vector $\theta \in \mathcal{R}^R$ corresponds to the most dominant eigenvector in the projection matrix Q. The index i of the weight vector θ contains the weight of the feature $K_r(i)$. We ignore the sign of individual coefficients in θ by taking its absolute. Finally, θ is used to obtain a sparse linear combination of different image set kernels.

2.3 Kernel Discriminant Analysis Based Classification

Since each K_r is symmetric, therefore; they can be converted to valid kernel matrices and subsequently used in a kernel based classification such as Kernel Linear Discriminant Analysis. Moreover, each K_r must be positive semidefinite to be a valid kernel matrix. This is not always guaranteed for each K_r. Therefore, we make K_r semipositive definite by simply adding a small perturbation to its

---

Algorithm 1. Sparse Kernel Learning Algorithm

Require: S_w and S_b from (2) and (3), C_t
Ensure: Weight vector θ
  $L \Leftarrow S_w - S_b$
  $L \Rightarrow \Psi \Sigma \Psi^\top$ {SVD of L}
  $D \Leftarrow \Psi \sqrt{abs(\Sigma)}\Psi^\top$
  $D \Rightarrow U \Lambda U^\top$ {SVD of D}
  $Q^* = \mathbf{0}^{R \times R}$, $\Delta Q = 10^5$, $\epsilon = 10^{-3}$, $c = 0$
  while $\Delta Q > \epsilon$ and $c < C_t$ **do**
    $Q_{old} = Q^*$
    $Q^* \equiv \min \|\Psi^\top D - UQ^\top D\|^2 + \sum_j \lambda_j \|q_j\|_1 + \alpha \|Q\|_2^2$ {Solve the Elastic Net problem}
    $LQ^* \Rightarrow Q\Omega V^\top$ {SVD of LQ^*}
    $U \Leftarrow QV^\top$
    $\Delta Q = max(abs(Q_{old}(:) - Q^*(:)))$
    $c = c + 1$
  end while
  $\theta \Leftarrow$ Dominant eigenvector in Q

---

diagonal (the absolute of its smallest non zero eigenvalue). After making all the K_r semipositive definite we can now linearly combine them in a weighted manner using θ to form a unified kernel matrix K

$$K = \sum_{r=1}^{R} \theta(r) K_r, \tag{6}$$

where θ is the sparse weight vector calculated using Algorithm 1. From the theory of Reproducing Kernel Hilbert Space (RKHS) it is well known that the superposition of two valid kernels gives a new valid kernel [21]. Therefore, the proposed unified kernel K can be used with any kernel based learning algorithm to perform classification.

In this paper, we perform Kernel Linear Discriminant Analysis for classification. Having obtained K, KLDA seeks to solve the following optimization problem

$$\alpha_{opt} = \arg\max \frac{\alpha^\top KWK\alpha}{\alpha^\top KK\alpha}, \tag{7}$$

where $\alpha = [\alpha_1, ..., \alpha_g]^\top$, and $\mathcal{W} \in \mathcal{R}^{g \times g}$ is a block diagonal matrix: $\mathcal{W} = diag\{\mathcal{W}_1, \mathcal{W}_2, ..., \mathcal{W}_c\}$, where $\mathcal{W}_j \in \mathcal{R}^{n_k \times n_k}$ is a matrix with all elements equal to $1/n_k$. The optimal α is given by the largest eigenvectors of the

$$(KK + \epsilon I)^{-1}(KWK)\alpha = \lambda\alpha, \tag{8}$$

Note that K is often a full rank matrix however, this is not guaranteed. Therefore, a regularization term ϵ is used to ensure that KK remains invertible. By selecting the $(c-1)$ dominant eigenvectors from the solution of (8), we obtain a transformation matrix $\hat{\alpha} = [\alpha_1, ..., \alpha_{c-1}]$. For a test image set X_t we first calculate $\mathcal{T}_t \in \mathcal{R}^{g \times R}$ where $\mathcal{T}_t(i) = K_i(G, X_t)$. The $c-1$ dimensional KLDA feature vector $\mathcal{Y}_t$ of $\mathcal{T}_t$ in the discriminant subspace is computed as

$$\mathcal{Y}_t = \hat{\alpha}^\top \mathcal{T}_t \theta. \tag{9}$$

Finally, to find the label of $\mathcal{Y}_t$ we use the nearest neighbour classifier in the KLDA feature space.

3   Image-Set Representations and Kernels

The proposed algorithm is generic and works with any number of kernels derived from different image set representations. In this paper we consider seven image set representations and their respective set to set distance measures i.e. $\{d_r\}_{r=1}^7$. The distance measures are brought to the kernel domain by the Gaussian function of (1) as discussed in Sect. 1. The proposed SKL algorithm then learns a unified kernel as the sparse linear combination of these kernels. A brief overview of each type of image set representation and its respective kernel function is given below.

i. Affine hull kernel (K_a) [3]: An image set is represented by the affine hull model computed from the set samples. The affine hull based set-to-set distance is computed using the method in [3]. Let U_i and U_j denote the subspace bases and μ_i and μ_j denote the mean of the two image sets X_i and X_j respectively. Defining $U \equiv [U_i \ -U_j]$, $\xi_i = \mu_i - U(U^T \mu_i)$ and $\xi_j = \mu_j - U(U^T \mu_j)$, the affine hull based image set kernel is given by

$$K_a(i,j) = e^{\left(\frac{-\|\xi_i - \xi_j\|_2}{\sigma_a^2}\right)} \tag{10}$$

ii. SANP kernel (K_s) [4]: An image set is represented by the affine hull model computed from the set samples and the samples themselves. Let U_i and U_j denote the subspace bases and μ_i and μ_j denote the mean of the two image sets X_i and X_j respectively. We compute the SANP kernel as

$$K_s(i,j) = e^{\left(\frac{(d_i + d_j)D^*}{\sigma_s^2}\right)} \tag{11}$$

where d_i and d_j are the dimensionalities of the subspaces U_i and U_j respectively (i.e. number of columns of U_i and U_j). D^* is the distance between the sparse approximated nearest points (SANP) of the two sets obtained by minimizing the following objective function [4]

$$D^* = \min_{\beta_i, \beta_j, v_i, v_j} \left(\|\mu_i + U_i v_i - (\mu_j + U_j v_j)\|_2^2 + \omega_1(\|\mu_i + U_i v_i - X_i \beta_i\|_2^2 \right.$$

$$\left. + \|\mu_j + U_j v_j - X_j \beta_j\|_2^2) + \omega_2 \|\beta_i\|_1 + \omega_3 \|\beta_j\|_1 \right) \tag{12}$$

iii. Mean kernel (K_m): An image set is represented by the first order statistics i.e. the mean of the set sample. Let μ_i and μ_j denote the mean of two image sets X_i and X_j respectively. We compute the mean image set kernel as

$$K_m(i,j) = e^{\left(\frac{-\|\mu_i - \mu_j\|_2}{\sigma_m^2}\right)} \tag{13}$$

iv. Subspace kernel (K_b): Let U_i and U_j denote the subspace bases of two image sets X_i and X_j respectively. We calculate the subspace based image set kernel as

$$K_b(i,j) = e^{\left(\frac{-\|U_i - U_j U_j^T U_i\|_F^2}{\sigma_b^2}\right)} \tag{14}$$

where $\| \cdot \|_F$ denotes the Frobenius norm.

v. Log Euclidean kernel (K_l): An image set X is represented by its sample covariance matrix $C = XX^T$. Note that X is first mean centred. Let C_i and C_j denote the sample covariance matrices of two image sets X_i and X_j. We compute the Log Euclidean image set kernel as

$$K_l(i,j) = e^{\left(\frac{-\|\log(C_i) - \log(C_j)\|_F^2}{\sigma_l^2}\right)} \tag{15}$$

where $\| \cdot \|_F$ denotes the matrix Frobenius norm. The logarithm of the SPD matrix C can be computed from its eigen-decomposition $C = USU^T$ by $\log(C) = U \log(S) U^T$ where $\log(S)$ is a diagonal matrix of the scaler logarithms of the eigenvalues of C.

vi. Cholesky kernel (K_c): A mean centered image set X is represented by its sample covariance matrix $C = XX^T$. Let C_i and C_j denote the sample covariance matrices of two image sets X_i and X_j. We compute the as

$$K_c(i,j) = e^{\left(\frac{-\|L_i - L_j\|_F^2}{\sigma_c^2}\right)} \tag{16}$$

where L_i is a lower triangular matrix of the Cholesky decomposition $C_i = L_i L_i^T$.

vii. MMD kernel (K_d): An image set is represented as a collection of linear patches on a manifold. The distance between two image sets X_i and X_j is computed by using the manifold to manifold distance (MMD) method presented in [2]. Specifically each image set is first clustered into multiple linear local models. Each local model is represented by a linear subspace and the mean of the local model. The MMD is then defined as the weighted sum of the subspace distance and the mean distance between the nearest local models. The MMD distance is then kernalized using (1).

These diverse image set representations encodes different characteristics of the underlying set data based on different assumptions. For example, the mean and covariance based representations show the position of the image set in high dimensional space and assume the set data to be Gaussian. The mean and covariance based representations may fail easily if the set data is multimodal. Similarly, the subspace based image set representation may not work well if the actual set data lie on complex manifolds.

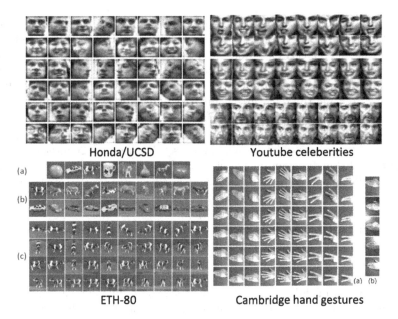

Fig. 3. Dataset Details. **HONDA/UCSD**: Each row represents images from a different image set. **Youtube celebrities:** Each row represents sample images from an image set. Two sets per subject are shown in this case. **ETH-80:** (a) Eight different object categories. (b) 10 different objects within each category. (c) Sample images from an image set of the cow category. **Cambridge Hand Gestures:** (a) Sample sequences from nine gesture classes. (b) Five different illumination conditions in the database.

4   Experimental Results

We perform extensive experiments on four standard datasets capturing a wide range of operating conditions for three image set classification applications: face recognition, object categorization and hand gesture recognition.

4.1   Dataset Details

The Honda/UCSD dataset [22] contains 59 video sequences of 20 different subjects. The faces in every frame of the video sequences are automatically detected using Viola and Jones algorithm [23], resized to 20×20 grayscale images and histogram equalized (Fig. 3).

The YouTube Celebrities dataset [24] is the most challenging dataset and contains 1910 video sequences of 47 celebrities (actors, actresses and politicians) which are collected from YouTube. Most videos are low resolution and recorded at high compression ratio, which leads to noisy and low-quality image frames. The clips contain different numbers of frames (from 8 to 400). Face image in each frame was first automatically detected by applying [23] and resized to a 20×20 (Fig. 3). We propose to compute the UoCTTI variant [25] of the histogram of oriented gradients (HOG) features using a cell size of 6 for each image. This results in a feature dimension $d = 279$ for each image. This simple and efficient pre-processing step has two advantages. Firstly, it reduces the feature dimension from 400 to 279 which significantly speeds up all the algorithms. Secondly, in our experiments we observed a significant increase in the accuracy of all the algorithms by using these features compared to using raw pixels values.

The ETH-80 dataset [26] contains images of 8 object categories where each category has 10 different objects of the same class. Each object has 41 images taken at different views which form an image set. We use 20×20 intensity images for the task of classifying an image set of an object into a known category. ETH-80 is a challenging database because it has fewer images per set, significant appearance variations across objects of the same class and larger viewing angle differences within each image set (Fig. 3).

The Cambridge Hand Gesture dataset [27] (Fig. 3) contains 900 image sequences of 9 gesture classes, which are defined by 3 primitive hand shapes and 3 primitive motions. Each class has 100 image sequences (5 different illuminations, 10 arbitrary motions, performed by 2 subjects). The recognition task involves the classification of different hand shapes as well as different hand motions at the same time. Following the experimental protocol of [28], the 100 videos of each gesture class are divided into five illumination sets (Set1, Set2, Set3, Set4 and Set5) where Set5 is chosen as the training images. The training set is further divided randomly into gallery and validation sets (10 sequences in the gallery and the other 10 sequences for validation). Since we do not use the validation set we discard it. Individual images are converted to grayscale and resized to 60×80. UoCTTI variant of HOG features with a cell size of 18 are calculated for each image resulting in a feature dimension $d = 372$. Details of all datasets used in our experiments are given in Table 1.

4.2 Experimental Setup

For each dataset the important parameters to compute the image set represen tations are selected according to the recommendations of the original authors. For the affine hull based image set representations we preserve 98 % total energy while computing the subspace bases for all the databases. For manifold representation K_d the parameters are configured as recommended in [2] for different data sets. The maximum canonical correlation is used in defining MMD. The number

Table 1. Dataset details including maximum, minimum and average images per set.

Dataset	Classes	Sets/class	Min images/set	Max images/set	Avg images/set
Honda/UCSD	20	1–5	13	782	267
Youtube Celeb	47	9	8	347	150
ETH-80	8	10	41	41	41
Cambridge	9	100	37	119	71

of connected nearest neighbours for computing geodesic distance in MMD is set to 12. For computing the Log Euclidean K_l and Cholesky kernels K_c the covariance matrix is first regularized by adding a small perturbation to its diagonal the (absolute of the smallest eigenvalue). The parameters of the MKLDR algorithm is configured according to the recommendations of the original authors [17]. For deriving the kernels, the optimal value of the Gaussian scale factor σ in (1) is selected automatically using the binary search algorithm of [17]. We set the parameter α to a small value of 10^{-6} when using the Elastic Net. The parameters λ_js can be automatically determined since the Elastic Net algorithm provides the optimal solution path of λ_js for given α [29].

For Honda dataset each subject has one image set in the gallery and the rest are used as probes. For the proposed SKL algorithm, at least two image sets per class are required in the gallery data. Therefore, when the gallery contained only one image set for a particular class, we randomly partitioned the set into two non-overlapping sub-sets. For Youtube dataset, the whole dataset is equally divided into five folds with minimal overlapping [4]. Each subject has 9 image sets. In each fold we use three image sets per class in the gallery and six image sets per class as probes. For ETH-80 dataset the gallery consists of 5 image sets per class and the remaining 5 image sets per class are used a probes. For Honda, ETH and Cambridge datasets, experiments are repeated 10-folds with different gallery probe combinations in each fold.

4.3   Results and Discussion

Table 2 summarizes our experimental results. Average recognition rates and standard deviations are reported for 10-fold experiments on Honda, ETH and Cambridge datasets and five fold experiments on the Youtube dataset.

On the Honda/UCSD dataset, the structure based image set representations perform better than the nearest sample based representations. Therefore the kernels derived from the subspace bases and the covariance representation (K_b, K_l, K_c) outperform the kernels derived from the affine hull representations (K_a, K_s, K_m) when used individually with KLDA. This is because there are enough samples available with adequate variations per set to accurately estimate the structure of the image set. The accuracy of the average kernel with KLDA is less than the maximum performing kernel K_b. This is because the lower performing kernels slightly degrade the performance of the overall mixture. Similarity, the MKLDR [17] method also uses all the kernels with different weights to compute the discriminative subspace and its performance is therefore affected by the poor performing kernels in this experiment. On the other hand the proposed SKL algorithm learns a sparse linear combination of only the most discriminative kernels to achieve the highest classification accuracy. Figure 2(a) shows the weights calculated by the proposed algorithm for the Honda dataset. The proposed algorithm automatically learns high weights for the subspace based kernel K_b and the log-Euclidean kernel K_l while the other kernels gets zero weights.

On the Youtube celebrities dataset, the kernels computed from the nearest neighbour based image set representations (K_a, K_s, K_m) perform better

Table 2. Comparison of average recognition rates and standard deviations (%).

Method	Kernel(s)	Honda	Youtube	ETH-80	Cambridge
KLDA	K_a	93.84 ± 2.47	72.51 ± 3.07	74.80 ± 2.83	36.68 ± 1.95
	K_s	95.33 ± 1.62	74.01 ± 4.10	72.38 ± 3.21	31.54 ± 1.89
	K_m	92.64 ± 2.71	69.19 ± 3.39	71.11 ± 4.67	48.56 ± 1.50
	K_b	100 ± 0.0	71.64 ± 4.42	90.25 ± 1.16	88.30 ± 0.08
	K_l	100 ± 0.0	67.54 ± 4.77	89.07 ± 1.72	90.04 ± 0.05
	K_c	96.26 ± 4.18	67.13 ± 4.01	90.65 ± 1.58	87.09 ± 1.65
	K_d	97.69 ± 2.54	66.23 ± 4.98	85.25 ± 3.12	64.41 ± 1.25
	Avg K	97.69 ± 1.45	72.12 ± 3.62	87.01 ± 5.94	87.19 ± 1.59
MKLDR [17]	All	98.71 ± 0.18	74.08 ± 4.62	90.70 ± 5.62	90.11 ± 1.80
Proposed SKL	Subset	**100 ± 0**	**77.07 ± 2.01**	**94.75 ± 0.31**	**92.43 ± 0.04**

than the kernels computed from the structure based image set representations (K_b, K_l, K_c). The reason being the useful variations in the image set data in this dataset is relatively low and the subspace or covariance structure cannot be estimated accurately. Our use of the HoG features also reduces the effects of illumination and pose variations which brings the individual samples belonging to the same classes closer. The accuracy of the MKLDR [17] is affected by the poor performing kernels. The proposed SKL algorithm achieves the highest accuracy by combing only the sample based kernels (K_a and K_s). Figure 2(b) shows that the MKLDR algorithm assigns almost equal weights to all the representations which degrade its overall accuracy. By learning a combination of only the best subset of kernel, the proposed SKL algorithm outperform the other algorithms.

On the ETH-80 dataset, the kernels derived from the sample based representations (K_a, K_s, K_m) perform poor. For this dataset, the locations of the individual samples in the sets cannot provide discriminative information due to the large intra-set pose variations and significant intra-class object appearance differences. In this case, the structure of the image set can describe the common properties of a class more accurately. Therefore, the kernels computed from the structure based representations show more accuracy on this dataset. Figure 2(c) shows that the propose weight learning algorithm has picked only the structure based kernels. The proposed SKL algorithm learns a combination of only the structure based kernels and hence outperforms all the others on this dataset.

On the Cambridge Hand Gestures dataset the sample based kernels K_a, K_s, K_m perform very poor when used individually with KLDA. For this dataset, the location of each individual sample cannot accommodate the hand gesture variations adequately. On the other hand the structure based kernels can capture the overall common properties of two gestures from the same class. Figure 2(d) shows that the proposed SKL algorithm selectively learns higher weights for the structure based kernels for this dataset. Thus the proposed SKL algorithm significantly outperforms the MKLDR algorithm. We also performed experiments to evaluate the performance of the proposed algorithm by setting $\lambda = 0$ and $\alpha = 0$. We noted

Table 3. Comparison with existing image set classification algorithms.

Algorithm	Honda	Youtube	ETH-80	Cambridge
DCC [5]	94.87 ± 2.24	66.75 ± 3.47	90.25 ± 3.06	88.31 ± 1.34
MMD [2]	94.87 ± 1.16	65.12 ± 4.36	69.72 ± 4.01	58.06 ± 2.71
MDA [6]	96.66 ± 1.73	68.12 ± 4.36	77.75 ± 6.17	26.63 ± 1.61
AHISD [3]	90.25 ± 3.97	71.92 ± 3.55	71.80 ± 8.61	35.91 ± 2.85
CHISD [3]	92.31 ± 2.12	72.83 ± 3.29	72.09 ± 8.11	37.25 ± 2.77
SANP [4]	94.34 ± 1.62	74.01 ± 3.48	72.15 ± 8.61	30.14 ± 1.35
CDL [7]	99.23 ± 1.23	68.96 ± 5.29	89.51 ± 3.68	90.18 ± 0.81
Proposed SKL	$\mathbf{100 \pm 0.0}$	$\mathbf{77.07 \pm 2.01}$	$\mathbf{94.75 \pm 0.31}$	$\mathbf{92.43 \pm 0.04}$

an accuracy drop from $\{100, 77.07, 94.75, 92.43\}\%$ to $\{98.00, 73.12, 92.0, 88.44\}\%$ for Honda, Youtube, ETH-80 and Cambridge datasets respectively. This confirms that the proposed sparsity constraints indeed improve the classification accuracy.

4.4 Comparison with Existing Image Set Classification Algorithms

The proposed SKL algorithm is also compared with seven state-of-the-art image set classification techniques including DCC [5], MMD [2], MDA [6], AHISD [3], CHISD [3], SANP [4] and CDL [7]. We have used the implementations from the original authors, except for MDA and CDL. For MDA, Hu's [4] implementation is used, while we have our own implementation of CDL. For a fair comparison, we follow the same protocol used previously by [3,4,6,7]. The existing image set classification algorithms consider only a single image set representation therefore the accuracies of these approaches vary for different properties of the image sets. Table 3 summarizes our results. Note that due to the use of HoG features the accuracy of the previous image set classification algorithms on the Youtube dataset has significantly increased. Also, the accuracy of AHISD and SANP algorithms is slightly lower compared to using the affine hull based kernel K_a and SANP kernel K_s used with KLDA. This is because AHISD and SANP algorithms do not perform any discriminant analysis after distance calculation, while our use of KLDA increases the inter-class similarity further. Because the proposed SKL algorithm combines only the best image set representations therefore it has shown the best accuracy on all the databases compared to the existing algorithms.

4.5 Computational Time

Table 4 shows the average execution times of all algorithms for 10-fold experiments on Honda dataset using a Pentium 3.4 GHz CPU with 8 GB RAM and MATLAB implementation. The computational complexity of the proposed algorithm involves the time to compute different kernel matrices plus the time of SKL and KLDA. In the training stage, the time taken to compute all the kernels is about 1100.02 s while the SKL takes 0.2 s. Note that in the testing phase

Table 4. Execution times of matching one probe image set with 20 gallery image sets of the Honda/UCSD

Algorithm	Training time (s)	Testing time (s)
DCC [5]	0.91	0.30
MMD [2]	184.57	38.10
MDA [6]	10.55	33.00
AHISD [3]	N/A	9.10
CHISD [3]	N/A	110.10
SANP [4]	N/A	5.01
CDL [7]	1.10	0.15
MKLDR [17]	>100	56.12
Proposed SKL	>100	1.01

we only compute the kernels which have non-zero weights which significantly reduces computation time compared to that of MKLDR.

5   Conclusion

We proposed a sparse kernel learning (SKL) algorithm for image set classification. By optimizing a sparse linear discriminant objective function, the proposed algorithm automatically learns the most discriminative subset of kernels from a large pool. Experimental results on four standard datasets showed that the proposed SKL algorithm outperforms current state of the art image set classification algorithms. The proposed algorithm also outperformed the standard feature combination methods such as MKLDR with significant improvement in the test set matching time.

Acknowledgement. This research work was supported by ARC grants DP1096801 and DP110102399.

References

1. Lu, J., Wang, G., Moulin, P.: Image set classification using holistic multiple order statistics features and localized multi-kernel metric learning. In: ICCV (2013)
2. Wang, R., Shan, S., Chen, X., Gao, W.: Manifold-manifold distance with application to face recognition based on image set. In: CVPR, pp. 1–8 (2008)
3. Cevikalp, H., Triggs, B.: Face recognition based on image sets. In: Computer Vsion and Pattern Recognition, pp. 2567–2573 (2010)
4. Hu, Y., Mian, A., Owens, R.: Face recognition using sparse approximated nearest points between image sets. IEEE Trans. PAMI **34**, 1992–2004 (2012)
5. Kim, T.K., Kittler, J., Cipolla, R.: Discriminative learning and recognition of image set classes using canonical correlations. IEEE PAMI **29**, 1005–1018 (2007)
6. Wang, R., Chen, X.: Manifold discriminant analysis. In: Computer Vsion and Pattern Recognition, pp. 429–436 (2009)

7. Wang, Guo, H., Davis, L., Dai, Q.: Covariance discriminative learning: a natural and efficient approach to image set classification. In: CVPR (2012)

8. Shakhnarovich, G., Fisher III, J.W., Darrell, T.: Face recognition from long-term observations. In: Heyden, A., Sparr, G., Nielsen, M., Johansen, P. (eds.) ECCV 2002, Part III. LNCS, vol. 2352, pp. 851–865. Springer, Heidelberg (2002)

9. Arandjelovic, O., Shakhnarovich, G., Fisher, J., Cipolla, R., Darrell, T.: Face recognition with image sets using manifold density divergence. In: CVPR (2005)

10. Uzair, M., Mahmood, A., Mian, A., McDonald, C.: A compact discriminative representation for efficient image-set classification with application to biometric recognition. In: ICB (2013)

11. Fukui, K., Yamaguchi, O.: The kernel orthogonal mutual subspace method and its application to 3D object recognition. In: Yagi, Y., Kang, S.B., Kweon, I.S., Zha, H. (eds.) ACCV 2007, Part II. LNCS, vol. 4844, pp. 467–476. Springer, Heidelberg (2007)

12. Gonen, M., Alpaydin, E.: Multiple kernel learning algorithms. JMLR 12, 2181–2238 (2011)

13. Varma, M., Ray, D.: Learning the discriminative power-invariance trade-off. In: ICCV, pp. 1–8 (2007)

14. Vedaldi, A., Gulshan, V., Varma, M., Zisserman, A.: Multiple kernels for object detection. In: ICCV, pp. 606–613 (2009)

15. Gehler, P., Nowozin, S.: On feature combination for multiclass object classification. In: ICCV, pp. 221–228 (2009)

16. Vemulapalli, R., Pillai, J., Chellappa, R.: Kernel learning for extrinsic classification of manifold features. In: CVPR (2013)

17. Lin, Y.Y., Liu, T.L., Fuh, C.S.: Multiple kernel learning for dimensionality reduction. IEEE Trans. PAMI 33, 1147–1160 (2011)

18. Yan, S., Xu, D., Zhang, B., Zhang, H.J., Yang, Q., Lin, S.: Graph embedding and extensions: a general framework for dimensionality reduction. IEEE PAMI 29, 40–51 (2007)

19. Li, X., Jiang, T., Zhang, K.: Efficient and robust feature extraction by maximum margin criterion. IEEE Trans. Neural Netw. 17, 157–165 (2006)

20. Lai, Z., Xu, Y., Yang, J., Tang, J., Zhang, D.: Sparse tensor discriminant analysis. IEEE Trans. Image Process. 22, 3904–3915 (2013)

21. Shawe-Taylor, J., Cristianini, N.: Kernel Methods for Pattern Analysis. Cambridge University Press, Cambridge (2004)

22. Lee, K.C., Ho, J., Yang, M.H., Kriegman, D.: Video-based face recognition using probabilistic appearance manifolds. In: CVPR, vol. 1, pp. I-313–I-320 (2003)

23. Viola, P., Jones, M.: Robust real-time face detection. IJCV 57, 137–154 (2004)

24. Kim, M., Kumar, S., Pavlovic, V., Rowley, H.: Face tracking and recognition with visual constraints in real-world videos. In: CVPR (2008)

25. Felzenszwalb, P., Girshick, R., McAllester, D., Ramanan, D.: Object detection with discriminatively trained part-based models. IEEE PAMI 32, 1627–1645 (2010)

26. Leibe, B., Schiele, B.: Analyzing appearance and contour based methods for object categorization. In: CVPR, vol. 2, pp. II-409–II-415 (2003)

27. Kim, T.K., Wong, K.Y.K., Cipolla, R.: Tensor canonical correlation analysis for action classification. In: Computer Vision and Pattern Recognition, pp. 1–8 (2007)

28. Kim, T.K., Cipolla, R.: Canonical correlation analysis of video volume tensors for action categorization and detection. IEEE PAMI 31, 1415–1428 (2009)

29. Zou, H., Hastie, T.: Regularization and variable selection via the elastic net. J. Royal Stat. Soc., Ser. B (Stat. Methodol.) 67, 301–320 (2005)

Automatic Feature Learning to Grade Nuclear Cataracts Based on Deep Learning

Xinting Gao[1][(✉)], Stephen Lin[2], and Tien Yin Wong[3]

[1] Agency for Science, Technology and Research,
Institute for Infocomm Research, Singapore, Singapore
xgao@i2r.a-star.edu.sg
[2] Microsoft Research, Beijing, People's Republic of China
[3] Singapore Eye Research Institute, Singapore, Singapore

Abstract. Cataracts are a clouding of the lens and the leading cause of blindness worldwide. Assessing the presence and severity of cataracts is essential for diagnosis and progression monitoring, as well as to facilitate clinical research and management of the disease. Existing automatic methods for cataract grading utilize a predefined set of image features that may provide an incomplete, redundant, or even noisy representation. In this work, we propose a system to automatically learn features for grading the severity of nuclear cataracts from slit-lamp images. Local filters learned from image patches are fed into a convolutional neural network, followed by a set of recursive neural networks to further extract higher-order features. With these features, support vector regression is applied to determine the cataract grade. The proposed system is validated on a large population-based dataset of 5378 images, where it outperforms the state-of-the-art by yielding with respect to clinical grading a mean absolute error (ε) of 0.322, a 68.6 % exact integral agreement ratio (R_0), a 86.5 % decimal grading error ≤ 0.5 ($R_{e0.5}$), and a 99.1 % decimal grading error ≤ 1.0 ($R_{e1.0}$).

1 Introduction

The lens of a human eye is optically transparent, consisting mostly of water and protein. Due to its shape, clarity and refractive index, the lens is able to focus light onto the retina, where the visual stimuli is transmitted through the optic nerve to the brain. Any clouding or loss of clarity in the lens is called a cataract, and the blockage of light results in impaired vision or even blindness [1]. Cataracts are the leading cause of visual impairment worldwide, accounting for more than 50 % of blindness in developing countries. As most cataracts are age-related, the global trend of aging populations is expected to increase the prevalence of cataracts, with the number of blind people projected to reach 75 million by 2020 [2]. Mass screening and timely treatment of cataracts in the elderly is thus essential to improve quality of life and reduce health care costs.

The lens can be anatomically divided into three layers: an outer layer called the capsule, a central compacted core called the nucleus, and the cortex which

© Springer International Publishing Switzerland 2015
D. Cremers et al. (Eds.): ACCV 2014, Part II, LNCS 9004, pp. 632–642, 2015.
DOI: 10.1007/978-3-319-16808-1_42

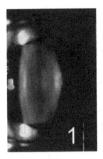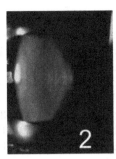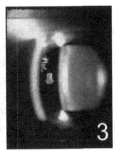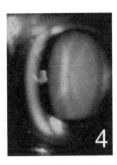

Fig. 1. Standard photographs of the Wisconsin grading system. The severity of the nuclear cataracts increases in the images from left to right, with greater brightness and lower contrast between anatomical landmarks. In addition, the color of the nucleus and posterior cortex exhibits more of a yellow tint due to brunescence.

surrounds the nucleus. Cataracts that occur in the nucleus are the most common type and will be the focus of this work. Since they appear as a homogeneous increase of opacification and coloration of the nucleus, they can be clearly seen in cross-sectional views of the lens in slit-lamp images [3].

For practical reasons, automatic methods for screening cataracts are needed, since manual examination, either directly through a slit-lamp microscope or indirectly through photographic comparisons to the Wisconsin grading protocol [4] (see Fig. 1), is time-consuming, expensive and subjective [5]. Though visually distinguishing grade 1 from grade 3 or 4 may be easy, it is difficult to determine precise grades on a continuous scale, which is critical for monitoring the progression of cataracts. In fact, human intra-grader agreement is only 70–80 %, and inter-grader agreement is about 65 % [4].

Existing techniques for automatic grading of nuclear cataracts utilize features designed according to the grading protocol [6–9]. These feature sets have the advantage of being low-dimensional; however, they may be incomplete, redundant, or even contain irrelevant (noisy) elements. For example, some earlier methods extract features from the whole lens [7,8], though it was later shown that the anterior cortex provides no information for nuclear cataract grading [9]. In [9], bag-of-features (BOF) descriptors are extracted from different parts of the lens, and group sparsity regression (GSR) is used to select the features, parameters and models simultaneously. Although the BOF model automatically learns a codebook and represents each image as a histogram of visual words, the local feature descriptors must be defined in advance. Furthermore, as a global representation of local features, the BOF model has limited ability to encode geometric information.

Different from previous techniques, we propose in this work to automatically learn features for nuclear cataract grading in slit-lamp images. Toward this end, we adopt the deep learning framework of convolutional-recursive neural networks (CRNNs) [10], which are able to extract discriminative higher-order features because of its hierarchical structure. With these features, we apply support vector regression (SVR) to obtain grading estimates. Experiments demonstrate that the learned features have greater discriminative power and the proposed system attains higher overall performance than previous methods.

Deep learning has been used in medical image processing for registration, segmentation and classification [11–16]. For our problem, we adopt the CRNN deep learning framework because of its ability to extract high-order semantic information from images of a realistic size (e.g., images of 1536 × 2048 resolution in our case). Although there exist many deep learning methods for learning features, most of them can handle only small images or local patches in practice [11–15], due to the considerable number of parameters that need to be learned for larger images. In the medical imaging domain, it is difficult if not infeasible to obtain a sufficiently large amount of data to effectively learn so many parameters (e.g., over one million parameters for supervised deep learning networks which typically consist of about seven layers). By contrast, the design of CRNNs allows for unsupervised learning within a hierarchical structure, which enables scaling up to realistic image sizes without requiring substantial training data [10,17]. In this paper, we leverage the unsupervised learning method of the CRNN framework to learn features automatically. This work represents the first application of deep learning for diagnosing large medical images, and it is shown to achieve better overall performance than the existing cataract grading techniques. With respect to clinical grading, our method yields a mean absolute error (ε) of 0.322, a 68.6 % exact integral agreement ratio (R_0), a 86.5 % decimal grading error ≤ 0.5 ($R_{e0.5}$), and a 99.1 % decimal grading error ≤ 1.0 ($R_{e1.0}$) on a large population-based dataset of 5378 images.

2   Method

In this section, we first introduce the CRNN deep learning framework and then the proposed automatic system which consists of three components: region of interest (ROI) and structure detection, feature learning and image representation, and grading.

2.1   Convolutional-Recursive Neural Networks

The unsupervised Convolutional-Recursive Neural Network (CRNN) method was proposed by Socher et al. [10]. It consists of three steps: pre-training CNN filters from randomly selected patches, generating local representations of each image by feeding the filters into a convolutional neural network (CNN) layer, and learning hierarchical feature representations using multiple recursive neural networks (RNNs) with random weights.

Pre-training CNN Filters. The CNN filters are learned from randomly selected image patches that have been normalized and whitened. There exist several methods for learning the filters, such as sparse auto-encoder, sparse restricted Boltzmann machine, k-means clustering, and Gaussian mixtures. Among them,

k-means clustering has been shown to achieve the best performance [18]. K-means clustering aims to minimize the sum of squared Euclidean distances between patches, represented as a vector x, and their nearest cluster centers m_k. The standard 1-of-K, hard-assignment coding scheme is as follows:

$$f_k(x) = \begin{cases} 1 & \text{if } k = argmin_j \|m_j - x\| \\ 0 & \text{otherwise.} \end{cases} \tag{1}$$

The learned K filters, $\{f_k, k = 1, 2...K\}$, will be used in the convolutional layer of the CNN.

Convolutional Neural Network. A convolutional neural network consists of a convolution layer and a pooling layer. In the convolution layer, the set of learned filters, f_k, is convolved with the entire image to yield K corresponding feature maps. In the pooling layer, each feature map is sub-sampled by average or max pooling, which makes the resulting features invariant to translation and small deformations.

Recursive Neural Networks. Recursive neural networks learn hierarchical feature representations by applying the same neural network recursively in a tree structure. The output of each neural network in an RNN is a parent vector computed from a set of child vectors, where the children at the bottom of the tree represent features generated by the CNN. Through this hierarchy, features of local image regions are merged into a higher-order, image-level feature representation. The RNN model can be trained through back-propagation [17]. In [10], Socher et al. demonstrated that a fixed tree structure can achieve good performance with the CNN as its preceding layer. Furthermore, multiple RNNs with random weights produce high quality features. As the learning is unsupervised, it is feasible to explore a large set of RNNs efficiently. It is particularly suitable for medical image processing applications where large amounts of labeled data are difficult or expensive to acquire.

2.2 Automatic Feature Learning to Grade Nuclear Cataracts

In applying the CRNN feature learning method to nuclear cataract grading, the lens structure is first detected and anatomical sections of the lens are segmented. Then CRNNs are applied to each section to learn a representation for that part of the lens. Finally, SVR is applied to the concatenated features to estimate the cataract grade. This procedure is illustrated in Fig. 2.

Lens Structure Detection. To detect the lens structure, we employ the method in [7], which uses an active shape model learned from a training set with manually annotated landmark points. We then extract the central part of the lens around the visual axis as done in [9], but remove the anterior cortex

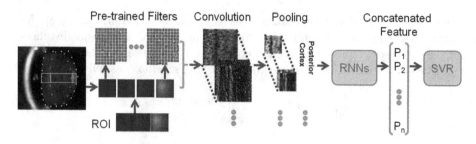

Fig. 2. Overview of deep learning based nuclear cataract grading. Regions of interest (ROIs) within detected lens structures are convolved with learned local filters, and then pooled for extracting higher-order features from recursive neural networks (RNNs). With the resulting feature vectors, final grading results are obtained using support vector regression (SVR).

section since it contains no information for nuclear cataract grading according to both the grading protocol [4] and the state-of-the-art grading technique [9]. Therefore, our region of interest contains only the posterior cortex and nucleus. After extracting the ROI, the posterior cortex section is resized to $n_s \times n_s$ and the nucleus is resized to $n_s \times (n_s \times 2)$ as done in [9]. The resized nucleus is further divided into three half-overlapping sections: the anterior nucleus, central nucleus and posterior nucleus. Features are learned and extracted from each of the $n_s \times n_s$ sections. By aligning these sections to specific anatomical structures that are geometrically similar among individuals, discriminative features can be more effectively extracted even with a relatively small amount of data.

Feature Learning. The features are learned for each section independently. First, we randomly extract local patches from a specific section of the training images for each grading category. Each patch has a spatial dimension of $n_p \times n_p$ and three color channels (R, G and B). Then, k-means clustering is used to generate the local filters from the randomly selected samples. Figure 2 shows the filters learned for the posterior cortex section and the anterior nucleus section, which capture standard edge and color features.

The local filters are used in the convolutional layer of the CNN, followed by rectification, local contrast normalization, and average pooling. The invariance of the obtained feature to translation and small deformations helps to compensate for inaccuracies in structure detection, bringing greater robustness to the system. Each section of size $n_s \times n_s \times 3$ is convolved with the K square filters of size $n_p \times n_p \times 3$. This results in K feature maps of size $(n_s - n_p + 1) \times (n_s - n_p + 1)$. In the pooling layer, each feature map is processed by average pooling over $n_a \times n_a$ regions with a stride size of n_l. The size of the final pooled feature map for each section is $n_c = ((n_s - n_p + 1) - n_a)/n_l + 1$. The CNN layer thus produces a $K \times n_c \times n_c$ dimensional 3D feature map, with each feature vector $c_i \in \mathbb{R}^K$.

To extract higher-order features from the low-level feature map $C \in \mathbb{R}^{K \times n_c \times n_c}$, multiple random RNNs are applied. For each RNN, the basic element is a 3D random matrix $W \in \mathbb{R}^{K \times b^2 \times K}$, where b is the block size which determines a set of local windows to merge into a parent vector $p \in \mathbb{R}^K$. The neural network is as follows:

$$p = g \left(W \begin{bmatrix} c_1 \\ \vdots \\ c_{b^2} \end{bmatrix} \right), \qquad (2)$$

where g is a nonlinear function such as $tanh$ and $c_i \in \mathbb{R}^K$ are the feature vectors obtained in the CNN layer. Equation 2 is recursively applied to the whole feature map without overlapping blocks to obtain a new layer R_1. Then Eq. 2 is applied again with the same weights W to the vectors in R_1, resulting in a second RNN layer R_2. The same procedure is repeated until only one parent vector is left. As the weight W is randomly generated without any supervised learning, multiple RNNs are needed to extract the higher-order features. Finally, each section is represented by the $N \times K$-dimensional vectors obtained through the N RNNs. We concatenate the feature vectors from all four of the sections to represent the image. The learned features are fed into an RBF ϵ-SVR [19] to obtain the final grading result.

3   Experiments

In this section, we first evaluate the proposed method by comparing it with the state-of-the-art nuclear cataract grading technique [9] using the dataset employed in their paper, ACHIKO-NC. Then, we compare the proposed learned features with the handcrafted features presented in [7] using the same learning method. The ACHIKO-NC dataset is comprised of 5378 images with decimal grading scores that range from 0.1 to 5.0. The scores are determined by professional graders based on the Wisconsin protocol [4], with higher decimal scores indicating greater severity of the cataract. The protocol takes the ceiling of each decimal grading score as the integral grading score, *i.e.*, a cataract with a decimal grading score of 1.2 has an integral grading score of 2. ACHIKO-NC contains 94 images of integral grade 1, 1874 images of integral grade 2, 2476 images of integral grade 3, 897 images of integral grade 4, and 37 images of integral grade 5. Since the unbalanced data distribution of ACHIKO-NC may skew a learned prediction model towards middle-grade estimates, we set the training sample size of each grade to 20 as done in [9].

3.1   Evaluation Criteria

In this work, we use the same four evaluation criteria as in [9] to measure grading accuracy, namely the exact integral agreement ratio (R_0), the percentage of decimal grading errors ≤ 0.5 ($R_{e0.5}$), the percentage of decimal grading errors ≤ 1.0 ($R_{e1.0}$), and the mean absolute error (ε), which are defined as

$$R_0 = \frac{|\lceil G_{gt} \rceil = \lceil G_{pr} \rceil|_0}{N}, \qquad R_{e0.5} = \frac{||G_{gt} - G_{pr}| \leq 0.5|_0}{N},$$

$$R_{e1.0} = \frac{||G_{gt} - G_{pr}| \leq 1.0|_0}{N}, \qquad \varepsilon = \frac{\sum |G_{gt} - G_{pr}|}{N}, \tag{3}$$

where G_{gt} denotes the ground-truth clinical grade, G_{pr} denotes the predicted grade, $\lceil \cdot \rceil$ is the ceiling function, $|\cdot|$ denotes the absolute value, $|\cdot|_0$ is a function that counts the number of non-zero values, and N is the number of testing images ($N = |G_{gt}|_0 = |G_{pr}|_0$).

The first metric (R_0) is based on grading protocol and has large quantization error, while the third metric ($R_{e1.0}$) also provides a relatively weak measure. On the other hand, the second ($R_{e0.5}$) and fourth (ε) metrics are more significant, since they measure performance at a finer scale and provide a better reflection of a method's utility in monitoring the progression of this disease. $R_{e0.5}$ has the most narrow tolerance among the four evaluation criteria, which makes it the most significant in evaluating the accuracy of grading.

3.2   Comparisons

We compare our method to the state-of-the-art technique, GSR [9], using the same dataset, experimental setting and reporting methods that they used. We also evaluate our method in relation to the method proposed in [7], which uses handcrafted features and RBF ϵ-SVR. Testing is conducted over twenty rounds. For each round, twenty images of each grade are selected randomly as the training data, and the remaining 5278 images are used for testing, which follows the training/testing sample ratio in [7,9]. In training, optimal parameters for SVR and GSR were selected for each method by cross-validation. For the proposed method, $n_s = 148$, $n_p = 9$, $n_a = 10$, $n_l = 5$, $K = 128$, $N = 64$, and $b = 3$, which results in a feature dimension for the four sections of $N \times K \times 4 = 64 \times 128 \times 4 = 32768$. The results are listed in Table 1 in terms of mean value and standard deviation of R_0, $R_{e0.5}$, $R_{e1.0}$ and ε over the twenty rounds. The evaluations of $R_{e0.5}$, $R_{e1.0}$ and ε were found to be statistically significant, with associated p-values of [0.0920, 2.0383e-10, 3.5271e-14, 9.8171e-11] for the four metrics.

As mentioned previously, the $R_{e0.5}$ and ε metrics measure performance at a finer scale, and thus offer a better indication of a method's utility in disease progression monitoring. For these important metrics, our method achieves an improvement of 3.7 % in $R_{e0.5}$ and 8.3 % in ε on the large population-based database (5378 images). These represent meaningful improvements in light of the impact of accurate diagnoses on cataract patients.

From the results, we also have the following observations. First, since our method and [7] both use RBF ϵ-SVR for regression, the better performance of our method indicates that our learned features obtained via the CRNN deep learning framework provide a better representation than the handcrafted features of [7]. Second, although GSR is able to reduce the noise and increase the

Table 1. Performance comparisons for nuclear cataract grading methods

Method	R_0	$R_{e0.5}$	$R_{e1.0}$	ε
Proposed	**0.686 ± 0.009**	**0.865 ± 0.010**	**0.991 ± 0.001**	**0.322 ± 0.009**
BOF + GSR [9]	0.682 ± 0.004	0.834 ± 0.005	0.985 ± 0.001	0.351 ± 0.004
RBF ε-SVR [7]	0.658 ± 0.014	0.824 ± 0.016	0.981 ± 0.004	0.354 ± 0.014
Our improvement over [9]	0.6 %	3.7 %	0.6 %	8.3 %

accuracy of structured BOF group features, its performance is still limited by the representation power of the BOF group features. The proposed learned features characterize the image well and furthermore encode high-level semantic information, which leads our method to better performance.

3.3 Computation Time

The proposed approach provides objective assessments at speeds comparable to state-of-the-art methods, making it useful for assisting and improving clinical management of the disease in the context of large-population screening. On a four-core 2.4 GHz PC with 24 GB RAM, the total training time using 100 images is about 1899 s, and it takes 17 s for prediction of one image. By comparison, the techniques of [7,9] run on the same computing platform at a speed of 20.45 and 25.00 s per image, respectively.

3.4 Analysis and Discussion

The features learned in the CRNN framework depend on the sections from which they are extracted in a lens image. We empirically studied the effect of different lens sectioning on our method by extracting features under the following settings: 2-sections (posterior cortex and full nucleus), 3-sections (posterior cortex, full nucleus, and anterior cortex), 4-sections (the current implementation with posterior cortex, posterior nucleus, central nucleus, and anterior nucleus), and 5-sections (same as 4-sections plus anterior cortex). We also examined the BOF + GSR method [9] under its original 3-section setting and with 5-sections. The results, listed in Table 2, show that for our CRNNs, including the anterior cortex always leads to lower performance, as seen by comparing 3-section CRNNs to 2-section CRNNs, and 5-section CRNNs to 4-section CRNNs, with either regression method. These results support the findings in [9] that the anterior cortex introduces noise into the classification. However, an examination of group weights when using CRNN features with GSR shows that GSR does not eliminate the CRNN features extracted from the anterior cortex, which suggests that GSR may not fully remove noisy elements from a feature set. The analysis of Table 2 additionally indicates that a finer partition of the nucleus leads to more discriminative CRNN and BOF features (comparing 4-sections vs. 2-sections, and 5-sections vs. 3-sections). In fact, it is seen that 5-section BOF outperforms the original 3-section BOF in [9].

Table 2. Analysis of different lens sectioning

Method	Feature	R_0	$R_{e0.5}$	$R_{e1.0}$	ε
RBF ϵ-SVR	2-section CRNNs	0.645 ± 0.013	0.819 ± 0.014	0.985 ± 0.003	0.358 ± 0.012
	3-section CRNNs	0.631 ± 0.013	0.801 ± 0.016	0.981 ± 0.003	0.372 ± 0.012
	4-section CRNNs	**0.686 ± 0.009**	**0.865 ± 0.010**	**0.991 ± 0.001**	**0.322 ± 0.009**
	5-section CRNNs	0.677 ± 0.008	0.857 ± 0.010	0.990 ± 0.002	0.329 ± 0.008
	3-section BOF [9]	0.615 ± 0.013	0.799 ± 0.012	0.980 ± 0.002	0.375 ± 0.011
	5-section BOF	0.654 ± 0.018	0.820 ± 0.019	0.976 ± 0.007	0.360 ± 0.017
GSR	2-section CRNNs	0.654 ± 0.021	0.823 ± 0.027	0.985 ± 0.005	0.355 ± 0.022
	3-section CRNNs	0.643 ± 0.024	0.808 ± 0.030	0.982 ± 0.005	0.366 ± 0.024
	4-section CRNNs	0.679 ± 0.011	**0.850 ± 0.015**	**0.989 ± 0.002**	**0.335 ± 0.012**
	5-section CRNNs	0.672 ± 0.009	0.843 ± 0.013	0.987 ± 0.002	0.341 ± 0.011
	3-section BOF [9]	0.682 ± 0.004	0.834 ± 0.005	0.985 ± 0.001	0.351 ± 0.004
	5-section BOF	**0.687 ± 0.009**	0.838 ± 0.011	0.987 ± 0.002	0.345 ± 0.008

For both CRNN and BOF features, k-means clustering is employed to learn local filters or a codebook. Besides being able to capture more global geometric and semantic information, CRNN differs from BOF in the representation of color, as BOF applies k-means to local patches in each color channel separately, while CRNN applies it to full color patches in a way that the learned filters characterize both standard edge features and color features. The ability to model correlated color information provides CRNN features with greater discriminative power.

4   Conclusion and Future Work

We have proposed a new method for nuclear cataract grading based on automatic feature learning. Difficulty in finding the right features has been a limiting factor in research on automatic cataract grading, and this work brings a new approach that directly addresses this issue in a systematic and general manner, in contrast to resorting to heuristic handpicked features. Through deep learning, discriminative features that characterize high-level semantic information are effectively extracted. In tests on the *ACHIKO-NC* dataset comprised of 5378 images, our system achieves a 68.6 % exact agreement ratio (R_0) against clinical integral grading, a 86.5 % decimal grading error ≤ 0.5 ($R_{e0.5}$), a 99.1 % decimal grading error ≤ 1.0 ($R_{e1.0}$), and 0.322 mean absolute error, which represents significant improvements over the state-of-the-art method.

This approach has the potential to be applied to other eye diseases. For example, different handcrafted features are used in optic cup/disc segmentation to assess the progression of glaucoma and to detect drusen for assessment of age-related macular degeneration (AMD). Features extracted through this type of deep learning approach may potentially lead to improved performance in these cases.

References

1. Kanski, J.: Clinical Ophthalmology: A Systematic Approach. Elsevier, New York (2007)
2. Vision 2020: International Agency for the Prevention of Blindness 2010 report (2010)
3. Wong, T., Loon, S., Saw, S.: The epidemiology of age related eye diseases in asia. Br. J. Ophthalmol. **90**, 506–511 (2006)
4. Klein, B., Klein, R., Linton, K., Magli, Y., Neider, M.: Assessment of cataracts from photographs in the beaver dam eye study. Ophthalmology **97**, 1428–33 (1990)
5. Thylefors, B., Chylack, L.T., Konyamia, K., Sasaki, K., Sperduto, R., Taylor, H.R., West, S.: A simplified cataract grading system - the WHO cataract grading group. Ophthalmic Epidemiol. **9**, 83–89 (2002)
6. Fan, S., Dyer, C.R., Hubbard, L., Klein, B.: An automatic system for classification of nuclear sclerosis from slit-lamp photographs. In: Ellis, R.E., Peters, T.M. (eds.) MICCAI 2003. LNCS, vol. 2878, pp. 592–601. Springer, Heidelberg (2003)
7. Li, H., Lim, J., Liu, J., Mitchell, P., Tan, A., Wang, J., Wong, T.: A computer-aided diagnosis system of nuclear cataract. IEEE Trans. Biomed. Eng. **57**, 1690–1698 (2010)
8. Huang, W., Chan, K., Li, H., Lim, J., Liu, J., Wong, T.: A computer assisted method for nuclear cataract grading from slit-lamp images using ranking. IEEE Trans. Med. Imaging **30**, 94–107 (2011)
9. Xu, Y., Gao, X., Lin, S., Wong, D.W.K., Liu, J., Xu, D., Cheng, C.Y., Cheung, C.Y., Wong, T.Y.: Automatic grading of nuclear cataracts from slit-lamp lens images using group sparsity regression. In: Mori, K., Sakuma, I., Sato, Y., Barillot, C., Navab, N. (eds.) MICCAI 2013, Part II. LNCS, vol. 8150, pp. 468–475. Springer, Heidelberg (2013)
10. Socher, R., Huval, B., Bhat, B., Manning, C., Ng, A.: Convolutional-recursive deep learning for 3d object classification. In: Advances in Neural Information Processing Systems (2012)
11. Cireşan, D.C., Giusti, A., Gambardella, L.M., Schmidhuber, J.: Mitosis detection in breast cancer histology images with deep neural networks. In: Mori, K., Sakuma, I., Sato, Y., Barillot, C., Navab, N. (eds.) MICCAI 2013, Part II. LNCS, vol. 8150, pp. 411–418. Springer, Heidelberg (2013)
12. Habibzadeh, M., Krzyżak, A., Fevens, F.: White blood cell differential counts using convolutional neural networks for low resolution images. In: Rutkowski, L., Korytkowski, M., Scherer, R., Tadeusiewicz, R., Zadeh, L.A., Zurada, J.M. (eds.) Artificial Intelligence and Soft Computing. LNCS, vol. 7895. Springer, Heidelberg (2013)
13. Wu, G., Kim, M., Wang, Q., Gao, Y., Liao, S., Shen, D.: Unsupervised deep feature learning for deformable registration of MR brain images. In: Mori, K., Sakuma, I., Sato, Y., Barillot, C., Navab, N. (eds.) MICCAI 2013, Part II. LNCS, vol. 8150, pp. 649–656. Springer, Heidelberg (2013)
14. Liao, S., Gao, Y., Oto, A., Shen, D.: Representation learning: a unified deep learning framework for automatic prostate MR segmentation. In: Mori, K., Sakuma, I., Sato, Y., Barillot, C., Navab, N. (eds.) MICCAI 2013, Part II. LNCS, vol. 8150, pp. 254–261. Springer, Heidelberg (2013)
15. Prasoon, A., Petersen, K., Igel, C., Lauze, F., Dam, E., Nielsen, M.: Deep feature learning for knee cartilage segmentation using a triplanar convolutional neural network. In: Mori, K., Sakuma, I., Sato, Y., Barillot, C., Navab, N. (eds.) MICCAI 2013, Part II. LNCS, vol. 8150, pp. 246–253. Springer, Heidelberg (2013)

16. Brosch, T., Tam, R.: Manifold learning of brain MRIs by deep learning. In: Mori, K., Sakuma, I., Sato, Y., Barillot, C., Navab, N. (eds.) MICCAI 2013. LNCS, vol. 8150. Springer, Heidelberg (2013)

17. Socher, R., Lin, C., Ng, A., Manning, C.: Parsing natural scenes and natural language with recursive neural networks. In: International Conference on Machine Learning (2011)

18. Coates, A., Lee, H., Ng, A.Y.: An analysis of single-layer networks in unsupervised feature learning. In: International Conference on Artificial Intelligence and Statistics (AISTATS) (2011)

19. Chang, C., Lin, C.: Libsvm: a library for support vector machines. ACM Trans. Intell. Syst. Technol. 2, 1–27 (2011)

Texture Classification Using Dense Micro-block Difference (DMD)

Rakesh Mehta[✉] and Karen Egiazarian

Tampere University of Technology, Tampere, Finland
`rakesh.mehta@tut.fi`

Abstract. The paper proposes a novel image representation for texture classification. The recent advancements in the field of patch based features compressive sensing and feature encoding are combined to design a robust image descriptor. In our approach, we first propose the local features, Dense Micro-block Difference (DMD), which capture the local structure from the image patches at high scales. Instead of the pixel we process the small blocks from images which capture the micro-structure from it. DMD can be computed efficiently using integral images. The features are then encoded using Fisher Vector method to obtain an image descriptor which considers the higher order statistics. The proposed image representation is combined with linear SVM classifier. The experiments are conducted on the standard texture datasets (KTH-TIPS-2a, Brodatz and Curet). On KTH-TIPS-2a dataset the proposed method outperforms the best reported results by 5.5 % and has a comparable performance to the state-of-the-art methods on the other datasets.

1 Introduction

Texture is an important attribute of an object or a material and has been widely utilized as a visual cue for image classification. A number of computer vision problems, such as material classification [1], face recognition [2], facial expression recognition [3], object detection [4] use the texture information from images. Therefore, the fundamental problem of texture classification is highly relevant. The texture classification system encounters the problems such as, the variations in scale, illuminations, rotation and the subtle difference in the different texture patterns. These challenges have not been addressed completely by the existing methods and require deeper analysis. This paper thoroughly studies above mentioned problem and proposes a method for texture classification by integrating the advancement in the field of key-points descriptors, image encoding approaches and compressive sensing.

A variety of approaches have been proposed for texture classification. A family of these algorithms represent an image using a subset of the features from an image patch. The examples of these algorithms include Co-occurring Histograms [5], Markov random Field [6], Gabor Filter Banks [7], Local Binary Patterns (LBP) [8] and Fractal Models [9]. The key idea behind these papers is that a discriminative information can be captured from the image patch. Different methods are used to capture this information from the patches, e.g. Xu et al. [9]

© Springer International Publishing Switzerland 2015
D. Cremers et al. (Eds.): ACCV 2014, Part II, LNCS 9004, pp. 643–658, 2015.
DOI: 10.1007/978-3-319-16808-1_43

use orientation histogram, LBP uses the sign of the difference of the pixel values, Gabor based methods [7] use the response of the Gabor filter banks, etc. These approaches consider texture as a local cue and global structure between the features is not taken into account. Another class of the texture classification methods are based on the Bag-of-Words (BoW) model of image representation [10–13]. The BoW model encodes both, the local structure by using the local features to form the texton dictionary, and the global appearance by computing certain statistics to represent the distribution of the textons. Due to its generalized structure it has been widely applied in a number of computer vision applications.

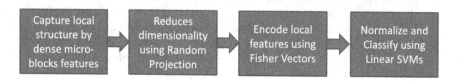

Fig. 1. The flowchart of proposed approach.

In this paper we present a texture descriptor by combining novel patch based local features with the advancement in the BoW model. We first propose the Dense Micro-block Difference (DMD), which are based on the idea that the texture image repetitively exhibit a specific local structure which can provide discriminative information about it. Although the idea is inspired from the success of the pattern based approaches, the proposed method in practice is very different and addresses various shortcomings of these approaches. DMD are patch based features which are computed by comparing the intensities of smaller regions in it. It has been shown that the texture images being repetitive are compressible, which is further exploited in the proposed approach. The features are very fast to compute using integral image and low in dimensionality. The proposed local features are then combined with the BoW model of image representation. We use advanced encoding approach that has recently shown very promising results in the classification tasks. The combination of the proposed features with efficient encoding from the BoW model results in a robust image descriptor. Finally, the descriptor is combined with the linear SVM classifier which achieves state-of-the-art performance on a number of standard texture datasets (KTH-TIPS-2a, CUReT and Brodatz). The flowchart of the proposed approach is shown in Fig. 1.

The rest of the paper is organized as follows. In Sect. 2, we discuss the related work on the local features and the BoW encoding methods. In Sect. 3, we present the proposed approach for the texture classification. In Sect. 4, we study the key parameter of the descriptor and evaluate the performance of the proposed approach on three texture datasets. Finally, the paper is concluded in Sect. 5.

2   Related Work and Its Analysis

Our work broadly draws inspiration from two different kind of approaches followed in texture classification. First, we call the local structure capturing features and the other is the Bag-of-Words based image representation model for feature encoding. In this section we provide a brief overview of the related work and analyse its shortcomings.

2.1   Local Feature

A number of patch based local features are based on the idea that the local region of the image exhibits a certain characteristic structure and various methods have been employed to capture that structure. Among these LBP [8] has shown very promising results, and a number of modifications of LBP have been proposed [14,15]. These features capture the local structure by taking the sign of the difference of image pixel values from the image patch in a circular geometry. The information provided by the magnitude of the difference is completely ignored, which results in the loss of the discriminative power of the features. To overcome this shortcoming, Tan et al. [16] compared the magnitude with a predefined threshold parameter, while Guo et al. [17] incorporated the magnitude by comparing it with a mean value of the image. The results from these approaches demonstrate that the magnitude provide a discriminative information which can be utilized in the patch based features.

Recently, Liu et al. [18] proposed Sorted Random Projection (SRP) which utilize the compressibility of the pixel intensity difference taken from a circular geometry. Sharma et al. [19] proposed Local Higher order Statistics (LHS), a descriptor that incorporates the high order statistics of the pixel difference from a patch. Approaches based on a pixel difference, such as LBP, SRP, LHS consider the circular geometry of the sampling points in the patch. Circular geometry can only capture the radial variation in the image patch as the difference is taken from the central pixel and its neighbours, all other directions are ignored. Although never applied in image classification, the geometry of the sampling points in the image patch has been studied in the binary key-point descriptors such as BRIEF [20], ORB [21]. Colander et al. [20] experimented with the five different kinds of geometries for sampling points and reported that random Gaussian sampling points outperforms the circular geometry and others. In ORB the sampling points are selected such that they have maximum variance in training samples and are uncorrelated.

The size of the patch is an important parameter for the patch based features. For LBP it was observed that the performance of the features improves with an increase in the patch size from 3×3 to 7×7. However, additional sampling points are required in large image patches to capture the intensity variations efficiently. The dimensionality of these descriptors grows exponentially with the number of sampling points considered in the image patch. Therefore, using this encoding scheme, the number of sampling points cannot be increased substantially, which in turn also puts a restriction on the size of the image patch. We aim to study the encoding techniques that can overcome these shortcomings.

2.2 Encoding

The BoW model has been extensively utilized in the texture classification task [10–13]. The main steps in this pipeline are: (1) Extract the features from the texture images, (2) Encode the features into an image descriptor, (3) Classify the image descriptor using a machine learning algorithm (e.g. Nearest Neighbour, Support Vector Machines (SVM)). While most of these papers use different kind of local features to capture the characteristic structure of the texture image, little importance is given to the feature encoding step. All these papers follow the encoding step of the vector quantization and hard assignment. In this step, first, the local features are extracted from the training images and, then exemplar features are chosen as the textons (using K-means clustering). These textons are used to label all the features from the training and the testing images. The local feature quantization, a common step in these approaches, is a lossy step as shown by Boiman [22]. Some attempts have been made to overcome this shortcoming. Farquhar et al. [23] applied soft assignment using Gaussian Mixture Models. Yang, et al. proposed sparse coding algorithm to replace the k-means which reduces the quantization error by applying less restrictive constraints. In this work we consider the Fisher kernel introduced by the Jaakola et al. [24] and applied to image categorization by Sanchez et al. [25]. It is an extension of BoW model as it not only encodes the zero order statistics but also the higher order statistics of the distribution of the local features.

3 Texture Classification

In this section we present the proposed approach for the texture classification. First, we introduce the local features DMD which captures the intensity variation in an image patch. Next, the compressible nature of the dense feature is utilized to reduce its dimensionality. Finally, the local features are combined with the efficient Fisher encoding scheme to obtain the image descriptor.

3.1 Dense Micro-block Difference

The proposed features are based on the idea that the small patches in the texture image exhibit a characteristic structure and if captured efficiently, discriminative information can be obtained from it. Based on the ample evidence from the related work we use the intensity difference from the image patch to capture the variations in it. Furthermore, we believe that the individual pixels are more susceptible to noise and do not capture regional information, therefore we use small blocks in the image patch instead of the raw pixel values.

To encode the local structure of the patch we take the pairwise intensity differences of smaller blocks in the image patch. We address these smaller square blocks as "micro-blocks" and their average intensity is considered for capturing variation in a patch. A image patch is usually of size 9×9 to 15×15 pixels and the micro-blocks are the smaller square region inside this patch. An illustration of the image patch and micro-blocks is provided in Fig. 2. The patch size is 21×21 and the micro-blocks are of sizes 2×2, 3×3 and 4×4. The micro-blocks pairs whose intensity difference is computed are shown color white and grey, and are connected with a line. For the sake of clarity here we show only eight micro-block pairs but in application we consider a much higher number. The high number of micro-block pairs assist in obtaining a rich and discriminative representation for a patch by capturing the variations in different directions and scales. It can be observed that the intensity difference is taken in different directions, unlike the LBP, SRP which only consider the radial direction. Furthermore, the distance between the micro-blocks is not constant, thus, the variations in patch are captured at different scales.

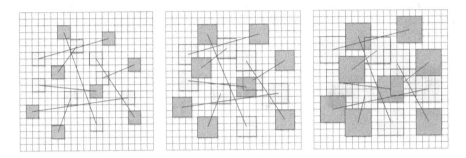

Fig. 2. The micro-blocks pairs in an image patch. Different micro-block sizes are shown (a) 2×2 (b) 3×3 and (c) 4×4.

Formally given a patch p of size $L \times L$ and two sets of image coordinates $X = \{\mathbf{x_1}, \mathbf{x_2}...\mathbf{x_N}\}, Y = \{\mathbf{y_1}, \mathbf{y_2}..., \mathbf{y_N}\}$ the DMD for the micro-blocks of size s is given as:

$$v(p) = \{M_s(\mathbf{x_1}) - M_s(\mathbf{y_1}), M_s(\mathbf{x_2}) - M_s(\mathbf{y_2}), ..., M_s(\mathbf{x_N}) - M_s(\mathbf{y_N})\} \quad (1)$$

where $M_s(\mathbf{x})$ is the average intensity of the pixel in micro-block located at position $\mathbf{x} = (a, b)^T$ in the patch and is given as

$$M_s(a, b) = \sum_{i=0}^{s-1} \sum_{j=0}^{s-1} p(a + i, b + j)/s^2, \quad (2)$$

and $p(a, b)$ denote the pixel intensity in patch p at location a, b.

The feature is completely specified by the following parameters: X, Y, L and s. The coordinate pair sets X and Y determine the location of sampling points in the patch and plays an important role in the design of the descriptor. Colander et al. studied five different spatial arrangements for selecting the sampling point for keypoint matching. We follow the similar approach to Colander et al. [20] and select the coordinates from isotropic Gaussian distribution i.e. $(X, Y) \sim$ i. i. d. $Gaussian(0, L^2/25)$. In this arrangement the coordinates are more densely distributed towards the center of the patch than towards its boundaries. Thus, larger weight is given to the center than to its boundaries, like SIFT features. The randomness in the sampling points coordinates help in capturing the variations at different scales because the distance between the sampling points $|x_i - y_i|$ is not constant. Moreover, we consider the magnitude of the difference without any thresholding, which helps in retaining the discriminative power of the features.

The computation of DMD for a image patch requires subtraction of N micro-blocks pairs. It involves the computation of the sum of the $2N$ micro-block. The micro-blocks sum can be efficiently implemented using the integral images. As summing a block using integral image requires 4 operation, for $2N$ micro-block $4 \times 2 \times N$ operations are required. Further, the computation of a feature requires N subtraction operations. The total number of operations required for a DMD feature computation is $9N$. Therefore, the complexity of the features computation is linear with the number of points considered in the image patch.

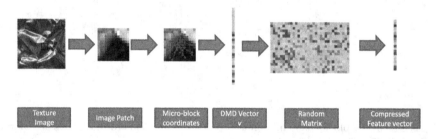

| Texture Image | Image Patch | Micro-block coordinates | DMD Vector v | Random Matrix | Compressed Feature vector |

Fig. 3. Feature extraction from a patch of texture image.

3.2 Utilizing Compressibility

Using the above feature we obtain a N dimensional representation for an image patch. To efficiently capture the intensity variations in the image patch, we select a large number of sampling points which results in high dimensional features. Considering the fact that image patches are sparse in nature, we aim to take advantage of this property of the texture images. To reduce the dimensionality of the vector $v(g)$ and to make it more compressed, we utilize the Random Projections (RP) [26]. The RP exhibit important properties of dimensionality reduction and information preservation. It is based on the idea that if the signal lies in a low dimensional manifold and is represented in a high dimensional ambient space, then, a small number of random projections of that signal preserve most of the information from it.

The random projection of the vector v is defined as:

$$d(g) = \Phi v(g) \tag{3}$$

where Φ is a $C \times N$ matrix, with $C << N$. With $C << N$ a loss in information is expected, however, if the signal is sparse and the matrix Φ exhibits the Restrictive Isometric Property (RIP) then the information is shown to be preserved during this transformation [27]. A number of matrices have shown to exhibit RIP property with high probability [27]. We use Gaussian random matrix as Φ (more details about it are provided in the implementation section). Figure 3 shows feature computation and compression for a single patch from a texture image. First, a patch is selected from the image and the DMD features are extracted using the set of coordinate pairs. Then, the DMD vector is projected using a random matrix to obtain the compressed feature vector. The projection is obtained by multiplying the DMD vector with the random matrix.

The projection using random matrix reduces the dimensionality from N to C. To analyse the impact of feature projection using random matrix on texture classification, we perform a test on the KTH-TIPS-2a dataset. KTH-TIPS-2a is a commonly used texture dataset and we follow the standard test protocol, where half of the images from each class are used for training and rest half for testing. We sample the 64 micro-blocks features from image patch of size 15×15 and apply random projection on it. The reduced dimensionality C is varied from 10 to 50. The classification accuracy is shown in Table 1. It can be observed that the classification accuracy increases with dimensionality of the compressed vector upto a point after which it becomes constant. As the dimensionality increases more information is captured from the features, however after a certain point due to redundancy in the dense DMD features the accuracy stays constant. It is also interesting to note that even with a fairly low dimensionality of 10, high accuracy is achieved. Based on these results, the dimensionality of the compressed feature vector is set to 40 in all our further tests and the number of sampling points are set to 64.

Table 1. Effect of Gaussian component on the accuracy of KTH-TIPS-2a dataset.

Dimension	10	20	30	40	50	No RP
Accuracy	76.83 %	77.23 %	77.87 %	78.54 %	77.67 %	77.31 %

3.3 Encoding

After computing the local features, we obtain a feature vector for each patch. Since we compute the features densely from an image, we get thousands of feature vector for an image. The features from a image have to be encoded to obtain a descriptor. Most of the early work on texture classification use the quantization/hard assignment for this purpose, however it leads to quantization error. Instead we use soft quantization by representing the feature distribution using Fisher Vector. It uses generative models for feature extraction by representing data by means of the gradient of the data log-likelihood w.r.t. the model parameters. The Fisher Vector use the Gaussian Mixture Models (GMM) to derive a probabilistic representation of the compressed features. The encoding captures the first and the second order differences between the image descriptors and the GMM centres. The higher order statistics that are learnt, provide a robust representation compared to other encoding methods such as histograms and kernel codebook.

The local features are modelled using GMM which is defined as:

$$p(\mathbf{d}|\theta) = \sum_{k=1}^{K} p(\mathbf{d}|\mu_k, \Sigma_k)\pi_k \tag{4}$$

where, $p(\mathbf{d}|\mu_k, \Sigma_k)$ is the multivariate Gaussian distribution with mean, μ_k, and covariance matrix, Σ_k, (assumed to be diagonal), π_k is the mixing coefficient of the Gaussian components and $\theta = (\pi_1, \mu_1, \Sigma_1 ... \pi_K, \mu_K, \Sigma_K)$ is the vector of the parameters for the model. K is the total number of Gaussian components assumed to be present while modelling the feature distribution. The parameters of the GMM are learned using Expectation Maximization (EM) using the features from the training samples.

Given the model, Fisher Vector is characterized by the gradient with respect to the parameter of the models. Thus, the gradient is computed with respect to the mean μ_k and the covariance Σ_k of the GMM. It is given as:

$$\frac{\partial \log p(\mathbf{d}|\theta)}{\partial \mu_k} = h_k \Sigma_k^{-1}(\mathbf{d} - \mu_k), \tag{5}$$

$$\frac{\partial \log p(\mathbf{d}|\theta)}{\partial \Sigma_k^{-1}} = \frac{h_k}{2}(\Sigma_k - (\mathbf{d} - \mu_k)^2), \tag{6}$$

where,

$$h_k = \frac{\pi_k p(\mathbf{d}|\mu_k, \Sigma_k)}{\sum_k \pi_k p(\mathbf{d}|\mu_k, \Sigma_k)}. \tag{7}$$

The Fisher encoding is obtained by concatenating the parametric gradient for all the K components of the GMM. Thus, the length of the feature vector is 2KC, where C is the dimensionality of the compressed features. After concatenation, we apply $l2$ and power normalization [25] on the feature vectors. The $l2$ normalization helps in compensating for the fact that different images contain different amount of relevant information. The power normalization ($z \leftarrow sign(z)|z|^\rho$) helps to 'unsparsify' the feature vector that becomes sparse when the number of Gaussian components in GMM are increased.

4   Experiments

To analyse the performance of the proposed descriptor, we conduct extensive experiments on three standard publicly available texture datasets: KTH-TIPS-2a, Brodatz and CUReT. We follow the standard protocol for testing.

The KTH-TIPS2-a texture dataset [1] contains 11 texture classes (e.g. cork, wool, linen, etc.) with 4,395 images. The images are 256×256 pixels in size, and they are transformed into 256 gray levels. Each texture class consists of images from four different samples. The images for each sample are taken at nine scales, under four different illumination directions, and three different poses. The variations in scales, illumination and pose makes it a challenging dataset.

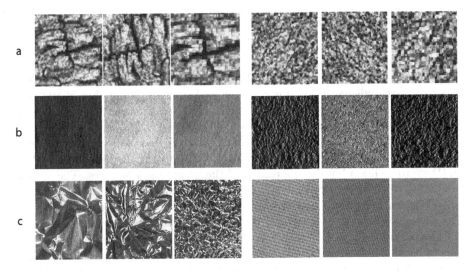

Fig. 4. The samples image from three different datasets, (a) Brodatz, (b) CUReT and (c) KTH-TIPS-2a.

We use the standard testing protocol [1, 28] where at each run the three sample sets are used for training and fourth samples images for testing.

The original Brodatz dataset [29] has 32 texture classes with 16 images per class. The images are of dimension 64 × 64. To make the test more challenging, three samples are generated from each image by (1) rotating (2) scaling and (3) both rotating and scaling the original images. The resulting images are resized to 200 × 200 pixels, converted to grayscale and histogram normalized. Therefore, the final test set-up consists of 2048 images with 64 images in each class. Following the usual protocol in our experiment [28], we randomly select 32 images from each class for training and rest are used for testing. The accuracy is reported on 5 fold cross validation.

CUReT database [30] consist of 61 classes each containing 205 images taken under range of viewing and lighting angles. Following the usual protocol we select only 92 images per class which afford the extraction of 200 × 200 pixels foreground region of a texture. It is a challenging set for classification because of intra-class variation in appearance resulting from the different illumination conditions. In our tests we varied the number of training samples in this dataset to observe the effect of varying number of training samples on the performance.

The samples images from these datasets are shown in Fig. 4. It shows three different images from two different classes of each dataset.

First, we provide details about our implementation, then, we study the effect of certain parameters involved in the descriptor on classification performance. Finally, we compare the obtained results with state-of-the-art approaches.

4.1   Implementation Details

The DMD features are extracted from the grid with a spacing of 3 pixels. It is observed that the performance of the features is maintained as long as the size of the grid does not exceed 5 pixels. With a larger grid size, the local structure is not captured efficiently and for a denser grid spacing the number of features becomes too large with no significant increase in performance. The number of sampling pairs in all our experiments is fixed to 64.

The matrix Φ is a Gaussian random matrix that is normalized to zero mean and unit variance. It is of dimension $C \times N$, where N is the dimension of the DMD vector while C is the dimension of the compressed features. The values of C is set to 40 in our experiments. The GMM parameters are estimated using 500,000 feature vectors that are randomly sampled from the training images. The center for GMM are initialized with k-mean clustering.

The parameter ρ is set to 0.5 for the power normalization. In all our experiments SVM classifier with linear kernels is used. The linear SVM requires less training time over types of kernels, during the testing it only requires a simple dot product. Another advantage of the linear kernel is that it directly operates on the feature, thus any improvement in the classification performance can be attributed to the features rather than the classifier.

Table 2. Recognition rate for KTH-TIPS-2a dataset

Micro-block size	Patch size			
	9×9	11×11	13×13	15×15
1×1	73.45 %	74.75 %	73.99 %	74.10 %
2×2	76.62 %	76.69 %	77.71 %	76.63 %
3×3	76.24 %	77.55 %	78.04 %	78.02 %
4×4	76.91 %	77.89 %	77.90 %	78.43 %
5×5	75.03 %	76.70 %	77.58 %	**78.54%**

4.2   Patch and Micro-block Size

In the proposed approach the information is being captured at two levels, first is the patch level and the other is the micro-blocks level. When we increase the micro-block size, the overlap between them also increases as shown in Fig. 2. If the patch size is small it would lead to repetitive overlap of the micro-blocks and consequently results in redundant and correlated features. Therefore the patch size should be big enough to allow sufficient degree of spatial freedom to micro-blocks. Since the patch size and micro-block size are dependent on each other, we vary these parameters jointly in our experiments. The size of the patch is varied from 9×9 to 15×15 with a step size of 2 and the micro-block size is varied from 1 to 5. The tests are performed on KTH-TIPS-2a and Brodatz dataset. The results for both these datasets are shown in Tables 2 and 3.

It can be observed from the results that for both these datasets there is an increase in the accuracy with an increase in the patch and micro-block size. The accuracy improves with increase in the micro-block size specially for large patch sizes. The observation supports our claim that the micro-block are more efficient element for capturing the information than pixels.

Table 3. Recognition rate for Brodatz dataset

Micro-block size	Patch size			
	9×9	11×11	13×13	15×15
1×1	98.96 %	99.24 %	99.22 %	99.24 %
2×2	98.71 %	99.18 %	**99.32%**	99.26 %
3×3	98.81 %	99.12 %	99.18 %	98.98 %
4×4	98.30 %	98.89 %	98.81 %	98.59 %
5×5	96.82 %	98.05 %	98.20 %	98.32 %

4.3 Number of Gaussian Components

The number of Gaussian Components used for modelling the features distribution plays an important role in the encoding step. With more Gaussian components the distribution can be modelled in a suitable manner, but, it also leads to an increase in the dimensionality. To analyse its role, we varied the number of components from 32 to 128 with the step size of 32 and performed the classification test on the KTH-TIPS-2a dataset. The accuracy for the dataset is shown in Table 4. As expected there is an increase in the accuracy with more Gaussian components due to better modelling of local features, however after a point the accuracy stays constant. Based on the results from these experiments in all our tests we use 128 Gaussian components. The Gaussian components can be further increased, however it will also result in an increase in the dimensionality of the descriptor, without any significant increase in the performance.

Table 4. Effect of Gaussian component on the accuracy of KTH-TIPS-2a dataset.

Gaussian component	32	64	96	128
Accuracy	76.26 %	77.19 %	77.89 %	78.54 %

4.4 Varying Number of Samples

We study the effect of different number of training samples on the proposed approach. To evaluate the performance, we conduct tests by varying the number of training samples in the CUReT dataset. We follow the protocol of [31], where the three different training scenarios are used. The number of training samples is set to 46, 23 and 3, while the rest of the images are used for testing. The block size for DMD is set to 13×13 and the micro-block size is fixed to 3×3. The results are shown in Table 5. The classification performance is compared with LBP, LBPV [14], LBPHF [32], MR8 [12], BIF [13] and recently proposed M-BIMF [31]. As expected, the performance drops with the less training samples. However, it is interesting to observe that accuracy decreases only by a few percents when samples are reduced from 46 to 23, however when the samples reduce to 3 from 23 the drop in accuracy is between 30 to 40 percent. It shows that with the 23 training samples the texture can be modelled considerable well, although it is not the case with 3 samples.

The proposed approach achieves the highest accuracy when the training samples are 46 and 3. When the number of samples is 23 then we achieve 93.66, which is second only to the M-BIMF features proposed recently. Even with the three samples we achieve an accuracy of 66.76 which is significantly higher than LBP, MR8, LBPHF methods.

Table 5. Recognition rate for CUReT dataset

Method	T_{46}	T_{23}	T_3
LBP	87.91	87.54	51.30
LBPV	78.83	73.71	42.03
LBP-HF	88.77	87.54	57.04
M-LBP	94.79	93.87	60.97
MR8	93.52	91.48	58.68
BIF	95.81	91.95	66.40
M-BIMF	95.62	**94.59**	65.11
Proposed	**97.32**	93.66	**66.76**

4.5 Comparison with State-of-the-art

In this section we compare our results on the Brodatz and KTH-TIPS-2a with a number of state-of-the-art texture classification approaches. The algorithms used for comparison are LBP, LTP, Local Quantized Patterns (LQP) [33], Weber Law Descriptor (WLD) [28], Caputo et al. [1] and Local Higher order Statistics (LHS) [19]. The LBP and LTP are computed by the binary and ternary thresholding of the pixel difference in the local circular neighbourhood and use histogram as the encoding method. LQP is also a pattern based descriptor, however the number of patterns sampled are very large, which are quantized using k-mean clustering. LHS performs the Fisher encoding of the pixel difference with LBP like geometry. WLD captures the local pattern from the gradient images. The results of all these approaches on the Brodatz and KTH-TIPS-2a dataset are shown in Table 6.

Table 6. Recognition rate for Brodatz and KTH-TIPS-2a datasets.

Method	KTH-TIPS-2a	Brodatz
WLD	64.7	97.5 ± 0.6
LQP	64.2	96.9
LBP	69.8 ± 6.9	87.2 ± 1.5
LTP	71.3 ± 5.3	95.0 ± 0.8
Caputo et al. [1]	71.0	-
LHS	73.0 ± 5.7	$\mathbf{99.3 \pm 0.3}$
Proposed	$\mathbf{78.5 \pm 4.6}$	$\mathbf{99.3 \pm 0.5}$

It can be observed from the results that the proposed features achieves the best results on KTH-TIPS-2a dataset. This is the highest accuracy reported on the KTH-TIPS-2a dataset to the best of our knowledge. It is interesting to note that the accuracy is still far from being perfect even for the best results. The first reason is that the variations in this dataset are much stronger than other texture datasets such as Brodatz, etc., for which nearly perfect accuracy can be achieved. Another reason for a lower accuracy on this dataset is the testing protocol for this dataset. Since the three samples are used for training and the fourth sample for testing, there is a considerable difference between the training and the testing images. The images from the three samples for two texture class are shown in Fig. 4. It can be seen that there is a significant difference in the images. Thus, to perform on this dataset the algorithm should have a generalization property. The high recognition rate of the proposed algorithm shows that it also has a generalization property and can easily adapt to the variations during training and testing.

The comparison of the accuracies on KTH-TIPS-2a, shows that the LBP and LTP are inferior to the state-of-the-art descriptor LHS. LTP achieves higher accuracy than LBP because it has three quantization levels compared to two levels of LBP. Since LHS has even more quantization levels than LTP, there is a further increase in the performance from LTP to LHS. Therefore, we can infer that with more quantization levels the pixel difference is modelled in a better way, hence an improvement in performance is observed. Although DMD and LHS both have same number of quantization levels, the gain of DMD over LHS can be attributed to the fact that DMD captures the information from the patches at the multiple scales rather than the single scale that is used in LHS. Also the compressed vectors of DMD, by means of random projection, capture the inherent structure of the patch in an effective way. The proposed method outperforms the LBP, LTP by 8.7 %, 7.2 % respectively. Compared to state-of-the-art descriptors, WLD, Caputo et al. [1] and LHS the proposed approach shows a significant improvement of 13.8 %, and 7.5 % and 5.5 % respectively.

For Brodatz dataset a near perfect recognition rate is shown by the LHS and DMD descriptors, which achieve more than 99 %. The proposed approach gains by more than 12 % over LBP and by 3 % over WLD. It can be seen that for Brodatz dataset all the descriptors achieve better recognition rate compared to the KTH-TIPS-2a dataset. The variation between the training and the testing samples are not as high as the previous dataset as the samples for both are taken from similar image samples. It is easier to model the texture samples and moreover it does not require the generalization property.

An important advantage of the DMD is its speed. We compare the computation time of DMD with the SIFT features. SIFT and other gradient based features are very frequently used for texture classification. The computation time for the DMD features for an image from KTH-TIPS-2a dataset is 0.28 s. For the same setting the computation time of the SIFT features is 25.67 s on a standard computer. The SIFT features are also densely computed with a grid of 3×3 pixels. The computation times for SIFT features is almost 100 times more than the DMD features, which make the proposed feature favourable for the real time applications.

5   Conclusion

We presented a novel approach for texture classification based on block based features and Fisher Vector encoding. The proposed DMD features capture the local structure from texture images with the help of micro-blocks. These are very fast to compute, easy to implement and discriminative in nature. When combined with efficient coding technique we obtain a robust texture descriptor. The tests performed on challenging datasets demonstrated the efficiency of the proposed approach.

Acknowledgement. The research leading to this paper partially received funding from TUT project Big Data 83255.

References

1. Hayman, E., Caputo, B., Fritz, M., Eklundh, J.-O.: On the significance of real-world conditions for material classification. In: Pajdla, T., Matas, J.G. (eds.) ECCV 2004. LNCS, vol. 3024, pp. 253–266. Springer, Heidelberg (2004)
2. Ahonen, T., Hadid, A., Pietikainen, M.: Face description with local binary patterns: application to face recognition. IEEE Trans. Pattern Anal. Mach. Intell. **28**, 2037–2041 (2006)
3. Shan, C., Gong, S., McOwan, P.W.: Facial expression recognition based on local binary patterns: a comprehensive study. Image Vis. Comput. **27**, 803–816 (2009)
4. Trefný, J., Matas, J.: Extended set of local binary patterns for rapid object detection. In: Proceedings of the Computer Vision Winter Workshop, vol. 2010 (2010)
5. Haralick, R.M., Shanmugam, K., Dinstein, I.H.: Textural features for image classification. IEEE Trans. Syst. Man Cybern. **3**, 610–621 (1973)
6. Cross, G.R., Jain, A.K.: Markov random field texture models. IEEE Trans. Pattern Anal. Mach. Intell. **5**, 25–39 (1983)

7. Bovik, A.C., Clark, M., Geisler, W.S.: Multichannel texture analysis using localized spatial filters. IEEE Trans. Pattern Anal. Mach. Intell. **12**, 55–73 (1990)

8. Ojala, T., Pietikainen, M., Maenpaa, T.: Multiresolution gray-scale and rotation invariant texture classification with local binary patterns. IEEE Trans. Pattern Anal. Mach. Intell. **24**, 971–987 (2002)

9. Xu, Y., Ji, H., Fermüller, C.: Viewpoint invariant texture description using fractal analysis. Int. J. Comput. Vision **83**, 85–100 (2009)

10. Lazebnik, S., Schmid, C., Ponce, J.: A sparse texture representation using local affine regions. IEEE Trans. Pattern Anal. Mach. Intell. **27**, 1265–1278 (2005)

11. Zhang, J., Marszałek, M., Lazebnik, S., Schmid, C.: Local features and kernels for classification of texture and object categories: a comprehensive study. Int. J. Comput. Vision **73**, 213–238 (2007)

12. Varma, M., Zisserman, A.: A statistical approach to texture classification from single images. Int. J. Comput. Vision **62**, 61–81 (2005)

13. Crosier, M., Griffin, L.D.: Using basic image features for texture classification. Int. J. Comput. Vision **88**, 447–460 (2010)

14. Guo, Z., Zhang, L., Zhang, D.: Rotation invariant texture classification using LBP variance (LBPV) with global matching. Pattern Recogn. **43**, 706–719 (2010)

15. Mehta, R., Egiazarian, K.: Rotated local binary pattern (RLBP) - rotation invariant texture descriptor. In: ICPRAM, pp. 497–502 (2013)

16. Tan, X., Triggs, B.: Enhanced local texture feature sets for face recognition under difficult lighting conditions. IEEE Trans. Image Process. **19**, 1635–1650 (2010)

17. Guo, Z., Zhang, D.: A completed modeling of local binary pattern operator for texture classification. IEEE Trans. Image Process. **19**, 1657–1663 (2010)

18. Liu, L., Fieguth, P., Kuang, G., Zha, H.: Sorted random projections for robust texture classification. In: 2011 IEEE International Conference on Computer Vision (ICCV), pp. 391–398. IEEE (2011)

19. Sharma, G., ul Hussain, S., Jurie, F.: Local higher-order statistics (LHS) for texture categorization and facial analysis. In: Fitzgibbon, A., Lazebnik, S., Perona, P., Sato, Y., Schmid, C. (eds.) ECCV 2012, Part VII. LNCS, vol. 7578, pp. 1–12. Springer, Heidelberg (2012)

20. Calonder, M., Lepetit, V., Strecha, C., Fua, P.: BRIEF: binary robust independent elementary features. In: Daniilidis, K., Maragos, P., Paragios, N. (eds.) ECCV 2010, Part IV. LNCS, vol. 6314, pp. 778–792. Springer, Heidelberg (2010)

21. Rublee, E., Rabaud, V., Konolige, K., Bradski, G.: ORB: an efficient alternative to sift or surf. In: 2011 IEEE International Conference on Computer Vision (ICCV), pp. 2564–2571. IEEE (2011)

22. Boiman, O., Shechtman, E., Irani, M.: In defense of nearest-neighbor based image classification. In: IEEE Conference on Computer Vision and Pattern Recognition, 2008, CVPR 2008, pp. 1–8. IEEE (2008)

23. Farquhar, J., Szedmak, S., Meng, H., Shawe-Taylor, J.: Improving "bag-of-keypoints" image categorisation: generative models and PDF-kernels (2005)

24. Jaakkola, T., Haussler, D., et al.: Exploiting generative models in discriminative classifiers. In: Advances in Neural Information Processing Systems, pp. 487–493 (1999)

25. Sánchez, J., Perronnin, F., Mensink, T., Verbeek, J.: Image classification with the fisher vector: theory and practice. Int. J. Comput. Vision **105**, 222–245 (2013)

26. Donoho, D.L.: Compressed sensing. IEEE Trans. Inf. Theor. **52**, 1289–1306 (2006)

27. Candes, E.J., Tao, T.: Decoding by linear programming. IEEE Trans. Inf. Theor. **51**, 4203–4215 (2005)

28. Chen, J., Shan, S., He, C., Zhao, G., Pietikainen, M., Chen, X., Gao, W.: WLD: a robust local image descriptor. IEEE Trans. Pattern Anal. Mach. Intell. **32**, 1705–1720 (2010)
29. Valkealahti, K., Oja, E.: Reduced multidimensional co-occurrence histograms in texture classification. IEEE Trans. Pattern Anal. Mach. Intell. **20**, 90–94 (1998)
30. Dana, K.J., Van Ginneken, B., Nayar, S.K., Koenderink, J.J.: Reflectance and texture of real-world surfaces. ACM Trans. Graph. (TOG) **18**, 1–34 (1999)
31. Pan, J.J., Tang, Y.Y.: Texture classification based on BIMF monogenic signals. In: Lee, K.M., Matsushita, Y., Rehg, J.M., Hu, Z. (eds.) ACCV 2012, Part II. LNCS, vol. 7725, pp. 177–187. Springer, Heidelberg (2013)
32. Ahonen, T., Matas, J., He, C., Pietikäinen, M.: Rotation invariant image description with local binary pattern histogram fourier features. In: Salberg, A.-B., Hardeberg, J.Y., Jenssen, R. (eds.) SCIA 2009. LNCS, vol. 5575, pp. 61–70. Springer, Heidelberg (2009)
33. Hussain, S., Triggs, B.: Visual recognition using local quantized patterns. In: Fitzgibbon, A., Lazebnik, S., Perona, P., Sato, Y., Schmid, C. (eds.) ECCV 2012, Part II. LNCS, vol. 7573, pp. 716–729. Springer, Heidelberg (2012)

Nuclear-L_1 Norm Joint Regression for Face Reconstruction and Recognition

Lei Luo, Jian Yang$^{(\boxtimes)}$, Jianjun Qian, and Ying Tai

Nanjing University of Science and Technology,
Nanjing 210094, People's Republic of China
csjyang@njust.edu.cn

Abstract. Recognizing a face with significant lighting, disguise and occlusion variations is an interesting and challenging problem in pattern recognition. To address this problem, many regression based methods, represented by sparse representation classifier (SRC), are presented recently. SRC uses the L_1-norm to characterize the pixel-level sparse noise but ignore the spatial information of noise. In this paper, we find that nuclear-norm is good for characterizing image-wise structural noise, and thus we use the nuclear norm and L_1-norm to jointly characterize the error image in regression model. Our experimental results demonstrate that the proposed method is more effective than state-of-the-art regression methods for face reconstruction and recognition.

1 Introduction

Face recognition is closely related to our life, which has been applied widely to information security, law enforcement and surveillance, smart cards, access control, etc. However, recognizing a face with significant lighting, disguiseand occlusion variations is still a challenging problem in pattern recognition.

Recently, a number of methods have been developed to address this problem. Among them, sparse Representation Coding (SRC) [1] is the most attractive and receiving more and more attention. In fact, SRC can be considered as a generalization of nearest feature classifiers, which strikes a balance between NN [2] and NFS [3]. Differing from these classifiers, the representation of SRC is global, using all the training data as a dictionary, and the classification is performed by checking which class yields the least coding error. Because of its simplicity and effectiveness, SRC has been applied and investigated extensively. In order to further improve the robustness of sparse coding, an extended SRC [4] and some re-weighted L_1 or L_2 minimization algorithms [5,6] were presented. Zhang et al. [7] have shown that it is the collaborative representation (CR) but not the L_1-norm sparse constraint that truly improves the FR performance. Yang et al. [8] re-examined the role of L_1-optimizer and found that for pattern recognition tasks, L_1-optimizer provides more meaningful classification information (e.g. closeness) than L_0-optimizer does. Meanwhile, integrating sparse coding with other methods is also a meaningful effort. For example, Yang et al. [9] proposed sparse representation classifier steered discriminative projection. Zheng et al. [10] performed SRC in low rank projection with discrimination.

© Springer International Publishing Switzerland 2015
D. Cremers et al. (Eds.): ACCV 2014, Part II, LNCS 9004, pp. 659–673, 2015.
DOI: 10.1007/978-3-319-16808-1_44

The characterization of the residual term plays a key role in regression model based face recognition Methods. Linear regression based classifier (LRC) [11] uses L_2- norm to characterize the coding residual, while SRC uses L_1- norm. Yang et al. [12] presented robust sparse coding (RSC), which uses an M-estimator to fit the general noises. He et al. [13] proposed a correntropy based sparse representation (CESR) scheme by virtue of the correntropy induced metric for describing residual. Essentially, the core idea of Yang et al. [12] and He et al. [13] is to use a robust estimator to generate the new variables in accordance with the known distributions. Li et al. [14] explored the structure of the error incurred by occlusion and measured errors by the weighted L_1 metric. K. Jia et al. [15] introduced a class of structured sparsity-inducing norms into the SRC framework to fit these structural noises. Yang et al. [16] used nuclear norm to describe the residual term and proposed a nuclear norm based matrix regression (NMR) model, which has been shown that NMR is robust to face recognition with occlusion and illumination changes.

From the probability distribution point of view, we know that L_1-norm provides an optimal characterization for errors with the Laplace distribution. Therefore, SRC (with L_1-norm) generally performs well for the sparse noise which on the whole follows the Laplace distribution. However, in practice, some noises caused by occlusions, disguise or illumination does not follow Laplacian distribution (see the example in Fig.1). Thus, L_1-norm is not enough for error characterization. In this paper, we find that the singular values of the error image fit Laplace distribution well in real-world disguises, occlusions, or illumination induced error images. Thus, we can use L_1-norm of the singular value vector, i.e., nuclear norm of the error image, to characterize this kind of structural noises. To handle the pixel-level sparse noise and image-level structural noise together, we will use two norms, i.e., nuclear norm and L_1-norm, to jointly characterize the error image in our regression model.

The proposed nuclear-L_1 norm joint regression model can be solved by using alternating direction method of multipliers (ADMM). In each step of the algorithm, a closed-form solution can be obtained by fixing the other variables. In general, the complexity of the proposed algorithm is much lower than SRC or RSC. In addition, nuclear norm is used as a metric to characterize the distance between test samples and classes, which is different from the previous methods using of the Euclidean (L_2)-norm. We perform experiments on the Extended Yale B and AR databases, the results demonstrate that the proposed method is more effective than state-of-the-art regression methods for face reconstruction and recognition.

The remainder of this paper is structured as follows: In Sect. 2, we first introduce our model, i.e., the nuclear-L_1 norm joint regression (NL_1R) model. In Sect. 3, we solve the proposed model by virtue of ADMM. In Sect. 4, we study the complexity of our algorithm. In Sect. 5, we design the NL_1R based classifier. In Sect. 6, we present a series of experiments to demonstrate the robustness effectiveness of the proposed algorithm. In Sect. 7, we conclude the paper with a brief conclusion.

2 Problem Formulation

Given a set of n observed 2D data matrices $\mathbf{A}_1, \cdots, \mathbf{A}_n \in R^{p \times q}$ and a matrix $\mathbf{D} \in R^{p \times q}$, let us represent $\mathbf{B}$ linearly using $\mathbf{A}_1, \cdots, \mathbf{A}_n$, i.e., $\mathbf{D} = x_1 \mathbf{A}_1 + x_2 \mathbf{A}_2 +, \cdots, + x_n \mathbf{A}_n + \mathbf{E}$, where $x_1, x_2, \cdots, x_n$ is a set of representation coefficients, $x_1 \mathbf{A}_1 + x_2 \mathbf{A}_2 +, \cdots, + x_n \mathbf{A}_n$ is the reconstructed image and $\mathbf{E}$ is the representation residual. Let us denote the following linear mapping from R^n to $R^{p \times q}$: $A(\mathbf{x}) = x_1 \mathbf{A}_1 + x_2 \mathbf{A}_2 +, \cdots, + x_n \mathbf{A}_n$, where $\mathbf{x} = [x_1, x_2, \cdots, x_n]^T$. Then, we will consider the following model

$$\min_{\mathbf{E}, \mathbf{x}} \|\mathbf{E}\| \quad \text{s.t.} \quad A(\mathbf{x}) - \mathbf{D} = \mathbf{E}, \tag{1}$$

where $\|\cdot\|$ is a norm.

It is crucial that which norm should be chosen to characterize the error matrix $\mathbf{E}$ better. It's well-known that if errors are independently and identically distributed with Laplacian(or Gaussian), then L_1(or L_2)-norm is optimal for characterizing the errors (a proof is in [12]). This means there must exist some close relationship between the error (or residual) metric and error distribution. Figure 1(a) shows an original image with scarf. One can decompose (a) into the recovered term (b) and noise term (c). Figure 2(a) delineates the empirical and fitted distributions of noise term $\mathbf{E}$ by using Gaussian or Laplacian distribution model. We can see that Gaussian and Laplacian distribution are far away from the empirical distribution. So, L_2-norm (or L_1-norm) based method can not describe the noise matrix effectively. Instead, Fig. 2(b) shows that singular values of noise matrix $\mathbf{E}$ follow Laplacian distribution well. And this trend becomes more stable and evident with the increase of the size of images. In addition, for other noises caused by occlusion and illumination, we obtain the similar result.

Thus, it's reasonable that we assume that the singular values of error matrix are independently and identically distributed with Laplacian distribution, i.e.,

$$\delta_i \sim p_\theta(\delta_i) = \frac{1}{2b} \exp(-|\delta_i - \mu|/b), \tag{2}$$

where $\delta_1 \geq \delta_2 \geq \cdots \geq \delta_n$ are the all singular values of error matrix $\mathbf{E}$, $\theta = (\mu, b)$. Thus, the likelihood function of the estimator is that

$$\prod_{i=1}^{n} p_\theta(\delta_i) = \frac{1}{(2b)^n} \exp(-\sum_{i=1}^{n} |\delta_i - \mu|/b). \tag{3}$$

By taking the logarithm, we obtain that

$$\ln \prod_{i=1}^{n} p_\theta(\delta_i) = -\sum_{i=1}^{n} |\delta_i - \mu|/b + \ln \frac{1}{(2b)^n}. \tag{4}$$

For convenience, we can assume $\mu = 0$, $b = 1$. According to the maximum likelihood criterion, we need to maximizing $\ln \prod_{i=1}^{n} p_\theta(\delta_i)$, which is equal to minimizing

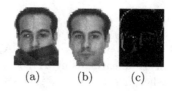

(a)   (b)   (c)

Fig. 1. (a) Original image; (b) recovered image; (c) noise image **E**

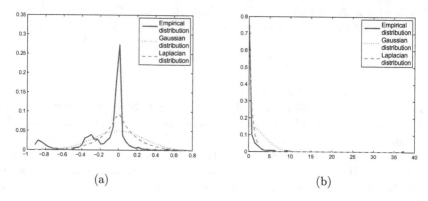

(a)   (b)

Fig. 2. (a) The empirical distribution and the fitted distribution of the noise image **E**; (b) The empirical distribution and the fitted distribution of the singular value vector of noise image **E**

$\sum_{i=1}^{n} |\delta_i|$, thus,

$$\min \sum_{i=1}^{n} |\delta_i| = \min |\boldsymbol{\delta}|_1 = \min \|\mathbf{E}\|_*. \qquad (5)$$

Therefore, under this assumption, nuclear norm can be chosen as a proper descriptor to characterize structural noises. Certainly, for some sparse noises, which follow Laplacian distribution, the L_1-norm is an optimal choice. In order to keep the advantage of L_1-norm, we can use L_1-norm as a regularized term to further improve the performance of nuclear norm, which yields the following model:

$$\min_{\mathbf{E},\mathbf{x}} \|\mathbf{E}\|_* + \alpha \|\mathbf{E}\|_1, \quad \text{s.t.} \quad A(\mathbf{x}) - \mathbf{D} = \mathbf{E}, \qquad (6)$$

where $\alpha > 0$ is a parameter. It is used to balance the nuclear norm and L_1-norm.

The advantage of this method is that the metric based on different norms can complement each other long for short, which prevents the limitation of the single metric. Thus, the collaborative effect of nuclear-L_1 norm will be suitable for characterizing the reconstruction error (or the difference between occluded face image and its ground truth) if we choose a proper parameter α. In Sect. 6, we will further see that the joint use of two norms is robust for the characterization of noises, and this method will fit more complicated noises.

Furthermore, borrowing the idea of the ridge regression, we would like to add a similar regularization term to Eq. (6) and obtain the regularized matrix regression model based on nuclear-L_1 norm:

$$\min_{\mathbf{E},\mathbf{x}} \|\mathbf{E}\|_* + \alpha\|\mathbf{E}\|_1 + \frac{1}{2}\beta\|\mathbf{x}\|_2^2, \quad \text{s.t.} \ \ \mathrm{A}(\mathbf{x}) - \mathbf{D} = \mathbf{E}. \tag{7}$$

The new objective function is non-smooth, but continuous and convex. For the convenience, we introduce an auxiliary variable $\mathbf{Z}$ for the splitting, thus, (7) is converted to the following equivalent problem:

$$\min_{\mathbf{E},\mathbf{Z},\mathbf{x}} \|\mathbf{E}\|_* + \alpha\|\mathbf{Z}\|_1 + \frac{1}{2}\beta\|\mathbf{x}\|_2^2, \quad \text{s.t.} \ \ \mathrm{A}(\mathbf{x}) - \mathbf{D} = \mathbf{E}, \ \mathbf{E} = \mathbf{Z}. \tag{8}$$

In (8), the new constraint $\mathbf{E} = \mathbf{Z}$ guarantees the identity of $\mathbf{E}$ and $\mathbf{Z}$, thus, $\mathbf{Z}$ can be regarded as a proxy for $\mathbf{E}$. We will discuss how to solve this model in the following section.

3 Proposed Algorithm

The alternating direction method of multipliers (ADMM) or the augmented La-grange multipliers (ALM) method was presented originally in [17,18], which has been studied extensively in the theoretical frameworks of Lagrangian functions [19]. Recently, ADMM has been applied to the nuclear norm optimization problems [20,21], which updates the variables alternately by minimizing the augmented Lagrangian function with respect to the variables in a Gauss-Seidel manner. Here, we provide the process of using ADMM to solve the problem (8), which is equal to minimizing the following augmented Lagrangian function:

$$\begin{aligned}
L_\mu = \quad & \|\mathbf{E}\|_* + \alpha\|\mathbf{Z}\|_1 + \frac{1}{2}\beta\|\mathbf{x}\|_2^2 + tr\left(\mathbf{Y}_1^T\left(\mathrm{A}(\mathbf{x}) - \mathbf{D} - \mathbf{E}\right)\right) \\
& + tr\left(\mathbf{Y}_2^T\left(\mathbf{E} - \mathbf{Z}\right)\right) + \frac{\mu}{2}\left(\|\mathrm{A}(\mathbf{x}) - \mathbf{D} - \mathbf{E}\|_F^2 + \|\mathbf{E} - \mathbf{Z}\|_F^2\right),
\end{aligned} \tag{9}$$

where μ is a penalty parameter, $\mathbf{Y}_1$ and $\mathbf{Y}_2$ are the Lagrange multipliers. We proceed by alternately fixing one variable and solving for the other, and iterating. Then, the detailed algorithm for solving nuclear-L_1 norm joint regression ($\mathrm{N}L_1\mathrm{R}$) model is summarized in Algorithm 1.

The key steps are to solve the optimization problems in step 2, 3 and 4. For step 4, by taking the derivative w.r.t $\mathbf{x}$ for the objective function, and setting the derivative to zero, we have the optimal solution of the sub-problem in step 4:

$$\mathbf{x} = (\mu\mathbf{M}^T\mathbf{M} + \beta\mathbf{I})^{-1}\mathbf{M}^T\mathrm{Vec}(\mu\mathbf{D} + \mu\mathbf{E} - \mathbf{Z}_1), \tag{10}$$

where $\mathbf{M} = [\mathrm{Vec}(\mathbf{A}_1), \cdots, \mathrm{Vec}(\mathbf{A}_n)]$, Vec is an operator converting a matrix into a vector.

Algorithm 1. Solving NL_1R by ADMM

Input: A set of matrices $\mathbf{A}_1, \cdots, \mathbf{A}_n$ and a matrix $\mathbf{D} \in R^{p \times q}$, the model parameters α, β and the value of μ.

while not converged **do**

1. Initialize $\mathbf{Z} = \mathbf{Y_1} = \mathbf{Y_2} = 0$, $\mathbf{x} = 0$;

2. fix the others and update $\mathbf{E}$ by

$$\mathbf{E} = \arg\min_{\mathbf{E}} \frac{1}{\mu}\|\mathbf{E}\|_* + \frac{1}{2}\left(\left\|\mathbf{E} - \left(A\left(\mathbf{x}\right) - \mathbf{D} + \frac{1}{\mu}\mathbf{Y_1}\right)\right\|_F^2 + \left\|\mathbf{E} - \left(\mathbf{Z} - \frac{1}{\mu}\mathbf{Y_2}\right)\right\|_F^2\right);$$

3. fix the others and update $\mathbf{Z}$ by

$$\mathbf{Z} = \arg\min_{Z} \frac{\alpha}{\mu}\|\mathbf{Z}\|_1 + \frac{1}{2}\left\|\mathbf{Z} - \left(\mathbf{E} + \frac{1}{\mu}\mathbf{Y_2}\right)\right\|_F^2;$$

4. fix the others and update $\mathbf{x}$ by

$$\mathbf{x} = \arg\min_{\mathbf{x}} \frac{1}{2}\beta\|\mathbf{x}\|_2^2 + \frac{\mu}{2}\left\|A\left(\mathbf{x}\right) - \mathbf{D} - \mathbf{E} + \frac{1}{\mu}\mathbf{Y_1}\right\|_F^2;$$

5. update the multipliers $\mathbf{Y}_1 = \mathbf{Y}_1 + \mu\left(A\left(\mathbf{x}\right) - \mathbf{D} - \mathbf{E}\right)$ and $\mathbf{Y}_2 = \mathbf{Y}_2 + \mu\left(\mathbf{E} - \mathbf{Z}\right)$.

end while

Output: Optimal representation coefficient $\mathbf{x}$ and $\mathbf{E}, \mathbf{Z}$

For step 3, we need to introduce the following soft-thresholding (shrinkage) operator:

$$S_\varepsilon[x] = \begin{cases} x - \varepsilon, & \text{if } x < \varepsilon, \\ x + \varepsilon, & \text{if } x > -\varepsilon, \\ 0, & \text{otherwise,} \end{cases} \tag{11}$$

where $x \in R$, and $\varepsilon > 0$, if we extend soft-thresholding operator to vectors or matrices, then we have

$$S_\varepsilon[\mathbf{W}] = \arg\min_{\mathbf{X}} \varepsilon\|\mathbf{X}\|_1 + \tfrac{1}{2}\|\mathbf{X} - \mathbf{W}\|_F^2. \tag{12}$$

That is, the optimal solution of the sub-problem in step 3 is that:

$$\mathbf{Z} = sgn(\mathbf{E} + \frac{1}{\mu}\mathbf{Y_2}) \circ max\{\left|\mathbf{E} + \frac{1}{\mu}\mathbf{Y_2}\right| - \frac{\alpha}{\mu}, 0\}, \tag{13}$$

where the symbolic function $sgn(\cdot)$ and the absolute value $|\cdot|$ act on the each element of the matrix $\mathbf{E} + \frac{1}{\mu}\mathbf{Y_2}$, and $\circ$ is the Hadamard product.

In the following, we consider how to solve the sub-problem in step 2.

Given a matrix $\mathbf{Q} \in R^{p \times q}$ of rank r, the singular value decomposition (SVD) of $\mathbf{X}$ is

$$\mathbf{Q} = \mathbf{U}_{p \times r}\mathbf{\Sigma}\mathbf{V}_{q \times r}^T, \quad \mathbf{\Sigma} = diag(\sigma_1, \cdots, \sigma_r), \tag{14}$$

where $\sigma_1, \cdots, \sigma_r$ are positive singular values, and $\mathbf{U}_{p \times r}$ and $\mathbf{V}_{q \times r}$ are corresponding matrices with orthogonal columns. For a given $\tau > 0$, the singular value shrinkage operator is defined as follows

$$D_\tau(\mathbf{Q}) = \mathbf{U}_{p \times r} \text{diag}\left(\{\max(0, \sigma_j - \tau)\}_{1 \le j \le r} \right) \mathbf{V}_{q \times r}^T. \tag{15}$$

Theorem 1. For each $\mathbf{A}, \mathbf{B} \in R^{p \times q}$ and $\tau > 0$, the singular value shrinkage operator in (15) obeys

$$\frac{1}{2} D_\tau(\mathbf{A} + \mathbf{B}) = \arg\min_E \tau \|\mathbf{E}\|_* + \frac{1}{2}\left(\|\mathbf{E} - \mathbf{A}\|_F^2 + \|\mathbf{E} - \mathbf{B}\|_F^2 \right). \tag{16}$$

Proof: Since the function $h_0(\mathbf{E}) = \tau\|\mathbf{E}\|_* + \frac{1}{2}\left(\|\mathbf{E} - \mathbf{A}\|_F^2 + \|\mathbf{E} - \mathbf{B}\|_F^2 \right)$ is strictly convex, it is easy to see that there exists a unique minimizer, and we thus need to prove that it is equal to $\frac{1}{2} D_\tau(\mathbf{A} + \mathbf{B})$. To do this, recall the definition of a sub-gradient of a convex function $f : R^{n_1 \times n_2} \to R$. We say that $\mathbf{J}$ is a sub-gradient of f at $\mathbf{E}_0$, denoted $\mathbf{J} \in \partial f(\mathbf{E}_0)$, if

$$f(\mathbf{E}) \ge f(\mathbf{E}_0) + \langle \mathbf{Z}, \mathbf{E} - \mathbf{E}_0 \rangle \tag{17}$$

for all $\mathbf{E}$. Now $\widehat{\mathbf{E}}$ minimizes h_0 if and only if 0 is a sub-gradient of the functional h_0 at the point $\widehat{\mathbf{E}}$, i.e.

$$0 \in \widehat{\mathbf{E}} - \mathbf{A} + \widehat{\mathbf{E}} - \mathbf{B} + \tau\partial\left\|\widehat{\mathbf{E}}\right\|_* = 2\widehat{\mathbf{E}} - (\mathbf{A} + \mathbf{B}) + \tau\partial\left\|\widehat{\mathbf{E}}\right\|_*, \tag{18}$$

where $\partial\left\|\widehat{\mathbf{E}}\right\|_*$ is the set of sub-gradients of the nuclear norm. Let $\mathbf{E} \in R^{n_1 \times n_2}$ be an arbitrary matrix and $\mathbf{U}\mathbf{\Sigma}\mathbf{V}^T$ be its SVD. It is known that

$$\partial\|\mathbf{E}\|_* \in \left\{ \mathbf{U}\mathbf{V}^T + \mathbf{W} : \mathbf{W} \in R^{n_1 \times n_2}, \mathbf{U}^T\mathbf{W} = 0, \mathbf{W}\mathbf{V} = 0, \|\mathbf{W}\|_2 \le 1 \right\}. \tag{19}$$

Set $\widehat{\mathbf{E}} = \frac{1}{2} D_\tau(\mathbf{A} + \mathbf{B})$ for short. In order to show that $\widehat{\mathbf{E}}$ obeys (17), decompose the SVD of $\mathbf{A} + \mathbf{B}$ as

$$\mathbf{A} + \mathbf{B} = \mathbf{U}_0 \mathbf{\Sigma}_0 \mathbf{V}_0^* + \mathbf{U}_1 \mathbf{\Sigma}_1 \mathbf{V}_1^*, \tag{20}$$

where $\mathbf{U}_0$, $\mathbf{V}_0$ (resp. $\mathbf{U}_1$, $\mathbf{V}_1$) are the singular vectors associated with singular values greater than τ (resp. smaller than or equal to τ). With these notations, we have

$$\widehat{\mathbf{E}} = \frac{1}{2}\mathbf{U}_0 (\mathbf{\Sigma}_0 - \tau\mathbf{I}) \mathbf{V}_0^*, \tag{21}$$

therefore,

$$\mathbf{A} + \mathbf{B} - 2\widehat{\mathbf{E}} = \tau (\mathbf{U}_0\mathbf{V}_0^* + \mathbf{W}), \mathbf{W} = \tau^{-1}\mathbf{U}_1\mathbf{\Sigma}_1\mathbf{V}_1^*. \tag{22}$$

By definition, $\mathbf{U}_0^*\mathbf{W} = 0$, $\mathbf{W}\mathbf{V}_0 = 0$ and since the diagonal elements of $\mathbf{\Sigma}_1$ have magnitudes bounded by τ, we also have $\|\mathbf{W}\|_2 \le 1$. Hence $\mathbf{A} + \mathbf{B} - 2\widehat{\mathbf{E}} \in \tau\partial\left\|\widehat{\mathbf{E}}\right\|_*$, which concludes the proof.

Therefore, for the sub-problem in step 2, the optimal solution is that:

$$\mathbf{E} = \frac{1}{2}\mathbf{D}_{\frac{1}{\mu}}\left(\mathbf{A}\left(\mathbf{x}\right) - \mathbf{D} + \frac{1}{\mu}\mathbf{Y}_1 + \mathbf{Z} - \frac{1}{\mu}\mathbf{Y}_2\right) \qquad (23)$$

It should be noted that (8) is different from low rank representation (LRR) [22], because both original variable $\mathbf{E}$ and the auxiliary variable $\mathbf{Z}$ brought in are all in the objective function for model (8). The aim of LRR is subspace segmentation, and the nuclear norm is the replacement of rank. But our model is based on face reconstruction and recognition, which is from the view of regression. And the nuclear norm is used to characterize the distribution of the singular values.

4   Complexity and Convergence Analysis

In this part, we discuss the time complexity of the proposed algorithm. It is easy to see that the main running time of the proposed algorithm is consumed by performing SVD on the small matrix of the size $p \times q$, and some matrix multiplications. In step 2, the time complexity of performing SVD is $O\left(pq^2\right)$ (we can assume that $q \leq p$). The time complexity of matrix multiplications is $O\left(npq + n^2\right)$. Thus, the total time complexity of the proposed algorithm is $O\left(pq^2 + npq + n^2\right)$. It is also reported that the commonly used L_1-minimization solvers have an empirical complexity of $O\left(p^2q^2n^{1.3}\right)$ and the complexity of RSC with $\beta = 1$ is about $O\left(p^2q^2n\right)$, where n is the sample number [12]. Now, we compare the complexity of RSC with Algorithm 1. Firstly, we can obtain that $\frac{pq^2+npq+n^2}{p^2q^2n} = \frac{1}{pn} + \frac{1}{pq} + \frac{n}{p^2q^2}$. In general, in the face recognition experiments, $pq \geq 10$, $pn \geq 10$, thus, if $\frac{n}{p^2q^2} \leq \frac{4}{5}$, i.e., $n \leq \frac{4}{5}p^2q^2$, then, our algorithm in this paper will have much lower complexity. It is evident that this condition $n \leq \frac{4}{5}p^2q^2$ can be easily satisfied, for example, in our experiments, $pq \geq 10$, $pn \geq 10$. This main reason for the lower complexity is that our model is based on matrix computation directly, e.g., in step 2, we don't need to convert the each sample of train image into a vector.

The convergence properties of the ADMM have been generally discussed. For more details, one may refer to [21,23]. But in this paper, it is enough that we only need to choose a proper termination parameters ε, and use the following termination conditions:

$$\left\|\mathbf{A}\left(\mathbf{x}\right) - \mathbf{D} - \mathbf{E}\right\|_\infty \leq \varepsilon \quad \text{and} \quad \left\|\mathbf{E} - \mathbf{Z}\right\|_\infty \leq \varepsilon. \qquad (24)$$

5   The Design of the Classifier

For the design of classifier, some new ideas should be noted, for example, Luan et al. [24] introduced two descriptors, i.e., sparsity and smoothness, to represent characteristic of the sparse error component, and applied them to face recognition. Li and Lu [25] proposed a new decision rule, i.e., sum of coefficient (SoC) to match better with SRC. That is, they make full use of the information of the objective function.

In this section, we will use nuclear norm as a metric to characterize the distance between test samples and classes. This is because nuclear norm is more robust than Frobenius (L_2)-norm as a distance metric [26]. Meanwhile, since reconstruction image of all training images can be regarded as the denoised image, thus, we use it as the reference image of classification. That is, we first use Algorithm 1 to obtain the optimal representation coefficients $\mathbf{x}^*$ for a test image $\mathbf{D}$, then use the reconstruction image $A(\mathbf{x}^*)$ of all training images as the new reference image of classification. In addition, let $\sigma_i : R^n \to R^n$ be the characteristic function that selects the coefficients associated with the i-th class. For $\mathbf{x} \in R^n$, $\sigma_i(\mathbf{x})$ is a vector whose only nonzero entries are the entries in $\mathbf{x}$ that are associated with Class i. Using the coefficients associated with the i-th class, one can get the reconstruction of $\mathbf{D}$ in class i as $\hat{\mathbf{D}}_i = A(\sigma_i(\mathbf{x}^*))$. Finally, the nuclear norm of the representation residual is used to characterize the distance between reconstruction image and classes, that is, $r_i(\mathbf{D}) = \|A(\mathbf{x}^*) - A(\sigma_i(\mathbf{x}^*))\|_*$ for $i = 1, \cdots k$. Thus, we can define the following decision rule: if $r_l(\mathbf{D}) = \min_i r_i(\mathbf{D})$, then $\mathbf{D}$ belongs to Class l.

6   Experiment and Analysis

In this Section, we perform experiments on public face image databases and compare the proposed model with state-of-the-art methods. Our aim is to demonstrate the robustness NL_1R to disguise, occlusion and illumination. Note that here in SRC and RSC, the matlab function "l_1-ls" [6] is used to calculate the sparse representation coefficients.

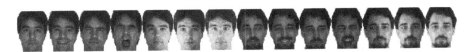

Fig. 3. Fourteen samples of cropped images of one person for training on AR database

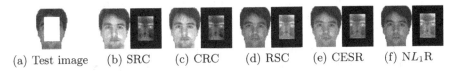

(a) Test image   (b) SRC   (c) CRC   (d) RSC   (e) CESR   (f) NL_1R

Fig. 4. Recovered clean image and occluded part via five methods for the image $\mathbf{B}$ with white block image

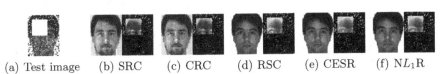

(a) Test image   (b) SRC   (c) CRC   (d) RSC   (e) CESR   (f) NL_1R

Fig. 5. Recovered clean image and occluded part via five methods for the image $\mathbf{B}$ with composite noise

Table 1. The comparison of the error rates(%) for face reconstruction via five methods for the image B with two different cases (a) and (b) corresponding to Figs. 4 and 5, respectively

Cases	SRC	CRC	RSC	CESR	NL$_1$R
(a)	33.43	33.42	0.38	15.30	3.5491×10^{-9}
(b)	31.84	31.84	0.18	4.02	8.7172×10^{-4}

6.1 Databases

The AR face database [27] contains over 4,000 color face images of 126 people (70 men and 56 women), including frontal views of faces with different facial expressions, lighting conditions and occlusions. The pictures of most persons were taken in two sessions (separated by two weeks). Each section contains 13 color images and 120 individuals (65 men and 55 women) participated in both sessions. The images of these 120 individuals were selected and used in our experiment. We manually cropped the face portion of the image and then normalized it to 50×40 pixels.

The extended Yale B face database [28] contains 38 human subjects under nine poses and 64 illumination conditions the light source direction and the camera axis. The 64 images of a subject in a particular pose are acquired at camera frame rate of 30 frames/s, so there is only small change in head pose and facial expression for those 64 images. All frontal-face images marked with P00 are used, and each image is resized to 96×84 pixels and 42×48 pixels (only in Sect. (6.4)), respectively.

6.2 Face Reconstruction

To evaluate the method proposed in this paper, some experiments for face reconstruction will perform on AR face database. Given fourteen face images selected from the AR face database, as shown in Fig. 3, which are used for training. We choose the first image from training images denoted by **B** as the original image. The original image with artificial occlusion is used as the testing image. For the artificial occlusion, we choose the cases: (a) white block image, (b) random sparse noise plus white block. For these cases, a comparison of Sparse representation (SRC), Collaborative representation based classification (CRC), Robust sparse coding (RSC), correntropy-based sparse representation (CESR), and our method is shown in Figs. 4 and 5, and the comparison of the reconstruction error rates is shown in Table 1. We compute the face reconstruction error rates by $E_{error} = \|\mathbf{X} - \mathbf{B}\|_F / \|\mathbf{B}\|_F$, where $\mathbf{X}$ is the reconstruction image. From Table 1, we can find that the reconstruction performance of NL$_1$R is superior to the other methods evidently.

Meanwhile, we can also see that SRC and CRC are not fit to recover the clean images for the images with block image or composite noise. Thus, a suitable error metric is very important for face reconstruction.

Table 2. The maximal recognition rates(%) of SRC, LRC, CRC, RSC, CESR and NL_1R on AR database

Cases	SRC	LRC	CRC	RSC	CESR	NL_1R
Clear	99.2	86.8	98.9	99.0	92.2	99.7
Glasses	95.1	93.2	92.9	96.7	95.0	96.7
Scarf	66.2	30.7	63.7	64.3	33.5	73.3

Table 3. The maximal recognition rates(%) of SRC, LRC, CRC, RSC, CESR and NL_1R on the extended Yale B face database

SRC	LRC	CRC	RSC	CESR	NL_1R
94.0	94.3	81.9	94.2	68.8	97.5

6.3 Recognition with Real Face Disguise

In this experiment, we mainly test the robustness of NL_1R in dealing with real disguise on the AR database. Twenty-six face images of these 120 individuals are selected and used in our experiment. Eight images of them are used for training, which vary as follows: (a) neutral expression, (b) smiling, (c) angry, (d) screaming, (e)–(h) are taken under the same conditions. Eighteen images of them are used for testing, but we will set three different cases: (1) **face images without occlusion** (or **clear images**): Images from the testing set vary as follows: (i) right light on (j) left light on (k) all sides light, (l)–(n) are taken under the same conditions. (2) **face images with glasses**: Images from the testing set vary as follows: (i) wearing sun glasses (j) wearing sun glasses and left light on (k) wearing sun glasses and right light on, and (l)–(n) are taken under the same conditions as (i)–(k). (3) **face images with scarf**: Images from the testing set vary as follows: (i) wearing scarf (j) wearing scarf and left light on (k) wearing scarf and right light on, and (l)–(n) are taken under the same conditions as (i)–(k). Thus, for each case, the total number of training samples is 840.

In all cases mentioned above, SRC, LRC, CRC, RSC, CESR and the NL_1R proposed are, respectively, used for image classification. Here, we can choose the balance factor $\alpha \in [0.00001, 0.5]$ and the regularized parameter $\beta \in [0.5, 3]$. The maximal recognition rate of each method is compared in Table 3, where the second, third and forth line correspond to the cases (1), (2) and (3), respectively. From Table 2, we can find that NL_1R gets the better performance than state-of-the-art methods. For example, CESR only achieves 33.5 % for the facial images with scarves, but our method is 73.3 %. This experiment means that nuclear-L_1 norm fits better to characterize real disguises.

6.4 Recognition with Illumination

In this Subsection we test the advantage of our algorithm for illumination. The first 16 images per subject are used for training, and the remaining images for testing on the extended Yale B face database, where α is 1 and the regularized parameter β is set to 0.05. Table 3 shows the results of some latest approaches and our method. We can find NL_1R achieves much higher recognition rates than the other methods. The maximal recognition rates of SRC, LRC, CRC, RSC, CESR and NL_1R are 94.0%, 94.3%, 81.9%, 94.2%, 68.8% and 97.5%, respectively. Compared to RSC, at least 3.3% improvement is achieved by NL_1R, which demonstrates NL_1R is more effective to illumination for face recognition.

6.5   Recognition with Different Random Occlusion

In the first experiment, we use the same experiment setting as in [8], [12] to test the robustness of NSC. Subsets 1 and 2 of Extended Yale B are used for training and subset 3 is used for testing. The face images are resized to 96×84. Subset 3 with the unrelated randomly block image is used for testing (see Fig. 6(a)). Here, α and β is set to 0.00001 and 0.05, respectively. Figure 6(c) shows recognition rates curve of SRC, CRC, RSC, CESR and NL_1R versus the various levels of occlusion (from 10 percent to 50 percent). From Fig. 6(c), we can see that the advantage of the proposed NL_1R is more evident with the level of occlusion increasing. Especially, when the occlusion percentage is 50%, NL_1R achieves the best recognition rate 95.2%, compared to 65.3% for SRC, 48.5% for CRC, 87.6% for RSC and 57.4% for CESR. And for other occlusion percents, RSC and our method achieve the similar results. But the performance of CESR and

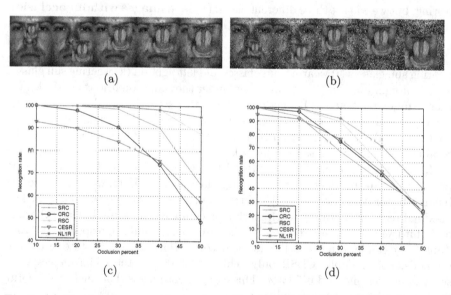

(a)   (b)

(c)   (d)

Fig. 6. (a) The face images with unrelated block occlusion; (b) the face images with Composite noise; (c) the recognition rates(%) of SRC, CRC, RSC, CESR and NL_1R under the unrelated block occlusion percentage from 10 to 50; (d) the recognition rates(%) of SRC, CRC, RSC, CESR and NL_1R under the composite noise percentage from 10 to 50.

CRC is very poor when the block is large, which shows these methods are not suit to deal with this block occlusion case.

In the second experiment, we use the composite noise (pixel corruption plus unrelated randomly block occlusion) (Fig. 6(b)) to further evaluate the robustness of our method. We choose the optimal $\alpha = 200$ and $\beta = 0.00005$, respectively. Figure 6(d) shows recognition rates curve of SRC, CRC, RSC, CESR and NL_1R versus the levels of composite noise (from 10 percent to 50 percent). From Fig. 6(d), we can see that when the occlusion percentage is 50 %, NL_1R achieves the best recognition rate 40.8 %, compared to 28.1 % for SRC, 24.1 % for CRC, 23.7 %for RSC and 22.1 % for CESR. The above experiments also illuminate that nuclear-L_1 norm is more suitable for large block occlusion and composite noise.

7   Conclusions

The characterization of noises is a significant problem in regression model based face recognition. This paper presents a nuclear-L_1 norm joint regression model. Since L_1-norm is good at characterizing sparse noises with the Laplace distribution, and nuclear norm is suitable for characterizing image-wise structural noises, our model fits more kinds of noises. This problem is solved by virtue of ADMM. In addition, nuclear norm is employed as a metric to characterize the distance between test samples and classes. Our experiments demonstrate that the proposed method is more effective than state-of-the-art regression methods for face reconstruction and recognition.

References

1. Wright, J., Yang, A., Ganesh, A., Sastry, S.S., Ma, Y.: Robust face recognition via sparse representation. IEEE PAMI **31**, 210–227 (2009)
2. Cover, T., Hart, P.: Nearest neighbor pattern classification. IEEE Trans. Inf. Theory **13**, 21–27 (1967)
3. Li, S., Lu, J.: Face recognition using the nearest feature line method. IEEE Trans. Neural Networks **10**, 439–443 (1999)
4. Lu, C.Y., Min, H., Gui, J., Zhu, L., Lei, Y.K.: Face recognition via weighted sparse representation. J. Vis. Commun. Image Represent **24**, 111–116 (2003)
5. Daubechies, I., Devore, R., Fornasier, M., Gunturk, C.: Iteratively re-weighted least squares minimization for sparse recovery. arXiv: 0807.0575 (2008)
6. Cands, E., Wakin, M., Boydg, S.: Enhancing sparsity by reweighted l1 minimization. J. Fourier Anal. Appl. **14**, 877–905 (2008)
7. Zhang, L., Yang, M., Feng, X.: Sparse representation or collaborative representation: which helps face recognition? In: ICCV (2011)
8. Yang, J., Zhang, L., Xu, Y., Yang, J.Y.: Beyond sparsity: the role of l1-optimizer in pattern classification. Pattern Recognit. **45**, 1104–1118 (2012)

9. Yang, J., Chu, D., Zhang, L., Xu, Y.: Sparse representation classifier steered discriminative projection with applications to face recognition. IEEE Trans. Neural Networks. Learn. Syst. **24**, 1023–1035 (2013)

10. Zheng, Z., Zhang, H., Jia, J., Zhao, J., Guo, L., Fu, F., Yu, M.: Low-rank matrix recovery with discriminant regularization. In: Pei, J., Tseng, V.S., Cao, L., Motoda, H., Xu, G. (eds.) PAKDD 2013, Part II. LNCS, vol. 7819, pp. 437–448. Springer, Heidelberg (2013)

11. Naseem, I., Togneri, R., Bennamoun, M.: Linear regression for face recognition. IEEE PAMI **32**, 2106–2112 (2010)

12. Yang, M., Zhang, L., Yang, J., Zhang, D.: Robust sparse coding for face recognition. In: CVPR (2011)

13. He, R., Zheng, W.S., Hu, B.G.: Maximum correntropy criterion for robust face recognition. IEEE PAMI **22**, 1753–1766 (2011)

14. Li, X.X., Dai, D.Q., Zhang, X.F., Ren, C.X.: Structured sparse error coding for face recognition with occlusion. IEEE Trans. Image Process. **22**, 1889–1990 (2013)

15. Jia, K., Chan, T.-H., Ma, Y.: Robust and practical face recognition via structured sparsity. In: Fitzgibbon, A., Lazebnik, S., Perona, P., Sato, Y., Schmid, C. (eds.) ECCV 2012, Part IV. LNCS, vol. 7575, pp. 331–344. Springer, Heidelberg (2012)

16. Yang, J., Qian, J.J., Luo, L., Zhang, F.L., Gao, Y.C.: Nuclear norm based matrix regression with applications to face recognition with occlusion and illumination changes. arXiv:1405.1207 (2014)

17. Gabay, D., Mercier, B.: A dual algorithm for the solution of nonlinear variational problems via finite element approximations. IEEE Trans. Image Process. **22**, 17–140 (1976)

18. Gabay, D.: Applications of the method of multipliers to variational inequalities. In: Fortin, M., Glowinski, R. (eds.) Augmented Lagrangian Methods: Applications to the Numerical Solution of Boundary-Value Problems, pp. 299–331. North-Holland, Amsterdam (1983)

19. Boyd, S., Parikh, N., Chu, E., Peleato, B., Eckstein, J.: Distributed optimization and statisticallearning via the alternating direction method of multipliers. Found. Trends Mach. Learn. **3**, 1–112 (2011)

20. Hansson, A., Liu, Z., Vandenberghe, L.: Subspace system identification via weighted nuclear norm optimization. In: CDC, pp. 3439–3444 (2012)

21. Lin, Z., Chen, M., Ma, Y.: Multiplier method for exact recovery of corrupted low-rank matrices. UIUC Technical Report UILU-ENG-09-2215 (2009)

22. Liu, G., Lin, Z., Yan, S., Sun, J., Yu, Y., Ma, Y.: Robust recovery of subspace structures by low-rank representation. IEEE Trans. Patt. Anal. Mach. Intell. **35**, 171–184 (2013)

23. He, B., Tao, M., Yuan, X.: Alternating direction method with gaussian back substitution for separable convex programming. SIAM J. Optim. **22**, 313–340 (2012)

24. Luan, X., Liu, B., Yang, L., Qian, J.: Extracting sparse error of robust pca for face recognition in the presence of varying illumination and occlusion. Pattern Recognit. **47**, 495–508 (2014)

25. Li, J., Lu, C.Y.: A new decision rule for sparse representation based classification for face recognition. Neurocomputing **116**, 265–271 (2013)

26. Gu, Z.H., Shao, M., Li, L.Y.: Discriminative metric: schatten norm vs. vector norm. In: ICPR 2012, Tsukuba, Japan

27. Martinez, A., benavente, R.: The ar face database. Tech-nical Report 24, CVC (1998)
28. Lee, K., Ho, J., Kriegman, D.: Acquiring linear subspaces for face recognition under variable lighting. IEEE PAMI **27**, 684–698 (2005)

Segmentation of X-ray Images by 3D-2D Registration Based on Multibody Physics

Jérôme Schmid[(✉)] and Christophe Chênes

Geneva School of Health, University of Applied Sciences
of Western Switzerland, Geneva, Switzerland
jerome.schmid@hesge.ch

Abstract. X-ray imaging is commonly used in clinical routine. In radio-therapy, spatial information is extracted from X-ray images to correctly position patients before treatment. Similarly, orthopedic surgeons assess the positioning and migration of implants after Total Hip Replacement (THR) with X-ray images. However, the projective nature of X-ray imaging hinders the reliable extraction of rigid structures in X-ray images, such as bones or metallic components. We developed an approach based on multibody physics that simultaneously registers multiple 3D shapes with one or more 2D X-ray images. Considered as physical bodies, shapes are driven by image forces, which exploit image gradient, and constraints, which enforce spatial dependencies between shapes. Our method was tested on post-operative radiographs of THR and thoroughly validated with gold standard datasets. The final target registration error was in average 0.3 ± 0.16 mm and the capture range improved more than 40% with respect to reference registration methods.

1 Introduction

The registration of pre-interventional 3D data to X-ray images is a challenging task due to the projective nature of the X-ray modality. Here, we address the registration problem by deriving 3D shapes from 3D data and by registering them to X-ray images. We express the shape registration as the evolution of shapes in a multibody physics framework – where shapes are driven by forces based on image information and by constraints to enforce spatial coherence.

X-ray imaging has many advantages such as availability, affordability and relatively low doses. These factors have favored its integration in clinical computer-assisted applications such as radiotherapy [1], interventional radiology [2] and orthopedic surgery [3–6]. In these applications, a single or multiple X-ray images are processed to extract spatial information to prepare or guide an intervention, or to analyze post-operative results.

Electronic supplementary material The online version of this chapter (doi:10. 1007/978-3-319-16808-1_45) contains supplementary material, which is available to authorized users. Videos can also be accessed at http://www.springerimages.com/ videos/978-3-319-16807-4.

D. Cremers et al. (Eds.): ACCV 2014, Part II, LNCS 9004, pp. 674–687, 2015.
DOI: 10.1007/978-3-319-16808-1_45

But X-ray images are difficult to process since their projective nature is associated with loss of image information, overlapping of structures and perspective deformations. Many applications rely on 3D-2D registration methods [7] to tackle this issue.

In 3D-2D registration methods, a pre-interventional 3D dataset is registered with intra-interventional [1,3] or post-interventional [6] 2D X-ray images – by optimizing the shape, position and orientation of the 3D dataset. The nature of the 3D dataset varies, it can be for instance a 3D shape (e.g., derived from statistical shape models [5,6] or CAD modeling [8]). Or a volumetric image such as Computed Tomography (CT) [4,9,10] or Magnetic Resonance (MR) [4,11,12].

Most approaches are based on Digitally Reconstructed Radiographs (DRR) [1,2,9,10,13], which are virtual radiographs created from volumetric images, commonly CT volumes. DRR-based registration methods find the optimal shape or transformation parameters that maximize a similarity metric between the computed DRRs and the corresponding X-ray images.

DRR-based approaches provide accurate results but have low capture ranges [7] due to their sensitivity to local optima in the objective function. Therefore, alternative strategies were imagined to avoid using DRR by directly exploiting gradients of the volumetric and X-ray images. Approaches are mainly classified based on the space in which gradients are compared [7], i.e., the X-ray [14,15] or the 3D data [3,4,12] space.

The registration of 3D data to a single X-ray image often results in "out-of-plane" errors occurring in the source to detector direction. For example, when 3D shapes are registered to a single X-ray image the registered shapes can present incorrect spatial adjacency – despite low image projection errors. This issue particularly affects the estimation of implant orientation [6] or joint kinematics [8].

We target the rigid 3D-2D registration of shapes derived from 3D data to one or several X-ray images. Shape registration is equivalent to finding the best transformation (position and orientation) that correctly projects the shape onto the X-ray images. Most shape-based approaches depend on the extraction of the shape silhouettes in the X-ray images – a segmentation task difficult to automate, time-consuming when performed manually and whose accuracy impacts the registration outcome [7,16].

Our work is original in computing the optimal transformation of shapes by considering the shapes as bodies evolving in a multibody physics framework. Multibody physics systems simulate the evolution of several bodies according to modeled Newtonian laws of motion. Rigid body motion is driven by user-defined external forces and subject to damping and inter-bodies constraints.

In [17], a similar approach was presented in which external forces were based on the minimization of distance between projected shape contours and extracted silhouettes from X-ray images. Our work avoids X-ray segmentation by using forces based on the similarity between DRRs and X-ray images. Despite the use of DRRs, our force-based method leads to large capture ranges by using an image similarity computation based on block matching.

Our approach is particularly novel in applying constraints between shapes to improve the simultaneous registration of multiple shapes. Constraints avoid non-plausible shape configuration such as inter-penetrations and provide robustness against out-of-plane errors. We demonstrate the good performances of our approach with publicly available gold standard datasets and preliminary data in the context of Total Hip Replacement (THR).

2   3D-2D Registration

Our approach targets the rigid 3D-2D registration of pre-interventional 3D data to one or several X-ray images. The 3D data can be composed of 3D models (e.g., CAD models of implants) or volumetric medical images – hereafter referred to as volumes to differentiate them from X-ray images. We derive 3D shapes from the pre-interventional 3D data, the registration problem is thus equivalent to registering the 3D shapes to the X-ray images.

2.1   Geometry and Shape Preparation

The geometry involved in our approach is depicted in Fig. 1. N X-ray images I^k ($k \in [1, N]$) are expressed in their local coordinate system (CS) $R(I^k)$ and are positioned with respect to a common world CS $R(W)$ based on rigid transformations $T_{R(W)}^{R(I^k)}$. We assume that the X-ray imaging system is calibrated – i.e., transformations and projective characteristics of X-ray images I^k (position of X-ray source O^k, pixel size) are known.

M shapes S^j ($j \in [1, M]$) are represented as triangular meshes and are expressed in their local CS $R(S^j)$. Each shape S^j is registered to the X-ray images I^k by optimizing the rigid transforms $T_{R(S^j)}^{R(W)} = T^j$ so that each shape is correctly

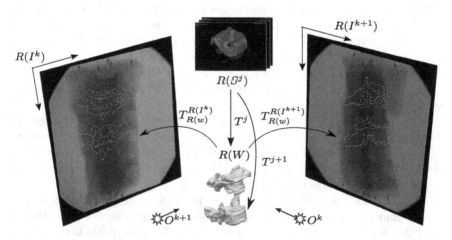

Fig. 1. Illustration of the 3D-2D registration with X-ray images from [3]. Shapes S^j and S^{j+1} share a same CS $R(S^j)$ as they were reconstructed from the same CT volume $V^j (= V^{j+1})$. The registration jointly optimizes the rigid transformations T^j and T^{j+1} so that shapes positioned in the world CS are correctly projected on images I^k and I^{k+1}.

projected onto the corresponding X-ray images. Shapes S^j are derived from the 3D pre-interventional data: CAD models are straightforwardly converted to triangular meshes, while volumes V^j are segmented to produce shapes after reconstruction.

2.2   Method Overview

Our 3D-2D registration starts with a Force-Based (FB) registration (Sect. 3), which repeats for each shape 3 major steps until convergence (Fig. 2): (i) point computation (Sect. 3.1), (ii) force calculation (Sect. 3.2) and (iii) shape position update (Sect. 3.3). After the FB registration, a registration based on gradient correlation, denoted as GCB, is applied to refine the results (Sect. 4). The overall process "FB followed by GCB" will be referred to as the Enhanced Force-Based method (EFB).

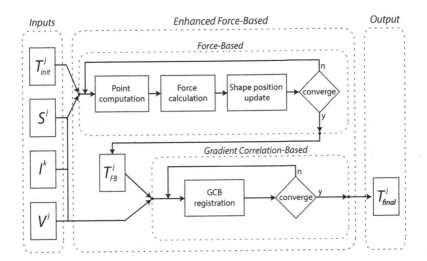

Fig. 2. Overview of our 3D-2D registration method: Enhanced Force-Based; Inputs: initial transformations for each shape (T^j_{init}), the shapes (S^j), the X-ray images (I^k) and the volumes (V^j); Intermediate output: FB result transformation T^j_{FB}; Output: final transformation T^j_{final}

3   Force-Based Registration

3.1   Point Computation

Based on the current transformation T^j of the shape S^j and an X-ray image I^k with corresponding projective properties, the associated volume V^j is used to generate a DRR D^{jk}. Since we use a ray-casting approach [9] to generate the DRR, we restrict our method to X-ray based modalities (e.g., 3D Rotational

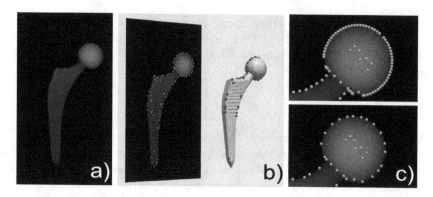

Fig. 3. DRR example and point selection. (a) DRR generated from an artificial volume of an implant model. (b) A silhouette criterion selects a subset of shape vertices (dark spheres) so that projected points (bright spheres) on the DRR image lie on strong edges. (c) The number of projected points is reduced by keeping a single point within image blocks.

X-ray Imaging or CT). For shapes not derived from medical volumes, we create artificial volumes by rasterizing the shapes into binary images and we apply the same DRR generation approach (Fig. 3a).

Vertices of the shape S^j are then filtered with a *silhouette criterion* such as in [5]. This criterion keeps vertices belonging to edges with front and back facing triangles with respect to a viewpoint located at the X-ray source position O^k (Fig. 3b). We chose the silhouette procedure to select points of interest that will exhibit a significant local gradient variation in the projected image.

The selected subset of vertices is then projected onto the image (Fig. 3b). We divide the image into a grid with blocks of $G \times G$ pixels and reduce all points falling into a block to a single point by choosing the closest point to the block point barycenter (Fig. 3c). This reduction process results in projected points p_i^{jk} corresponding to *source* shape vertices y_i^{jk} ($i \in [1, L^{jk}]$).

For each projected point p_i^{jk} defined in DRR image D^{jk} we look for a position in the corresponding X-Ray image I^k which maximizes a local similarity criterion. A block d_i^{jk} of $B \times B$ pixels is defined around each projected point p_i^{jk} in D^{jk} (Fig. 4b). Similarly, we specify a search window w_i^{jk} of $W \times W$ pixels for each projected point in I^k (Fig. 4a).

A block matching procedure is subsequently applied by finding the block b_i^{*jk} within the search window that matches at best each block d_i^{jk} (Fig. 4a). *Target* projected points q_i^{jk} are chosen as the center positions of the resulting blocks b_i^{*jk}. The block matching technique increases the capture range of registrations method [18] and speeds up the DRR computation since we can restrict its computation within the blocks only.

We chose the Gradient Correlation (GC) [9] for the similarity metric due to its good performance in DRR-based 3D-2D registration [10,13]. $GC(b, d)$ maximizes

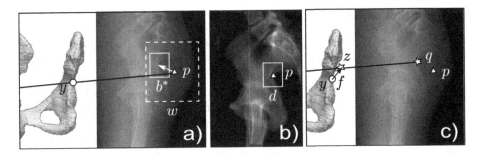

Fig. 4. Force-based registration. (a) A silhouette shape point y ($\bullet$) is projected on p ($\triangle$) in the X-ray image I and (b) on the DRR D. In I, a block b^* is found within a search window w such that it matches at best the block d in D. (c) Based on the ray (O, q), where O is the position of the X-ray source and q ($\star$) is the center of b^*, a new shape point z ($\star$) is computed to produce the image force f.

the alignment of gradient vectors in blocks b and d normalized by the mean gradient vector of the corresponding block. A gradient-based metric is adequate to capture the gradient variations near the projected silhouette points.

3.2 Force Calculation

The optimization of the transformations T^j is indirectly performed by controlling the motion of the shapes S^j that evolve in a system built upon Newtonian laws of motion. Each shape S^j is modeled as a rigid body with mass m^j driven by Newtonian dynamics and subjected to external forces and constraints, as well as damping γ.

We devise external forces to alter the position of shapes in the world CS so that transformations T^j are optimized. *Image* forces enforce at the point level the similarity between local areas of the DRRs and the X-Ray images. Given a source point y_i^{jk} of a shape S^j selected at the point selection stage, we compute a force f_i^{jk} at y_i^{jk} that follows the Hooke's law of a spring with stiffness l^j:

$$f_i^{jk} = l^j * (z_i^{jk} - y_i^{jk}) \tag{1}$$

where a target point z_i^{jk} is computed as the projection of y_i^{jk} on the ray passing through the X-ray source O^k and the target projected point q_i^{jk} resulting from the block matching (Fig. 4c). This force "attracts" the shape to a position where the image similarity is maximized – i.e., a location satisfying the 3D-2D registration problem. Given a shape S^j, forces calculated for each image I^k are back-transformed in the world CS and summed at vertex level – providing a natural way to consider multiple X-ray images:

$$f_i^j = \sum_{k=1}^{N} (T_{R(w)}^{R(I^k)})^{-1} f_i^{jk} \tag{2}$$

3.3 Shape Position Update

A simulation step of the physics system updates the position of the rigid bodies based on their current state (velocity, position), the external forces and the damping γ (which produces a resisting force with an amplitude proportional to body velocity). This is performed by a numerical integration scheme which solves a set of algebraic and differential equations. The resulting position of a shape S^j is eventually used to update the transformation T^j.

A simulation step also considers constraints that model dependencies between shapes. Examples of constraints are collision response to avoid colliding bodies and the modeling of joints with various degrees of freedom. For instance, a pivot constraint can be defined between two bodies to have them rotate around a relative rotation center.

The simulation runs until shape motion reaches an equilibrium – a state which balances respect of constraints and image similarity maximization. In practice, a perfect equilibrium is not always observed since joint constraints can be over restrictive yielding a small "oscillation" of the shape position around the equilibrium. This issue is addressed by "softening" the constraints to allow small violations, like an inter-penetration threshold between bodies or a small distance between pivot centers.

The equilibrium is also affected by the accuracy of the block matching. A subpixel accuracy cannot be reached with block matching since the computation of block positions is restricted to integer pixel locations. Consequently, image forces at some vertices can contribute to the position instability around the equilibrium.

The variation of shapes could be analyzed between two successive steps to stop the simulation when the Euclidean distance between the shape vertices is below a threshold. However, choosing an adequate threshold value is not an easy task since e.g. a too big value can lead to premature termination. An alternative approach is to run the simulation for a fixed number of steps n – such value being selected based on experiments.

4   Enhanced Force-Based Registration by Gradient Correlation Refinement

After completion of the force-based registration FB, the GCB refinement is performed to improve the accuracy of our block-based approach. This refined registration does not rely anymore on the physics system but instead it optimizes the transformation T^j of a shape S^j by maximizing the sum of the GC similarities between the DRRs D^{jk} and X-ray images I^k [10]. Similarly to the block matching process, we only compute the sum of similarities Φ^j inside blocks d_i^{jk}:

$$\Phi^j = \sum_{k=1}^{N} \sum_{i=1}^{L^{jk}} GC(b_i^{jk}, d_i^{jk}) \tag{3}$$

where blocks b_i^{jk} and d_i^{jk} are computed for the X-ray image I^k and the DRR D^{jk}, and are centered on the filtered projected points p_i^{jk} with the same selection procedure of the FB method (Sect. 3.1).

As suggested by [10], we used a Powell-Brent optimizer for which we automatically compute the parameter scales. For an average translation step of t mm, we choose an angular step α such as $tan(\alpha) = t/r$, where r is the radius of the enclosing sphere of the shape. Isotropic translation and rotation scales are finally set to $1/t$ and $1/\alpha$. The rotation center of the rigid transformation T^j is set to the gravity center of the shape S^j.

The rationale behind using the GCB is that after FB we are close to the final solution so that constraints are not necessary at this stage. A way to consider constraints in Eq. 3 would depend on the type of constraints. For instance, we could add a penalty term to minimize the distance between pivot centers for pivot constraints.

5 Experiments

We tested our FB and EFB methods with two experiments. The first experiment uses gold standard 3D-2D registration datasets and exemplifies the use of multiple X-ray images. In the second experiment, we registered multiple shapes to a single post-THR X-ray image.

Multibody physics were implemented with Bullet Physics library[1], while block-matching and image similarity optimization were implemented with ITK[2]. We used a computer with i7 core and 6GB RAM running Windows 7. Table 1 reports the values of the different parameters.

Table 1. Experiment parameters for the FB first and second passes, and for the GCB refinement.

Parameters			FB first pass	FB second pass	GCB
block size	B	(Sects. 3.1, 4)	15 px	11 px	9 px
window size	W	(Sect. 3.1)	20 px	10 px	-
reduction block size	G	(Sect. 3.1)	10 px	10 px	10 px
mass	m^j	(Sect. 3.2)	1 kg	1 kg	-
stiffness	l^j	(Sect. 3.2)	0.2 N.m^{-1}	0.2 N.m^{-1}	-
damping	γ	(Sect. 3.3)	0.99 N.s.m^{-1}	0.99 N.s.m^{-1}	-
# steps	n	(Sect. 3.3)	40	40	-
translation step	t	(Sect. 4)	-	-	1 mm

We applied a multi-resolution strategy with two consecutive passes in the FB method. In the first pass, the sizes of the search window W and block B were

---

[1] http://www.bulletphysics.org.
[2] http://www.itk.org.

chosen to ensure large capture ranges and improve robustness against image arti-facts. In the second pass, the sizes were reduced to improve accuracy and speed.

Same physical parameters were set for all shapes. We experimentally defined a number of 40 simulation steps per pass – the value being an upper limit as sometimes we observed earlier convergence to a stable equilibrium. The values of the image parameters B, G and W were chosen for an average pixel size of 0.5 mm and for standard clinical usage of X-ray imaging (e.g., average source to detector distance of 1200 mm).

5.1   Validation on Gold Standard Datasets

We used two gold standard datasets *Dataset A* [3] and *Dataset B* [4], which contain CT images with 8 and 5 human vertebrae. Datasets include calibrated X-ray images registered to a world CS. For each vertebra, a gold standard trans-formation from the CT CS to the world CS is provided.

Corresponding works [3,4] describe tests for objective evaluation, which include pairs of quasi-perpendicular X-ray images, starting positions and ref-erence points to compute mean Target Registration Error (mTRE) [3]. We used the same testing conditions and data except for the size of X-ray images in *Dataset B* which was divided by 2 to speed-up DRR generation and satisfy block parameters reported in Table 1. Additionally, we coarsely reconstructed the shapes of vertebrae from CT volumes.

We ran a total of 3850 (1600 on *Dataset A* and 2250 on *Dataset B*) tests to validate our methods – with a test taking about 5 min to complete. A sin-gle vertebra was optimized during a test, hence constraints were not necessary. Our FB and EFB methods were compared against the following approaches: Intensity-Based (IB) [9], Gradient-Based (GB) [4], Reconstruction-Based (RB) [11] and Robust Gradient Reconstruction-Based extension (RGRBe) [12].

The accuracy of registration was assessed with the mTRE. Success criteria was set to $mTRE \leq 2$ mm and Capture Range (CR) was defined as the distance from the reference position for which 95 % of the registrations were success-ful [12]. Success Rate (SR) was defined as the percentage of successful tests.

Table 2 reports the results of compared methods for both datasets. For *Dataset A* figures were copied from [12]. For *Dataset B* data was only available for the GB method, from which we computed the metrics.

The performances of the FB method were satisfactory. The CR was almost as good as the reference method RGRBe on *Dataset A* (10.3 vs. 11 mm) and larger than GB on *Dataset B*. However, FB was less accurate than RGRBe on *Dataset A* (0.65 vs. 0.32) and *GB* on *Dataset B* (0.77 vs. 0.32). SR was in average greater than 70 %.

The use of GCB improved the results of the FB method for both datasets (e.g., Fig. 5 for *Dataset A*) – with improvements in CR and SR values and a significant difference in accuracy (p-value < 1e-16, Wilcoxon matched pairs test). We tested a direct application of the GCB on *Dataset A* which produced poor results (accuracy of 0.6 mm, SR of 21.6 %). This upholds the use of our EFB method which combines the force-based method with the GCB method.

Table 2. Comparison of our 3D-2D registration methods Force-Based (FB) and Enhanced Force-Based (EFB) with existing methods: Intensity-Based (IB) [9], Gradient-Based (GB) [4], Reconstruction-Based (RB) [11] and Robust Gradient Reconstruction-Based extension (RGRBe) [12]; A = Accuracy (mm), CR = Capture Range (mm) and SR = Success Rate (%)

	Dataset A						Dataset B		
	IB	GB	RB	RGRBe	**FB**	**EFB**	GB	**FB**	**EFB**
A	0.65	0.38	0.43	0.32	**0.65**	**0.22**	0.32	**0.77**	**0.39**
CR	3.00	6.00	5.00	11.00	**10.30**	**15.70**	4.20	**6.40**	**7.40**
SR	-	56.00	65.00	92.00	**73.20**	**80.00**	51.40	**71.90**	**74.10**

With our EFB method, we measured a CR 42 % higher than the reference method on *Dataset A* with an improvement in accuracy (0.22 vs. 0.32 mm). Though our SR (80 %) was below RGRBe (92 %), the greater CR of the EFB method (15.7 mm) compared to RGRBe (11 mm) highlighted the better consistency of our method.

The EFB approach also yielded better results on *Dataset B*. CR and SR were improved by 76 % and 44 %. Accuracy significantly decreased (p-value < 0.0001) to a low value of 0.39 mm but it remained greater than the accuracy of GC method (p-value < 0.0001).

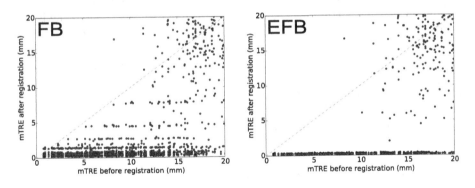

Fig. 5. Registration results on *Dataset A* for FB and EFB methods.

5.2 Experiment on Total Hip Replacement Data

We tested our EFB method on THR post-operative data by registering shapes of hip implants and hip bone to a single anteroposterior (AP) X-ray image. This experiment investigates the use of our 3D-2D registration to compute the anteversion (RA) and inclination (RI) angles. These angles quantify the cup orientation with respect to the hip bone and are essential for evaluation of outcome after THR [6].

After ethical approval, we acquired post-operative CT images and AP radiographs from 3 patients who underwent THR. The manufacturer provided the shapes of implants which we carefully registered to the CT volumes, while the hip bone was manually segmented in the CT dataset. Based on the reconstructed hip, we computed the RA and RI angles according to the radiographic convention [19].

A hip implant is composed of two parts which are mechanically linked by a pivot joint. The femoral implant is made of the stem and head while the acetabular implant includes the cup and the liner. For each part, we created a shape derived from the implant CAD models of the manufacturer.

We conducted an experiment to register the implants and hip bone to the AP radiograph – by keeping the same parameters as in previous experiment (Table 1). To remove the bias of using the post-operative CT volume with implants, we built for each implant shape an artificial binary volume with isotropic spacing of 0.5 mm (Sect. 3.1). Similarly, shapes were not initialized from the configuration of the post-operative CT, but were instead initialized based on manually placed landmarks.

We modeled pivot constraints between the femoral and acetabular shapes by using the rotation center provided by the manufacturer and defined in the CS of each shape. An additional pivot constraint was defined between the hip bone and the acetabular implant. The pivot center of the hip bone was estimated as the center of the sphere, with same radius as the cup, which fitted at best the acetabulum area of the bone.

To account for inaccuracies in estimating the pivot centers, we relaxed constraints by allowing slight deviations from constrained states. We used the Error Reduction Parameter (ERP) of Bullet library – where an ERP value < 1 softens the joint, while a value of 1 yields a perfect joint. We chose an ERP value of 0.8.

Pixel size and source-to-detector distance of X-ray images were known. But compared to the previous experiment a gold-standard transformation from CT to X-ray CS was not available. Thus, we assessed the relative positioning of the cup with respect to the hip bone.

We measured a Surface Distance error [20] (SD in mm) between acetabular implants in CT and X-ray images. We also computed Absolute Differences (AD in °) between expected (CT) and computed (X-ray) RA and RI angles. Results for FB and EFB methods are reported in Table 3.

Table 3. Results of our Enhanced Force-Based method (EFB) on THR data with and without the use of constraints; Measures are the Absolute Differences (AD) for the anteversion (RA) and inclination (RI) angles, and the Surface Distance error (SD).

	AD RA	AD RI	SD
EFB with pivot constraints	$0.57 \pm 0.50°$	$2.37 \pm 2.29°$	0.61 ± 0.59 mm
EFB without pivot constraints	$3.95 \pm 4.96°$	$9.09 \pm 8.04°$	2.03 ± 2.05 mm

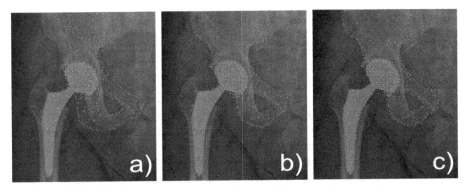

Fig. 6. Example of projected points onto X-ray images for one patient. **(a)** The initialization is approximate but the points appear well projected in the final results **(b)** without and **(c)** with the use of pivot constraints.

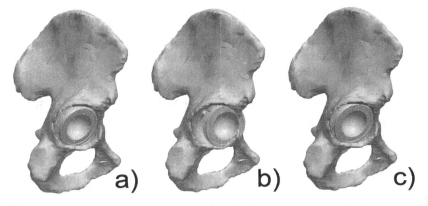

Fig. 7. Illustration of the performances in using constraints for one patient. The positioning of the acetabular implant looks quite similar between the **(a)** expected and **(c)** the result with constraints. **(b)** Without constraints, the acetabular implant is clearly in the wrong location.

When using constraints we observed a good projection of shapes after registration (e.g., Fig. 6c) and measured an average SD of 0.61 ± 0.59 mm – despite an approximate initialization (e.g., Fig. 6a). The AD was low for the RA ($0.57 \pm 0.50°$) but was high for the RI – due to a large AD of $5°$ computed for one patient. By removing this patient's data, the AD improved about 50 % for both angles.

When constraints were not used, we measured a large increase of the distance and angle errors (e.g., 0.57 to 3.95 for the AD of RA). We observed out-of-plane errors illustrated in Fig. 7b in which the cup left the acetabular socket in the detector-to-source direction – despite a good projection of points on the X-ray image (Fig. 6b).

Despite a low number of subjects in this experiment, results were very promising. They highlighted the EFB strong potential to accurately segment multiple shapes from a single X-ray image.

6 Discussion and Conclusion

Based on Markelj et al.'s classification [7], we devised a novel hybrid approach mixing projection (block-matching coupled with DRR) and back-projection (force driven optimization) techniques. Our approach relies on a multibody physics system that provides a natural and efficient way to tackle the simultaneous registration of several shapes with multiple X-ray images.

Compared to other existing methods, our approach generally returned more accurate results with a larger capture range in gold standard benchmarks using two radiographs. In particular, the block-based matching improved the capture range compared to direct DRR-based approaches. Physical constraints brought robustness to the registration of multiple shapes to a single X-ray image, but additional testing is necessary to assess its viability in clinical use (e.g., cup orientation computation [6] or joint tracking by fluoroscopy [8]).

A limitation of our approach is the need of shapes of the patient, which may require some 3D segmentation. However, we observed that our approach was not very sensitive to the segmentation quality, which is not the case for techniques based on 2D X-ray segmentations [16]. Nevertheless, current work focuses on creating forces based on statistical shape models, like [21], to remove this dependency of patient-specific shapes as in [5,6].

Similarly, we plan to avoid the use of invasive CT scans by adding new image forces which do not require DRR and support MR images. It could be based on the back projected gradients [12]. By adding new forces, we can easily extend our framework while preserving its advantages such as constraints.

Acknowledgment. This work is funded by the Swiss CTI project MyHip (no. 13573.1). Authors would like to thank E. Ambrosetti, J. Marquis and the MyHip consortium. The CT and Xray images and gold standard registration were provided by the Laboratory of Imaging Technologies, University of Ljubljana, Slovenia [4] and the Image Sciences Institute, Utrecht, Netherlands [3].

References

1. Fu, D., Kuduvalli, G.: A fast, accurate, and automatic 2D–3D image registration for image-guided cranial radiosurgery. Med Phys. **35**, 2180–2194 (2008)
2. Hurvitz, A., Joskowicz, L.: Registration of a CT-like atlas to fluoroscopic X-ray images using intensity correspondences. IJCARS **3**, 493–504 (2008)
3. van de Kraats, E., Penney, G., Tomazevic, D., van Walsum, T., Niessen, W.: Standardized evaluation methodology for 2-D-3-D registration. IEEE Trans. Med. Image **24**, 1177–1189 (2005)
4. Tomazevic, D., Likar, B., Slivnik, T., Pernus, F.: 3-D/2-D registration of CT and MR to X-ray images. IEEE Trans. Med. Image **22**, 1407–1416 (2003)
5. Benameur, S., Mignotte, M., Parent, S., Labelle, H., Skalli, W., de Guise, J.: 3D/2D registration and segmentation of scoliotic vertebrae using statistical models. Comput. Med. Image Graph. **27**, 321–337 (2003)

6. Zheng, G., von Recum, J., Nolte, L.P., Grützner, P.A., Steppacher, S.D., Franke, J.: Validation of a statistical shape model-based 2D/3D reconstruction method for determination of cup orientation after THA. IJCARS **7**, 225–231 (2012)

7. Markelj, P., Tomazevic, D., Likar, B., Pernus, F.: A review of 3D/2D registration methods for image-guided interventions. Med. Image Anal. **16**, 642–661 (2010)

8. Koyanagi, J., Sakai, T., Yamazaki, T., Watanabe, T., Akiyama, K., Sugano, N., Yoshikawa, H., Sugamoto, K.: In vivo kinematic analysis of squatting after total hip arthroplasty. Clin. Biomech. **26**, 477–483 (2011)

9. Penney, G., Weese, J., Little, J., Desmedt, P., Hill, D.L.G., Hawkes, D.: A comparison of similarity measures for use in 2-D-3-D medical image registration. IEEE Trans. Med. Image **17**, 586–595 (1998)

10. van der Bom, I., Klein, S., Staring, M., Homan, R., Bartels, L., Pluim, J.: Evaluation of optimization methods for intensity-based 2D–3D registration in x-ray guided interventions. In: Proceedings of SPIE 7962, Medical Imaging, pp. 796223–796238 (2011)

11. Tomazevic, D., Likar, B., Pernus, F.: 3-D/2-D registration by integrating 2-D information in 3-D. IEEE Trans. Med. Image **25**, 17–27 (2006)

12. Markelj, P., Tomazevic, D., Pernus, F., Likar, B.: Robust gradient-based 3-D/2-D registration of CT and MR to X-Ray images. IEEE Trans. Med. Image **27**, 1704–1714 (2008)

13. Kubias, A., Deinzer, F., Feldmann, T., Paulus, D., Schreiber, B., Brunner, T.: 2D/3D image registration on the GPU. Pattern Recogn. Image Anal. **18**, 381–389 (2008)

14. Livyatan, H., Yaniv, Z., Joskowicz, L.: Gradient-based 2-D/3-D rigid registration of fluoroscopic X-ray to CT. IEEE Trans. Med. Image **22**, 1395–1406 (2003)

15. Wein, W., Roeper, B., Navab, N.: 2D/3D registration based on volume gradients. Proc. SPIE **5747**, 144–150 (2005)

16. Mahfouz, M.R., Hoff, W.A., Komistek, R.D., Dennis, D.A.: Effect of segmentation errors on 3D-to-2D registration of implant models in X-ray images. J. Biomech. **38**, 229–239 (2005)

17. Kurazume, R., Nakamura, K., Okada, T., Sato, Y., Sugano, N., Koyama, T., Iwashita, Y., Hasegawa, T.: 3D reconstruction of a femoral shape using a parametric model and two 2D fluoroscopic images. Comput. Vis. Image Underst. **113**, 202–211 (2009)

18. Ourselin, S., Roche, A., Prima, S., Ayache, N.: Block matching: a general framework to improve robustness of rigid registration of medical images. In: Delp, S.L., DiGoia, A.M., Jaramaz, B. (eds.) MICCAI 2000. LNCS, vol. 1935, pp. 557–566. Springer, Heidelberg (2000)

19. Murray, D.: The definition and measurement of acetabular orientation. J. Bone Joint Surg. **75**, 228–232 (1993)

20. Roy, M., Foufou, S., Truchetet, F.: Mesh comparison using attribute deviation metric. Int. J. Image Graph. **4**, 127–140 (2004)

21. Schmid, J., Magnenat-Thalmann, N.: MRI bone segmentation using deformable models and shape priors. In: Metaxas, D., Axel, L., Fichtinger, G., Székely, G. (eds.) MICCAI 2008, Part I. LNCS, vol. 5241, pp. 119–126. Springer, Heidelberg (2008)

View-Adaptive Metric Learning for Multi-view Person Re-identification

Canxiang Yan[1,2], Shiguang Shan[1(✉)], Dan Wang[1,2], Hao Li[1,2], and Xilin Chen[1]

[1] Key Lab of Intelligent Information Processing of Chinese Academy
of Sciences (CAS), Institute of Computing Technology, CAS,
Beijing 100190, China
{sgshan,xlchen}@ict.ac.cn, hao.li.ict@gmail.com
[2] University of Chinese Academy of Sciences, Beijing 100049, China
{canxiang.yan,dan.wang}@vipl.ict.ac.cn

Abstract. Person re-identification is a challenging problem due to drastic variations in viewpoint, illumination and pose. Most previous works on metric learning learn a global distance metric to handle those variations. Different from them, we propose a view-adaptive metric learning (VAML) method, which adopts different metrics adaptively for different image pairs under varying views. Specifically, given a pair of images (or features extracted), VAML firstly estimates their view vectors (consisting of probabilities belonging to each view) respectively, and then adaptively generates a specific metric for these two images. To better achieve this goal, we elaborately encode the automatically estimated view vector into an augmented representation of the input feature, with which the distance can be analytically learned and simply computed. Furthermore, we also contribute a new large-scale multi-view pedestrian dataset containing 1000 subjects and 8 kinds of view-angles. Extensive experiments show that the proposed method achieves state-of-the-art performance on the public VIPeR dataset and the new dataset.

1 Introduction

Person re-identification is the technique to identify an individual across spatially disjoint cameras. It is believed to have deep potential applications such as suspect tracking and lost children finding in next-generation intelligent video surveillance. With the ever growing requirements in public security, such techniques are becoming more and more urgently required in order to automatically locate and track wanted persons, or at least dramatically reduce the workload of human operators checking the large-scale recorded surveillance videos.

However, even if it is assumed that the person does not change clothes across the network of cameras, person re-identification suffers from two technical difficulties: first, the appearance of the same person can vary dramatically in different cameras because of both intrinsic and extrinsic variations, including poses, lighting (especially in outdoor scenario), viewpoints, etc. The second difficulty is that there might be a large number of similar individuals, such as, many people wearing dark coats of similar color in winter. Essentially, these two difficulties can be

© Springer International Publishing Switzerland 2015
D. Cremers et al. (Eds.): ACCV 2014, Part II, LNCS 9004, pp. 688–702, 2015.
DOI: 10.1007/978-3-319-16808-1_46

cast to the general pattern recognition challenges: large within-class variations and small between-class variations.

Because of the above-mentioned application values and theoretical challenges, person re-identification has attracted more and more research efforts in recent years. Similar to most methods for pattern recognition problems, existing technologies for person re-identification either seek good features or pursue good distance metrics. Previous methods [1–11] seeking good features attempt to extract features that are not only robust to variations, but are also discriminative for different persons. Gray and Tao [7] proposed a boosting-based approach to find the best feature representation for the viewpoint invariant person recognition. However, such selection may not be globally optimal because features are selected independently from the original feature space in which different classes can be heavily overlapped. In [2], co-occurrence metric is used to capture the spatial structure of the colors in each divided region. Farenzena et al. [3] proposed three localized features under symmetric-driven principles to achieve the robustness to pose, viewpoint and illumination variations. Cheng et al. [6] adopted a part-based model to handle pose variation. However, It is not flexible enough and has strong dependence on the performance of the pose estimators. More recently, Zhao et al. [11] proposed a saliency matching method, which used patch saliency to find the distinctive local patches and recognized same persons by minimizing the salience matching cost. These handcrafted appearance descriptors mostly worked on person matching from close views, but it is not necessarily true for large viewpoint variations, e.g., front view vs. back view. Directly feature matching in corresponding region may derive false distance when existing large view gap.

In contrast to the above feature extraction method, metric learning emphasizes the similarity/dissimilarity measurement, given a pair of images or features extracted using above methods. For instance, LMNN [12] learned a distance metric for kNN classification with the goal that k-nearest neighbors are from the same class as that of input one while instances from different classes should be separated by a large margin. Davis et al. [13] formulated metric learning problem as that of minimizing the differential relative entropy between two multivariate Gaussians distance distribution under the given constraints on the distance function. They integrated a regularization step to avoid over-fitting. Zheng et al. [14] proposed Relative Distance Comparison (RDC) to deal with large appearance changes. In their model, the likelihood of image pairs of the same person having relatively smaller distance than that of different persons is maximized to obtain the optimal similarity measure. Recently, Köstinger [15] proposed a simple strategy to learn a distance metric from equivalence constraints, based on a statistical inference perspective. Pedagadi et al. [16] proposed a supervised dimensionality reduction method based on Fisher Discriminant Analysis. Li et al. [17] learned a decision function with locally adaptive thresholding rule to deal with appearance variations.

All above metric learning methods learn a global distance metric for matching across different views. However, since the discriminatory power of the input features might vary between different image pairs under varying views, learning a global metric cannot fit well the distance over the multi-view image pairs.

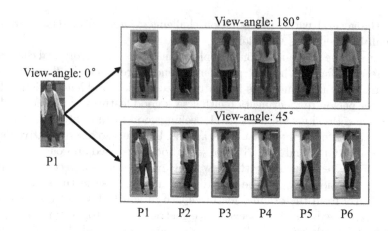

Fig. 1. An example of multi-view person re-identification. Given a probe image with view-angle 0° and two gallery sets with view-angle 45° and 180° respectively, it is easier to find the target image (with green bounding box) from the gallery set with view-angle 45° because more common appearances are shared between images with smaller view gap (Color figure online).

As shown in Fig. 1, given a probe image with view-angle 0°, it is more difficult to recognize its target image with larger view gap (180°) than that with smaller view gap (45°). Thus, it is necessary and reasonable to learn different metrics for different view pairs. For instance, the Multi-view CCA (MCCA) [18] obtains one common space for multiple views. In MCCA, several view-specific transforms, each for one person view-angle, are obtained by maximizing total correlations between any pair of views. However, it not only neglects discriminant information when training but also needs to know view-angle of each image when testing.

To explicitly address the multi-view person re-identification problem, we propose a view-adaptive metric learning (VAML) method. Different from traditional metric learning methods, VAML adopts different metrics adaptively for different image pairs, according to their views. Specifically, given a pair of images (or features extracted), VAML firstly estimates their view vectors (consisting of probabilities belonging to each view) respectively, and then adaptively generates a specific metric for these two images. To learn single unified discriminant common space, the view vector is encoded into an augmented representation of the input feature. Then, all the view-specific metrics are jointly optimized by maximizing between-class variations while minimizing within-class variations from both inter-view and intra-view. This optimization problem can be solved analytically by using generalized eigenvalue decomposition. Extensive comparisons to state of the art methods on VIPeR dataset [19] show that the proposed method achieves better performance. To advance the multi-view person re-identification problem, we further collect a new large-scale **Multi-view** pedestrian dataset (MV), simulating video surveillance scenario. In this dataset, there are 1000 subjects, each with 8 discrete view-angles quantified from the full range of 360°. To our best knowledge, this dataset is the largest one of the same type (at least in terms of the number of persons and view-angles). On this new dataset, the proposed VAML achieves higher performance than the state-of-the-art methods.

The rest of the paper is organized as follows: Sect. 2 describes the proposed approach. Section 3 introduces the MV dataset. Experiments on VIPeR and MV dataset are presented in Sect. 4. Finally, we conclude and summarize the paper in Sect. 5.

2   View-Adaptive Metric Learning

We define the multi-view person re-identification problem as follows: suppose we have a gallery set G consisting of N persons, each has one or multiple images captured from any of V views. Given a probe image $\mathbf{x}_i$, our goal is to find the image of the same person in a different view from G. To make images with different views comparable, we assume that there is a common metric space. In this common space, the matching of all the image pairs can be done by applying a view-adaptive Mahalanobis metric, which is learned to maximize between-class variation while minimizing within-class variation, as shown in Fig. 2. To better achieve this goal, we first extract feature and estimate view vector (consisting of the probabilities of the image belonging to each view) for any input image. Then, the estimated view vector is encoded into an augmented representation of the feature.

In the next, we first introduce the formulation of the VAML. Then, describe the process of feature augmentation in detail. Finally, we describe how to learn the metric analytically.

2.1   Formulation

Recently, metric learning methods [15,20] have been proposed for person re-identification. They learn a global distance metric for image matching across different views. However, since the discriminatory power of the image features varies a lot between different image pairs under varying views, learning a global metric cannot fit well the distance over the multi-view image pairs. Thus, the goal of this paper is to introduce a view-adaptive metric, which adopts different metrics adaptively for different image pairs and can be derived in the following.

The most widely used approach for metric learning is Mahalanobis distance learning. Given data points $\mathbf{x}_i$ and $\mathbf{x}_j \in \mathbb{R}^D$, Mahalanobis distance metric between the two data points is

$$d(\mathbf{x}_i, \mathbf{x}_j) = (\mathbf{x}_i - \mathbf{x}_j)^\top \mathbf{M}(\mathbf{x}_i - \mathbf{x}_j) \tag{1}$$

where $\mathbf{M} \succeq 0$ is a positive semi-define matrix. $\mathbf{M}$ can also be decomposed to $\mathbf{M} = \mathbf{L}\mathbf{L}^\top$. Then,

$$d(\mathbf{x}_i, \mathbf{x}_j) = (\mathbf{x}_i - \mathbf{x}_j)^\top \mathbf{L}\mathbf{L}^\top (\mathbf{x}_i - \mathbf{x}_j) = \left\| \mathbf{L}^\top (\mathbf{x}_i - \mathbf{x}_j) \right\|^2 \tag{2}$$

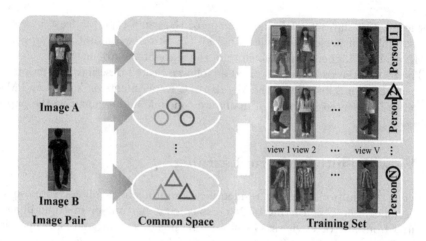

Fig. 2. The overview of VAML. Image pairs with different views are matched in a common metric space. In this common space, images in one class with different views are close to each other, while images in different classes with different views are far away from each other. According to the view information (e.g. view vector) of input image pair, a specific metric can be adaptively generated to measure the dissimilarity of the pair.

Note that Eq. (2) uses a global metric to match all image pairs with different views. Here we introduce a view-adaptive metric, which is adaptive to different image views. Suppose there are V views, a new distance between a pair of images is defined as the sum of Mahalabonis distances over all the views:

$$d_{mv}(\mathbf{x}_i, \mathbf{x}_j) = \sum_{v=1}^{V}(\mathbf{x}_{iv} - \mathbf{x}_{jv})^{\top}\mathbf{M}_v(\mathbf{x}_{iv} - \mathbf{x}_{jv}) = \sum_{v=1}^{V}\left\|\mathbf{L}_v^{\top}(\mathbf{x}_{iv} - \mathbf{x}_{jv})\right\|^2 \quad (3)$$

where $\mathbf{M}_v = \mathbf{L}_v\mathbf{L}_v^{\top}$ is positive semi-define and is the metric matrix for vth view; $\mathbf{x}_{iv}$ and $\mathbf{x}_{jv}$ are features under the vth view. However, it's hard to extract all the view-specific features $\{\mathbf{x}_{iv}\}_{v=1}^{V}$ from single image because only part of person appearances are visible. Instead, we introduce a view vector $\mathbf{p}_i = [p_{i1}, p_{i2}, \ldots, p_{iv}, \ldots, p_{iV}]^{\top}$, where p_{iv} measures the ability of $\mathbf{x}_i$ to represent person appearance under the vth view, to weigh the image feature $\mathbf{x}_i$ and make it view-specific. Thus, let $\mathbf{x}_{iv} = p_{iv}\mathbf{x}_i$, the Eq. (3) can be re-written as

$$d_{mv}(\mathbf{x}_i, \mathbf{x}_j) = \sum_{v=1}^{V}\left\|\mathbf{L}_v^{\top}(p_{iv}\mathbf{x}_i - p_{jv}\mathbf{x}_j)\right\|^2 \quad (4)$$

By expanding Eq. (4), we can get the view-adaptive metric as follows:

$$\begin{aligned} d_{mv}(\mathbf{x}_i, \mathbf{x}_j) &= (\mathbf{p}_i \otimes \mathbf{x}_i - \mathbf{p}_j \otimes \mathbf{x}_j)^{\top}\mathbf{M}_{mv}(\mathbf{p}_i \otimes \mathbf{x}_i - \mathbf{p}_j \otimes \mathbf{x}_j) \\ &= (\mathbf{x}_i^* - \mathbf{x}_j^*)^{\top}\mathbf{M}_{mv}(\mathbf{x}_i^* - \mathbf{x}_j^*) \end{aligned} \quad (5)$$

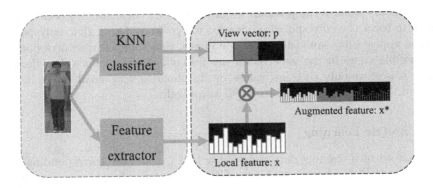

Fig. 3. Feature augmentation. The view vector of input image is estimated using the kNN-classifier. Then the view vector is encoded into an augmented representation of the image feature using Kronecker multiplication operation.

where $\mathbf{M}_{mv}$ is a new positive semi-define matrix, which contains V positive semi-define matrices; '$\otimes$' is a Kronecker multiplication operator, and $\mathbf{x}^* = \mathbf{p} \otimes \mathbf{x}$ is an augmented representation of the original feature $\mathbf{x}$ (see Sect. 2.2 for details). Thus, Eq. (5) is a kind of parameter metric learning methods. The view adaptive property is achieved by the parameter vector $\mathbf{p}_i$ and $\mathbf{p}_j$.

2.2   Feature Augmentation

Figure 3 illustrates the process of feature augmentation. To obtain the augmented feature, we extract texture and color features to generate $\mathbf{x}$ and use kNN-based view estimation to get the view vector $\mathbf{p}$. We describe the details of feature extraction and view estimation in the following:

Feature Extraction. We use texture and color features to represent the input image. Haralick et al. [21] proposed gray level co-occurrence matrix (GLCM) as the distribution of co-ocurring values at a given offset vector (angle and distance) and extracted texture features based on it. In our method, we first separate the images into horizontal strips of size 8×48 and control the overlapping stride to be 4 in the vertical direction. Then local GLCMs are calculated from each strip with 4 offset vectors: $[0°; 1]$, $[45°; 1]$, $[90°; 1]$ and $[135°; 1]$. We also calculate GLCMs between any two strips, which describe frequencies of co-ocurring color pair. For each GLCM, entropy and homogeneity [22] are used to generate the texture features. Then in each strip, HSV histogram is extracted from three color channels with $(8, 8, 4)$ bins respectively. Finally, texture and color features extracted from all strips are concatenated to generate the representation $\mathbf{x}$ for the input image.

View Estimation. We treat the view estimation problem as a multi-class classification problem by grouping data with different view-angles into different classes. Then kNN classifier is learned from a training set with labeled view and used to estimate the possibilities of input image belonging to each view in order to form the corresponding view vector $\mathbf{p}$. Considering that only part of person appearances are visible in single image, thus some entries corresponding to invisible views in the view vector are insignificant. To reduce the effects of those noises, we only keep few values by thresholding very small values in $\mathbf{p}$ to be zero. We set the threshold to be 0.2 empirically.

2.3 Metric Learning

Given a set of n training data points $\chi = \{\mathbf{x}_i\}_{i=1}^n$, and the corresponding class label $\mathcal{L} = \{l_i\}_{i=1}^n$, where $l_i \in \{1, 2, ..., C\}$, and corresponding binary view vector $\mathcal{P} = \{\mathbf{p}_i\}_{i=1}^n$, in which $\mathbf{p}_i$ consists of V binary values and only one of them that corresponds to the labeled view-angle is 1, we describe the process of view-adaptive metric learning in the following.

Denote that $\mathbf{L}_{mv} = [\mathbf{L}_1^\top \mathbf{L}_2^\top \cdots \mathbf{L}_V^\top]^\top$, $\mathbf{M}_{mv}$ in Eq. (5) can be decomposed to $\mathbf{M}_{mv} = \mathbf{L}_{mv}\mathbf{L}_{mv}^\top$. Thus, Eq. (5) can be equivalently written as:

$$d_{mv}(\mathbf{x}_i, \mathbf{x}_j) = (\mathbf{x}_i^* - \mathbf{x}_j^*)^\top \mathbf{L}_{mv}\mathbf{L}_{mv}^\top(\mathbf{x}_i^* - \mathbf{x}_j^*)$$
$$= \left\| \mathbf{L}_{mv}^\top \mathbf{x}_i^* - \mathbf{L}_{mv}^\top \mathbf{x}_j^* \right\|^2 \tag{6}$$

Based on the derivation of view-adaptive Mahalanobis distance above, we then define our objective function by considering two aspects in the new metric space: the separability of distances between images from different classes and the compactness of distances between images from the same class.

The separability, which describes the between-class variation, is defined as

$$J_S = \sum_{i=1}^C \frac{n_i}{n} d_{mv}(\boldsymbol{\mu}_i, \boldsymbol{\mu}) = \mathrm{Tr}(\mathbf{L}_{mv}^\top S_b \mathbf{L}_{mv}), \tag{7}$$

where $\boldsymbol{\mu}_i$ and n_i are the mean and the number of the data points belonging to the ith class, and $\boldsymbol{\mu}$ is the mean of all the data points in the transformed space $\mathbf{L}_{mv}$. $\mathrm{Tr}(\cdot)$ is trace operator; $S_b = \sum_{i=1}^C (n_i)/(n)(\boldsymbol{\mu}_i - \boldsymbol{\mu})(\boldsymbol{\mu}_i - \boldsymbol{\mu})^\top$ is the between-class covariance matrix.

From another aspect, we use compactness to represent the intra-class variation. Let J_C denoted the compactness, which can be calculated as the sum of distances of images from the same class:

$$J_C = \sum_{i=1}^n \frac{n_{l_i}}{n} d_{\mathbf{L}}(\mathbf{x}_i^*, \boldsymbol{\mu}_{l_i}) = \mathrm{Tr}(\mathbf{L}_{mv}^\top S_w \mathbf{L}_{mv}), \tag{8}$$

where the within-class covariance matrix $S_w = \sum_{i=1}^n (n_{l_i})/(n)(\mathbf{x}_i^* - \boldsymbol{\mu}_{l_i})(\mathbf{x}_i^* - \boldsymbol{\mu}_{l_i})^\top$.

To obtain the optimal $\mathbf{L}_{mv}$, the following objective function should be maximized:

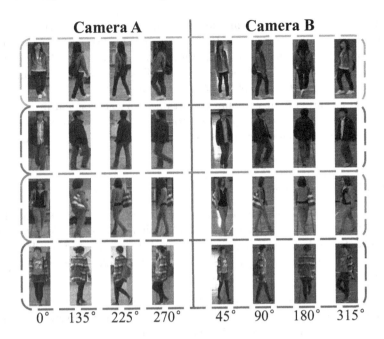

Fig. 4. Examples of multi-view images from MV dataset. Pose, viewpoint and illuminance variations can be observed across camera views.

$$\mathbf{L}^*_{mv} = \underset{\mathbf{L}_{mv}}{\text{argmax}} \ \text{Tr}(\mathbf{L}^\top_{mv}\mathbf{S}_b\mathbf{L}_{mv})$$

$$s.t. \quad \mathbf{L}^\top_{mv}\mathbf{S}_w\mathbf{L}_{mv} = \mathbf{I} \tag{9}$$

This problem can be efficiently solved by generalized eigenvalue decomposition $\mathbf{S}_b\theta_k = \beta_k\mathbf{S}_w\theta_k$, where β_k is the kth largest generalized eigenvalue. The matrix $\mathbf{L}^*_{mv}$ is then constituted of the corresponding eigenvalues θ_k, $k = 1, 2, \dots, d$.

3   MV Dataset and Evaluation Protocol

MV is a new multi-view pedestrian dataset we constructed for the research on the multi-view person re-identification problem. To our best knowledge, MV is the largest dataset in terms of the number of persons and annotated view-angles. The following subsection will describe the construction and evaluation protocol of the MV dataset.

3.1   Construction of MV Dataset

The dataset is collected from two HD (1920×1080) cameras in different locations of a sport square. 1000 participants from the local university or residents walk along the same 'S'-type route in the sport square. We record video clips for each person using the two cameras simultaneously. Then we perform background substraction [23] to locate the person. With estimation of the walking direction at each location, we can get full range of views. We quantify the range and define 8 discrete view-angles: $0°$, $45°$, $90°$, $135°$, $180°$, $225°$, $270°$ and $315°$. To cover the variations of an individual, we sampled 5 frames for each person in each of the 8 different view-angles and cropped them out from background with resolution of 48×128. Figure 4 shows examples with different view-angles from the two cameras.

3.2   Evaluation Protocol

To allow consistent comparison of different methods, we define a standard evaluation protocol about dataset splitting and evaluation. We randomly split the dataset into two sets of 500 persons each, one for training and one for testing. This process is carried out 10 times. For each splitting, there are two testing scenarios:

- S2S (single-shot vs single-shot). In the testing set, we select one view from **Camera A** as gallery set P and another view from **Camera B** as probe set G. Totally, there are 4 combinations of P and G: $(0°, 180°)$, $(135°, 315°)$, $(225°, 45°)$ and $(270°, 90°)$. In each combination, P and G both have size of 500 images, each represents a different individual and its corresponding view-angle is considered to be unknown. This is a general setting which can be found in [2,7,24].
- M2M (multi-shot vs multi-shot). The only difference from S2S scenario is that each person is described by multiple images in both gallery set G and probe set P, following previous work [3,25]. In this scenario, the number of images of each person are set to 3.

There are several established evaluation methods for evaluating person re-identification system. Among them, cumulative matching characteristic (CMC) curve is used to indicate performance of various methods. In our evaluation protocol, we average the multi-view recognition results of the 4 combinations of probe set and gallery set to present **average CMC curve**. To measure the performance of multi-view person re-identification, we also propose **average recognition rate (ARR)** which results from averaging recognition rates of all combinations.

4   Experiments

We evaluate our approach on MV dataset and the public VIPeR dataset. The reason we choose VIPeR is that it is the most widely used dataset for evaluation and it provides most of the challenges faced in real-world person re-identification applications, e.g., viewpoint, pose, different background, illumination variation, low resolution, occlusions, etc. Experimental results are shown in terms of recognition rate, by the Cumulative Matching Characteristic (CMC) curve.

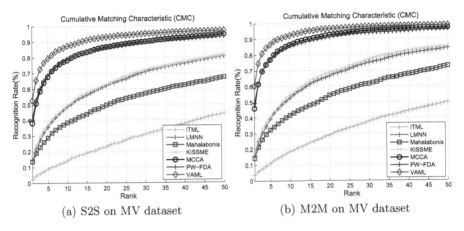

(a) S2S on MV dataset   (b) M2M on MV dataset

Fig. 5. Comparisons to metric learning method on MV dataset under S2S and M2M protocol using CMC curve. The rank-1 ARR of VAML is much higher than others. It indicates that VAML achieves state-of-the-art performance.

4.1 MV Dataset

We randomly split the dataset as described in the protocol. The color and texture features are extracted from images with resolution of 48×128. Then, we use PCA to reduce the feature dimension by keeping 90 % energy for all the metric learning methods. For view estimation, we set the parameter k, the number of nearest neighbors in kNN Classifier, to be 100. This process repeats 10 times.

Cross-view experiments are conducted under the S2S and M2M scenarios. We select images from one view as probe set and images from another view as gallery set(totally 4 combinations). In Fig. 5 we report the average CMC curve under S2S and M2M scenarios for LMNN [12], ITML [13], KISSME [15], MCCA [18], our method(VAML), the Mahalabonis distance of the similar pairs and pairwise Fisher Discriminant Analysis (PW-FDA) [26] as baseline. Note that PW-FDA and MCCA use the view-angle of input image when testing. It is obvious that using the proposed VAML metric leads to a large performance gain over traditional metric learning methods and that VAML also outperforms the two methods using labeled view.

Moreover, in Table 1 we show the result of rank-1 recognition rate on each cross-view combination. It can be seen that our VAML under two scenarios is significantly better than other methods reported results on MV dataset. Specifically under S2S scenario, rank-1 ARR is 51.1 % for VAML, versus 38.4 % for MCCA [18], 16.1 % for LLADF [17], 14.8 % for LFDA [16], 7.2 % for SM [11], 17.1 % for KISSME [15], 14.5 % for LMNN [12], 2.3 % for ITML [13], 13.7 % for Mahalabonis and 6.2 % for SDALF [3]. In particular, VAML outperforms the rank-1 ARR of the second best PW-FDA [26] by 10.5 %. This improvement is due to our view-adaptive strategy, which can make full use of multi-view information from the same class and is robust to viewpoint change and pose variations. In M2M, set-to-set distance is introduced because each person in probe and

Table 1. Rank-1 recognition rates in % on MV dataset under S2S and M2M scenarios respectively.

(a) Rank-1 recognition rate in % on MV dataset under S2S scenario

Method	$0° \Rightarrow 180°$	$135° \Rightarrow 315°$	$225° \Rightarrow 45°$	$270° \Rightarrow 90°$	ARR
VAML	**53.4**	**48.5**	**47.1**	**55.3**	**51.1**
MCCA[18]	40.6	36.4	33.4	43.0	38.4
PW-FDA	39.8	37.2	39.8	45.4	40.6
KISSME[15]	22.2	16.4	15.0	14.8	17.1
LMNN[12]	18.2	13.2	14.6	11.8	14.5
ITML[13]	2.0	1.8	2.0	3.4	2.3
Mahalabonis	16.8	11.2	15.6	11.0	13.7
SDALF[3]	7.4	5.2	5.8	6.2	6.2
LLADF[17]	21.0	12.2	13.2	17.8	16.1
LFDA[16]	18.2	11.2	11.6	18.0	14.8
SM[11]	9.2	5.0	6.2	8.5	7.2
P-VAML	53.9	47.9	47.2	55.0	51.0

(b) Rank-1 recognition rate in % on MV dataset under M2M scenario

Method	$0° \Rightarrow 180°$	$135° \Rightarrow 315°$	$225° \Rightarrow 45°$	$270° \Rightarrow 90°$	ARR
VAML	**60.6**	**57.4**	**58.0**	**65.0**	**60.3**
MCCA[18]	49.2	42.2	41.8	51.4	46.2
PW-FDA	48.8	45.4	49.0	54.0	49.3
KISSME[15]	21.8	16.6	20.0	14.8	18.3
LMNN[12]	20.2	14.8	16.6	11.8	15.9
ITML[13]	4.6	3.2	3.4	3.6	3.7
Mahalabonis	19.2	11.0	17.0	10.4	14.4
SDALF[3]	8.8	5.4	7.8	7.2	7.3
P-VAML	61.2	56.8	58.2	64.6	60.2

gallery set contains 3 images. To recognize one person, we compare the distance of each possible pair from different persons, associating the person to the one from gallery set with lowest distance. In Table 1(b), all the methods have performance gain under M2M compared to that under S2S. Specifically, rank-1 ARR of VAML is improved by 9.2 %, versus 7.8 % for MCCA [18] and 8.7 % for PW-FDA [26]. In particular, the rank-1 ARR difference between our method and KISSME is increased to 42.0 %. By comparing the results of all methods on different combinations, it also can be observed that $(135°, 315°)$ and $(225°, 45°)$ are the most challenge combinations because worst performance of most methods are reported on them.

Based on this analysis, VAML outperforms all other metric learning methods significantly. The main reason for VAML to obtain the best performance is that latent relationship between different views of the same person is learned successfully and robustness to large viewpoint variations is improved by exploiting the view-adaptive metric.

Table 2. Recognition rates in [%] at different ranks r on VIPeR dataset.

Method	r = 1	10	25	50
VAML	**26**	**63**	**82**	**92**
ELF [7]	12	43	66	81
SDALF [3]	20	49	70	83
CPS [6]	22	57	76	87
DDC [25]	19	52	69	80
ERSVM [8]	13	50	71	85
SM [11]	25	52	72	87
RDC [14]	16	54	76	87
KISSME [15]	21	60	81	92
LMNN [12]	19	53	74	87
ITML [13]	16	51	77	90
LLADF [17]	29	78	92	97
LFDA [16]	23	66	84	93
Mahalabonis	17	49	69	82
P-VAML	29	68	84	94

4.2   VIPeR Dataset

VIPeR [19] is the first publicly available dataset for person re-identification consisting of 632 people captured outdoor with two images for each person with size at 128×48 pixels. The biggest challenges in VIPeR are viewpoint and illuminance variations, which may cause the change of appearance largely. For each person, corresponding individuals have viewpoint change up to 90 degrees.

Our setting for the splitting of training/testing set is same to SDALF [3], by which VIPeR dataset is splitted into two set with equal size (316 persons), one as training set and another as testing set. Then we estimate the view vector of each image by kNN classifier using 20,000 images from MV dataset as training data. Different from the setting of MV, only three most dominant estimated view-angles are kept. Thus, the view vector of each data in VIPeR have only 3 dimensions. The whole evaluation procedure is carried out 10 times.

We compare the performance of proposed VAML in the ranging of first 50 ranks to various state of the arts, as illustrated in Table 2. It is noted that our method outperforms all other appearance-based methods. Specifically, SM [11] achieves second best results compared to the other appearance-based methods, like CPS [6], SDALF [3], ELF [7], DDC [25] and ERSVM [8]. However its recognition rate is 1 % lower than ours at rank-1 and have a difference of 11 %, 10 %, 5 % at rank-10, rank-25 and rank-50 respectively. It shows that our method can handle the appearance variations caused by viewpoint change better than traditional appearance-based methods. Moreover, we also analyze the performance of popular metric learning methods [12–17]. Our VAML has much better

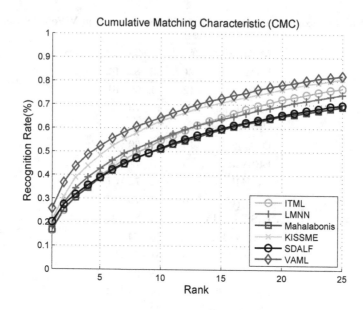

Fig. 6. Average Cumulative Matching Characteristic (CMC) curves of metric learning methods.

performance compared to LMNN [12], ITML [13], KISSME [15],LFDA [16] and RDC [14], and shows comparable performance with that of LLADF [17]. The performance of top-25 ranks is also represented with CMC curve in Fig. 6.

The Effect of View Estimation. One factor affecting the performance is the accuracy of view estimation. The average accuracy of kNN-based view classification is 70 % on VIPeR dataset and 90 % on MV dataset respectively. In order to evaluate the contribution of view estimation, we propose a 'perfect' VAML (P-VAML), in which we use labeled view vector (100 % accuracy) to form the augmented feature. Tables 1 and 2 show the results of P-VAML on VIPeR and MV datasets respectively. It is observed that better performance can be achieved along with the increasement of classification accuracy on VIPeR while the improvement is not obvious on MV dataset.

5   Conclusion

In this paper, we have proposed view-adaptive metric learning to learn a metric which can be adaptive to the views of matching pair for multi-view person re-identification. Both separability of instances from different classes and compactness of instances with different views from same class are exploited in our method. Meanwhile, a multi-view dataset MV, which consists of 1000 persons and has explicit annotation of view-angles, have been released with our expectation to advance the research of multi-view person re-identification. Compared with existing competitive methods, the extensive experiments show that our approach achieves the state-of-the-art results over MV and VIPeR datasets. In the future, we would like to develop the VAML by considering the symmetry of views.

Acknowledgement. The work is partially supported by Natural Science Foundation of China(NSFC) under contracts Nos. 61222211, 61272321, 61402430 and 61025010; and the China Postdoctoral Science Foundation 133366.

References

1. Gheissari, N., Sebastian, T., Hartley, R.: Person reidentification using spatiotemporal appearance. In: CVPR, pp. 1528–1535 (2006)
2. Wang, X., Doretto, G., Sebastian, T., Rittscher, J., Tu, P.: Shape and appearance context modeling. In: ICCV, pp. 1–8 (2007)
3. Farenzena, M., Bazzani, L., Perina, A., Murino, V., Cristani, M.: Person re-identification by symmetry-driven accumulation of local features. In: CVPR, pp. 2360–2367 (2010)
4. Bak, S., Corvee, E., Bremond, F., Thonnat, M.: Multiple-shot human re-identification by mean riemannian covariance grid. In: AVSS, pp. 179–184 (2011)
5. Bazzani, L., Cristani, M., Perina, A., Farenzena, M., Murino, V.: Multiple-shot person re-identification by HPE signature. In: ICPR, pp. 1413–1416 (2010)
6. Cheng, D., Cristani, M., Stoppa, M., Bazzani, L., Murino, V.: Custom pictorial structures for re-identification. In: BMVC (2011)
7. Gray, D., Tao, H.: Viewpoint invariant pedestrian recognition with an ensemble of localized features. In: Forsyth, D., Torr, P., Zisserman, A. (eds.) ECCV 2008, Part I. LNCS, vol. 5302, pp. 262–275. Springer, Heidelberg (2008)
8. Prosser, B., Zheng, W.S., Gong, S., Xiang, T.: Person re-identification by support vector ranking. In: BMVC (2010)
9. Ma, B., Su, Y., Jurie, F.: Bicov: a novel image representation for person re-identification and face verification. In: BMVC (2012)
10. Schwartz, W., Davis, L.: Learning discriminative appearance-based models using partial least squares. In: SIBGRAPI, pp. 322–329 (2009)
11. Zhao, R., Ouyang, W., Wang, X.: Person re-identification by salience matching. In: ICCV, pp. 2528–2535 (2013)
12. Weinberger, K.Q., Blitzer, J., Saul, L.K.: Distance metric learning for large margin nearest neighbor classification. In: NIPS (2006)
13. Davis, J.V., Kulis, B., Jain, P., Sra, S., Dhillon, I.S.: Information-theoretic metric learning. In: ICML, pp. 209–216 (2007)
14. Zheng, W.S., Gong, S., Xiang, T.: Re-identification by relative distance comparison. PAMI **35**, 653–668 (2013)
15. Köstinger, M., Hirzer, M., Wohlhart, P., Roth, P.M., Bischof, H.: Large scale metric learning from equivalence constraints. In: CVPR (2012)
16. Pedagadi, S., Orwell, J., Velastin, S., Boghossian, B.: Local fisher discriminant analysis for pedestrian re-identification. In: CVPR, pp. 3318–3325 (2013)
17. Li, Z., Chang, S., Liang, F., Huang, T., Cao, L., Smith, J.: Learning locally-adaptive decision functions for person verification. In: CVPR, pp. 3610–3617 (2013)
18. Rupnik, J., Shawe-Taylor, J.: Multi-view canonical correlation analysis. In: SiKDD, pp. 1–4 (2010)

19. Gray, D., Brennan, S., Tao, H.: Evaluating appearance models for recognition, reacquisition, and tracking. In: PETS (2007)
20. Zheng, W.S., Gong, S., Xiang, T.: Person re-identification by probabilistic relative distance comparison. In: CVPR (2011)
21. Haralick, R., Shanmugam, K., Dinstein, I.: Textural features for image classification. SMC **3**, 610–621 (1973)
22. Howarth, P., Rüger, S.: Evaluation of texture features for content-based image retrieval. In: IVR, pp. 326–334 (2004)
23. Zivkovic, Z.: Improved adaptive gaussian mixture model for background subtraction. In: ICPR, pp. 28–31 (2004)
24. Lin, Z., Davis, L.: Learning pairwise dissimilarity profiles for appearance recognition in visual surveillance. In: AVC, pp. 23–24 (2008)
25. Hirzer, M., Beleznai, C., Roth, P.M., Bischof, H.: Person re-identification by descriptive and discriminative classification. In: Heyden, A., Kahl, F. (eds.) SCIA 2011. LNCS, vol. 6688, pp. 91–102. Springer, Heidelberg (2011)
26. Belhumeur, P., Hespanha, J., Kriegman, D.: Eigenfaces vs. fisherfaces: recognition using class specific linear projection. PAMI **19**, 711–720 (1997)

Author Index

Printed in the United States
By Bookmasters